Biomarkers in Drug Discovery and Disease Diagnosis

Biomarkers in Drug Discovery and Disease Diagnosis

Editor: Holly Lambert

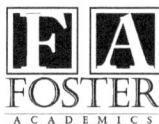

FOSTER
ACADEMICS

www.fosteracademics.com

www.fosteracademics.com

FA
FOSTER
ACADEMICS

Cataloging-in-Publication Data

Biomarkers in drug discovery and disease diagnosis / edited by Holly Lambert.
    p. cm.
Includes bibliographical references and index.
ISBN 978-1-63242-835-6
1. Biochemical markers. 2. Drug development. 3. Drugs--Design.
4. Diagnosis. 5. Pharmaceutical chemistry. 6. Biopharmaceutics. I. Lambert, Holly.
RS420 .B56 2019
615.19--dc23

Foster Academics,
118-35 Queens Blvd., Suite 400,
Forest Hills, NY 11375, USA

ISBN 978-1-63242-835-6 (Hardback)

Contents

Preface

This book aims to highlight the current researches and provides a platform to further the scope of innovations in this area. This book is a product of the combined efforts of many researchers and scientists, after going through thorough studies and analysis from different parts of the world. The objective of this book is to provide the readers with the latest information of the field.

A biological marker or biomarker is a measurable indicator of a biological state or condition. Biomarkers are evaluated to investigate pharmacologic responses to a therapeutic intervention or to examine biological and pathogenic processes. In medicine, a biomarker may be used to examine organ function or other health aspects. They can be prognostic or predictive. Prostate-specific antigen (PSA) is a common biomarker that is used in medicine. Biomarkers are used in the molecular diagnosis of colon, breast and lung cancer, melanoma and chronic myeloid leukemia. Effective and robust biomarkers can be instrumental in improving diagnosis of diseases, monitoring drug activity and guiding the development of targeted therapies for varied chronic conditions. This book is compiled in such a manner, that it will provide in-depth knowledge about biomarkers. It aims to present researches that have advanced the understanding of biomarkers and their role in drug discovery and disease diagnosis. The readers would gain knowledge that would broaden their perspective about biological markers.

I would like to express my sincere thanks to the authors for their dedicated efforts in the completion of this book. I acknowledge the efforts of the publisher for providing constant support. Lastly, I would like to thank my family for their support in all academic endeavors.

Editor

Paediatric acute myeloid leukaemia with the t(7;12)(q36;p13) rearrangement

Sabrina Tosi[1*], Yasser Mostafa Kamel[1], Temitayo Owoka[1], Concetta Federico[2], Tony H. Truong[3] and Salvatore Saccone[2]

Abstract

The presence of chromosomal abnormalities is one of the most important criteria for leukaemia diagnosis and management. Infant leukaemia is a rare disease that affects children in their first year of life. It has been estimated that approximately one third of infants with acute myeloid leukaemia harbour the t(7;12)(q36;p13) rearrangement in their leukaemic blasts. However, the WHO classification of acute myeloid leukaemia does not yet include the t(7;12) as a separate entity among the different genetic subtypes, although the presence of this chromosomal abnormality has been associated with an extremely poor clinical outcome. Currently, there is no consensus treatment for t(7;12) leukaemia patients. However, with the inferior outcome with the standard induction therapy, stem cell transplantation may offer a better chance for disease control. A better insight into the chromosome biology of this entity might shed some light into the pathogenic mechanisms arising from this chromosomal translocation, that at present are not fully understood. Further work is needed to improve our understanding of the molecular and genetic basis of this disorder. This will hopefully open some grounds for possible tailored treatment for this subset of very young patients with inferior disease outcome. This review aims at highlighting the cytogenetic features that characterise the t(7;12) leukaemias for a better detection of the abnormality in the diagnostic setting. We also review treatment and clinical outcome in the cases reported to date.

Keywords: Acute myeloid leukaemia, Paediatric leukaemia, t(7;12) translocation, Chromosomal abnormalities, HLXB9 gene, Clinical outcome

Introduction

Leukaemia is the most common type of cancer in childhood (Fig. 1). Among acute leukaemias, one in five is represented by acute myeloid leukaemia (AML), whereas four fifths are acute lymphoblastic leukaemia (ALL). Cancer statistics from the National Registry of Childhood Tumours show a peak at age 2–3 years for the insurgence of ALL, whereas AML is more common within the first year of life and after age 10, with an incidence of 16 cases per million in the United Kingdom. The incidence of AML decreases in children older than 2 years of age, but rises in adolescence when it stays stable until adulthood, reaching its peak in older individuals [1]. Similar statistics have been encountered in the populations of the United States [2, 3].

In the past three decades, there has been a considerable improvement in the cure of childhood leukaemia, reaching a long term survival rate of more than 90 % in ALL and approximately 70 % in AML [3, 4]. However, certain categories of childhood leukaemia are still considered high risk, and this level of risk is dictated by the presence of cytogenetic and molecular genetic markers. The amended world health organization (WHO) leukaemia classification includes the most relevant chromosomal rearrangements to allow proper risk stratification of leukaemia patients [5]. To date, the t(7;12)(q36;p13) rearrangement found in infant AML has not been incorporated in the WHO classification, although it has been

* Correspondence: sabrina.tosi@brunel.ac.uk
[1]Leukaemia and Chromosome Research Laboratory, Division of Biosciences, Brunel University London, Middlesex UB8 3PH, UK
Full list of author information is available at the end of the article

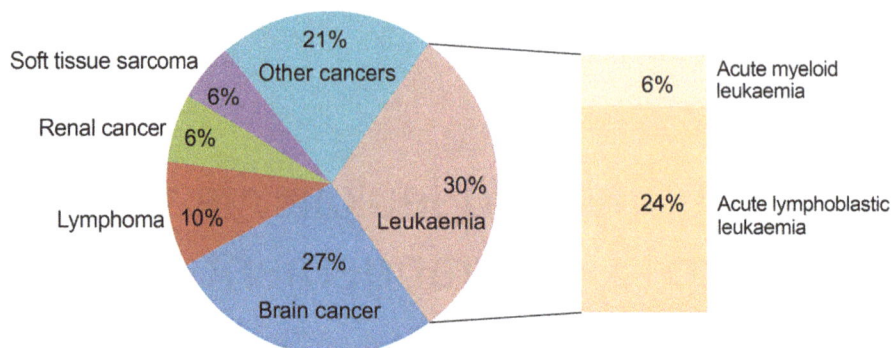

Fig. 1 Main types of childhood cancers. The ideogram shows the different proportions of cancers affecting paediatric patients. Acute leukaemia is the most commonly reported cancer in children, with ALL affecting approximately 80 % of patients and AML diagnosed in 15–20 % of patients. Forms of chronic leukaemia and myelodysplastic syndromes are very rare in children and their incidence has been omitted from this graph (based on cancers statistics collected from the National Registry of Childhood Tumours, years 2009–2011, accessed through the Cancer Research UK website)

associated with poor clinical outcome [3, 6]. This cytogenetic entity has not been associated with a particular morphologic or immunophenotypic subtype [6, 7], but has been found in a range of AML types as well as a case of myelodysplastic syndrome [8]. The scope of this review is to give the reader a comprehensive understanding of the t(7;12) rearrangement at the chromosomal level and the available methods for the detection of this cytogenetic marker for an improved diagnosis and a better estimate of the real incidence of this type of leukaemia. We also review the clinical outcome and the therapeutic approaches that have been adopted in the cases reported to date.

Review

The t(7;12) rearrangement: chromosomal appearance and cytogenetic features

The t(7;12) rearrangement typically involves the long arm of chromosome 7 at band q36 and the short arm of chromosome 12 at band p13 (Fig. 2). These chromosomal regions reside towards the end of the chromosomes, near the telomeres and involve fragments of similar sizes. The banding patterns of these subtelomeric regions are typically fairly homogeneous and not distinctive of a specific chromosome. For these reasons the t(7;12) rearrangement is a difficult cytogenetic entity to detect microscopically, using conventional methods of chromosome banding. Nevertheless, early reports demonstrate identification of t(7;12) based on banding analysis only [9–11]. Furthermore, the t(7;12) has been found associated with deletions of the long arm of chromosome 7, therefore the der(7) in these cases might be misinterpreted as a del(7q). Fluorescence in situ hybridisation in one del(7)(q22) case, helped revising this abnormality as a der(7)del(7)(q22q36)t(7;12)(q22;p13) [7, 8, 12].

Translocation breakpoints

In the t(7;12)(q36;p13), the breakpoints on chromosome 12 are consistently at the 5′ end of *ETV6*, between exons 1 and 3, whereas the breakpoints on chromosome 7 are quite heterogeneous affecting band q36 in regions proximal to the Homeobox HB9 (*HLXB9)* gene [6, 12, 13], also known as *MNX1* (motor neuron and pancreas homeobox 1). There have been descriptions of breakpoints in 7q31 [10], 7q32 [14, 15], and 7q35–36 [8]. However, some of these findings were not validated using fluorescence in situ hybridisation (FISH). Informative FISH probes spanning 7q would have been helpful towards achieving a more accurate definition of the breakpoints in these cases.

Cryptic and complex rearrangements

To date, three cases of complex rearrangements harbouring the t(7;12) have been reported [16, 17]. These three way translocations were characterised by FISH and described as (i) t(5;7;12)(q31;q36;p13) [16]; (ii) t(1;7;12)(q25;q36;p13) [16] and (iii) t(7;12;16)(q36;p13;q12) [17] respectively. Due to the breakpoints affecting the terminal regions of both chromosomes 7 and 12, the t(7;12)(q36;p13) is considered a cryptic rearrangement. The use of appropriate FISH probes would surely improve the detection of this abnormality and might uncover a higher proportion of t(7;12) translocations masked by more complex rearrangements, as in the cases of the three way translocations previously described.

Additional abnormalities

Interestingly, the majority of t(7;12) cases have been reported in association with specific aneusomies. A recent review of the literature reported that only 2 out of 44 cases harboured the t(7;12) as a sole abnormality [17]. In particular, the presence of one or more additional copies of chromosomes 8, 19 and/or 22 have been recurrently

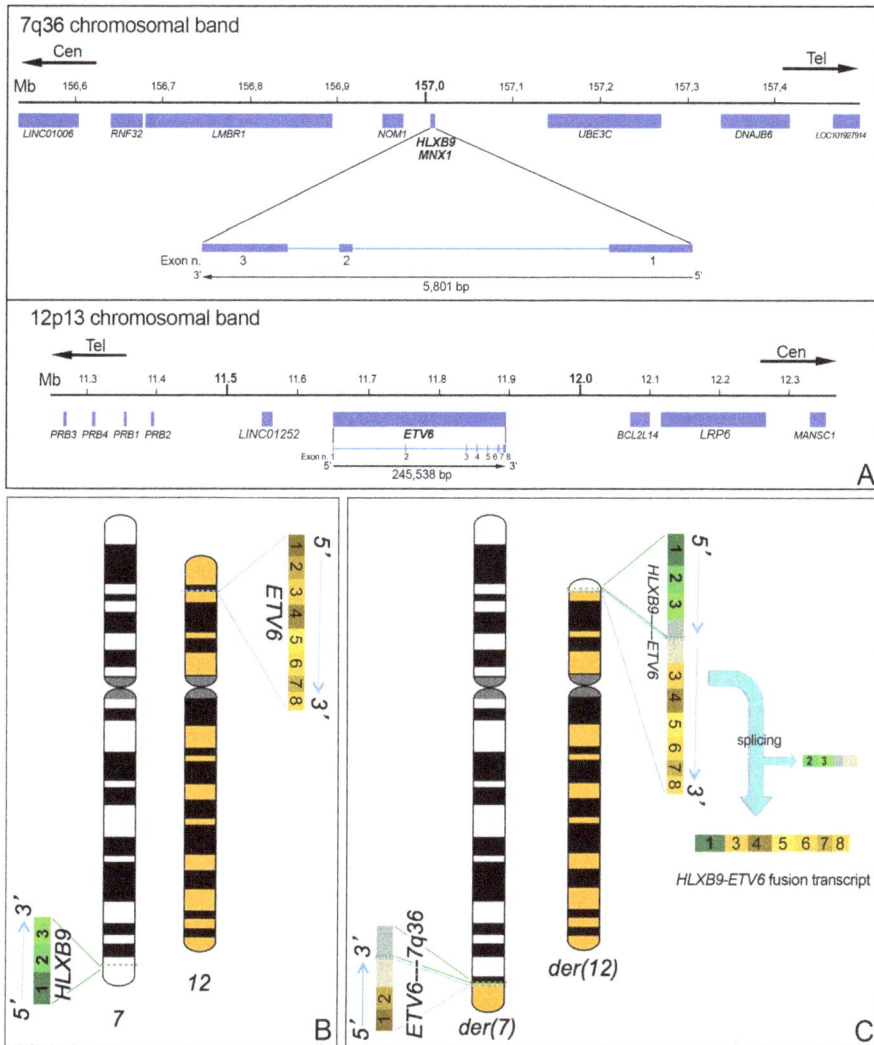

Fig. 2 Schematic representation of the t(7;12)(q36;p13) and fusion transcript formation. **a** Representation of the 7q36 and 12p13 regions spanning 1 Mb around the genes of interests. The breakpoints are proximal to the *HLXB9* gene on chromosome 7 and at the 5′ end of the *ETV6* gene on chromosome 12. *HLXB9* is a small gene composed of three exons. *ETV6* is a larger gene composed of eight exons. In both cases the direction of transcription is from the telomeric to the centromeric end. **b** The gene location and direction of transcription of both *HLXB9* and *ETV6* are shown on the ideograms of chromosomes 7 and 12. For each gene all the exons are indicated. **c** Derivative chromosomes 7 and 12: the der(12) harbours the whole *HLXB9* gene and the 3′ portion of *ETV6* including exons 3–8. If a fusion transcript arose from this translocation, splicing of *HLXB9* exons 2 and 3 as well as any genomic material from chromosome 7 downstream to *HLXB9* that was translocated on the der(12) should take place

described [6, 7, 15]. The presence of these additional abnormalities has been reported in samples at diagnosis and/or at relapse, indicating that the acquired aneusomies might be sign of clonal evolution and important for the establishment and the survival of the leukaemic clone.

Molecular mechanisms

Is there a fusion gene?

A well-established driver of haematological malignancy when a chromosomal translocation is present, is the formation of an oncogenic fusion gene such as *BCR-ABL* resulting from the t(9;22)(q34; q11) in chronic myeloid leukaemia or *ETV6-RUNX1* in t(12;21)(p13;q22) positive ALL [18]. As a consequence of these gene fusions, a fusion transcript is produced with subsequent generation of a chimeric protein whose altered properties have an impact on the onset of the disease. Reverse transcriptase-polymerase chain reaction (RT-PCR) to identify the fusion transcript in t(7;12) patients showed a fusion of exon 1 of the *HLXB9* gene to either exons 2 or 3 of the *ETV6* gene resulting in two different *HLXB9-ETV6* fusion transcripts: an out of frame longer variant (exon 1 of *HLXB9* to exon

2 of *ETV6*) or an in-frame shorter variant (exon 1 of *HLXB9* to exon 3 of *ETV6*), both fusion transcripts contain the first exon of the *HLXB9* gene as well as the ETS domain (DNA and protein binding domain) and the pointed N terminal domain (PNT) (protein-protein binding domain) of the *ETV6* gene [6, 19–21]. However, the presence of an *HLXB9-ETV6* fusion transcript has been shown only in approximately 50–60 % of t(7;12) patients reported to date (Table 1), whereas the reciprocal *ETV6-HLXB9* transcript has never been observed. This is understandable when looking at the details of the translocation breakpoints at the chromosomal/genomic level. Although the breakpoints on chromosome 12 are well defined and disrupt the *ETV6* gene in a precise location at its 5′ end, on chromosome 7 the breakpoints are scattered in different regions proximal to the *HLXB9* gene. This implies that the whole *HLXB9* gene is transferred onto the der(12), but there is no disruption of the gene itself. Moreover, between *HLXB9* and *ETV6* on the der(12) there should be genomic material of variable extent from 7q, depending on the location of the 7q breakpoint (Fig. 2). This means that an *HLXB9-ETV6* fusion transcript would be generated due to some form of long range splicing. Depending on how efficient this mechanism is, the fusion transcript might fail to be present in all t(7;12) patients. Importantly, there has been no report on the presence of a HLXB9-ETV6 protein to date, therefore the production of a chimeric protein as an oncogenic trigger for the t(7;12) leukaemias is debatable.

HLXB9 over-expression

As a fusion transcript is detected in only approximately fifty per cent of t(7;12) AML patients, it is debatable that the formation of the fusion gene is the only contributor to leukaemogenesis in these cases. What all the t(7;12) leukaemias have in common is the over-expression of the

Table 1 Proportion of patients showing an *HLXB9-ETV6* fusion transcript

No. of t(7;12) patients considered	No. of patients with *HLXB9-ETV6* fusion transcript	Percentage of patients with *HLXB9-ETV6* fusion transcript	Reference
2	2	100	[21]
7	4	57	[6]
2	1	50	[13]
1	1	100	[19]
7	4	57	[20]
6	6	100	[50]

Notes: The majority of patients considered in this table were reported as having the t(7;12) in the karyotype of their leukaemic cells. However, in 4 cases [13, 50, 56] the fusion transcript was described in patients with abnormalities of 7q and or 12p, implying that the t(7;12) might have been present, but underestimated in these cases

HLXB9 gene, suggesting that this, rather than the formation of a fusion gene, might be the driver of leukaemogenesis in these patients. Expression of other genes mapping at 7q36 near the breakpoint has also been evaluated and quantified in t(7;12) patients. However, this analysis showed that expression of *NOM1, LMBR1* and *RNF32* in 7q36 as well as *ETV6* on 12p13 was not different from that observed in AML patients without the t(7;12) and in normal bone marrow [6].

The expression of *HLXB9* in healthy progenitor blood cells in the bone marrow has been investigated by several groups. Early expression studies performed in 1991 showed that bone marrow enriched for CD34-positive cells highly expressed *HLXB9*, whereas unfractionated bone marrow cells expressed *HLXB9* in low levels, and bone marrow cells depleted of CD34-positive cells did not show detectable levels of *HLXB9* [22]. Later on, the same authors reported increased levels of *HLXB9* expression in acute leukaemias that were not seen in the leukaemia patients at remission. These studies suggested a link between *HLXB9* over-expression and leukaemogenesis [23]. Other authors reported a relatively low *HLXB9* expression in normal bone marrow by real time quantitative PCR (RT-Q-PCR) and did not observe *HLXB9* expression in healthy CD34-positive bone marrow cells, but described increased levels in the bone marrow of leukaemia patients with the t(7;12) rearrangement [6, 24]. Observations from our group and by others confirmed elevated *HLXB9* expression in t(7;12) leukaemias as well as in some patients with acute myeloid leukaemia with chromosomal abnormalities other than the t(7;12) [20, 25]. *HLXB9* expression has been associated with hypo-methylation of its promoter in a series of paediatric AMLs. However, in the same study it was found that in childhood ALL the *HLXB9* promoter was hyper-methylated leading to down-regulation of this gene. The authors suggest that *HLXB9* might act as an oncogene in AML, whereas it would act as a tumour suppressor gene in ALL [26]. Over-expression of *HLXB9* has been also reported in lymphoma [27, 28] and cancer types other than haematological malignancies, such as breast cancer [29], testicular cancer [30, 31] and hepatocarcinoma [32]. These studies support the idea that *HLXB9* involvement might be pivotal in other tumours as well as leukaemia. Limited studies have been carried out on the HLXB9 expression at the protein level, whose presence has been demonstrated in bone marrow smear of leukaemia patients with the t(7;12) by immunohistochemistry [16]. Further studies on leukaemia as well as other cancer types are needed in order to clarify whether the presence of elevated *HLXB9* transcript corresponds to proportionate levels of the corresponding protein, or whether translation is regulated by RNA interference pathways [31].

HLXB9 over-expression and genome organisation

An increasing number of studies currently focus on gene expression in the context of the three dimensional (3D) genome organisation in the interphase nucleus [33]. Gene positioning within the different areas of the cell nucleus has been associated with different levels of gene activity, with the general assumption that transcriptionally active genes are localised in the nuclear interior, whereas less active genes tend to be positioned towards the periphery of the nucleus [34–37]. It has also been shown that gene positioning in the nucleus is not fixed, but may change according to different stages of development [38, 39] and in pathologies [40]. It has been demonstrated that the chromosome 3D structure within the interphase nucleus has an influence on the transcriptional activities of specific genes due to a position effect mechanism. For instance, gene expression at a specific locus can be controlled in *cis* by enhancer elements localised at a distance from it, via formation of active chromatin hubs (ACH) [41–43]. Several studies have been conducted to observe the behaviour of cancer loci in the interphase nuclei using different cellular models and some authors proposed that the altered nuclear topography of genes could be used as diagnostic tool in oncology [44, 45]. Studies on cancer fusion genes have shown nuclear repositioning of chromosomes and genes after a translocation event [46–48] and this repositioning has been shown to have an impact on expression profiling [49]. We have observed the behaviour of 7q and 12p loci in the interphase nuclei of leukaemia cells carrying the t(7;12) in a number of patients and shown that the

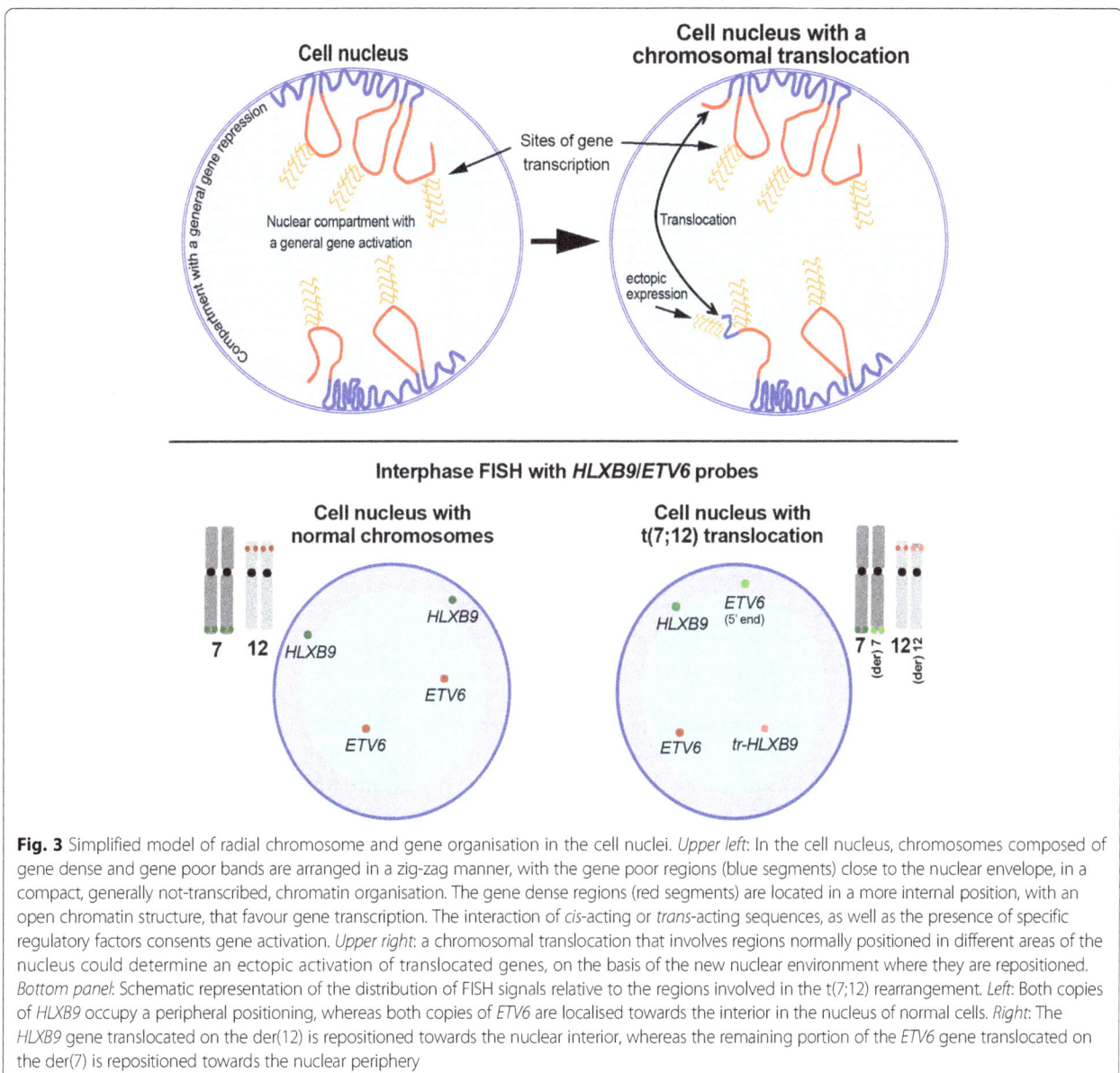

Fig. 3 Simplified model of radial chromosome and gene organisation in the cell nuclei. *Upper left*: In the cell nucleus, chromosomes composed of gene dense and gene poor bands are arranged in a zig-zag manner, with the gene poor regions (blue segments) close to the nuclear envelope, in a compact, generally not-transcribed, chromatin organisation. The gene dense regions (red segments) are located in a more internal position, with an open chromatin structure, that favour gene transcription. The interaction of *cis*-acting or *trans*-acting sequences, as well as the presence of specific regulatory factors consents gene activation. *Upper right*: a chromosomal translocation that involves regions normally positioned in different areas of the nucleus could determine an ectopic activation of translocated genes, on the basis of the new nuclear environment where they are repositioned. *Bottom panel*: Schematic representation of the distribution of FISH signals relative to the regions involved in the t(7;12) rearrangement. *Left*: Both copies of *HLXB9* occupy a peripheral positioning, whereas both copies of *ETV6* are localised towards the interior in the nucleus of normal cells. *Right*: The *HLXB9* gene translocated on the der(12) is repositioned towards the nuclear interior, whereas the remaining portion of the *ETV6* gene translocated on the der(7) is repositioned towards the nuclear periphery

translocation leads to repositioning of the loci of interest (Fig. 3) [20]. What does this imply in terms of gene transcription? We have shown the presence of *HLXB9* transcripts in the same samples with the t(7;12) rearrangement by RT-PCR, however, we did not investigate the origin of the transcript. We assume that the nascent transcript would originate from the der(12), due to the juxtaposition of the *HLXB9* gene to the downstream region of *ETV6*. This would facilitate new interactions between active *cis* elements and the *HLXB9* promoter, leading to the formation of active chromatin hubs and repositioning of the chromatin in the cell nucleus. Alternatively, active *trans* sequences from different chromosomes could activate *HLXB9* by a bridge formation in the new nuclear environment.

Gene expression signature of t(7;12) leukaemias and HLXB9 targets

The first study to investigate expression profiling of t(7;12) leukaemias was conducted by Wildenhain et al. [50], who compared leukaemic blasts of patients positive for the presence of the *HLXB9/ETV6* fusion transcript with those with *MLL* rearrangements. It has to be said that these represent the two most common chromosomal rearrangements found in very young AML patients, including infants and mainly children younger than 2 years of age. The authors found that genes expressed in the *MLL* group of patients, were significantly down-regulated in the *HLXB9/ETV6* positive patients. These included HOX genes and genes characteristic for the *MLL*-induced transformation process such as *MEIS1*, *HOXA9* and *C-MYB*. On the other hand, together with over-expression of *HLXB9*, the *HLXB9/ETV6* positive patients showed up-regulation of genes implicated in cell–cell interactions and cell adhesion such as *EDIL3*, *CNTNAP5*, *ANGPT1*, *DSG2*, *ITGA9*, *ITGAV*, *KDR* and *SIGLEC6*. These are known to be implicated in the maintenance of quiescent haematopoietic stem cells (HSC) and homeostasis of the HSC niche. Overall, this study implies that the mechanisms of leukaemogenesis in these two types of childhood leukaemia are fundamentally very different. Evidence would suggest that the *HLXB9/ETV6* positive leukaemias might be initiated through an alterations of interactions between the HSC and the HSC niche. Balgobind et al. [51] used expression microarrays to examine a large cohort of samples from paediatric patients with AML including seven samples from patients with the t(7;12). The authors built a classifier based on 59 genes that enabled them to identify very specific expression profiling signatures predictive of cytogenetic and molecular subtypes. This classification tool, based on the genetic heterogeneity of paediatric AML, is of great diagnostic potential although its feasibility and implementation in the

diagnostic setting will have to be further explored. The significance and the impact of *HLXB9* up-regulation in the t(7;12) leukaemias merits further studies. These would shed some light on the pathways triggered by this chromosomal rearrangement. The only report to date to explore possible targets for HB9 (the transcription factor coded by the *HLXB9* gene) in haematopoietic cells was performed on the HL-60 myeloid cell line using ChiP-on-chip and expression profiling analyses [24]. This study describes binding of HB9 to the prostaglandin E receptor 2 (*PGTER2*) promoter resulting in down-regulation of *PGTER2* and consequent reduction of intracellular cAMP level. This down-regulatory effect on *PGTER2* expression was also observed in t(7;12) patients. Together with repression of *PGTER2*, Wildenhain et al. [24], found that HLXB9 expression in the HL60 cell line had mostly a down-regulatory effect on other genes, particularly *ZYX* and *ETS1*. Physiologically, expression of *PGTER2* modulates differentiation of osteoclasts. Up-regulation of *PTGER2* has been shown in immature myeloid precursors. *PTGER2* becomes subsequently down-regulated after the cells have differentiated into osteoclasts [52]. Further work is needed to clarify the implications of *PTGER2* down-regulation on the bone marrow niche and on the differentiation of immature pre-leukaemic cells.

Diagnostic tools
Chromosome banding
The t(7;12)(q36;p13) rearrangement affects the subtelomeric regions of chromosomes 7 and 12 respectively. Due to the small size of the genomic fragments translocated, this rearrangement is difficult to detect using the conventional methods of chromosome banding.

Fluorescence in situ hybridisation
Fluorescence in situ hybridisation (FISH) has been fundamental for the identification of the t(7;12) as a non-random rearrangement [7]. Initially, probes covering the entire *ETV6* gene in conjunction with 7q36 probes have been used for the screening of a relatively large number of paediatric patients. This screening enabled us to estimate the incidence of this translocation of approximately one third of patients with infant leukaemia [7]. It has to be noted that the breakpoints on 7q36 in the t(7;12) patients were found to be heterogeneous and generally proximal to *HLXB9* without disrupting the gene itself [12]. A three colour FISH assay with probes flanking the *HLXB9* gene was developed specifically for the detection of the t(7;12) (q36;p13) (Fig. 4). This assay enabled us to successfully identify cryptic and more complex t(7;12) rearrangements [17]. Commercially available FISH probes for the detection of the t(12;21) translocation are also suitable for the detection of the t(7;12), where a

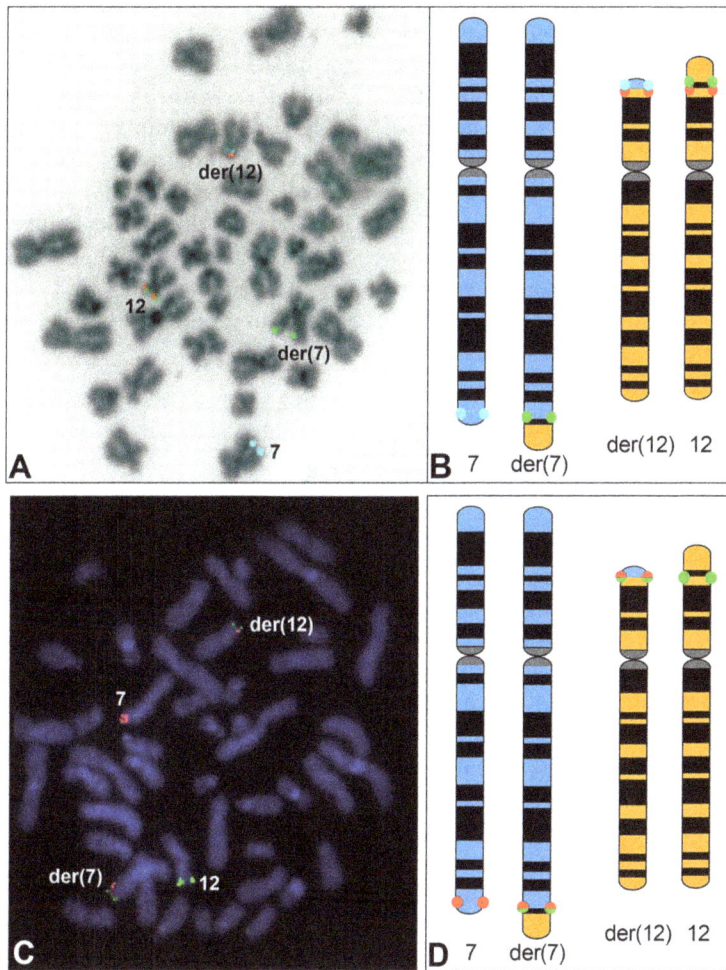

Fig. 4 Fluorescence *in situ* hybridisation (FISH) performed on metaphase chromosomes harbouring the t(7;12)(q36;p13). **a** FISH using a three colour approach enables the detection of both normal chromosomes 7 (harbouring only blue hybridisation signals) and 12 (harbouring green and orange fluorescent signals) and their derivatives (green signals on the der(7) and blue and orange signals on the der(12)). The DAPI counterstaining of the chromosomes has been converted into grey scale to simulate a G-banding pattern (figure taken from Naiel et al., 2013 [17]). **b** Schematic representation showing localisation and colour-code of the FISH probes relative to the three colour probe set used. **c** FISH using a two colour approach enables the detection of both normal chromosomes 7 (harbouring only orange hybridisation signals) and 12 (harbouring only green fluorescent signals) and their derivatives carrying orange and green fusion signals. **d** Schematic representation showing localisation and colour-code of the FISH probes relative to the two colour probe set used. It should be noted that the two colour set does not allow to discriminate between the two derivatives based on colour pattern only. The size and morphology of chromosomes 7 and 12 compared to their respective derivatives are very similar, making the identification of the rearrangement difficult without the aid of FISH. Both probe sets have been provided by MetaSystems Gmbh, Altlussheim, Germany

split *ETV6* signal is found on the der(7) and on the der(12). Dual colour whole or partial chromosome painting may also reveal the t(7;12)(q36;p13). However, visualisation of the rearrangement on one or both derivatives might be impaired due to the small size of the translocated fragments.

Reverse transcription polymerase chain reaction
Specific primers have been designed for the detection of the *HLXB9/ETV6* fusion at the cDNA level by reverse transcription polymerase chain reaction (RT-PCR) [21]. However, the presence of a fusion transcript by RT-PCR

has been identified only in approximately 50 % of t(7,12) leukaemia patients (Table 1). For this reason RT-PCR does not represent a reliable method for the detection of the t(7,12) rearrangements at diagnosis. However, in those patients positive for the *HLXB9/ETV6* fusion transcript, RT-PCR would prove useful for the monitoring of minimal residual disease [53].

Expression profiling
Studies based on expression microarrays have shown that the leukaemic cells of patients carrying the t(7,12) have a distinctive expression pattern that allows to discriminate

this specific cytogenetic subgroup from other [51]. Micro-array based technologies combined with appropriate classifiers constitute potentially a very powerful diagnostic approach, although in a routine diagnostic laboratory the availability of specialised equipment and costs involved might impact on the choice of method.

Incidence

A literature search has shown that at least 47 leukaemia patients with the t(7;12) have been reported to date, based on the presence of the chromosomal translocation and/or the fusion transcript [17]. To date, there are a very limited number of studies to address the incidence of this translocation, with a quite comprehensive investigation considering a total of 345 paediatric patients [6]. In this study, patients were subdivided in 289 ALL, of which 99 were infants, and 59 AML, of which 18 were infants. It emerged that 5 out of 18 infant AMLs (age 0–12 months) harboured the t(7;12) rearrangement, making the incidence of this rearrangement near one third of infant AML. In addition to the above, the t(7;12) was also found in one infant with ALL and one 18 month old child with AML. A previous study was conducted on a more selected series of leukaemia patients, chosen on the basis of age <20 months and the presence of additional copies of chromosomes 8 and/or 19, as well as abnormalities of 7q and/or 12p [7]. This study showed that 10 out of 23 patients harboured a translocation between 7q and 12p. However, in only 7 cases *ETV6* was involved in the translocation and of these, 6 cases had breakpoint in 7q36 and one in 7q22. Later studies confirmed that the incidence of t(7;12)(q36;p13) was low when considering AML paediatric patients enrolled for clinical trials. These studies reported four t(7;12) cases out of 729 enrolled in the UK MRC AML10 and AML 12; one case out of 454 in AML-BFM 98 and 8 cases out of 981 enrolled in the COG trial AAML0531 [54–56].

Prognostic significance and treatment options
Prognostic significance and clinical outcome
Cytogenetic and molecular markers are important factors to be taken in consideration when stratifying patients into high risk/low risk categories and are of guidance for making treatment choices. The WHO system for the classification of myeloid neoplasms and acute leukemia has been amended to include such information [5]. At present, the t(7;12)(q36;p13) is not included in the WHO classification, although it is recommended that it be considered as a separate entity when assessing infant leukaemia [3]. Review of published data on the clinical outcome of the t(7;12) AMLs reveals inferior outcome with 3 years probabilities of event free survival (EFS) of 0–14 % and overall survival

(OS) of 0–28 % (Table 2) [6, 13, 14, 16, 56]. However, one report of a paediatric patient with acute megakaryocytic leukaemia and t(7;12) described achievement of complete remission with chemotherapy alone for 60 months at time of publication [19]. Papers from different clinical trial groups such as the Children's Oncology Group (COG) [56], UK MRC AML 10 and 12 [53] and the Berlin-Frankfurt-Munich (BFM) [55] included the t(7;12)(q36;p13) in the group of patients with 12p abnormalities and confirmed their association with poor prognosis. It was also stressed the need to

Table 2 Summary of reports of t(7;12) leukaemias with treatments and clinical outcome

Reference	Study group	No. of patients	CNS status	Treatment/Course/Outcome
[15]	DCLSG/ POG	10	5	Treatment N/S
				6 died of leukemia
				1 died of leukemia and infection
				1 died of infection
				1 died of treatment related toxicity
				1 alive, 22 months after BMT in CR1
[13]	CCG	2	2	1 relapsed in bone marrow with bilateral chloromas on the hips. Treated with radiation and BMT, but later died due to disease
				1 relapsed twice, treated with BMT, alive after 2 years
[6]	DCOG	6	N/S	Treatment N/S
				Median EFS: 9 months
				3-year EFS: 0 %
				3-year OS: 0 %
[19]	Japan	1	N/S	Alive after 5 years, treated with chemotherapy only
[16]	Korea	3	N/S	1 received cord blood transplantation at 11 months, relapsed 4 months later, then died at 16 months
				1 died during induction chemotherapy from multiple organ failure
				1 achieved remission, but relapsed at 10 months, and died at 16 months
[56]	COG	8	N/S	Treatment N/S
				3-year EFS: 14 %
				3-year OS: 28 %
				2 of 7 evaluable patients are alive (1 after chemotherapy, 1 after BMT) (personal communication)

Notes: *DCLSG* Dutch Childhood Leukemia Study Group; *POG* Pediatric Oncology Group; *CCG* Children's Cancer Group; *COG* Children Oncology Group; *DCOG* Dutch Childhood Oncology Group; *N/S* not specified; *BMT* bone marrow transplantation; *CR1* first complete remission; *EFS* event-free survival; *OS* overall survival

consider these patients as a high risk group based on the cytogenetic classification of AML.

Standard treatment

Standard treatment for paediatric patients with AML includes induction chemotherapy (remission induction) with an anthracycline based regimen which also contains cytarabine. The choice of the anthracycline drug used, as well as the total doses of chemotherapy differ between different centres and collaborative study groups. Most children achieve complete remission with rates of 80–90 % after 2 induction courses and the toxic death rate is in the region of 5 %, with the failures being due to resistant disease [4]. Consolidation or Intensification chemotherapy (post-remission therapy) is essential for cure. It includes the administration of high dose cytarabine possibly in combination with other drugs. Doses, duration, number of drugs as well as scheduling differ between collaborative groups. Currently, treatment related death rates in AML paediatric patients, with the improvement of supportive care and the administration of treatment in experienced units, are now less than 10 % [4].

Stem cell transplantation

Haematopoietic stem cell transplantation (HSCT) is considered an effective therapy for treatment of high risk leukaemia. However, the high toxicity which includes a mortality rate reaching up to 20 % in some series, makes it not a standard therapy in the first line treatment of AML patients with favourable cytogenetics, where a high cure rate is achieved with chemotherapy alone. For patients with unfavourable cytogenetics, although the benefit of HSCT is still to be fully explored, HSCT is considered by many groups as the standard of care [57, 58]. When patients relapse, the most important prognostic factors that will determine the outcome of the salvage therapy are the length of first remission and cytogenetics. In the United Kingdom, HSCT is generally used as consolidation therapy as part of salvage treatment with a survival rate of around 40 % achieved irrespective of the source of stem cells. However, it is important to better understand molecular markers and cytogenetics of the disease to identify patients who would most likely benefit from this modality of treatment [59]. To date, although there are no published guidelines about the management of this group, there is increasing interest among paediatric haematologists/study groups to consider intensification of therapy with allogeneic stem cell transplantation in first complete remission [13, 15, 16, 56]. Further study of this important subgroup of infant AML as well as the incorporation of t(7;12) in future risk stratification schemas are needed to better understand the best treatment approach.

Conclusions

The t(7;12)(q36;p13) is a rare cytogenetic abnormality in paediatric AML and difficult to identify using conventional karyotyping. The use of FISH with appropriate probe sets would enable diagnostic laboratories to identify this cytogenetic entity confidently and to give a better estimate of its occurrence. The incidence of t(7;12) leukaemias is low in overall paediatric AML, but significant in infant leukaemia. There are no published management guidelines for those patients, but it is now acknowledged as a high risk group with poor prognosis and accordingly many are being treated with HSCT in first complete remission. Better understanding of the genetic mechanisms at the basis of t(7;12) leukaemias and the role of *HLXB9* in the establishment of this malignancies would provide grounds for possible tailored therapy.

Competing interests
The authors declare that they have no competing interests.

Authors' contributions
ST designed and wrote the review. YMK and THT contributed the clinical part of the review. TO contributed the molecular mechanisms section and CF and SS contributed the genome organisation part. ST and SS generated the figures. All authors read and approved the manuscript.

Author details
[1]Leukaemia and Chromosome Research Laboratory, Division of Biosciences, Brunel University London, Middlesex UB8 3PH, UK. [2]Dipartimento di Scienze Biologiche, Geologiche e Ambientali, Sezione di Biologia Animale, University of Catania, Catania, Italy. [3]Division of Pediatric Oncology, Blood and Marrow Transplant, Alberta Children's Hospital, University of Calgary, Calgary, Canada.

References
1. Cancer statistics for the UK: Cancer research UK. [http://www.cancerresear chuk.org/cancer-info/cancerstats/].
2. Howlader N, Noone AM, Krapcho M, Garshell J, Neyman N, Altekruse SF, et al. SEER Cancer Statistics Review, 1975–2010, Bethesda, MD; National Cancer Institute. http://seer.cancer.gov/csr/1975_2010/
3. De Rooij J, Zwaan C, van den Heuvel-Eibrink M. Pediatric AML: from biology to clinical management. J Clin Med. 2015;4:127–49.
4. Ward E, DeSantis C, Robbins A, Kohler B, Jemal A. Childhood and adolescent cancer statistics, 2014. CA Cancer J Clin. 2014;64:83–103.
5. Vardiman JW, Thiele J, Arber DA, Brunning RD, Borowitz MJ, Porwit A, et al. The 2008 revision of the World Health Organization (WHO) classification of myeloid neoplasms and acute leukemia: rationale and important changes. Blood. 2009;114:937–51.
6. Von Bergh ARM, van Drunen E, van Wering ER, van Zutven LJCM, Hainmann I, Meijerink JP, et al. High Incidence of t (7; 12)(q36; p13) in infant AML but not in infant ALL, with a dismal outcome and ectopic expression of HLXB9. Genes Chromosomes Cancer. 2006;45:731–9.
7. Tosi S, Harbott J, Teigler-Schlegel A, Haas OA, Pirc-Danoewinata H, Harrison CJ, et al. t(7;12)(q36;p13), a new recurrent translocation involving ETV6 in infant leukemia. Genes Chromosomes Cancer. 2000;29:325–32.
8. Tosi S, Giudici G, Mosna G, Harbott J, Specchia G, Grosveld G, et al. Identification of new partner chromosomes involved in fusions with the ETV6 (TEL) gene in hematologic malignancies. Genes Chromosom Cancer. 1998;21:223–9.
9. Hagemeijer A, Halen K, Abels J. Cytogenetic follow-up of patients with nonlymphocytic leukemia. II. Acute nonlymphocytic leukemia. Cancer Genet Cytogenet. 1981;3:109–24.
10. Slater RM, Behrendt H, De Waal FC. Chromosome studies on acute nonlymphocytic leukemia in children. Pediatr Res. 1983;17:398–405.

11. Heim S, Békàssy A, Garwicz S, Heldrup J, Wiebe T, Kristoffersson U, et al. New structural chromosomal rearrangements in congenital leukemia. Leukemia. 1987;1:16–23.

12. Tosi S, Hughes J, Scherer SW, Nakabayashi K, Harbott J, Haas OA, et al. Heterogeneity of the 7q36 breakpoints in the t(7;12) involving ETV6 in infant leukemia. Genes Chromosomes Cancer. 2003;38:191–200.

13. Simmons HM, Oseth L, Nguyen P, O'Leary M, Conklin KF, Hirsch B. Cytogenetic and molecular heterogeneity of 7q36/12p13 rearrangements in childhood AML. Leuk Off J Leuk Soc Am Leuk Res Fund UK. 2002;16:2408–16.

14. Satake N, Maseki N, Nishiyama M, Kobayashi H, Sakurai M, Inaba H, et al. Chromosome abnormalities and MLL rearrangements in acute myeloid leukemia of infants. Leuk Off J Leuk Soc Am Leuk Res Fund UK. 1999;13:1013–7.

15. Slater RM, von Drunen E, Kroes WG, Weghuis DO, Berg E Van Den, Smit EM, et al. t(7;12)(q36;p13) and t(7;12)(q32;p13)-translocations involving ETV6 in children 18 months of age or younger with myeloid disorders. Leukemia. 2001;15:915–20.

16. Park J, Kim M, Lim J, Kim Y, Han K, Lee J, et al. Three-way complex translocations in infant acute myeloid leukemia with t(7;12)(q36;p13): the incidence and correlation of a HLXB9 overexpression. Cancer Genet Cytogenet. 2009;191:102–5.

17. Naiel A, Vetter M, Plekhanova O, Fleischman E, Sokova O, Tsaur G, et al. A novel three-colour fluorescence in situ hybridization approach for the detection of t(7;12)(q36;p13) in acute myeloid leukaemia reveals new cryptic three way translocation t(7;12;16). Cancers (Basel). 2013;5:281–95.

18. Zheng J. Oncogenic chromosomal translocations and human cancer (review). Oncol Rep. 2013;30:2011–9.

19. Taketani T, Taki T, Sako M, Ishii T, Yamaguchi S, Hayashi Y. MNX1-ETV6 fusion gene in an acute megakaryoblastic leukemia and expression of the MNX1 gene in leukemia and normal B cell lines. Cancer Genet Cytogenet. 2008;186:115–9.

20. Ballabio E, Cantarella CD, Federico C, Di Mare P, Hall G, Harbott J, et al. Ectopic expression of the HLXB9 gene is associated with an altered nuclear position in t(7;12) leukaemias. Leuk Off J Leuk Soc Am Leuk Res Fund UK. 2009;23:1179–82.

21. Beverloo HB, Panagopoulos I, Isaksson M, Wering E Van, van Drunen E Van, Klein A De, et al. Advances in Brief Fusion of the Homeobox Gene HLXB9 and the ETV6 Gene in Infant Acute Myeloid Leukemias with the t (7 ; 12)(q36 ; p13) 1. Cancer Res. 2001;61:5374–7.

22. Deguchi Y, Kehrl JH. Selective expression of two homeobox genes in CD34-positive cells from human bone marrow. Blood. 1991;78:323–8.

23. Deguchi Y, Yamanaka Y, Theodossiou C, Najfeld V, Kehrl J. High expression of two diverged homeobox genes, HB24 and HB9, in acute leukemias: molecular markers of hematopoietic cell immaturity. Leukemia. 1993;7:446–51.

24. Wildenhain S, Ingenhag D, Ruckert C, Degistirici Ö, Dugas M, Meisel R, et al. Homeobox protein HB9 binds to the prostaglandin E receptor 2 promoter and inhibits intracellular cAMP mobilization in leukemic cells. J Biol Chem. 2012;287:40703–12.

25. Nagel S, Kaufmann M, Scherr M, Drexler HG, MacLeod RA. Activation of HLXB9 by juxtaposition with MYB via formation of t(6;7)(q23;q36) in an AML-M4 cell line (GDM-1). Genes Chromosomes Cancer. 2005;42:170–8.

26. Ferguson S, Gautrey H, Strathdee G. The dual role of HLXB9 in leukemia. Pediatr Blood Cancer. 2011;56:349–52.

27. Nagel S, Scherr M, Quentmeier H, Kaufmann M, Zaborski M, Drexler HG, et al. HLXB9 activates IL6 in Hodgkin lymphoma cell lines and is regulated by PI3K signalling involving E2F3. Leuk Off J Leuk Soc Am Leuk Res Fund UK. 2005;19:841–6.

28. Nagel S, Ehrentraut S, Meyer C, Kaufmann M, Drexler HG, MacLeod RAF. Oncogenic deregulation of NKL homeobox gene MSX1 in mantle cell lymphoma. Leuk Lymphoma. 2014;55:1893–903.

29. Neufing PJ, Kalionis B, Horsfall DJ, Ricciardelli C, Stahl J, Vivekanandan S, et al. Expression and localization of homeodomain proteins DLX4/HB9 in normal and malignant human breast tissues. Anticancer Res. 2003;23:1479–88.

30. Almstrup K, Leffers H, Lothe RA, Skakkebaek NE, Sonne SB, Nielsen JE, et al. Improved gene expression signature of testicular carcinoma in situ. Int J Androl. 2007;30:292–302. discussion 303.

31. Novotny GW, Nielsen JE, Sonne SB, Skakkebaek NE, Rajpert-De Meyts E, Leffers H. Analysis of gene expression in normal and neoplastic human testis: new roles of RNA. Int J Androl. 2007;30:316–7.

32. Wilkens L, Jaggi R, Hammer C, Inderbitzin D, Giger O, von Neuhoff N. The homeobox gene HLXB9 is upregulated in a morphological subset of poorly differentiated hepatocellular carcinoma. Virchows Arch. 2011;458:697–708.

33. Pombo A, Dillon N. Three-dimensional genome architecture: players and mechanisms. Nat Rev Mol Cell Biol. 2015;16:245–57.

34. Boyle S, Gilchrist S, Bridger J, Mahy N, Ellis J, Bickmore W. The spatial organization of human chromosomes within the nuclei of normal and emerin-mutant cells. Hum Mol Genet. 2001;10:211–9.

35. Bolzer A, Kreth G, Solovei I, Koehler D, Saracoglu K, Fauth C, et al. Three-dimensional maps of all chromosomes in human male fibroblast nuclei and prometaphase rosettes. PLoS Biol. 2005;3, e157.

36. Misteli T. Beyond the sequence: cellular organization of genome function. Cell. 2007;128:787–800.

37. Federico C, Cantarella CD, Di Mare P, Tosi S, Saccone S. The radial arrangement of the human chromosome 7 in the lymphocyte cell nucleus is associated with chromosomal band gene density. Chromosoma. 2008;117:399–410.

38. Szczerbal I, Foster HA, Bridger JM. The spatial repositioning of adipogenesis genes is correlated with their expression status in a porcine mesenchymal stem cell adipogenesis model system. Chromosoma. 2009;118:647–63.

39. Leotta CG, Federico C, Brundo MV, Tosi S, Saccone S. HLXB9 gene expression, and nuclear location during in vitro neuronal differentiation in the SK-N-BE neuroblastoma cell line. PLoS One. 2014;9, e105481.

40. Bourne G, Moir C, Bikkul MU, Ahmed Hassan M, Eskiw CH, Kill IR, et al. Interphase Chromosome Behaviour in Normal and Diseased Cells. In: Yurov Y, Vorsanova S, Iourov I, editors. Human Interphase Chromosomes: the Biomedical Aspects. Springer-Verlag New York; 2013. p. 9–33

41. De Laat W. Long-range DNA contacts: romance in the nucleus? Curr Opin Cell Biol. 2007;19:317–20.

42. Palstra R-J, Tolhuis B, Splinter E, Nijmeijer R, Grosveld F, de Laat W. The beta-globin nuclear compartment in development and erythroid differentiation. Nat Genet. 2003;35:190–4.

43. Zlatanova J, Caiafa P. CCCTC-binding factor: to loop or to bridge. Cell Mol Life Sci. 2009;66:1647–60.

44. Meaburn KJ, Gudla PR, Khan S, Lockett SJ, Misteli T. Disease-specific gene repositioning in breast cancer. J Cell Biol. 2009;187:801–12.

45. Wiech T, Timme S, Riede F, Stein S, Schuricke M, Cremer C, et al. Human archival tissues provide a valuable source for the analysis of spatial genome organization. Histochem Cell Biol. 2005;123:229–38.

46. Kozubek S, Lukasova E, Mareckova A, Skalnikova M, Kozubek M, Bartova E, et al. The topological organization of chromosomes 9 and 22 in cell nuclei has a determinative role in the induction of t(9,22) translocations and in the pathogenesis of t(9,22) leukemias. Chromosoma. 1999;108:426–35.

47. Lukasova E, Kozubek S, Kozubek M, Kjeronska J, Ryznar L, Horakova J, et al. Localisation and distance between ABL and BCR genes in interphase nuclei of bone marrow cells of control donors and patients with chronic myeloid leukaemia. Hum Genet. 1997;100:525–35.

48. Taslerová R, Kozubek S, Lukásová E, Jirsová P, Bártová E, Kozubek M. Arrangement of chromosome 11 and 22 territories, EWSR1 and FLI1 genes, and other genetic elements of these chromosomes in human lymphocytes and Ewing sarcoma cells. Hum Genet. 2003;112:143–55.

49. Harewood L, Schutz F, Boyle S, Perry P, Delorenzi M, Bickmore WA, et al. The effect of translocation-induced nuclear reorganization on gene expression. Genome Res. 2010;20:554–64.

50. Wildenhain S, Ruckert C, Röttgers S, Harbott J, Ludwig W-D, Schuster FR, et al. Expression of cell-cell interacting genes distinguishes HLXB9/TEL from MLL-positive childhood acute myeloid leukemia. Leuk Off J Leuk Soc Am Leuk Res Fund UK. 2010;24:1657–60.

51. Balgobind BV, van den Heuvel-Eibrink MM, De Menezes RX, Reinhardt D, Hollink IHI, Arentsen-Peters STJCM, et al. Evaluation of gene expression signatures predictive of cytogenetic and molecular subtypes of pediatric acute myeloid leukemia. Haematologica. 2011;96:221–30.

52. Kobayashi Y, Take I, Yamashita T, Mizoguchi T, Ninomiya T, Hattori T, et al. Prostaglandin E2 receptors EP2 and EP4 are down-regulated during differentiation of mouse osteoclasts from their precursors. J Biol Chem. 2005;280:24035–42.

53. Hauer J, Tosi S, Schuster FR, Harbott J. Graft Versus Leukemia Effect After Haploidentical HSCT in a MLL-Negative Infant AML With HLXB9 / ETV6 Rearrangement. Pediatr Blood Cancer. 2007;50:921–23.

54. Harrison CJ, Hills RK, Moorman AV, Grimwade DJ, Hann I, Webb DKH, et al. Cytogenetics of childhood acute myeloid leukemia: United Kingdom Medical Research Council Treatment trials AML 10 and 12. J Clin Oncol. 2010;28:2674–81.

55. Von Neuhoff C, Reinhardt D, Sander A, Zimmermann M, Bradtke J, Betts DR, et al. Prognostic impact of specific chromosomal aberrations in a large

group of pediatric patients with acute myeloid leukemia treated uniformly according to trial AML-BFM 98. J Clin Oncol. 2010;28:2682–9.

56. Hirsch B, Alonzo T, Gerbing R, Kahwash S, Heerema-McKenney A, Aplenc R, et al. 612 Abnormalities Of 12p Are Associated With High-Risk Acute Myeloid Leukemia : A Children's Oncology Group Report. In: 55th ASH annual meeting and exposition. 2013. https://ash.confex.com/ash/2013/webprogram/Paper62375.html

57. Cornelissen JJ, Breems D, van Putten WLJ, Gratwohl AA, Passweg JR, Pabst T, et al. Comparative analysis of the value of allogeneic hematopoietic stem-cell transplantation in acute myeloid leukemia with monosomal karyotype versus other cytogenetic risk categories. J Clin Oncol. 2012;30:2140–6.

58. Koreth J, Schlenk R, Kopecky KJ, Honda S, Sierra J, Djulbegovic BJ, et al. Allogeneic stem cell transplantation for acute myeloid leukemia in first complete remission: systematic review and meta-analysis of prospective clinical trials. JAMA. 2009;301:2349–61.

59. Webb DK. Acute Myeloid leukemia and Myelodysplastic Disorders. In: Pediatric Haematology and Oncology. 1st ed. Wiley-Blackwell: Oxford; 2010;95–108.

Tissue MicroRNA profiles as diagnostic and prognostic biomarkers in patients with resectable pancreatic ductal adenocarcinoma and periampullary cancers

Dan Calatayud[1,11]* ⓘ, Christian Dehlendorff[2], Mogens K. Boisen[3], Jane Preuss Hasselby[4], Nicolai Aagaard Schultz[1], Jens Werner[5], Heike Immervoll[6,7], Anders Molven[6,8], Carsten Palnæs Hansen[1] and Julia S. Johansen[3,9,10]

Abstract

Background: The aim of this study was to validate previously described diagnostic and prognostic microRNA expression profiles in tissue samples from patients with pancreatic cancer and other periampullary cancers.

Methods: Expression of 46 selected microRNAs was studied in formalin-fixed paraffin-embedded tissue from patients with resected pancreatic ductal adenocarcinoma ($n = 165$), ampullary cancer ($n=59$), duodenal cancer ($n = 6$), distal common bile duct cancer ($n = 21$), and gastric cancer ($n = 20$); chronic pancreatitis ($n = 39$); and normal pancreas ($n = 35$). The microRNAs were analyzed by PCR using the Fluidigm platform.

Results: Twenty-two microRNAs were significantly differently expressed in patients with pancreatic cancer when compared to healthy controls and chronic pancreatitis patients; 17 miRNAs were upregulated (miR-21-5p, −23a-3p, −31-5p, −34c-5p, −93-3p, −135b-3p, −155-5p, −186-5p, −196b-5p, −203, −205-5p, −210, −222-3p, −451, −492, −614, and miR-622) and 5 were downregulated (miR-122-5p, −130b-3p, −216b, −217, and miR-375). MicroRNAs were grouped into diagnostic indices of varying complexity. Ten microRNAs associated with prognosis were identified (let-7 g, miR-29a-5p, −34a-5p, −125a-3p, −146a-5p, −187, −205-5p, −212-3p, −222-5p, and miR-450b-5p). Prognostic indices based on differences in expression of 2 different microRNAs were constructed for pancreatic and ampullary cancer combined and separately (30, 5, and 21 indices).

Conclusion: The study confirms that pancreatic cancer tissue has a microRNA expression profile that is different from that of other periampullary cancers, chronic pancreatitis, and normal pancreas. We identified prognostic microRNAs and microRNA indices that were associated with shorter overall survival in patients with radically resected pancreatic cancer.

Keywords: Ampullary cancer, Biomarkers, microRNA, Pancreatic ductal adenocarcinoma, Pancreatic cancer

Background

Pancreatic cancer (PC) is the fourth most common cause of cancer-related death in the Western world, although it only represents 3% of all new cancer cases [1, 2]. Most cases are pancreatic ductal adenocarcinomas (PDAC). Due to locally advanced or metastatic disease, only 20% of all patients diagnosed with PC are accessible to radical surgical treatment, and thereby have the potential for long-term survival [3, 4]. However, even in this group, the 5-year survival is only 20% due to the high recurrence rate [5, 6].

PC located in the head of the pancreas constitutes the majority (60–70%) of the group of cancers in the region, which also includes of ampullary adenocarcinomas (A-AC), accounting for 15–25%; and duodenal cancers (DC); and distal common bile duct (CBD) cancers, each accounting for approximately 10%[6].

* Correspondence: dan.calatayud@gmail.com
[1]Department of Surgical Gastroenterology and Transplantation, Rigshospitalet, Copenhagen University Hospital, Copenhagen, Denmark
[11]Department of Oncology, Herlev University Hospital, Herlev Ringvej 75, DK-2730 Herlev, Denmark
Full list of author information is available at the end of the article

The distribution of the different types of the periampullary cancers is variously reported, probably due to the complexity of the periampullary anatomy and histopathology. The 5-year survival rate after surgery is 45–55% for A-AC and DC [7, 8] and approximately 25% for distal CBD cancers [6].

Cancer antigen 19–9 (CA 19–9, also named carbohydrate antigen 19–9 and sialylated Lewis antigen) is the most widely used biomarker for patients with PC. Serum CA19-9 alone is insufficient as a diagnostic biomarker, although it may have prognostic value in the absence of cholestasis [9]. There is an obvious need for better biomarkers in PC, and microRNAs (miRNAs, miRs) could be interesting in this regard.

MiRNAs are small (18–24 nucleotides) non-coding RNAs that regulate gene expression post-transcriptionally by binding to messenger RNA molecules through nucleotide complementarity [10, 11]. MiRNAs regulate critical cellular processes such as differentiation, proliferation, apoptosis, and metastasis [12–16]. MiRNAs are stable and analyzable in formalin-fixed paraffin-embedded (FFPE) tissue, which is suitable for analysis [17, 18]. So far, 2603 human miRNA sequences have been discovered and the number is increasing [19].

The expression patterns of miRNAs can be combined into profiles that are specific for a given type of tissue or disease. Several specific miRNA expression profiles in PC tissue have been described, with a promising consistency between studies and different array or PCR platforms. The expressions of miR-15b, –21, –95, –103, –107, –122, –135b, –148a, –155, –190, –196a, –200, –203, –210, –216b, –217, –221, –222, and miR-375 differ between PC and normal pancreas or chronic pancreatitis [20–28]. Furthermore, miRNA expression profiling indicates a close relationship between PDAC and A-AC [27]. Specific miRNAs have also been suggested as prognostic biomarkers in several cancers, including PC [23, 29–32].

The aim of the present study was to validate previously described diagnostic and prognostic miRNA expression profiles for PDAC and A-AC in FFPE specimens.

Methods

Patients

Diagnostic miRNA study

FFPE tumor specimens ($n = 359$ including an internal control) were obtained from patients who underwent resection with radical intent for the following diagnoses: PDAC ($n = 165$), A-AC ($n = 59$), DC ($n = 6$), distal CBD cancer ($n = 21$), chronic pancreatitis (CP) ($n = 39$), gastric cancer (GC) ($n = 20$), serous cyst adenoma ($n = 2$), and no cancer ($n = 4$; cysts or fibrosis that could not be classified as normal pancreas or pancreatitis and did not

have any malignant foci) and healthy subjects (HS) ($n = 35$). The pancreatic and periampullary specimens came from patients who had undergone pancreaticoduodenectomy, distal pancreatectomy, or total pancreatectomy between 2004 and 2011 in Denmark (Herlev Hospital $n = 9$; Rigshospitalet $n = 198$), Germany (Heidelberg $n = 69$), and Norway (Bergen $n = 55$). The chronic pancreatitis specimens came from Copenhagen ($n = 5$) and Heidelberg ($n = 34$). All normal pancreas tissue was obtained from Heidelberg from organ donors or patients with traumatic pancreatic lesions leading to resection of healthy pancreatic tissue. The Danish patients were included in the BIOPAC Study (BIOmarkers in patients with Pancreatic Cancer). The gastric cancers came from patients who had undergone surgery at Gentofte Hospital. An experienced pathologist reassessed all samples to select the most representative part of the specimen, and tumors were classified and graded according to the World Health Organization criteria [33].

Prognostic miRNA study

One hundred fifty-seven FFPE tumor specimens were analyzed from patients who underwent surgery with radical intent for PDAC ($n = 103$) and A-AC ($n = 54$). The patients were included in the BIOPAC Study at Rigshospitalet in Denmark. Inclusion criteria were age ≥ 18 years and histologically verified PC in a resected specimen. After surgery, the majority of the patients (87%) were treated with adjuvant gemcitabine for 6 months or until disease recurrence.

Patient characteristics are shown in Table 1.

MiRNA purification from FFPE tissues

One FFPE block was selected from each patient for miRNA analysis. From each of these blocks, 3 10-μm sections were cut for miRNA extraction without microdissection. As method control, 9×3 sections were cut from a specimen from 1 of the PDAC patients. MiRNAs were extracted using Qiagen miRNeasy FFPE kit, Cat No./ID: 217504. Briefly, the sections were deparaffinized in xylene and ethanol and then treated with proteinase K, and RNA was isolated using the one-column spin column protocol for total RNA. The concentration of small RNAs was assessed by absorbance spectrometry on a DTX 880 (Beckman Coulter).

MiRNA analysis

The following 46 miRNAs were selected for analysis: miR-21-5p, –23a-3p, –29a-5p, –31-5p, –34a-5p, –34c-5p, –93-3p, –122-5p, –125a-3p, –130b-3p, –135b-3p, –136-3p, –146a-5p, –148a-3p, –148a-5p, –155-5p, –186-5p, –187-3p, –194-3p, –196b-5p, –198, –203, –205-5p, –210, –212-3p, –216b, –217, –222-3p, –222-5p, –375, –411-5p, –431-5p, –450b-5p, –451a, –490-3p, –492,

Table 1 Characteristics of the Danish patients

Characteristic	PDAC N = 110	A-AC N = 59	Duodenal cancer N = 6	Distal CBD cancer N = 21	Chronic pancreatitis N = 5	Serous cystadenoma and other benign diagnosis N = 6
Age, years median (range)	65.7 (37.4-81.3)	64.9 (38.3-80.5)	69.0 (54.3-74.4)	64.7 (38.6-74.6)	56.4 (43.8-68.2)	60.6 (46.7-84.7)
Gender						
Male	60 (55%)	37 (63%)	5 (83%)	11 (52%)	5 (100%)	2 (33%)
Female	50 (45%)	22 (37%)	1 (17%)	10 (48%)	0	4 (67%)
ASA score						
1	12 (11%)	9 (15%)	0	2 (10%)	1 (20%)	0
2	58 (53%)	38 (66%)	5 (83%)	15 (75%)	2 (40%)	4 (80%)
3	30 (27%)	11 (19%)	1 (17%)	3 (15%)	2 (40%)	1 (20%)
4	0	0		0	0	0
TNM-Stage						
IA	9 (8%)	4 (7%)	1 (17%)	1 (5%)		
IB	3 (3%)	7 (12%)	1 (17%)	1 (5%)		
IIA	27 (25%)	6 (10%)	2 (33%)	7 (52%)		
IIB	67 (65%)	24 (41%)	2 (33%)	11 (33%)		
III	0	16 (27%)	0	1 (5%)		

Values are N (%). Numbers may not add up due to missing values
No clinical information is available from the patients with gastric cancer and the patients and healthy subjects from Heidelberg and Bergen

−509-5p, −571, −614, −622, −625-5p, −675-5p, −769-5p, −939, −944, and let-7 g. The selection was based on the previously described relationship of the miRNAs to PC in particular and to cancer biology in general (Detailed information on each specific miRNA is available in "Additional file 1").

The miRNAs were analyzed in triplicate using the Fluidigm BioMark System™. This system can perform multiple simultaneous real-time PCR measurements running gold-standard Taqman® assays in nanolitre quantities. The instructions from Fluidigm were followed in all details (https://www.fluidigm.com). The analyses were performed at AROS Applied Biotechnology A/S (www.arosab.com, Aarhus, Denmark).

Statistical analysis

Differences in miRNA expression according to diagnosis were tested by univariate logistic regression including the raw miRNA expression level as continuous variables on the cycle threshold scale. Odds ratios (OR) per interquartile increase and 95% confidence intervals were computed for both PC vs. HS and PC vs. HS and CP.

Diagnostic indices were identified in 3 different ways among the significant miRNAs: (1) As a manually defined index by including 2 miRNA with OR > 1 and 2 with OR < 1 (indices I and IV);(2) As a computer generated index found by backwards elimination of a model with miRNAs chosen from 18 miRNAs described in an previous index (the so-called LASSO-classifier: miR-23a, 34c-5p, −122, −135b-3p, −136-3p, −186, −196b, −198,

−203, −222-3p, −451, −490, −492, −509-5p, −571, −614, −622, and miR-93 [27]) which were significant at a 1% significance level, to account for multiple testing and with less than 10% missing values (indices II and V) and (3) as a computer generated index like (2) but based on all significant miRNAs (indices III and VI). A total of 6 indices were identified: I, II, and III developed for the PC vs. HS comparison and IV, V, and VI developed for the PC vs. HS + CP comparison. The indices were evaluated by means of boxplots, and their performance was evaluated by computing sensitivity, specificity, accuracy, area under curve (AUC), true positives (TP), true negatives (TN), false positives (FP), and false negatives (FN). The indices were also tested on other cancer types. For each index, we first found a suitable cut-off by requiring a sensitivity of 85% in the PC vs. HS or vs. HS + CP comparison. Subsequently, this cut-off point was applied in all other comparisons.

It was not possible to stratify our patients according to TNM due to the very uneven distribution of cancer stages and resulting small subgroups.

For the prognostic study, the association between overall survival (OS) and miRNA expression was illustrated by Kaplan–Meier curves by dichotomizing the miRNA expression into below and above the median expression for each miRNA. The association was tested by means of univariate Cox proportional hazards regression both on the continuous variables and on the dichotomized variables, and presented as hazard ratios (HR) and corresponding 95% confidence intervals (CIs). In addition, analyses adjusted for age, sex, tumor stage, ASA score, and tumor differentiation were performed. Finally, we considered differences between 2 miRNAs at a time as a continuous variable in the Cox models (unadjusted and adjusted) for OS. Analyses were made for the diagnoses PDAC and A-AC together and separately.

In all analysis, the software package R version 3.1.1 (R Core Team 2014; R: A language and environment for statistical computing. R Foundation for Statistical Computing, Vienna, Austria. www.R-project.org) was used, and *P*-values below 5% were considered statistically significant.

Results

Diagnosis – Pancreatic cancer vs. healthy subjects

The following 14 miRNAs were upregulated in PC compared to HS: miR-21-5p, –23a-3p, –31-5p, –34c-5p, –93-3p, –135b-3p, –155-5p, –196b-5p, –203, –205-5p, –210, –222-3p, –451, and miR-622. The following 5 miRNAs were downregulated in PC: miR-122-5p, –130b-3p, –216b, – 217, and miR-375 (Table 2).

Three indices of miRNA expression, index I, II, and III, were identified to separate PC from HS (i.e., normal pancreas tissue):

(I) A manually defined index: miR-375 + miR-130b-3p – miR-451 – miR34c-5p.

(II) A computer-generated index based on univariate significant miRNAs chosen from 18 miRNAs describes in a previous index with less than 10% missing: 292.6458– 3.0539×miR-34c-5p + 4.007×miR-203–10.4×miR-222-3p– 3.6057×miR-451–4.3015×miR-622.

The potential miRNAs for index II were miR-34c-5p, –135-3p, –203, –222-3p, –451,and miR-622.

(III) A computer-generated index based on all univariate significant miRNAs with less than 10% missing values: 118.7249 + 77.2459×miR-130b-3p–23.7911×miR-34c-5p–49.923×miR-451.

The potential miRNAs for index III were miR-31-5p, –34c-5p,-93-3p, –130b-3p, –135b-3p, –155-5p, –203, –205-5p, –210, –216b, –217, –222-3p, –375, –451,and miR-622.

The performances of these indices are illustrated in box plots in Fig. 1 and Table 3 (upper part). The manually calculated index I was able to separate PC from HS with a sensitivity of 84.9 (CI 78.5–90.0), but could also differentiate the other malignant diagnoses from HS, with a sensitivity varying from 66.7 (distal CBD cancer) to 100.0 (DC and GC). The computer-generated index II performed in the same way with regard to PC vs. HS, but was inferior for separating the other malignancies from HS except for distal CBD cancer, where it performed better than index I. The computer-generated index III performed slightly better than index II with

regard to separating A-AC and DC cancer from HS, but was inferior for separating distal CBD cancer and GC.

Diagnosis - Pancreatic cancer vs. healthy subjects + chronic pancreatitis

The following 17 miRNAs were upregulated in PDAC compared with benign specimens (HS and CP combined): miR-21-5p, –23a-3p, –31-5p, –34c-5p, –93-3p, –135b-3p, –155-5p, –186-5p, –196b-5p, –203, –205-5p, –210, –222-3p, –451, –492, –614, and miR-622. The following 5 miRNAs were downregulated in PDAC compared to benign specimens (HS and CP combined): miR-122-5p, –130b-3p, –216b, –217, and miR-375 (Table 2).

Three indices, IV, V, and VI, of miRNA expression to separate PC from benign tissue (i.e., HS and CP combined) were identified.

(IV) A manually defined index: miR-375 + miR-130b-3p – miR-451 – miR-34c-5p.

(V) A computer-generated index based on significant miRNAs chosen from 18 miRNAs described in a previous index with less than 10% missing values: 20.5487–1.5899×miR-222-3p–0.4006×miR-451– 0.3864×miR-203–0.5056×miR-622+ 1.203×miR-186-5p.

The potential miRNAs for index V weremiR-34c-5p, –135b-3p, –186-5p, –203, –222-3p, –451, and miR-622.

(VI) A computer-generated index based on all significant miRNAs with less than 10% missing values: 7.1834– 0.5175×miR-210 + 1.3893×miR-93-3p – 0.7423×miR-375– 2.6184×miR-222-3p – 0.3414×miR-451–0.3852×miR-203– 0.5316×miR-622 + 1.822×miR-186-5p.

The potential miRNAs for index VI were miR-31-5p, –34c-5p, –93-3p, –130b-3p, –135b-3p, –155-5p, –186-5p, –203, –210, –216b, –217, –222-3p, –375, –451, and miR-622.

The performances of these indices are illustrated in box plots in Fig. 1 and in Table 3 (lower part). Index IV could separate HS from the other diagnoses. Indices V and VI were able to separate CP from the malignant diagnoses.

Diagnostic miRNA indices previously identified for pancreatic cancer

We have previously described the following 4 different diagnostic miRNA indices in FFPE cancer tissues consisting of 2 different miRNAs [27]: (1) miR-196b-5p – miR-217; (2) miR-411 – miR-198; (3) miR-614 – miR-122-5p; and (4) miR-614 – miR-93-3p. The performance of the 4 indices in the present cohort was tested using the Fluidigm method. Since many samples had non-detectable miRNAs, we only used observations that were non-missing, i.e., not imputed by a large C_t-value. Index 1 had 97 samples with at least 1miRNA missing, index 2 had 122 samples with

Table 2 Significantly deregulated microRNAs

microRNA upregulated in PC compared to healthy subjects

miRNA	OR (CI)	p-value	PC	HS	Missing
miR-21-5p	0.11 (0.03–0.25)	0.0000	134	13	53
miR-23a-3p	0.36 (0.13–0.67)	0.0100	156	5	39
miR-31-5p	0.38 (0.28–0.50)	0.0000	165	35	0
miR-34c-5p	0.17 (0.09–0.28)	0.0000	165	35	0
miR-93-3p	0.14 (0.06–0.26)	0.0000	165	34	1
miR-135b-3p	0.31 (0.20–0.44)	0.0000	165	30	5
miR-155-5p	0.11 (0.03–0.23)	0.0000	165	33	2
miR-196b-5p	0.14 (0.02–0.45)	0.0151	147	3	50
miR-203	0.37 (0.25–0.51)	0.0000	165	35	0
miR-205-5p	0.71 (0.59–0.82)	0.0000	148	21	31
miR-210	0.12 (0.05–0.22)	0.0000	165	34	1
miR-222-3p	0.06 (0.02–0.15)	0.0000	165	35	0
miR-451	0.14 (0.06–0.27)	0.0000	165	35	0
miR-622	0.57 (0.41–0.76)	0.0003	165	34	1

microRNA downregulated in PC compared to healthy subjects

miRNA	OR (CI)	p-value	PC	HS	Missing
miR-122-5p	2.08 (1.40–3.51)	0.0014	30	18	152
miR-130b-3p	5.34 (3.17–9.98)	0.0000	165	35	0
miR-216b	6.30 (3.36–14.24)	0.0000	149	35	16
miR-217	2.94 (2.03–4.69)	0.0000	142	35	23
miR-375	26.10 (9.48–90.22)	0.0000	165	35	0

microRNA upregulated in PC compared to healthy subjects and chronic pancreatitis

miRNA	OR (CI)	p-value	PC	HS + CP	Missing
miR-21-5p	0.24 (0.14–0.36)	0.0000	134	42	63
miR-23a-3p	0.54 (0.38–0.74)	0.0003	156	31	52
miR-31-5p	0.50 (0.41–0.59)	0.0000	165	74	0
miR-34c-5p	0.33 (0.25–0.43)	0.0000	165	74	0
miR-93-3p	0.27 (0.17–0.40	0.0000	165	73	1
miR-135b-3p	0.31 (0.22–0.41	0.0000	165	58	16
miR-155-5p	0.46 (0.37–0.56	0.0000	165	72	2
miR-186-5p	0.71 (0.55–0.89	0.0041	165	74	0
miR-196b-5p	0.53 (0.39–0.70	0.0000	147	20	72
miR-203	0.36 (0.26–0.46	0.0000	165	74	0
miR-205-5p	0.79 (0.71–0.88	0.0000	148	46	45
miR-210	0.27 (0.18–0.36	0.0000	165	73	1
miR-222-3p	0.23 (0.16–0.32	0.0000	165	74	0
miR-451	0.44 (0.35–0.54	0.0000	165	74	0
miR-492	0.46 (0.22–0.78	0.0097	57	4	178
miR-614	0.75 (0.57–0.94	0.0219	110	14	115
miR-622	0.52 (0.41–0.66	0.0000	165	72	2

Table 2 Significantly deregulated microRNAs *(Continued)*

microRNA downregulated in PC compared to healthy subjects and chronic pancreatitis					
miRNA	OR (CI)	*p*-value	PC	HS + CP	Missing
miR-122-5p	1.99 (1.46–2.98)	0.0001	30	40	169
miR-130b-3p	1.71 (1.33–2.23)	0.0001	165	74	0
miR-216b	1.55 (1.34–1.84)	0.0000	149	73	17
miR-217	1.46 (1.28–1.69)	0.0000	142	71	26
miR-375	2.22 (1.62–3.15)	0.0000	165	74	0

at least 1 miRNA missing, index 3 had 213 samples with at least 1 miRNA missing, and index 4 had 115 samples with at least 1miRNA missing. For indices 2 and 3, it was not possible to consider HS alone. The performances of these indices are shown in box plots in Fig. 2. Index 1 could separate HS from PC patients but could not separate CP from A-AC. Index 1 could separate GC from all other diagnoses with high accuracy. Indices 2, 3, and 4 could not separate samples with benign from malignant diagnoses. Further information is given in the "Additional file 2".

Prognostic miRNAs – PDAC and A-AC patients combined

In all, 157 patients with either PDAC or A-AC were available for the survival analysis, and 112died during the follow-up period. Table 4 illustrates that low expression of 6 miRNAs (miR-29a-5p, miR-34a-5p, miR-125a-3p, miR-146a-5p, miR-205-5p, and miR-212-3p) was associated with short OS, both with and without adjustment for age, sex, tumor stage/differentiation, and ASA-score. When patients were divided into 2 groups for each miRNA (defined as expression under or above the median level), low miR-34a-5p, miR-205-5p, miR-212-

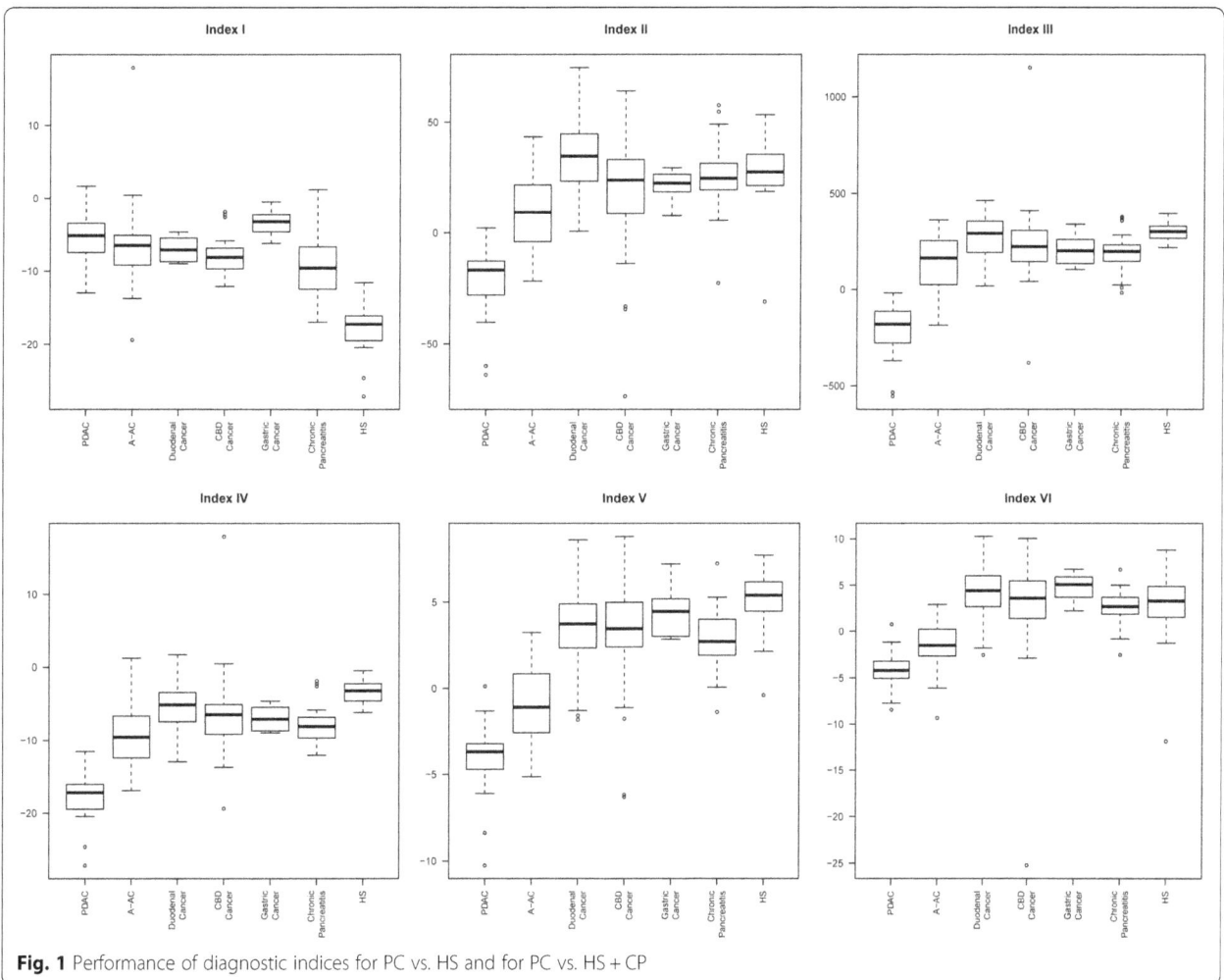

Fig. 1 Performance of diagnostic indices for PC vs. HS and for PC vs. HS + CP

Table 3 Performance of diagnostic indices

Study	Index	Designed sensitivity	cutoff	Sensitivity (CI)	Specificity (CI)	Accuracy (CI)	AUC (CI)	TP	TN	FP	FN
Performance of diagnostic indices developed on PC vs. HS											
PC vs. HS	I	0.85	−9.13	84.85 (78.45–89.95)	100.00 (90.00–100.00)	87.50 (82.10–91.74)	1.00 (1.00–1.00)	140	35	0	25
A-AC vs. HS	I		−9.13	74.58 (61.56–85.02)	100.00 (90.00–100.00)	84.04 (75.05–90.78)	0.99 (0.96–1.00)	44	35	0	15
DC vs. HS	I		−9.13	100.00 (54.07–100.00)	100.00 (90.00–100.00)	100.00 (91.40–100.00)	1.00 (1.00–1.00)	6	35	0	0
CBD vs. HS	I		−9.13	66.67 (43.03–85.41)	100.00 (90.00–100.00)	87.50 (75.93–94.82)	1.00 (0.99–1.00)	14	35	0	7
A-AC, DC, CBD vs. HS	I		−9.13	74.42 (63.87–83.22)	100.00 (90.00–100.00)	81.82 (73.78–88.24)	0.99 (0.97–1.00)	64	35	0	22
GC vs. HS	I		−9.13	100.00 (83.16–100.00)	100.00 (90.00–100.00)	100.00 (93.51–100.00)	1.00 (1.00–1.00)	20	35	0	0
PC vs. HS	II	0.85	16.68	84.85 (78.45–89.95)	100.00 (90.00–100.00)	87.50 (82.10–91.74)	1.00 (1.00–1.00)	140	35	0	25
A-AC vs. HS	II		16.68	67.80 (54.36–79.38)	100.00 (90.00–100.00)	79.79 (70.25–87.37)	0.94 (0.89–0.98)	40	35	0	19
DC vs. HS	II		16.68	83.33 (35.88–99.58)	100.00 (90.00–100.00)	97.56 (87.14–99.94)	1.00 (1.00–1.00)	5	35	0	1
CBD vs. HS	II		16.68	80.95 (58.09–94.55)	100.00 (90.00–100.00)	92.86 (82.71–98.02)	0.97 (0.90–1.00)	17	35	0	4
A-AC, DC, CBD vs. HS	II		16.68	72.09 (61.38–81.23)	100.00 (90.00–100.00)	80.17 (71.94–86.86)	0.95 (0.91–0.99)	62	35	0	24
GC vs. HS	II		16.68	95.00 (75.13–99.87)	100.00 (90.00–100.00)	98.18 (90.28–99.95)	0.96 (0.87–1.00)	19	35	0	1
PC vs. HS	III	0.85	149.10	84.85 (78.45–89.95)	100.00 (90.00–100.00)	87.50 (82.10–91.74)	1.00 (1.00–1.00)	140	35	0	25
A-AC vs. HS	III		149.10	72.88 (59.73–83.64)	100.00 (90.00–100.00)	82.98 (73.84–89.95)	0.98 (0.95–1.00)	43	35	0	16
DC vs. HS	III		149.10	66.67 (22.28–95.67)	100.00 (90.00–100.00)	95.12 (83.47–99.40)	1.00 (1.00–1.00)	4	35	0	2
CBD vs. HS	III		149.10	71.43 (47.82–88.72)	100.00 (90.00–100.00)	89.29 (78.12–95.97)	1.00 (0.99–1.00)	15	35	0	6
A-AC, DC, CBD vs. HS	III		149.10	72.09 (61.38–81.23)	100.00 (90.00–100.00)	80.17 (71.94–86.86)	0.99 (0.97–1.00)	62	35	0	24
GC vs. HS	III		149.10	100.00 (83.16–100.00)	100.00 (90.00–100.00)	100.00 (93.51–100.00)	1.00 (1.00–1.00)	20	35	0	0
Performance of diagnostic indices developed on PC vs. HS + CP											
PC vs. HS + CP	IV	0.85	−9.13	84.85 (78.45–89.95)	75.68 (64.31–84.90)	82.01 (76.54–86.66)	0.89 (0.84–0.94)	140	56	18	25
A-AC vs. HS + CP	IV		−9.13	74.58 (61.56–85.02)	75.68 (64.31–84.90)	75.19 (66.96–82.26)	0.83 (0.76–0.90)	44	56	18	15
DC vs. HS + CP	IV		−9.13	100.00 (54.07–100.00)	75.68 (64.31–84.90)	77.50 (66.79–86.09)	0.85 (0.76–0.93)	6	56	18	0
4 vs. HS + CP	IV		−9.13	66.67 (43.03–85.41)	75.68 (64.31–84.90)	73.68 (63.65–82.19)	0.80 (0.71–0.88)	14	56	18	7
A-AC, DC, CBD vs. HS + CP	IV		−9.13	74.42 (63.87–83.22)	75.68 (64.31–84.90)	75.00 (67.55–81.50)	0.83 (0.76–0.89)	64	56	18	22
CG vs. HS + CP	IV		−9.13	100.00 (83.16–100.00)	75.68 (64.31–84.90)	80.85 (71.44–88.24)	0.97 (0.93–1.00)	20	56	18	0
PC vs. HS + CP	V	0.85	1.38	84.85 (78.45–89.95)	91.89 (83.18–96.97)	87.03 (82.10–91.01)	0.96 (0.94–0.98)	140	68	6	25
A-AC vs. HS + CP	V		1.38	77.97 (65.27–87.71)	91.89 (83.18–96.97)	85.71 (78.59–91.17)	0.93 (0.87–0.97)	46	68	6	13
DC vs. HS + CP	V		1.38	100.00 (54.07–100.00)	91.89 (83.18–96.97)	92.50 (84.39–97.20)	1.00 (0.98–1.00)	6	68	6	0
CBD vs. HS + CP	V		1.38	85.71 (63.66–96.95)	91.89 (83.18–96.97)	90.53 (82.78–95.58)	0.94 (0.89–0.98)	18	68	6	3
A-AC, DC, CBD vs. HS + CP	V		1.38	81.40 (71.55–88.98)	91.89 (83.18–96.97)	86.25 (79.93–91.18)	0.94 (0.89–0.97)	70	68	6	16
GC vs. HS + CP	V		1.38	95.00 (75.13–99.87)	91.89 (83.18–96.97)	92.55 (85.26–96.95)	0.99 (0.96–1.00)	19	68	6	1
PC vs. HS + CP	VI	0.85	1.46	84.85 (78.45–89.95)	93.24 (84.93–97.77)	87.45 (82.57–91.37)	0.97 (0.95–0.99)	140	69	5	25

Table 3 Performance of diagnostic indices (Continued)

						TP	TN	FP	FN
A-AC vs. HS + CP	VI	1.46	72.88 (59.73–83.64)	93.24 (84.93–97.77)	84.21 (76.88–89.95)	0.92 (0.87–0.96)	43	69	5	16
DC vs. HS + CP	VI	1.46	100.00 (54.07–100.00)	93.24 (84.93–97.77)	93.75 (86.01–97.94)	0.99 (0.97–1.00)	6	69	5	0
CBD vs. HS + CP	VI	1.46	76.19 (52.83–91.78)	93.24 (84.93–97.77)	89.47 (81.49–94.84)	0.93 (0.87–0.98)	16	69	5	5
A-AC, DC, CBD vs. HS + CP	VI	1.46	75.58 (65.13–84.20)	93.24 (84.93–97.77)	83.75 (77.10–89.10)	0.93 (0.89–0.96)	65	69	5	21
GC vs. HS + CP	VI	1.46	75.00 (50.90–91.34)	93.24 (84.93–97.77)	89.36 (81.30–94.78)	0.91 (0.80–0.98)	15	69	5	5

AUC Area under Curve, TP True positive, TN True negative, FP False positive, FN False negative, PC Pancreatic Cancer, A-AC Ampullary Adenocarcinoma, DC Duodenal Cancer, CBD Common bile duct cancer, GC Gastric cancer, HS Healthy subjects

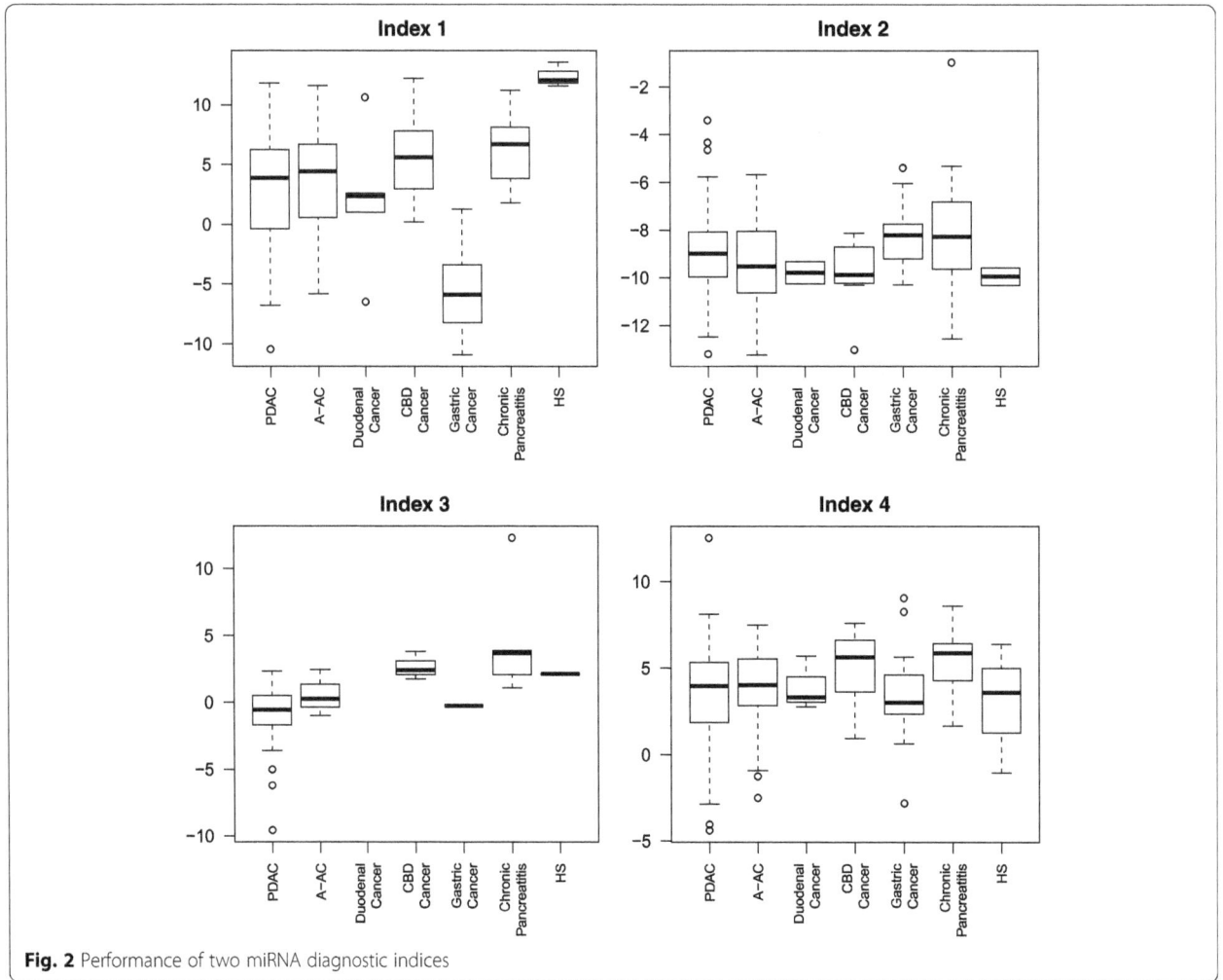

Fig. 2 Performance of two miRNA diagnostic indices

3p, and miR-222-5plevels were significantly associated with short OS. After adjusting for age, sex, tumor stage/differentiation, and ASA-score, let-7 g, miR-29a-5p, miR-34a-5p, miR-205-5p, and miR-212-3p were associated with short OS. Figure 3 illustrates Kaplan–Meier curves for the6 miRNAs reaching a significance level below 0.01.

Table 5 shows 30 and 27 combinations of 2 miRNAs significantly associated with short OS in an unadjusted and an adjusted analysis in PDAC and A-AC in combination.th=tlb=

Prognostic miRNAs - PDAC

One hundred three patients with PDAC were available for the survival analysis, and 83 died during the follow-up period. In both the unadjusted and the adjusted (age, sex, tumor stage/differentiation, ASA-score) analyses, low expression of 2 miRNAs was associated with short OS prognosis:miR-34a-5p: HR = 0.72(CI: 0.56–0.93) (unadjusted) and HR = 0.70(CI: 0.52–0.93) (adjusted); and miR-212-3p HR = 0.83(CI: 0.71–0.99) (unadjusted)

and HR = 0.82(CI: 0.68–0.99) (adjusted). Dividing the patients into 2 groups for each miRNA (defined as expression under or above the median level), low miR-34a-5p and miR-212-3p levels were associated with short OS. Figure 4 shows Kaplan–Meier curves for the miRNAs reaching a significance level below 0.01.

Table 5 shows 5 and 12 combinations of 2 miRNAs significantly associated with short OS in an unadjusted and an adjusted analysis in PDAC.

Prognostic miRNAs – A-AC

Fifty-four patients with A-AC were available for the survival analysis, and 29 died during the follow-up period. In the unadjusted analysis, 4 miRNAs were significantly associated with prognosis: let-7 g: HR = 0.74(CI: 0.58–0.93), miR-34a-5p: HR = 0.66(CI: 0.46–0.94), miR-187: HR = 1.51(CI: 1.01–2.24), and miR-205-5p: HR = 0.74(CI: 0.63–0.86). In the adjusted analysis (age, sex, tumor stage/differentiation, ASA-score), low expression of miR-34a-5p: HR = 0.58(CI: 0.38–0.89) and miR-450b-5p: HR = 0.48(CI: 0.23–0.99) and high expression of miR-187:

Table 4 Prognostic miRNAs in patients with PC + A-AC, PC and A-AC

PDAC and A-AC

CT-expression (per IQR increase)

miRNA	Unadjusted			Adjusted		
	HR (CI)	P	N	HR (CI)	P	N
miR-29a-5p	0.87 (0.76–0.99)	0.0302	156	0.85 (0.74–0.98)	0.0212	145
miR-34a-5p	0.66 (0.54–0.81)	<0.0001	156	0.64 (0.52–0.79)	<0.0001	145
miR-125a-3p	0.83 (0.73–0.95)	0.0051	153	0.83 (0.72–0.95)	0.0077	142
miR-146a-5p	0.87 (0.76–0.99)	0.0296	157	0.85 (0.74–0.97)	0.0191	146
miR-205-5p	0.91 (0.86–0.96)	4e-04	130	0.92 (0.87–0.97)	0.0037	120
miR-212-3p	0.81 (0.72–0.91)	4e-04	156	0.80 (0.71–0.91)	4e-04	145

Under median vs. over median

miRNA	Unadjusted			Adjusted		
	HR (CI)	P	N	HR (CI)	P	N
let-7 g	NS			0.62 (0.41–0.93)	0.0220	145
miR-29a-5p	NS			0.64 (0.42–0.96)	0.0314	145
miR-34a-5p	0.46 (0.31–0.67)	<0.0001	156	0.47 (0.31–0.71)	0.0003	145
miR-205-5p	0.37 (0.25–0.57)	<0.0001	130	0.44 (0.28–0.69)	0.0003	120
miR-212-3p	0.51 (0.35–0.74)	5e-04	156	0.53 (0.35–0.79)	0.0021	145
miR-222-5p	0.68 (0.47–1.00)	0.0495	152	NS		

PDAC

CT-expression (per IQR increase)

miRNA	Unadjusted			Adjusted		
	HR (CI)	P	N	HR (CI)	P	N
miR-34a-5p	0.72 (0.56–0.93)	0.0104	103	0.70 (0.52–0.93)	0.0144	93
miR-212-3p	0.83 (0.71–0.99)	0.0328	103	0.82 (0.68–0.99)	0.0350	93

Under median vs. over median

miRNA	Unadjusted			Adjusted		
	HR (CI)	P	N	HR (CI)	P	N
miR-34a-5p	0.49 (0.31–0.77)	0.0020	103	0.53 (0.32–0.89)	0.0151	93
miR-212-3p	0.64 (0.41–0.98)	0.0417	103	0.59 (0.36–0.97)	0.0358	93

A-AC

CT-expression (per IQR increase)

miRNA	Unadjusted			Adjusted		
	HR (CI)	P	N	HR (CI)	P	N
let-7 g	0.74 (0.58–0.93)	0.0100	53	NS		
miR-34a-5p	0.66 (0.46–0.94)	0.0218	53	0.58 (0.38–0.89)	0.0121	52
miR-187	1.51 (1.01–2.24)	0.0439	24	2.34 (1.22–4.48)	0.0104	24
miR-205-5p	0.73 (0.63–0.86)	0.0001	37	NS		
miR-450b-5p	NS			0.48 (0.23–0.99)	0.0458	26

Under median vs. over median

miRNA	Unadjusted			Adjusted		
	HR (CI)	P	N	HR (CI)	P	N
miR-34a-5p	0.40 (0.19–0.86)	0.0183	53	0.36 (0.16–0.85)	0.0195	52

NS Not significant

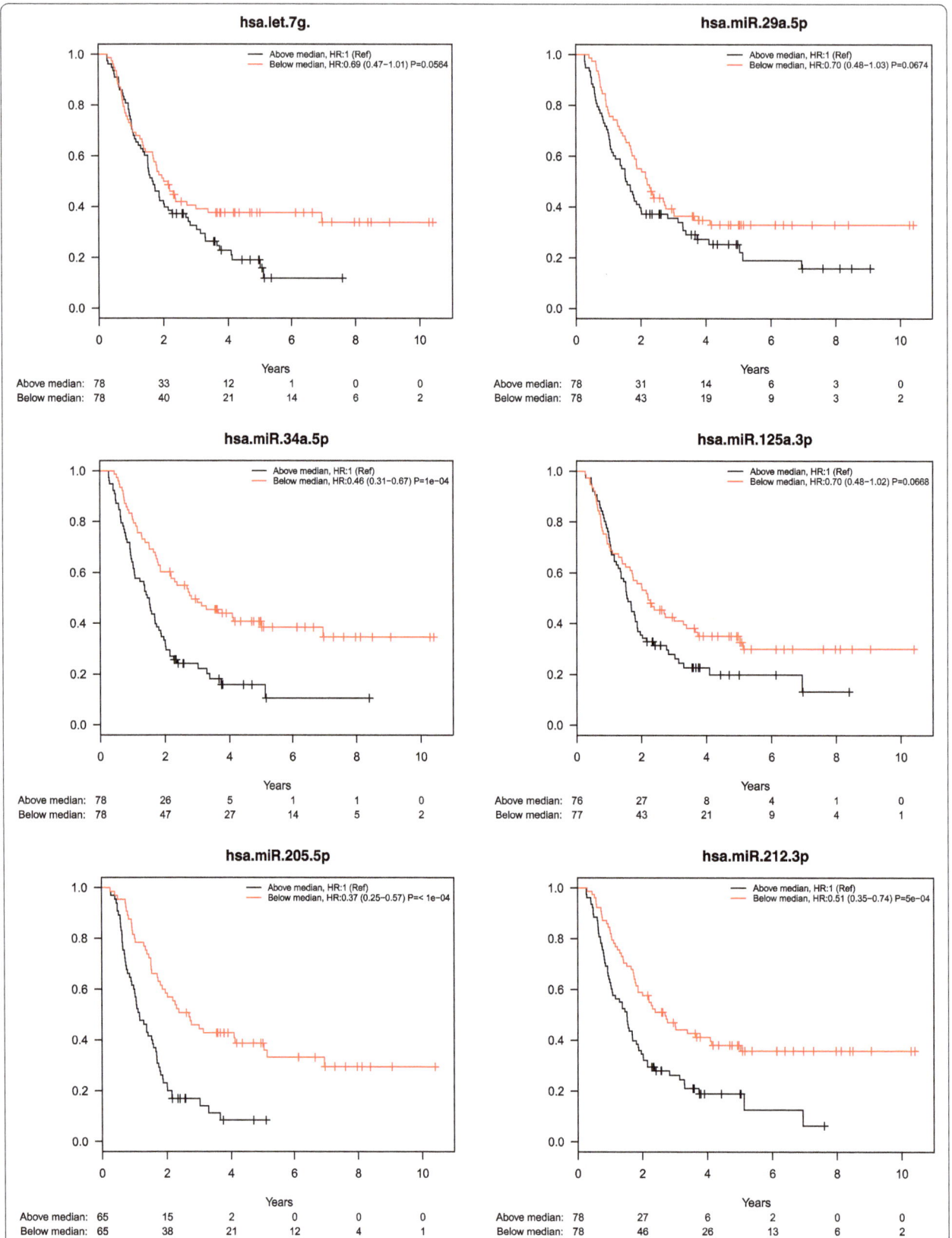

Fig. 3 Kaplan–Meier curves for miRNAs significantly associated to survival in patients with PC + A-AC

Table 5 Differences of miRNA

Unadjusted effects on differences					Adjusted effects on differences				
miRNA1	miRNA2	HR (CI)	P	N	miRNA1	miRNA2	HR (CI)	P	N
PDAC + AAC									
miR-148a	miR-212-3p	1.20 (1.09–1.33)	0.0002	155	miR-34a-5p	miR-148a	0.82 (0.73–0.92)	0.0011	144
miR-205-5p	miR-769-5p	0.90 (0.85–0.95)	0.0003	129	miR-205-5p	miR-769-5p	0.91 (0.85–0.96)	0.0015	119
miR-148a	miR-205-5p	1.08 (1.04–1.13)	0.0004	130	miR-146a-5p	miR-212-3p	1.33 (1.11–1.60)	0.0017	145
miR-34a-5p	miR-148a	0.83 (0.75–0.92)	0.0009	155	miR-34a-5p	miR-187	0.67 (0.52–0.88)	0.0038	44
miR-34a-5p	miR-187	0.64 (0.50–0.83)	0.0009	47	miR-148a	miR-205-5p	1.07 (1.02–1.12)	0.004	120
miR-146a-5p	miR-212-3p	1.32 (1.12–1.57)	0.0013	156	miR-29a-5p	miR-205-5p	1.08 (1.03–1.15)	0.0046	119
miR-187	miR-212-3p	1.55 (1.18–2.04)	0.0016	47	miR-125a-3p	miR-769-5p	0.81 (0.69–0.94)	0.0071	140
miR-34a-5p	miR-769-5p	0.74 (0.62–0.89)	0.0017	154	miR-187	miR-212-3p	1.47 (1.11–1.96)	0.0078	44
miR-212-3p	miR-769-5p	0.81 (0.70–0.92)	0.0020	154	let-7 g	miR-187	0.74 (0.59–0.93)	0.0085	44
miR-205-5p	miR-625-5p	0.91 (0.86–0.97)	0.0023	72	miR-146a-5p	miR-205-5p	1.08 (1.02–1.14)	0.0097	120
miR-205-5p	miR-450b-5p	0.91 (0.86–0.97)	0.0031	94	miR-205-5p	miR-222-5p	0.93 (0.87–0.99)	0.0152	117
miR-146a-5p	miR-205-5p	1.08 (1.03–1.14)	0.0033	130	miR-29a-5p	miR-769-5p	0.81 (0.68–0.96)	0.0171	143
miR-205-5p	miR-222-5p	0.92 (0.86–0.97)	0.0034	127	let-7 g	miR-205-5p	1.07 (1.01–1.13)	0.018	120
let-7 g	miR-205-5p	1.08 (1.02–1.14)	0.0048	130	miR-29a-5p	miR-194-3p	0.68 (0.50–0.94)	0.0188	46
miR-194-3p	miR-205-5p	1.26 (1.07–1.48)	0.0062	36	miR-125a-3p	miR-187	0.76 (0.61–0.96)	0.0188	43
miR-29a-5p	miR-205-5p	1.07 (1.02–1.13)	0.0072	129	let-7 g	miR-212-3p	1.14 (1.02–1.28)	0.0233	144
miR-125a-3p	miR-205-5p	1.08 (1.02–1.15)	0.0074	128	miR-125a-3p	miR-205-5p	1.07 (1.01–1.14)	0.0236	118
let-7 g	miR-187	0.82 (0.70–0.95)	0.0093	47	miR-205-5p	miR-450b-5p	0.93 (0.87–0.99)	0.024	85
miR-34a-5p	miR-205-5p	1.07 (1.02–1.13)	0.0125	130	miR-34a-5p	miR-194-3p	0.64 (0.43–0.94)	0.0262	45
miR-125a-3p	miR-148a	0.90 (0.83–0.98)	0.0139	152	miR-194-3p	miR-212-3p	1.39 (1.04–1.85)	0.0273	45
miR-125a-3p	miR-769-5p	0.84 (0.73–0.97)	0.0146	151	miR-212-3p	miR-625-5p	0.86 (0.75–0.98)	0.0298	74
miR-125a-3p	miR-187	0.80 (0.66–0.96)	0.0155	46	miR-34a-5p	miR-205-5p	1.07 (1.01–1.13)	0.0307	120
miR-212-3p	miR-625-5p	0.87 (0.77–0.98)	0.0194	79	miR-194-3p	miR-205-5p	1.21 (1.02–1.45)	0.0326	33
let-7 g	miR-212-3p	1.12 (1.01–1.25)	0.0332	155	miR-625-5p	miR-944	1.51 (1.03–2.22)	0.0339	20
miR-187	miR-194-3p	1.41 (1.02–1.96)	0.0366	21	miR-125a-3p	miR-148a	0.91 (0.84–1.00)	0.0383	141
miR-205-5p	miR-212-3p	0.95 (0.90–1.00)	0.0410	130	miR-146a-5p	miR-769-5p	0.84 (0.71–1.00)	0.0394	144
miR-34a-5p	miR-625-5p	0.88 (0.78–1.00)	0.0443	79	miR-34a-5p	miR-625-5p	0.87 (0.75–1.00)	0.0478	74
miR-146a-5p	miR-187	0.79 (0.63–1.00)	0.0452	47					
miR-187	miR-205-5p	1.12 (1.00–1.26)	0.0468	38					
miR-34a-5p	miR-146a-5p	0.83 (0.68–1.00)	0.0488	156					
PDAC									
miR-148a	miR-212-3p	1.18 (1.04–1.33)	0.0077	103	miR-34a-5p	miR-769-5p	0.63 (0.47–0.84)	0.002	92
miR-34a-5p	miR-148a	0.86 (0.76–0.97)	0.0156	103	miR-29a-5p	miR-187	1.99 (1.20–3.29)	0.0072	20
miR-34a-5p	miR-769-5p	0.75 (0.59–0.96)	0.0199	102	miR-187	miR-769-5p	0.54 (0.33–0.87)	0.0111	20
miR-146a-5p	miR-212-3p	1.26 (1.01–1.56)	0.0371	103	miR-187	miR-205-5p	0.72 (0.56–0.94)	0.0138	19
miR-34a-5p	miR-146a-5p	0.74 (0.56–0.99)	0.0427	103	miR-212-3p	miR-769-5p	0.75 (0.60–0.95)	0.0153	92
					miR-148a	miR-212-3p	1.18 (1.03–1.34)	0.016	93
					miR-450b-5p	miR-944	1.56 (1.06–2.30)	0.0243	24
					miR-34a-5p	miR-148a	0.86 (0.75–0.99)	0.0341	93
					miR-146a-5p	miR-212-3p	1.29 (1.02–1.63)	0.0343	93
					miR-148a	miR-431-5p	1.32 (1.02–1.72)	0.0364	34
					miR-146a-5p	miR-187	1.57 (1.01–2.44)	0.0438	20
					miR-222-5p	miR-769-5p	0.84 (0.70–1.00)	0.0491	92

Table 5 Differences of miRNA *(Continued)*

A-AC

miR-205-5p	miR-769-5p	0.71 (0.60–0.84)	<0.0001	36		miR-34a-5p	miR-769-5p	0.51 (0.32–0.81)	0.0043	51
miR-34a-5p	miR-187	0.44 (0.27–0.72)	0.0011	24		miR-125a-3p	miR-187	0.37 (0.18–0.75)	0.0055	23
miR-148a	miR-205-5p	1.25 (1.09–1.44)	0.0018	37		miR-34a-5p	miR-187	0.48 (0.28–0.82)	0.0067	24
miR-125a-3p	miR-187	0.69 (0.54–0.88)	0.0032	23		miR-148a	miR-187	0.59 (0.40–0.87)	0.0074	24
miR-187	miR-205-5p	1.35 (1.10–1.66)	0.0041	17		miR-29a-5p	miR-769-5p	0.65 (0.48–0.89)	0.0077	52
miR-187	miR-212-3p	2.22 (1.29–3.82)	0.0042	24		miR-222-5p	miR-450b-5p	2.12 (1.18–3.81)	0.0123	25
miR-205-5p	miR-450b-5p	0.73 (0.59–0.91)	0.0045	22		miR-187	miR-769-5p	2.09 (1.16–3.78)	0.0148	24
let-7 g	miR-205-5p	1.28 (1.07–1.52)	0.006	37		miR-29a-5p	miR-187	0.62 (0.42–0.91)	0.0154	24
miR-146a-5p	miR-205-5p	1.19 (1.05–1.34)	0.0065	37		miR-187	miR-212-3p	2.23 (1.16–4.30)	0.016	24
let-7 g	miR-769-5p	0.74 (0.59–0.93)	0.0083	52		miR-146a-5p	miR-187	0.54 (0.33–0.90)	0.0175	24
miR-34a-5p	miR-769-5p	0.66 (0.48–0.91)	0.0122	52		miR-148a	miR-450b-5p	2.12 (1.14–3.96)	0.0181	26
miR-34a-5p	miR-205-5p	1.22 (1.04–1.43)	0.0126	37		miR-450b-5p	miR-769-5p	0.31 (0.12–0.84)	0.0214	26
let-7 g	miR-187	0.77 (0.62–0.95)	0.017	24		miR-34a-5p	miR-625-5p	0.71 (0.52–0.96)	0.0267	30
let-7 g	miR-625-5p	0.74 (0.58–0.95)	0.0175	31		miR-125a-3p	miR-769-5p	0.75 (0.58–0.97)	0.0283	49
miR-125a-3p	miR-205-5p	1.21 (1.03–1.43)	0.0227	36		miR-29a-5p	miR-625-5p	0.74 (0.56–0.99)	0.0408	30
let-7 g	miR-222-5p	0.80 (0.67–0.97)	0.0242	50		miR-205-5p	miR-222-5p	0.81 (0.66–0.99)	0.0436	33
miR-29a-5p	miR-187	0.74 (0.56–0.97)	0.0272	24						
miR-205-5p	miR-212-3p	0.86 (0.75–0.98)	0.0289	37						
miR-146a-5p	miR-187	0.67 (0.46–0.96)	0.0308	24						
miR-187	miR-769-5p	1.47 (1.02–2.11)	0.0367	24						
miR-450b-5p	miR-769-5p	0.59 (0.35–1.00)	0.0489	27						

HR = 2.34(CI: 1.22–4.48) were associated with short OS. When patients were divided into 2 groups for each miRNA (defined as expression under or above the median level), low expression of miR-34a-5p was associated with short OS. Figure 4 shows Kaplan–Meier curves for the miRNAs reaching a significance level below 0.01.

Table 5 shows 21 and 16 combinations of 2 miRNAs in A-AC FFPE tissue significantly associated with short OS in both an unadjusted and an adjusted analysis.

Discussion

In the present study, our aim was to validate previously described tissue miRNA expression profiles as diagnostic and prognostic biomarkers of PC and other periampullary cancers [20–32]. We used non-microdissected FFPE tissue from 165 patients who had undergone surgery for PDAC and from 86 patients who had undergone resection for other periampullary cancers.

Many of the diagnostic miRNAs described in the literature [20, 21, 34] could be validated. We found the following miRNAs either upregulated or downregulated in PC tissue compared to tissue from CP and/or normal pancreas, upregulated miRNAs: miR-21-5p, −23a-3p, −31-5p, −34c-5p, −93-3p, −135b-3p, −155-5p, −186-5p, −196b-5p, −203, −205-5p, −210, −222-3p, −451, −492, −614, and miR-622; and downregulated miRNAs: miR-

122-5p, −130b-3p, −216b, −217, and miR-375. Furthermore, we validated the two-miRNA index "miR-196b − miR-217" [27], and suggested new diagnostic indices for separating patients with PC vs. HS and PC vs. HS and CP combined. We found that these indices were useful in discriminating other upper gastrointestinal cancers (duodenal cancer, common bile duct cancer and gastric cancer) from normal pancreas and CP.

In addition to the diagnostic miRNAs, we demonstrated the association of 10 miRNAs with prognosis and constructed several indices based on differences of 2 miRNA associated with poor prognosis.

A major limitation of the study was the high number of non-detectable miRNAs using the Fluidigm BioMark System™. Even though we purified the miRNAs from FFPE by the same method as in our previous studies [27, 31] and repeated the analysis several times, we still experienced a high number of undetectable miRNAs. At present, we have no explanation for this problem apart from possible platform sensitivity limitations.

We consider it a strength of the study that non-microdissected samples were used, since this will also be the case in a clinical setting. The tumor microenvironment is a highly dynamic component of PC, often constitutes the bulk of the tumor, and should therefore be

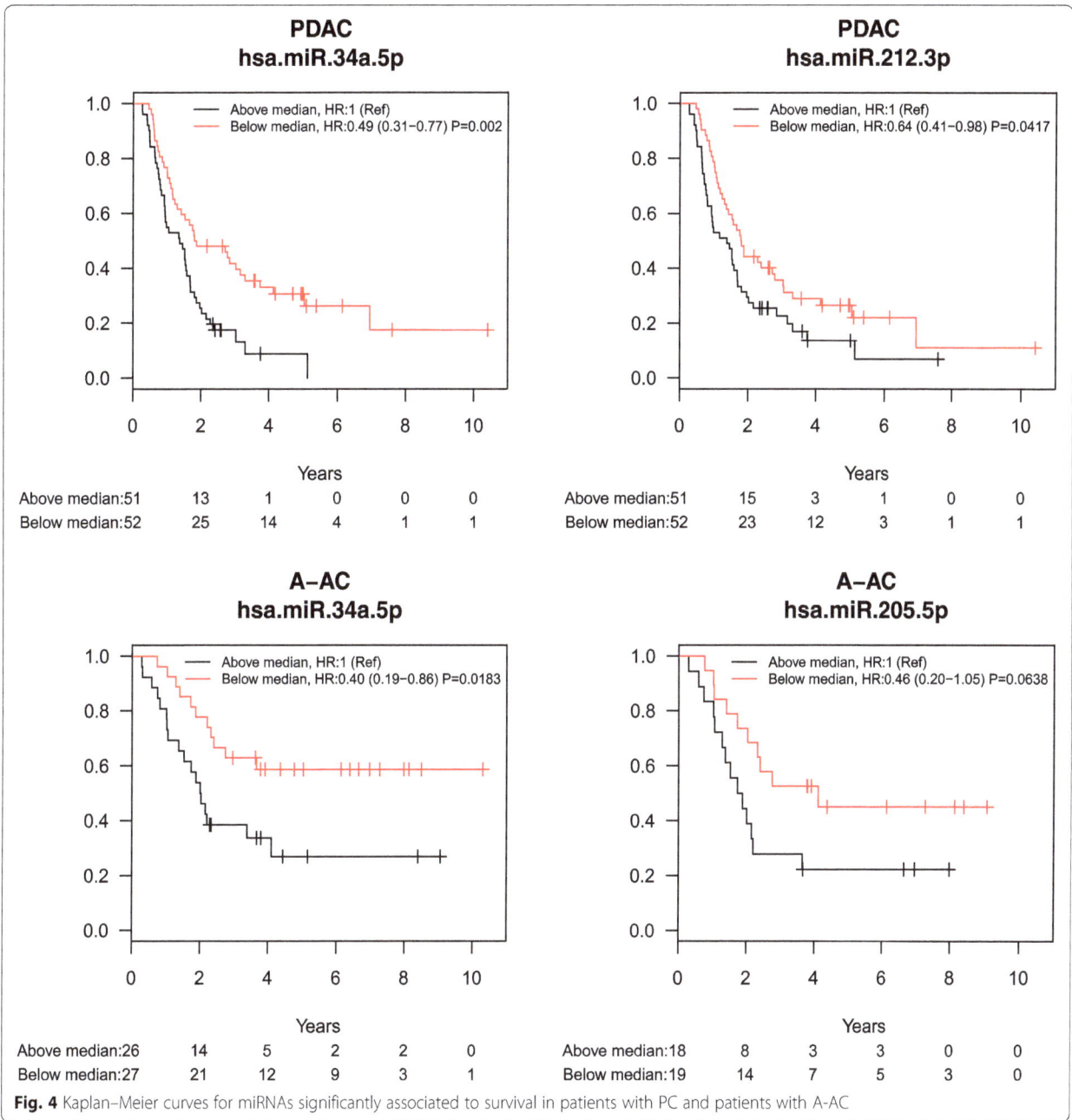

Fig. 4 Kaplan–Meier curves for miRNAs significantly associated to survival in patients with PC and patients with A-AC

taken into account. The extracellular stroma participates in paracrine signaling that promotes PDAC cell survival and metastasis, and the dense extracellular matrix characteristic of PDAC acts as a physical barrier to infiltrating immune cells and the diffusion of chemotherapy [35–37]. MicroRNAs are involved in the regulation of the extracellular components in different tissues [38, 39]. Since many studies regarding miRNAs in PC are performed on microdissected tissue or cell lines the miRNAs originating from the extracellular stroma are less elucidated. The following miRNAs significantly deregulated in the present study are known to be related to the

extracellular compartment of PC: miR-21, –29, –130b, –210, and-451 [40–43].

Among the validated miRNAs, high expression of miR-21, miR-31, and miR-155 and low expression of miR-217 and miR-375are the most consistently described dysregulated miRNAs in PC. Several studies have found miR-155to be upregulated in PC [20–22, 28, 32, 44, 45]. miR-155 functions as an onco-miRNA in different types of cancer,e.g., breast, cervix, colon, and lung cancer, and high miR-155 expression in cancer tissue is associated with poor prognosis in PC and lung cancer [30, 46–49]. The oncogenic effect of miR-155 maybe caused by the targeting of anti-inflammatory signal pathways such as Sh2 domain-containing inositol phosphatase-1 (Ship1) or from suppression of cytokine signaling 1 (Socs1) [50, 51].

miR-21 is also an onco-miR involved in PC tumorigenesis, invasion, metastasis, and chemoresistance [20, 21, 23, 27, 32, 44, 45, 52–57]. miR-21 is primarily upregulated in the extracellular stroma, which is considered a dynamic component of PC, and high expression is associated with poor prognosis [40]. Our study was conducted on non-microdissected tissue and thus also detects miRNAs in the extracellular stroma.miR-21 targets tumor suppressors like PTEN, PDCD4, and TIMP3, components of the p53 pathway, and modulates TGF-b signaling, thus promoting cell proliferation, survival, and migration/invasion [45, 58–60].

miR-31 is upregulated in PC [21, 27, 28, 45, 61]. miR-31 targets human mutL homolog 1 (a mismatch repair protein) [62] and activates the RAS pathway by inhibiting RAS p21 GTPase activating protein 1 (RASA1) in colorectal cancer [63].

miR-217 is downregulated in PC and in pancreatic intraepithelial neoplasm (PanIN) [21, 27, 28, 32, 45, 64]. This finding has also been replicated in studies using fine needle aspirates from PC [24, 65].miR-217 acts as a tumor suppressor in PC by targeting *KRAS* [66] and is involved in epithelial-mesenchymal-transition (EMT) in PC and CP via the miR-217-SIRT1 pathway, which can be triggered by TGF-β1 in inflammatory processes [67].

miR-375 is downregulated in PC compared to normal pancreas, is associated with prognosis, and can differentiate between pancreatobiliary and intestinal subtypes in ampullary adenocarcinoma [20, 21, 27, 28, 32, 68]. miR-375 is also downregulated in esophageal, gastric, breast, lung, colorectal, and cervical cancers [69–74]. miR-375 plays a role in the development and maintenance of the α- and β-cell mass in the normal pancreas and is upregulated in patients with type 2 diabetes [75, 76].miR-375 targets 3-phosphoinositide-dependent protein kinase-1 (PDK1) in PC and inhibits PC cell proliferation in vitro [77, 78].

In the literature, the following miRNAs are described as prognostic after PC resection:Let-7 g, miR-21, miR-29a-5p, miR-34a-5p, miR-146a, miR-155, miR-196a, miR-203, miR-205, miR-210, miR-212, miR-222, miR-450b-5p, and miR-675 [23, 29–32]. We have previously described prognostic indices using combinations of high expression of miR-212 and miR-675 and low expression of miR-148a-5p (previous ID: miR-148a*), miR-187 and let-7 g-3p (previous ID: let-7 g*) in FFPE tissue from patients operated for PC [31]. Only a few of these patients received adjuvant chemotherapy after surgery. In the present study, patients with PDAC and A-AC were all treated with adjuvant gemcitabine for 6 months or until disease recurrence. In this population, we could validate let-7 g, miR-29a-5p, miR-34a-5p, miR-146a-5p, miR-205-5p, and miR-212-3pas prognostic biomarkers after radical resection for PC.

The let-7 family of miRNAs includes tumor suppressor miRNAs, the expression of which is prognostic in HCC, gastric, and ovarian cancers [79–81]. Let-7 g is involved in pathways essential for the development of cancer. It targets Fas and is involved in Fas-mediated apoptosis [82]. Silencing of let-7b/g activates AKT signaling and promotes carcinogenesis in gastric cancer [83]. Let-7 inhibits cell motility in breast cancer by regulating genes in the cytoskeleton pathway and silencing of let-7 promotes metastases [84]. Let-7 inhibits proliferation in HCC by downregulation of c-Myc and upregulation of p16(INK4A) [85].

In PC, miR-29a-5p induces EMT, stimulates pancreatic stellate cells to accumulate protein in the extracellular matrix, and increases resistance to gemcitabine through the Wnt/beta-catenin pathway [41, 86, 87]. miR-34a is upregulated in cervical and colorectal cancers and downregulated in breast, prostate, renal and lung cancer [49, 88].

The miR-34 family miRNAs are described as tumor suppressor miRNAs, and miR-34a/c suppresses breast cancer invasion and metastasis by targeting Fos-related antigen-1 [89]. PC mouse models show that miR-146a acts through EGFR signaling [90]. miR-205 is involved in EMT and acts through the anti-apoptotic protein Bcl-2 (in prostate cancer) and HER3 (in breast cancer) [91–93]. We found that low expression of miR-125a-3p was associated with short OS in patients with PC, and this is a novel observation.miR-125a-3p has been described as a tumor suppressor miRNA in several cancers [94, 95].

In the present study, miR-130b was found to be downregulated in PDAC compared to benign specimens. Interestingly, this miRNA is upregulated in the stroma compared to carcinoma cells [42].

Further information about the 46 miRNAs analyzed in the present study is given in "Additional file 1".

Conclusions

In conclusion, we could validate miRNAs selected from the literature as diagnostic and/or prognostic biomarkers in patients radically resected for PC. No microdissection of the tumors was done, and some of the miRNAs most likely originated from the stroma and not the cancer cells. The diagnostic ability of these miRNAs was also tested on duodenal cancer, common bile duct cancer, and gastric cancer – diagnoses that represent a considerable diagnostic challenge in separating from PC in a clinical setting. Hopefully, this study can contribute to the understanding of pancreatic and periampullary cancers and improve the diagnosis, prognosis, and ultimately treatment of patients with these conditions. For example, this could be achieved by allocating young patients with a miRNA expression profile suggestive of poor prognosis to a more aggressive chemotherapy regimen, or elderly patients with a more promising prognostic profile could be spared from adjuvant therapy.

Abbreviations
A-AC: Ampullary adenocarcinoma; CBD: Common bile duct; CP: Chronic pancreatitis; DC: Duodenal cancer; FFPE: Formalin-fixed paraffin-embedded; GC: Gastric cancer; HS: Healthy subjects; miR: microRNA; miRNA: microRNA; PC: Pancreatic cancer; PDAC: Pancreatic ductal adenocarcinoma

Acknowledgements
We thank Dr. Nathalia A. Giese, MD, PhD, Heidelberg, Germany, for providing tissue samples for this study.

Funding
Professor Molven received a grant from Western Norway Regional Health Authority (Helse Vest).

Authors' contributions
DC designed the study, collected the specimens from Denmark and the corresponding clinical data, interpreted the calculations wrote the manuscript; CD performed all calculations and contributed to the manuscript; MKB contributed to the manuscript; JPH re-assessed all the specimens from Denmark; NAS contributed to data interpretation and to the manuscript; JW contributed with the German specimens; HI contributed with the Norwegian specimens; AM contributed with the Norwegian specimens and contributed to the manuscript; CPH contributed with clinical data and contributed to the manuscript. JSJ designed the study, contributed with collection of specimens, clinical data, interpretation of the calculations, preparation of the manuscript and funding. All authors read and approved the final manuscript.

Competing interests
The authors declare that they have no competing interests.

Author details
[1]Department of Surgical Gastroenterology and Transplantation, Rigshospitalet, Copenhagen University Hospital, Copenhagen, Denmark. [2]Danish Cancer Society Research Center, Danish Cancer Society, Copenhagen, Denmark. [3]Department of Oncology, Herlev and Gentofte Hospital, Copenhagen University Hospital, Herlev, Denmark. [4]Department of Pathology, Rigshospitalet, Copenhagen University Hospital, Copenhagen, Denmark. [5]Department of General, Visceral, and Transplant Surgery, LMU, University of Munich, Munich, Germany. [6]Gade Laboratory for Pathology, Department of Clinical Medicine, University of Bergen, Bergen, Norway. [7]Department of Pathology, Ålesund Hospital, Ålesund, Norway. [8]Department of Pathology, Haukeland University Hospital, Bergen, Norway. [9]Department of Medicine, Herlev and Gentofte Hospital, Copenhagen University Hospital, Herlev, Denmark. [10]Institute of Clinical Medicine, Faculty of Health and Medical Sciences, University of Copenhagen, Copenhagen, Denmark. [11]Department of Oncology, Herlev University Hospital, Herlev Ringvej 75, DK-2730 Herlev, Denmark.

References
1. Ryan DP, Hong TS, Bardeesy N. Pancreatic adenocarcinoma. N Engl J Med. 2014;371(11):1039–49.
2. Siegel RL, Miller KD, Jemal A. Cancer statistics, 2016. CA Cancer J Clin. 2016; 66(1):7–30.
3. Yeo CJ, Cameron JL, Lillemoe KD, Sitzmann JV, Hruban RH, Goodman SN, Dooley WC, Coleman J, Pitt HA. Pancreaticoduodenectomy for cancer of the head of the pancreas. 201 patients. Ann Surg. 1995;221(6):721–31. discussion 731–723.
4. Cancer Research UK. Cancer mortality: UK Statistics. In.; 2009. http://www. cancerresearchuk.org/health-professional/cancer-statistics/statistics-by-cancer-type/pancreatic-cancer/mortality. (Accessed 15th Mar 2016).
5. Hartwig W, Hackert T, Hinz U, Gluth A, Bergmann F, Strobel O, Buchler MW, Werner J. Pancreatic cancer surgery in the new millennium: better prediction of outcome. Ann Surg. 2011;254(2):311–9.
6. He J, Ahuja N, Makary MA, Cameron JL, Eckhauser FE, Choti MA, Hruban RH, Pawlik TM, Wolfgang CL. 2564 resected periampullary adenocarcinomas at a single institution: trends over three decades. HPB (Oxford). 2014;16(1):83–90.
7. Bettschart V, Rahman MQ, Engelken FJ, Madhavan KK, Parks RW, Garden OJ. Presentation, treatment and outcome in patients with ampullary tumours. Br J Surg. 2004;91(12):1600–7.
8. Struck A, Howard T, Chiorean EG, Clarke JM, Riffenburgh R, Cardenes HR. Non-ampullary duodenal adenocarcinoma: factors important for relapse and survival. J Surg Oncol. 2009;100(2):144–8.
9. Seufferlein T, Bachet JB, Van Cutsem E, Rougier P. Pancreatic adenocarcinoma: ESMO-ESDO Clinical Practice Guidelines for diagnosis, treatment and follow-up. Ann Oncol. 2012;23 Suppl 7:vii33–40.
10. Waldman SA, Terzic A. Translating MicroRNA discovery into clinical biomarkers in cancer. JAMA. 2007;297(17):1923–5.
11. Nelson KM, Weiss GJ. MicroRNAs and cancer: past, present, and potential future. Mol Cancer Ther. 2008;7(12):3655–60.
12. Ambros V. The functions of animal microRNAs. Nature. 2004;431(7006):350–5.
13. Hwang HW, Mendell JT. MicroRNAs in cell proliferation, cell death, and tumorigenesis. Br J Cancer. 2006;94(6):776–80.
14. Li M, Marin-Muller C, Bharadwaj U, Chow KH, Yao Q, Chen C. MicroRNAs: control and loss of control in human physiology and disease. World J Surg. 2009;33(4):667–84.
15. Bartel DP. MicroRNAs: target recognition and regulatory functions. Cell. 2009;136(2):215–33.
16. Almeida MI, Reis RM, Calin GA. MicroRNA history: discovery, recent applications, and next frontiers. Mutat Res. 2011;717(1–2):1–8.
17. Li J, Smyth P, Flavin R, Cahill S, Denning K, Aherne S, Guenther SM, O'Leary JJ, Sheils O. Comparison of miRNA expression patterns using total RNA extracted from matched samples of formalin-fixed paraffin-embedded (FFPE) cells and snap frozen cells. BMC Biotechnol. 2007;7:36.
18. Zhang X, Chen J, Radcliffe T, Lebrun DP, Tron VA, Feilotter H. An array-based analysis of microRNA expression comparing matched frozen and formalin-fixed paraffin-embedded human tissue samples. J Mol Diagn. 2008;10(6):513–9.
19. MirBase [http://www.mirbase.org]. Accessed 15th Mar 2016.
20. Bloomston M, Frankel WL, Petrocca F, Volinia S, Alder H, Hagan JP, Liu CG, Bhatt D, Taccioli C, Croce CM. MicroRNA expression patterns to differentiate

pancreatic adenocarcinoma from normal pancreas and chronic pancreatitis. JAMA. 2007;297(17):1901–8.

21. Szafranska AE, Davison TS, John J, Cannon T, Sipos B, Maghnouj A, Labourier E, Hahn SA. MicroRNA expression alterations are linked to tumorigenesis and non-neoplastic processes in pancreatic ductal adenocarcinoma. Oncogene. 2007;26(30):4442–52.

22. Lee EJ, Gusev Y, Jiang J, Nuovo GJ, Lerner MR, Frankel WL, Morgan DL, Postier RG, Brackett DJ, Schmittgen TD. Expression profiling identifies microRNA signature in pancreatic cancer. Int J Cancer. 2007;120(5):1046–54.

23. Dillhoff M, Liu J, Frankel W, Croce C, Bloomston M. MicroRNA-21 is overexpressed in pancreatic cancer and a potential predictor of survival. J Gastrointest Surg. 2008;12(12):2171–6.

24. Szafranska AE, Doleshal M, Edmunds HS, Gordon S, Luttges J, Munding JB, Barth Jr RJ, Gutmann EJ, Suriawinata AA, Marc Pipas J, et al. Analysis of microRNAs in pancreatic fine-needle aspirates can classify benign and malignant tissues. Clin Chem. 2008;54(10):1716–24.

25. Habbe N, Koorstra JB, Mendell JT, Offerhaus GJ, Ryu JK, Feldmann G, Mullendore ME, Goggins MG, Hong SM, Maitra A. MicroRNA miR-155 is a biomarker of early pancreatic neoplasia. Cancer Biol Ther. 2009;8(4):340–6.

26. Zhang Y, Li M, Wang H, Fisher WE, Lin PH, Yao Q, Chen C. Profiling of 95 microRNAs in pancreatic cancer cell lines and surgical specimens by real-time PCR analysis. World J Surg. 2009;33(4):698–709.

27. Schultz NA, Werner J, Willenbrock H, Roslind A, Giese N, Horn T, Wojdemann M, Johansen JS. MicroRNA expression profiles associated with pancreatic adenocarcinoma and ampullary adenocarcinoma. Mod Pathol. 2012;25(12):1609–22.

28. Bauer AS, Keller A, Costello E, Greenhalf W, Bier M, Borries A, Beier M, Neoptolemos J, Buchler M, Werner J, et al. Diagnosis of pancreatic ductal adenocarcinoma and chronic pancreatitis by measurement of microRNA abundance in blood and tissue. PLoS One. 2012;7(4), e34151.

29. Ikenaga N, Ohuchida K, Mizumoto K, Yu J, Kayashima T, Sakai H, Fujita H, Nakata K, Tanaka M. MicroRNA-203 expression as a new prognostic marker of pancreatic adenocarcinoma. Ann Surg Oncol. 2010;17(12):3120–8.

30. Greither T, Grochola LF, Udelnow A, Lautenschlager C, Wurl P, Taubert H. Elevated expression of microRNAs 155, 203, 210 and 222 in pancreatic tumors is associated with poorer survival. Int J Cancer. 2010;126(1):73–80.

31. Schultz NA, Andersen KK, Roslind A, Willenbrock H, Wojdemann M, Johansen JS. Prognostic microRNAs in cancer tissue from patients operated for pancreatic cancer–five microRNAs in a prognostic index. World J Surg. 2012;36(11):2699–707.

32. Jamieson NB, Morran DC, Morton JP, Ali A, Dickson EJ, Carter CR, Sansom OJ, Evans TR, McKay CJ, Oien KA. MicroRNA molecular profiles associated with diagnosis, clinicopathologic criteria, and overall survival in patients with resectable pancreatic ductal adenocarcinoma. Clin Cancer Res. 2012; 18(2):534–45.

33. Aaltonen LA, Hamilton SR, World Health Organization, International Agency for Research on Cancer. Pathology and genetics of tumours of the digestive system. Lyon, Oxford: IARC Press; Oxford University Press (distributor); 2000.

34. Frampton AE, Giovannetti E, Jamieson NB, Krell J, Gall TM, Stebbing J, Jiao LR, Castellano L. A microRNA meta-signature for pancreatic ductal adenocarcinoma. Expert Rev Mol Diagn. 2014;14(3):267–71.

35. Neesse A, Algul H, Tuveson DA, Gress TM. Stromal biology and therapy in pancreatic cancer: a changing paradigm. Gut. 2015;64(9):1476–84.

36. Hwang RF, Moore T, Arumugam T, Ramachandran V, Amos KD, Rivera A, Ji B, Evans DB, Logsdon CD. Cancer-associated stromal fibroblasts promote pancreatic tumor progression. Cancer Res. 2008;68(3):918–26.

37. Xu Z, Vonlaufen A, Phillips PA, Fiala-Beer E, Zhang X, Yang L, Biankin AV, Goldstein D, Pirola RC, Wilson JS, et al. Role of pancreatic stellate cells in pancreatic cancer metastasis. Am J Pathol. 2010;177(5):2585–96.

38. Chou J, Shahi P, Werb Z. microRNA-mediated regulation of the tumor microenvironment. Cell Cycle. 2013;12(20):3262–71.

39. Zhang Y, Yang P, Wang XF. Microenvironmental regulation of cancer metastasis by miRNAs. Trends Cell Biol. 2014;24(3):153–60.

40. Kadera BE, Li L, Toste PA, Wu N, Adams C, Dawson DW, Donahue TR. MicroRNA-21 in pancreatic ductal adenocarcinoma tumor-associated fibroblasts promotes metastasis. PLoS One. 2013;8(8), e71978.

41. Kwon JJ, Nabinger SC, Vega Z, Sahu SS, Alluri RK, Abdul-Sater Z, Yu Z, Gore J, Nalepa G, Saxena R, et al. Pathophysiological role of microRNA-29 in pancreatic cancer stroma. Sci Rep. 2015;5:11450.

42. Sandhu V, Bowitz Lothe IM, Labori KJ, Skrede ML, Hamfjord J, Dalsgaard AM, Buanes T, Dube G, Kale MM, Sawant S, et al. Differential expression of miRNAs in pancreatobiliary type of periampullary adenocarcinoma and its associated stroma. Mol Oncol. 2016;10(2):303–16.

43. Takikawa T, Masamune A, Hamada S, Nakano E, Yoshida N, Shimosegawa T. miR-210 regulates the interaction between pancreatic cancer cells and stellate cells. Biochem Biophys Res Commun. 2013;437(3):433–9.

44. Panarelli NC, Chen YT, Zhou XK, Kitabayashi N, Yantiss RK. MicroRNA expression aids the preoperative diagnosis of pancreatic ductal adenocarcinoma. Pancreas. 2012;41(5):685–90.

45. Nagao Y, Hisaoka M, Matsuyama A, Kanemitsu S, Hamada T, Fukuyama T, Nakano R, Uchiyama A, Kawamoto M, Yamaguchi K, et al. Association of microRNA-21 expression with its targets, PDCD4 and TIMP3, in pancreatic ductal adenocarcinoma. Mod Pathol. 2012;25(1):112–21.

46. Volinia S, Calin GA, Liu CG, Ambs S, Cimmino A, Petrocca F, Visone R, Iorio M, Roldo C, Ferracin M, et al. A microRNA expression signature of human solid tumors defines cancer gene targets. Proc Natl Acad Sci U S A. 2006;103(7):2257–61.

47. Yanaihara N, Caplen N, Bowman E, Seike M, Kumamoto K, Yi M, Stephens RM, Okamoto A, Yokota J, Tanaka T, et al. Unique microRNA molecular profiles in lung cancer diagnosis and prognosis. Cancer Cell. 2006;9(3):189–98.

48. Saito M, Schetter AJ, Mollerup S, Kohno T, Skaug V, Bowman ED, Mathe EA, Takenoshita S, Yokota J, Haugen A, et al. The association of microRNA expression with prognosis and progression in early-stage, non-small cell lung adenocarcinoma: a retrospective analysis of three cohorts. Clin Cancer Res. 2011;17(7):1875–82.

49. Gocze K, Gombos K, Juhasz K, Kovacs K, Kajtar B, Benczik M, Gocze P, Patczai B, Arany I, Ember I. Unique MicroRNA expression profiles in cervical cancer. Anticancer Res. 2013;33(6):2561–7.

50. Jiang S, Zhang HW, Lu MH, He XH, Li Y, Gu H, Liu MF, Wang ED. MicroRNA-155 functions as an OncomiR in breast cancer by targeting the suppressor of cytokine signaling 1 gene. Cancer Res. 2010;70(8):3119–27.

51. Ji Y, Wrzesinski C, Yu Z, Hu J, Gautam S, Hawk NV, Telford WG, Palmer DC, Franco Z, Sukumar M, et al. miR-155 augments CD8+ T-cell antitumor activity in lymphoreplete hosts by enhancing responsiveness to homeostatic gammac cytokines. Proc Natl Acad Sci U S A. 2015;112(2):476–81.

52. Giovannetti E, Funel N, Peters GJ, Del Chiaro M, Erozenci LA, Vasile E, Leon LG, Pollina LE, Groen A, Falcone A, et al. MicroRNA-21 in pancreatic cancer: correlation with clinical outcome and pharmacologic aspects underlying its role in the modulation of gemcitabine activity. Cancer Res. 2010;70(11): 4528–38.

53. Frampton AE, Castellano L, Colombo T, Giovannetti E, Krell J, Jacob J, Pellegrino L, Roca-Alonso L, Funel N, Gall TM, et al. MicroRNAs cooperatively inhibit a network of tumor suppressor genes to promote pancreatic tumor growth and progression. Gastroenterology. 2014; 146(1):268–77. e218.

54. Hwang JH, Voortman J, Giovannetti E, Steinberg SM, Leon LG, Kim YT, Funel N, Park JK, Kim MA, Kang GH, et al. Identification of microRNA-21 as a biomarker for chemoresistance and clinical outcome following adjuvant therapy in resectable pancreatic cancer. PLoS One. 2010;5(5):e10630.

55. Moriyama T, Ohuchida K, Mizumoto K, Yu J, Sato N, Nabae T, Takahata S, Toma H, Nagai E, Tanaka M. MicroRNA-21 modulates biological functions of pancreatic cancer cells including their proliferation, invasion, and chemoresistance. Mol Cancer Ther. 2009;8(5):1067–74.

56. Zhang S, Hao J, Xie F, Hu X, Liu C, Tong J, Zhou J, Wu J, Shao C. Downregulation of miR-132 by promoter methylation contributes to pancreatic cancer development. Carcinogenesis. 2011;32(8):1183–9.

57. Tavano F, di Mola FF, Piepoli A, Panza A, Copetti M, Burbaci FP, Latiano T, Pellegrini F, Maiello E, Andriulli A, et al. Changes in miR-143 and miR-21 expression and clinicopathological correlations in pancreatic cancers. Pancreas. 2012;41(8):1280–4.

58. Niwa R, Slack FJ. The evolution of animal microRNA function. Curr Opin Genet Dev. 2007;17(2):145–50.

59. Papagiannakopoulos T, Shapiro A, Kosik KS. MicroRNA-21 targets a network of key tumor-suppressive pathways in glioblastoma cells. Cancer Res. 2008; 68(19):8164–72.

60. Tili E, Michaille JJ, Croce CM. MicroRNAs play a central role in molecular dysfunctions linking inflammation with cancer. Immunol Rev. 2013;253(1):167–84.

61. Piepoli A, Tavano F, Copetti M, Mazza T, Palumbo O, Panza A, di Mola FF, Pazienza V, Mazzoccoli G, Biscaglia G, et al. Mirna expression profiles identify drivers in colorectal and pancreatic cancers. PLoS One. 2012;7(3), e33663.

62. Zhong Z, Dong Z, Yang L, Chen X, Gong Z. MicroRNA-31-5p modulates cell cycle by targeting human mutL homolog 1 in human cancer cells. Tumour Biol. 2013;34(3):1959–65.

63. Sun D, Yu F, Ma Y, Zhao R, Chen X, Zhu J, Zhang CY, Chen J, Zhang J. MicroRNA-31 activates the RAS pathway and functions as an oncogenic MicroRNA in human colorectal cancer by repressing RAS p21 GTPase activating protein 1 (RASA1). J Biol Chem. 2013;288(13):9508–18.

64. Xue Y, Abou Tayoun AN, Abo KM, Pipas JM, Gordon SR, Gardner TB, Barth Jr RJ, Suriawinata AA, Tsongalis GJ. MicroRNAs as diagnostic markers for pancreatic ductal adenocarcinoma and its precursor, pancreatic intraepithelial neoplasm. Cancer Genet. 2013;206(6):217–21.

65. Hong TH, Park IY. MicroRNA expression profiling of diagnostic needle aspirates from surgical pancreatic cancer specimens. Ann Surg Treat Res. 2014;87(6):290–7.

66. Zhao WG, Yu SN, Lu ZH, Ma YH, Gu YM, Chen J. The miR-217 microRNA functions as a potential tumor suppressor in pancreatic ductal adenocarcinoma by targeting KRAS. Carcinogenesis. 2010;31(10):1726–33.

67. Deng S, Zhu S, Wang B, Li X, Liu Y, Qin Q, Gong Q, Niu Y, Xiang C, Chen J, et al. Chronic pancreatitis and pancreatic cancer demonstrate active epithelial-mesenchymal transition profile, regulated by miR-217-SIRT1 pathway. Cancer Lett. 2014;355(2):184–91.

68. Kalluri Sai Shiva UM, Kuruva MM, Mitnala S, Rupjyoti T, Guduru Venkat R, Botlagunta S, Kandagaddala R, Siddapuram SP, Sekaran A, Chemalakonda R, et al. MicroRNA profiling in periampullary carcinoma. Pancreatology. 2014;14(1):36–47.

69. Gu J, Wang Y, Wu X. MicroRNA in the pathogenesis and prognosis of esophageal cancer. Curr Pharm Des. 2013;19(7):1292–300.

70. Ding L, Xu Y, Zhang W, Deng Y, Si M, Du Y, Yao H, Liu X, Ke Y, Si J, et al. MiR-375 frequently downregulated in gastric cancer inhibits cell proliferation by targeting JAK2. Cell Res. 2010;20(7):784–93.

71. Luo D, Wilson JM, Harvel N, Liu J, Pei L, Huang S, Hawthorn L, Shi H. A systematic evaluation of miRNA:mRNA interactions involved in the migration and invasion of breast cancer cells. J Transl Med. 2013;11:57.

72. Li Y, Jiang Q, Xia N, Yang H, Hu C. Decreased expression of microRNA-375 in nonsmall cell lung cancer and its clinical significance. J Int Med Res. 2012;40(5):1662–9.

73. Dai X, Chiang Y, Wang Z, Song Y, Lu C, Gao P, Xu H. Expression levels of microRNA-375 in colorectal carcinoma. Mol Med Rep. 2012;5(5):1299–304.

74. Bierkens M, Krijgsman O, Wilting SM, Bosch L, Jaspers A, Meijer GA, Meijer CJ, Snijders PJ, Ylstra B, Steenbergen RD. Focal aberrations indicate EYA2 and hsa-miR-375 as oncogene and tumor suppressor in cervical carcinogenesis. Genes Chromosomes Cancer. 2013;52(1):56–68.

75. Poy MN, Hausser J, Trajkovski M, Braun M, Collins S, Rorsman P, Zavolan M, Stoffel M. miR-375 maintains normal pancreatic alpha- and beta-cell mass. Proc Natl Acad Sci U S A. 2009;106(14):5813–8.

76. Zhao H, Guan J, Lee HM, Sui Y, He L, Siu JJ, Tse PP, Tong PC, Lai FM, Chan JC. Up-regulated pancreatic tissue microRNA-375 associates with human type 2 diabetes through beta-cell deficit and islet amyloid deposition. Pancreas. 2010;39(6):843–6.

77. Zhou J, Song S, Cen J, Zhu D, Li D, Zhang Z. MicroRNA-375 is downregulated in pancreatic cancer and inhibits cell proliferation in vitro. Oncol Res. 2012;20(5–6):197–203.

78. Song SD, Zhou J, Zhou J, Zhao H, Cen JN, Li DC. MicroRNA-375 targets the 3-phosphoinositide-dependent protein kinase-1 gene in pancreatic carcinoma. Oncol Lett. 2013;6(4):953–9.

79. Ueda T, Volinia S, Okumura H, Shimizu M, Taccioli C, Rossi S, Alder H, Liu CG, Oue N, Yasui W, et al. Relation between microRNA expression and progression and prognosis of gastric cancer: a microRNA expression analysis. Lancet Oncol. 2010;11(2):136–46.

80. Chen KJ, Hou Y, Wang K, Li J, Xia Y, Yang XY, Lv G, Xing XL, Shen F. Reexpression of Let-7 g microRNA inhibits the proliferation and migration via K-Ras/HMGA2/snail axis in hepatocellular carcinoma. Biomed Res Int. 2014;2014:742417.

81. Lu L, Katsaros D, Shaverdashvili K, Qian B, Wu Y, de la Longrais IA, Preti M, Menato G, Yu H. Pluripotent factor lin-28 and its homologue lin-28b in epithelial ovarian cancer and their associations with disease outcomes and expression of let-7a and IGF-II. Eur J Cancer. 2009;45(12):2212–8.

82. Wang S, Tang Y, Cui H, Zhao X, Luo X, Pan W, Huang X, Shen N. Let-7/miR-98 regulate Fas and Fas-mediated apoptosis. Genes Immun. 2011;12(2):149–54.

83. Kang W, Tong JH, Lung RW, Dong Y, Yang W, Pan Y, Lau KM, Yu J, Cheng AS, To KF. let-7b/g silencing activates AKT signaling to promote gastric carcinogenesis. J Transl Med. 2014;12:281.

84. Hu X, Guo J, Zheng L, Li C, Zheng TM, Tanyi JL, Liang S, Benedetto C, Mitidieri M, Katsaros D, et al. The heterochronic microRNA let-7 inhibits cell motility by regulating the genes in the actin cytoskeleton pathway in breast cancer. Mol Cancer Res. 2013;11(3):240–50.

85. Lan FF, Wang H, Chen YC, Chan CY, Ng SS, Li K, Xie D, He ML, Lin MC, Kung HF. Hsa-let-7 g inhibits proliferation of hepatocellular carcinoma cells by downregulation of c-Myc and upregulation of p16(INK4A). Int J Cancer. 2011;128(2):319–31.

86. Nagano H, Tomimaru Y, Eguchi H, Hama N, Wada H, Kawamoto K, Kobayashi S, Mori M, Doki Y. MicroRNA-29a induces resistance to gemcitabine through the Wnt/beta-catenin signaling pathway in pancreatic cancer cells. Int J Oncol. 2013;43(4):1066–72.

87. Chen J, Li Q, An Y, Lv N, Xue X, Wei J, Jiang K, Wu J, Gao W, Qian Z, et al. CEACAM6 induces epithelial-mesenchymal transition and mediates invasion and metastasis in pancreatic cancer. Int J Oncol. 2013;43(3):877–85.

88. Di Leva G, Garofalo M, Croce CM. MicroRNAs in cancer. Annu Rev Pathol. 2014;9:287–314.

89. Yang S, Li Y, Gao J, Zhang T, Li S, Luo A, Chen H, Ding F, Wang X, Liu Z. MicroRNA-34 suppresses breast cancer invasion and metastasis by directly targeting Fra-1. Oncogene. 2012.

90. Ali S, Ahmad A, Aboukameel A, Ahmed A, Bao B, Banerjee S, Philip PA, Sarkar FH. Deregulation of miR-146a expression in a mouse model of pancreatic cancer affecting EGFR signaling. Cancer Lett. 2014;351(1):134–42.

91. Gregory PA, Bracken CP, Bert AG, Goodall GJ. MicroRNAs as regulators of epithelial-mesenchymal transition. Cell Cycle. 2008;7(20):3112–8.

92. Verdoodt B, Neid M, Vogt M, Kuhn V, Liffers ST, Palisaar RJ, Noldus J, Tannapfel A, Mirmohammadsadegh A. MicroRNA-205, a novel regulator of the anti-apoptotic protein Bcl2, is downregulated in prostate cancer. Int J Oncol. 2013;43(1):307–14.

93. Iorio MV, Casalini P, Piovan C, Di Leva G, Merlo A, Triulzi T, Menard S, Croce CM, Tagliabue E. microRNA-205 regulates HER3 in human breast cancer. Cancer Res. 2009;69(6):2195–200.

94. Jiang L, Huang Q, Chang J, Wang E, Qiu X. MicroRNA HSA-miR-125a-5p induces apoptosis by activating p53 in lung cancer cells. Exp Lung Res. 2011;37(7):387–98.

95. Ma Y, Zhang P, Yang J, Liu Z, Yang Z, Qin H. Candidate microRNA biomarkers in human colorectal cancer: systematic review profiling studies and experimental validation. Int J Cancer. 2012;130(9):2077–87.

Expression of IFITM1 as a prognostic biomarker in resected gastric and esophageal adenocarcinoma

David Borg[*], Charlotta Hedner, Alexander Gaber, Björn Nodin, Richard Fristedt, Karin Jirström, Jakob Eberhard and Anders Johnsson

Abstract

Background: There is an increasing amount of reports on IFITM1 (interferon-inducible transmembrane protein 1) in various malignancies. The aim of this study was to examine the expression of IFITM1 and its prognostic significance in gastroesophageal adenocarcinoma.

Methods: Tissue samples were obtained from a consecutive cohort of 174 patients surgically treated between 2006 and 2010 for gastroesophageal (gastric, gastroesophageal junction and esophageal) adenocarcinoma, not subjected to neoadjuvant therapy. Expression of IFITM1 was examined using immunohistochemistry on tissue microarrays of primary tumors and paired samples of adjacent normal epithelium, intestinal metaplasia and lymph node metastases.

Results: Expression of IFITM1 was significantly elevated in primary tumors and lymph node metastases compared to adjacent normal epithelium and intestinal metaplasia, regardless of tumor location. Overexpression of IFITM1 was associated with M0-disease (no distant metastases). In gastric cancer IFITM1 expression was significantly associated with improved TTR (time to recurrence) in Kaplan-Meier analysis and Cox regression, both in the unadjusted analysis (HR 0.33, 95 % CI 0.12-0.88) and in the adjusted analysis (HR 0.32, 95 % CI 0.12-0.87) but there was no significant impact on OS (overall survival). In esophageal adenocarcinoma expression of IFITM1 had no impact on TTR or OS in Kaplan-Meier-analyses, but in the adjusted Cox regression IFITM1 expression had a negative impact on both TTR (HR 3.05, 95 % CI 1.09-8.53) and OS (HR 2.71, 95 % CI 1.11-6.67).

Conclusions: IFITM1 was overexpressed in gastroesophageal adenocarcinoma and associated with M0-disease. In gastric cancer IFITM1 expression had a positive impact on TTR but in esophageal cancer it seemed to have an adverse impact on survival.
The reason for the diverging prognostic impact of IFITM1 in esophageal and gastric cancer is unclear and warrants further studies.

Keywords: Esophageal neoplasms, Stomach neoplasms, Adenocarcinoma, Prognosis, *IFITM1*

Background

Gastroesophageal adenocarcinoma is the 5th most common cancer worldwide [1]. The incidence of esophageal and GE (gastroesophageal) junction adenocarcinoma has drastically increased in many Western countries for the last four decades [2, 3]. Suggested factors to explain this increase are gastroesophageal reflux disease, obesity and decreased prevalence of *Helicobacter pylori* infection

[4, 5]. In contrast, the incidence of gastric adenocarcinoma has declined globally for several decades [6], possibly due to decreased prevalence of *Helicobacter pylori* infection and improved dietary conditions [7].

The prognosis of gastroesophageal adenocarcinoma is generally poor, at least in Western populations. For operable patients with resectable tumors recent studies have shown that the addition of neoadjuvant and/or adjuvant chemotherapy or chemoradiotherapy improves the 5-year survival rate with 10–15 % [8–11]. To further improve the overall survival in gastroesophageal

* Correspondence: david.borg@med.lu.se
Department of Clinical Sciences Lund, Division of Oncology and Pathology, Lund University, Skåne University Hospital, 221 85 Lund, Sweden

Table 1 Patient and tumor characteristics

Factor	Entire cohort ($n = 174$) n (%)	Esophagus ($n = 60$) n (%)	GE junction ($n = 45$) n (%)	Stomach ($n = 69$) n (%)
Age (years)				
Mean	70.2	67.9	69.9	72.4
Median	70.0	66.0	68.7	73.9
(Range)	(42.6-94.4)	(48.2-88.5)	(48.7-88.6)	(42.6-94.4)
Sex				
Women	40 (23.0)	6 (10.0)	12 (26.7)	22 (31.9)
Men	134 (77.0)	54 (90.0)	33 (73.3)	47 (68.1)
T stage				
T1	19 (10.9)	9 (15.0)	3 (6.7)	7 (10.1)
T2	32 (18.4)	10 (16.7)	4 (8.9)	18 (26.1)
T3	93 (53.4)	34 (56.7)	33 (73.3)	26 (37.7)
T4	27 (15.5)	6 (10.0)	4 (8.9)	17 (24.6)
Unknown	3 (1.7)	1 (1.7)	1 (2.2)	1 (1.4)
N stage				
N0	59 (33.9)	15 (25.0)	12 (26.7)	32 (46.4)
N1	30 (17.2)	11 (18.3)	7 (15.6)	12 (17.4)
N2	41 (23.6)	15 (25.0)	14 (31.1)	12 (17.4)
N3	44 (25.3)	19 (31.7)	12 (26.7)	13 (18.8)
Number of examined nodes				
Mean	30.3	36.6	29.7	24.3
Median	29.0	33.5	28.0	22.0
Range	1–112	10–72	8–48	1–112
Unknown	14	2	1	11
M stage				
M0	152 (87.4)	52 (86.7)	40 (88.9)	60 (87.0)
M1	22 (12.6)	8 (13.3)	5 (11.1)	9 (13.0)
R classification				
R0	121 (69.5)	38 (63.3)	30 (66.7)	53 (76.8)
R1	43 (24.7)	21 (35.0)	13 (28.9)	9 (13.0)
R2	10 (5.7)	1 (1.7)	2 (4.4)	7 (10.1)
Differentiation grade				
High	8 (4.6)	4 (6.7)	1 (2.2)	3 (4.3)
Intermediate	53 (30.5)	26 (43.3)	13 (28.9)	14 (20.3)
Low	113 (64.9)	30 (50.0)	31 (68.9)	52 (75.4)
Lauren classification				
Intestinal	120 (69.0)	54 (90.0)	31 (68.9)	35 (50.7)
Mixed	9 (5.2)	4 (6.7)	3 (6.7)	2 (2.9)
Diffuse	45 (25.9)	2 (3.3)	11 (24.4)	32 (46.4)
Intestinal metaplasia background				
No	101 (58.0)	37 (61.7)	34 (75.6)	30 (43.5)
Yes	73 (42.0)	23 (38.3)	11 (24.4)	39 (56.5)
Adjuvant therapy				
No	161 (92.5)	55 (91.7)	42 (93.3)	64 (92.8)
Chemoradiotherapy	11 (6.3)	3 (5.0)	3 (6.7)	5 (7.2)
Chemotherapy	1 (0.6)	1 (1.7)		
Radiotherapy	1 (0.6)	1 (1.7)		
Follow-up (years)				
Mean	3.25	3.36	3.06	3.28
Median	2.28	2.47	2.17	2.09
Range	0.01-8.95	0.26-8.95	0.01-8.89	0.01-8.85

Table 1 Patient and tumor characteristics *(Continued)*

Recurrence				
No	62 (35.6)	20 (33.3)	15 (33.3)	27 (39.1)
Yes	78 (44.8)	29 (48.3)	22 (48.9)	27 (39.1)
Unknown/Not applicable	34 (19.5)	11 (18.3)	8 (17.8)	15 (21.7)
Vital status				
Alive	48 (27.6)	21 (35.0)	8 (17.8)	19 (27.5)
Dead	126 (72.4)	39 (65.0)	37 (82.2)	50 (72.5)

adenocarcinoma, a deepened understanding of the tumor biology is required. Moreover, identification of prognostic and response predictive biomarkers is warranted to optimize and personalize the treatment strategies.

IFITM1 (interferon-inducible transmembrane protein 1), also known as 9–27, Leu-13 or CD225, is a cell surface 17-kDa membrane protein that is encoded on the short arm of chromosome 11. It is mainly known as an inhibitor of viral entry and replication [12], but it has also been associated with angiogenesis [13], inflammatory bowel disease [14] and osteogenesis [15].

There are now emerging data on IFITM1 and its role in malignancy. An upregulation of IFITM1 in different types of cancer and promotion of tumorigenesis by enhancing tumor cell migration, invasion and proliferation has been reported in several studies [16–23] but the opposite has also been shown [24–26]. Overexpression of IFITM1 has been reported to correlate with improved survival in glioma and chronic myeloid leukemia [17, 27] but in a South Korean study on gastric cancer, there was a trend towards worse survival in patients with high expression of IFITM1 [23]. Apart from the latter study, the knowledge on IFITM1 in gastroesophageal cancer survival is very limited, especially in Western populations. Therefore, the current study was designed to explore the expression and prognostic significance of IFITM1 in adenocarcinoma of the esophagus, GE junction and stomach in a consecutive cohort of patients from southern Sweden, that were treated 2006–2010, prior to the wide implementation of (neo-)adjuvant oncological treatment.

Methods

Study design and participants

The study comprises a consecutive cohort of 174 patients with chemo-/radiotherapy-naive gastroesophageal (gastric, GE junction and esophageal) adenocarcinoma subjected to surgical resection at the University Hospitals of Lund and Malmö between January 1, 2006 and December 31, 2010. This patient cohort has been used in several previous reports on other biomarkers [28–32]. Data on survival and recurrence were updated until December 31 2014. Tumor location was based on endoscopy findings. Classification of tumor stage was done according to UICC/AJCC TNM edition 7. Residual tumor status was classified as: R0 = no residual tumor, R1 = microscopic residual tumor, R2 = macroscopic residual tumor. The vast majority of the patients were operated on with a curative intent but three patients with metastatic disease were resected to palliate symptoms from the primary tumor. In 16 patients, M1-disease (distant metastases) was revealed either during surgery or in the resected specimens. All patients had surgery up-front, without neoadjuvant oncological therapy and a minority (7.5 %) of the patients received adjuvant treatment (chemo-/radiotherapy). Clinical data, recurrence status and vital status were obtained retrospectively

from medical records. Clinicopathological data and follow-up data are described in Table 1. The study was approved by the regional ethics committee at Lund University (ref nr 445/07).

Tissue microarrays

Using a semi-automated arraying device (TMArrayer™, Pathology Devices, Westminster, MD, USA) tissue microarrays (TMAs) were constructed. From all 174 primary tumors duplicate cores (1 mm) were obtained from areas with morphologically viable cancer in different blocks. In 81 cases lymph node metastases were sampled

Table 2 Associations of IFITM1 expression in primary tumors with clinicopathological data

Factor	Entire cohort median (range)	p-value	Esophagus median (range)	p-value	GE junction median (range)	p-value	Stomach median (range)	p-value
Age								
≤ average	1.75 (0.00-10.50)	0.103	2.00 (0.00-10.50)	0.363	2.50 (0.00-9.80)	0.693	0.00 (0.00-9.00)	0.001
>average	2.00 (0.00-12.00)		1.00 (0.00-7.50)		2.50 (0.00-12.00)		2.50 (0.00-12.00)	
Sex								
Female	2.50 (0.00-11.00)	0.207	4.00 (1.00-6.50)	0.080	2.50 (0.00-6.50)	1.000	2.00 (0.00-11.00)	0.588
Male	1.00 (0.00-12.00)		1.00 (0.00-10.50)		2.00 (0.00-12.00)		1.00 (0.00-12.00)	
T-stage								
T1	1.75 (0.00-10.00)	0.805	2.00 (0.00-8.00)	0.400	1.75 (0.00-3.50)	0.669	1.00 (0.00-10.00)	0.883
T2	2.00 (0.00-12.00)		2.25 (0.00-7.50)		0.50 (0.00-4.00)		3.00 (0.00-12.00)	
T3	1.75 (0.00-12.00)		1.25 (0.00-9.80)		2.50 (0.00-12.00)		1.25 (0.00-11.00)	
T4	1.00 (0.00-12.00)		0.50 (0.00-7.00)		2.50 (2.00-8.00)		1.00 (0.00-12.00)	
N-stage								
N0	2.00 (0.00-12.00)	0.585	2.25 (0.00-8.00)	0.471	2.50 (0.00-12.00)	0.694	1.25 (0.00-12.00)	0.504
N1	2.00 (0.00-12.00)		2.00 (0.00-6.50)		3.00 (0.00-11.00)		2.50 (0.00-12.00)	
N2	1.00 (0.00-12.00)		0.75 (0.00-9.80)		1.25 (0.00-8.00)		2.00 (0.00-12.00)	
N3	1.75 (0.00-10.50)		1.50 (0.00-10.50)		2.75 (0.00-9.80)		0.50 (0.00-6.00)	
M-stage								
M0	2.00 (0.00-12.00)	0.033	1.75 (0.00-10.50)	0.528	2.50 (0.00-12.00)	0.693	2.00 (0.00-12.00)	0.011
M1	0.50 (0.00-6.50)		1.25 (0.00-5.50)		2.00 (0.00-6.50)		0.00 (0.00-2.00)	
R-classification								
R0	2.00 (0.00-12.00)	0.055	2.00 (0.00-10.50)	0.444	3.00 (0.00-12.00)	0.252	2.00 (0.00-12.00)	0.225
R1	1.00 (0.00-9.80)		1.00 (0.00-9.80)		2.00 (0.00-7.00)		0.50 (0.00-4.50)	
R2	0.00 (0.00-10.00)		0.00 (0.00-0.00		0.125 (0.00-0.30)		0.25 (0.00-10.00)	
Differentiation grade								
High	2.00 (0.00-3.00)	0.759	2.00 (1.00-2.00)	0.629	2.50 (2.50-2.50	0.586	0.50 (0.00-3.00)	0.324
Intermediate	2.00 (0.00-12.00)		2.00 (0.00-10.50)		1.50 (0.00-5.50)		3.00 (0.00-12.00)	
Low	1.50 (0.00-12.00)		1.00 (0.00-8.00)		2.50 (0.00-12.00)		1.00 (0.00-12.00)	
Lauren classification								
Intestinal	2.00 (0.00-12.00)	0.150	1.75 (0.00-10.50)	0.191	2.00 (0.00-12.00)	0.565	3.00 (0.00-12.00)	0.008
Mixed	1.00 (0.00-6.50)		1.875 (0.00-6.50)		3.00 (0.00-3.00)		0.25 (0.00-0.50)	
Diffuse	0.50 (0.00-12.00)		0.00 (0.00-0.00)		3.50 (0.00-12.00)		0.38 (0.00-10.00)	
Intestinal metaplasia background								
No	1.00 (0.00-12.00)	0.083	1.00 (0.00-10.50)	0.446	2.00 (0.00-12.00)	0.090	0.75 (0.00-12.00)	0.271
Yes	2.25 (0.00-12.00)		2.00 (0.00-7.00)		4.25 (0.00-12.00)		1.75 (0.00-12.00)	
Location								
Esophagus	1.50 (0.00-10.50)	0.829						
GE junction	2.50 (0.00-12.00)							
Stomach	1.00 (0.00-12.00)							

in duplicate cores. In addition 1–3 cores from intestinal metaplasia (gastric intestinal metaplasia or Barrett's esophagus) were sampled in 73 cases. Single core samples from adjacent normal gastric mucosa (131 cases) and normal squamous epithelium of the esophagus (96 cases) were also retrieved. All samples were paired.

Immunohistochemistry

For immunohistochemical analysis of IFITM1 expression, 4 μm TMA-sections were automatically pre-treated using the PT Link system and then stained in an Autostainer Plus (DAKO; Glostrup, Copenhagen, Denmark) with the rabbit polyclonal anti-IFITM1 antibody HPA004810 (Atlas Antibodies AB, Stockholm, Sweden) diluted 1:250. The specificity of the antibody has been validated [33]. Staining was assessed by two different observers (DB and AG) blinded to clinical and outcome data. Scoring discrepancies were discussed to reach consensus. IFITM1

staining was mainly detected in the cytoplasm, with an accentuation towards the membrane. The fraction of stained tumor cells was scored as: 0 (0–1 %), 1 (2–25 %), 2 (26–50 %), 3 (51–75 %) or 4 (>75 %). Staining intensity was scored as: 0 (negative), 1 (weak), 2 (moderate) or 3 (strong). By multiplying fraction and intensity a combined score (0–12) was constructed.

Statistical analysis

The Mann–Whitney U test was applied to compare the distribution of IFITM1 expression in different tissues (Fig. 2) and also to describe the relationship between IFITM1 expression and clinicopathological factors (Table 2). Time to recurrence (TTR) was defined as time from date of surgery to date of biopsy or radiology proven recurrent disease. Overall survival (OS) was defined as time from date of surgery to date of death. TTR and OS were analysed for resected M0-patients with no macroscopic residual tumor

Table 3 Hazard ratios for recurrence and death M0 R0-1

| | | Time to recurrence | | | | |
| | | Unadjusted | | Adjusted[a] | |
	n (events)	HR (95 % CI)	p-value	HR (95 % CI)	p-value
Esophagus					
IFITM1					
Low	23 (13)	1.00	0.836	1.00	0.034
High	16 (9)	1.09 (0.47-2.56)		3.05 (1.09-8.53)	
GE junction					
IFITM1					
Low	16 (10)	1.00	0.852	1.00	0.400
High	17 (10)	1.09 (0.45-2.62)		1.50 (0.59-3.82)	
Stomach					
IFITM1					
Low	30 (19)	1.00	0.026	1.00	0.026
High	20 (5)	0.33 (0.12-0.88)		0.32 (0.12-0.87)	
		Overall survival				
		Unadjusted		Adjusted[b]	
	n (events)	HR (95 % CI)	p-value	HR (95 % CI)	p-value
Esophagus					
IFITM1					
Low	31 (20)	1.00	0.976	1.00	0.029
High	18 (11)	0.99 (0.47-2.07)		2.71 (1.11-6.67)	
GE junction					
IFITM1					
Low	19 (15)	1.00	0.995	1.00	0.937
High	19 (16)	1.00 (0.49-2.03)		0.97 (0.44-2.15)	
Stomach					
IFITM1					
Low	32 (22)	1.00	0.592	1.00	0.539
High	24 (15)	0.83 (0.43-1.62)		0.80 (0.39-1.64)	

[a]Adjusted for: T-stage, N-stage, R-classification
[b]Adjusted for: age, T-stage, N-stage, R-classification, differentiation grade

(R0-1). To determine the optimal prognostic cut-off for IFITM1 expression in the primary tumors, ROC-curves were used. Differences in Kaplan-Meier survival curves were calculated by log-rank test (Fig. 3). Unadjusted and adjusted hazard ratios for survival were determined using Cox proportional-hazards regression (Table 3). The adjusted model for TTR included T-stage, N-stage and R-classification. For OS, the adjusted model included age, T-stage, N-stage, R-classification and differentiation grade. All tests were 2-sided and a p-value <0.05 was considered significant. IBM® SPSS® Statistics version 22.0.0.1 for Mac was used for all statistical analyses.

Results
Expression of IFITM1 in normal epithelium, intestinal metaplasia, primary tumors and lymph node metastases
Immunohistochemical expression of IFITM1 could be assessed in 91/96 (95 %) samples with esophageal squamous epithelium, 122/131 (93 %) samples with gastric mucosa, 56/73 (77 %) samples with intestinal metaplasia (gastric intestinal metaplasia or Barrett's esophagus), 169/174 (97 %) samples with primary tumors, and 77/81 (95 %) samples with lymph node metastases. Sample images are shown in Fig. 1. The distribution of immunohistochemical expression of IFITM1 in the different tissue types is shown in Fig. 2. Expression of IFITM1 was significantly elevated in primary tumors and lymph node metastases compared to adjacent normal epithelium and intestinal metaplasia (Fig. 2). There were no significant differences of IFITM1 expression in primary tumors grouped by tumor location (Table 2).

Associations of IFITM1 expression in primary tumors with clinicopathological data
Table 2 describes the expression of IFITM1 in primary tumors in relationship to clinicopathological data for the entire cohort and for the separate tumor locations. In the entire cohort, IFITM1 was significantly elevated in

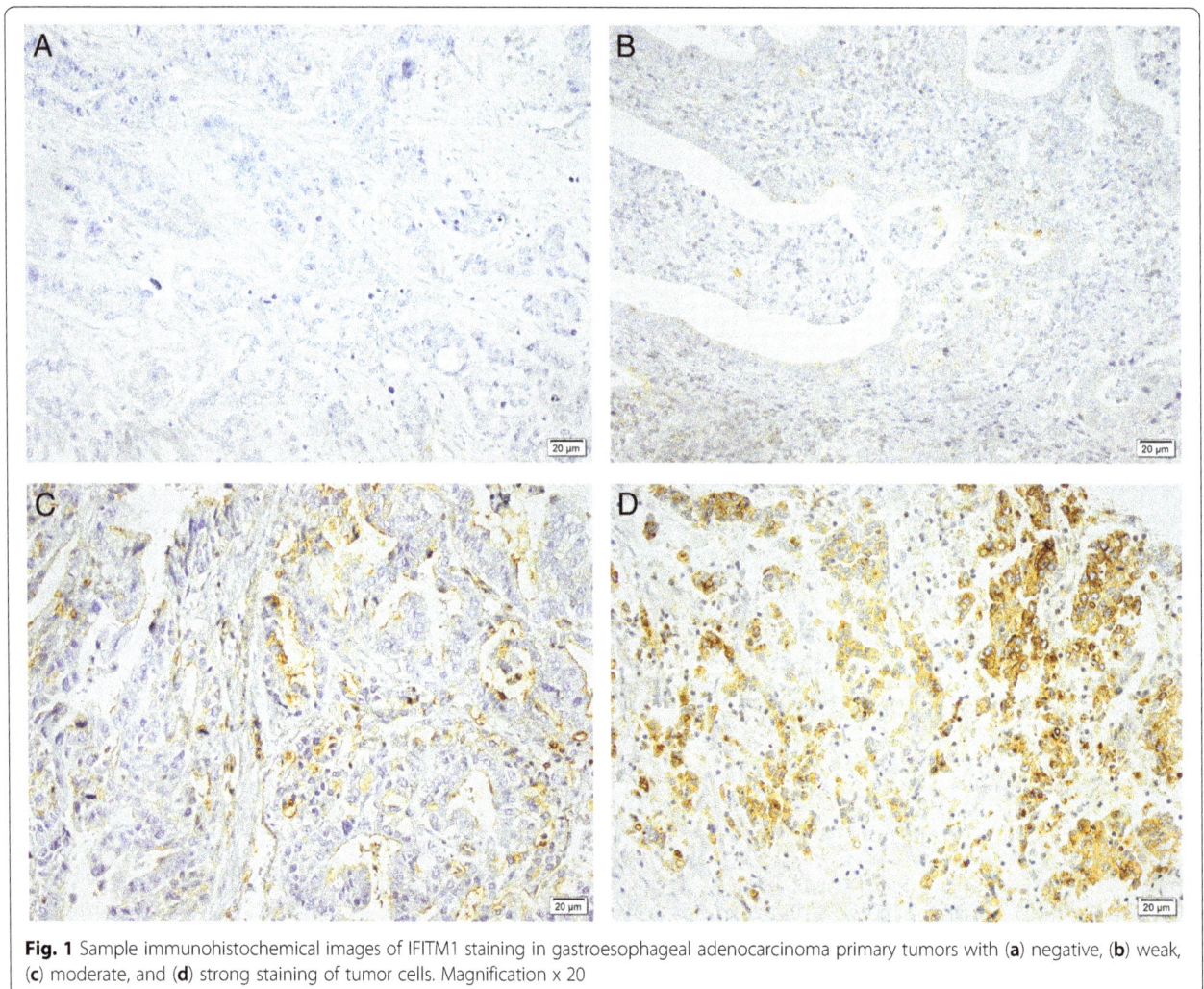

Fig. 1 Sample immunohistochemical images of IFITM1 staining in gastroesophageal adenocarcinoma primary tumors with (**a**) negative, (**b**) weak, (**c**) moderate, and (**d**) strong staining of tumor cells. Magnification x 20

Expression of IFITM1 as a prognostic biomarker in resected gastric and esophageal...

35

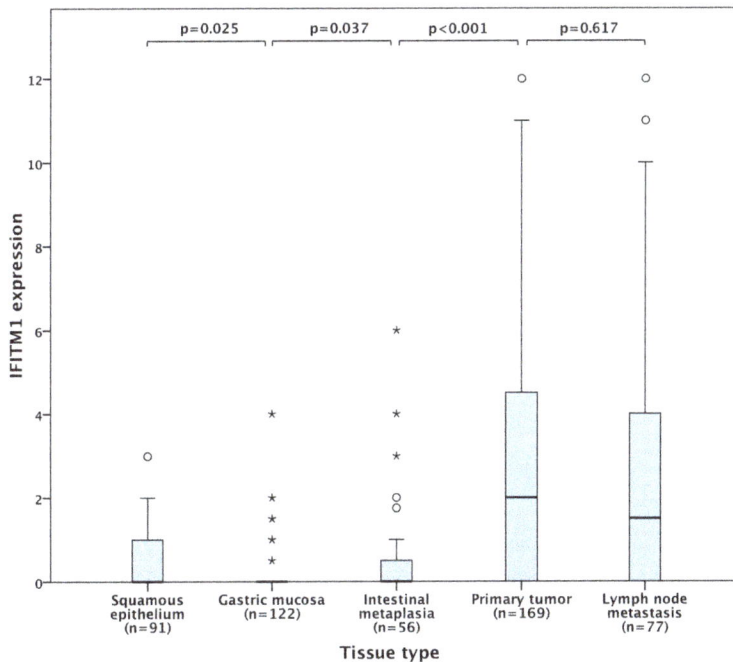

Fig. 2 Box plots visualizing the distribution of immunohistochemical IFITM1 expression (fraction x intensity) in normal squamous epithelium, normal gastric mucosa, intestinal metaplasia (Barrett's esophagus or gastric intestinal metaplasia), primary tumors and lymph node metastases in the entire cohort. The whiskers represent the largest values within 1.5 x interquartile range, the circles and asterisks represent outliers and extremes, respectively

M0-disease, most notably in gastric cancer. There was a trend towards higher IFITM1 expression in primary tumors with a background of intestinal metaplasia. In the subset of gastric tumors there were significant associations of high IFITM1 expression with age and Lauren's intestinal type, respectively.

Impact of IFITM1 expression on survival
Survival analyses were performed on patients with M0-disease and no macroscopic residual tumor (R0-1). Using ROC-curves, both for the separate primary tumor locations and for the entire cohort and with regard to TTR as well as OS, an optimal cut-off at 3 (IFITM1 low < 3, IFITM1 high 3–12) was identified and subsequently used for both TTR and OS, irrespectively of tumor location. In esophageal adenocarcinoma, expression of IFITM1 had no impact on TTR and OS in the Kaplan-Meier-analyses (Fig. 3a, d), but in the adjusted Cox regression analyses (Table 3 and Additional file 1: Table S1)) high IFITM1 expression had a negative impact on both TTR (HR 3.05, 95 % CI 1.09-8.53, $p = 0.034$) and OS (HR 2.71, 95 % CI 1.11-6.67, $p = 0.029$). IFITM1 expression in GE junction tumors did not correlate with TTR or OS in neither Kaplan-Meier (Fig. 3b, e) nor Cox regression analyses (Table 3 and Additional file 1: Table S2). In gastric cancer, high IFITM1 expression was significantly associated with improved TTR in the Kaplan-Meier analyses (Fig. 3c, f) and Cox regression (Table 3 and Additional file 1:

Table S3), both in the unadjusted analysis (HR 0.33, 95 % CI 0.12-0.88, $p = 0.026$) and in the adjusted analysis (HR 0.32, 95 % CI 0.12-0.87, $p = 0.026$) but there was no significant impact on OS.

Of note, considering the association of high IFITM1 with Lauren's intestinal type in gastric cancer (Table 2), we also tested to replace IFITM1 with Lauren classification in the adjusted Cox regression model but the hazard ratio of Lauren classification for TTR was not significant (data not shown) and when we added Lauren classification to the model with IFITM1 the hazard ratio of IFITM1 on TTR remained significant (data not shown). Thus, we do not believe that IFITM1 is just a marker for Lauren's intestinal type.

Of the 78 patients that developed recurrent disease during the follow-up period, 36 patients received palliative treatment with chemotherapy and/or radiotherapy. To what extent palliative therapy may have affected the outcome is unclear, but due to a considerable heterogeneity regarding treatment type, doses and duration as well as to avoid selection bias (patients offered active palliative treatment usually have better performance status and prognosis) we decided not to include palliative oncological treatment after recurrence as a variable in the survival analyses.

Discussion
The current study showed a significantly increased expression of IFITM1 in gastroesophageal adenocarcinoma

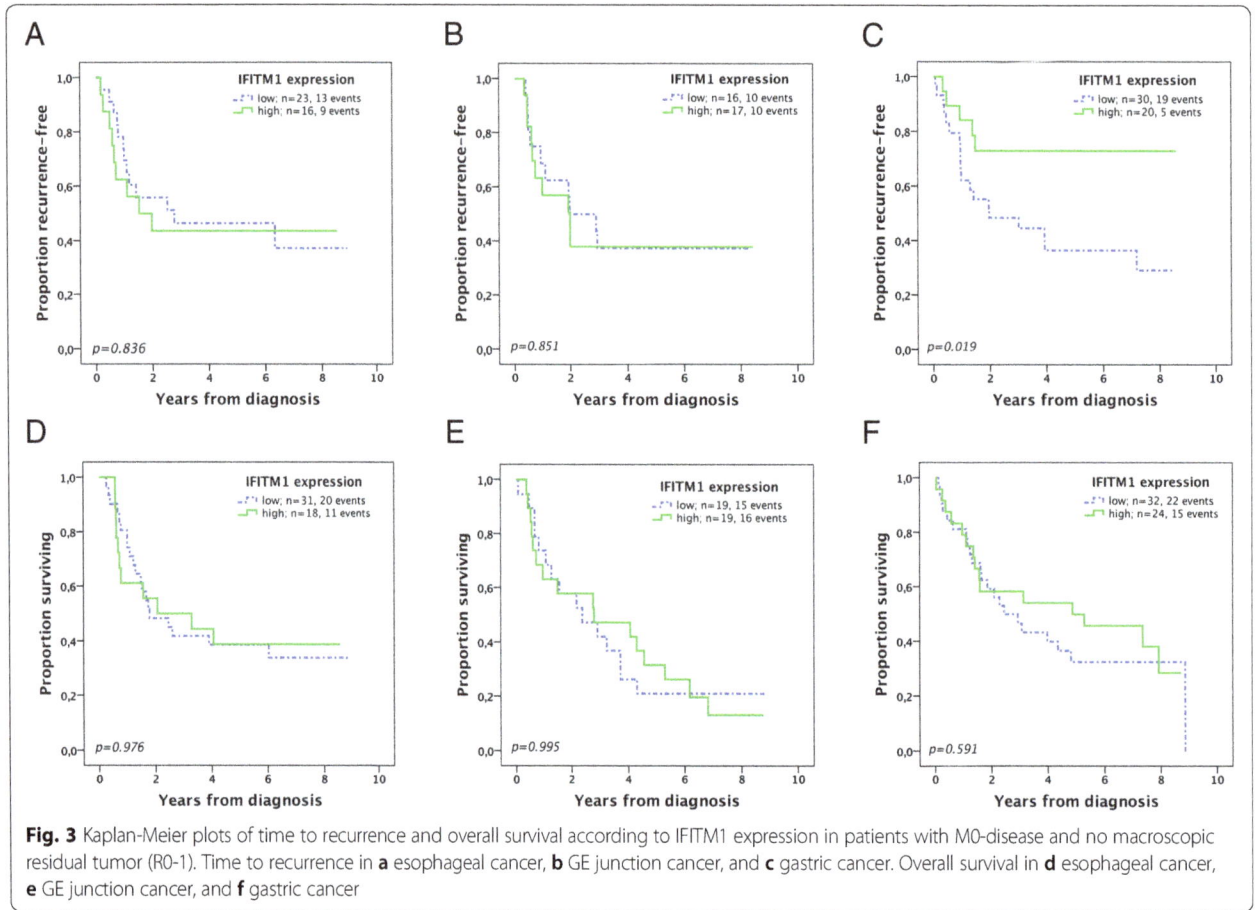

Fig. 3 Kaplan-Meier plots of time to recurrence and overall survival according to IFITM1 expression in patients with M0-disease and no macroscopic residual tumor (R0-1). Time to recurrence in **a** esophageal cancer, **b** GE junction cancer, and **c** gastric cancer. Overall survival in **d** esophageal cancer, **e** GE junction cancer, and **f** gastric cancer

compared to adjacent normal epithelium. This finding is in accordance with other reports on IFITM1 in gastric and colorectal adenocarcinoma [23, 34, 35]. The association of high IFITM1 expression and M0-disease, particularly seen in gastric cancer, has to our knowledge not been described previously.

In gastric cancer with high expression of IFITM1, we have demonstrated consistent findings of a beneficial effect on TTR. However, we could not demonstrate any significant relationship between IFITM1 and OS in gastric cancer, and one possible explanation for this could be the older age in these patients. It has previously been suggested that IFITM1 may have an adverse impact on OS in gastric cancer [23] but, even though our data on OS were non-significant, the association of elevated IFITM1 with M0-disease and the favorable impact on TTR implies that high expression of IFITM1 could rather be a positive prognostic factor in gastric cancer. It may seem like a paradox that the overexpression of IFITM1 in gastric cancer, which in other malignancies has been shown to promote tumorigenesis, was associated with M0-disease and a favorable TTR. A possible explanation might be that gastric tumorigenesis associated with elevated IFITM1 confers a less malignant

phenotype. Support for this is the observed association of high IFITM1 expression and the prognostically favorable Lauren's intestinal type demonstrated both in this study and by others [23]. A similar contradiction has been described in glioma cells where knockdown of IFITM1 was demonstrated to inhibit proliferation, migration and invasion [17, 18], whereas reduced expression of IFITM1 correlated with shorter survival in a cohort of 30 glioma patients [17].

The proposed negative impact of IFITM1 on TTR and OS in esophageal adenocarcinoma has to be interpreted with caution since it was only demonstrated in the adjusted Cox regression analysis. However, if true, this would suggest the involvement of a different tumorigenic pathway than in gastric cancer. Esophageal and gastric cancers are indeed different malignancies, with diverging incidence trends and different risk factors. For instance, *Helicobacter pylori* infection is associated with gastric cancer [7] but may be a protective factor for esophageal cancer [5].

The exact function of IFITM1 in malignancy is poorly understood and its role might differ depending on tumor cell type and context. IFITM1 has been demonstrated to promote malignant progression in gastric cancer cells by increasing invasion and migration and by suppressing natural killer cell activity [23, 35]. It has been shown that IFITM1 expression is regulated by DNA methylation of its promoter region [23]. Furthermore, expression of a transcript of CDH1 (E-cadherin) intron 2 (CDH1a) has been shown to increase gastric cancer cell invasion and angiogenesis and this increase correlated with IFITM1 expression [36]. The downstream effectors of IFITM1 on tumorigenesis are largely unknown but one possible mechanism of promoting invasion could be the upregulation of matrix metalloproteinases [20].

An association between high IFITM1 expression and sensitivity to cisplatin has been described in esophageal squamous cell carcinoma [37] whereas in gastric cancer, overexpression of IFITM1 may confer resistance to cisplatin [38]. Thus, future studies, on patient cohorts treated with neoadjuvant or palliative chemotherapy, would be of interest to further assess the possible role of IFITM1 as a predictive biomarker for response to platinum-based chemotherapy.

A limitation of our study is the retrospective design. However, all available surgically resected tumors were included consecutively, which decreases the risk of selection bias, and all clinical and histopathological data have been thoroughly re-examined. Another possible limitation is the use of the TMA technique, but since duplicate cores were obtained from different donor blocks, the risk of sampling bias should be low. Moreover, analyzing the data grouped by tumor location reduces the sample size and number of events and thus limits the possibility to adjust for multiple possible confounders in the Cox regression analyses. Due to the exploratory nature of the study, our results should mainly be regarded as hypothesis-generating, providing a basis for further exploration of IFITM1 as a biomarker in gastroesophageal adenocarcinoma.

Conclusion

In summary, we have shown that the immunohistochemical expression of IFITM1 was elevated in gastroesophageal adenocarcinoma and that it was associated with M0-disease. In gastric cancer, IFITM1 had a positive impact on TTR, whereas in esophageal cancer, data indicates an adverse impact on survival, suggesting that the role of IFITM1 may differ depending on the tumorigenic pathway. The mechanistic basis for this observation merits further study, and validatory studies on tumors from additional patient cohorts are warranted.

Ethics approval

The study was approved by the regional ethics committee at Lund University (ref nr 445/07), whereby the committee waived the need for consent other than by the option to opt out.

Abbreviations

CI: confidence interval; GE: gastroesophageal; HR: hazard ratio; IFITM1: interferon-inducible transmembrane protein 1; OS: overall survival; ROC: receiver operating characteristic; TMA: tissue microarray; TTR: time to recurrence.

Competing interests

The authors declare that they have no competing interests.

Authors' contributions

DB evaluated the immunohistochemical stainings, re-examined clinicopathological data, updated survival data, performed the statistical analyses and drafted the manuscript. CH collected and re-examined clinicopathological data and assisted with TMA construction. AG evaluated the immunohistochemical stainings and assisted with the statistical analysis. BN constructed the TMA and performed the IHC stainings. RF contributed with intellectual input. KJ, JE and AJ conceived of the study. All authors read and approved the final manuscript.

Funding

This study was supported by grants from the Knut and Alice Wallenberg Foundation, the Swedish Cancer Society, the Crafoord Foundation, the Olle Engkvist Foundation, Anna Lisa and Sven-Eric Lundgren's Foundation, Lund University Faculty of Medicine and Skåne University Hospital Funds and Donations.

References

1. Ferlay J, Soerjomataram I, Ervik M, Dikshit R, Eser S, Mathers C, et al. GLOBOCAN 2012 v1.0, Cancer Incidence and Mortality Worldwide: IARC CancerBase No. 11 [Internet]. Lyon, France. 2013. Available from: http://globocan.iarc.fr. Accessed 08 Feb 2016.
2. Edgren G, Adami H-O, Weiderpass E, Nyrén O. A global assessment of the oesophageal adenocarcinoma epidemic. Gut. 2013;62:1406–14.
3. Buas MF, Vaughan TL. Epidemiology and Risk Factors for Gastroesophageal Junction Tumors: Understanding the Rising Incidence of This Disease. Semin Radiat Oncol. 2013;23(1):3–9.
4. Carr JS, Zafar SF, Saba N, Khuri FR, El-Rayes BF. Risk Factors for Rising Incidence of Esophageal and Gastric Cardia Adenocarcinoma. J Gastrointest Cancer. 2013;44(2):143–51.
5. Nie S, Chen T, Yang X, Huai P, Lu M. Association of Helicobacter pylori infection with esophageal adenocarcinoma and squamous cell carcinoma: a meta-analysis. Dis Esophagus. 2014;27(7):645–53.
6. Ferro A, Peleteiro B, Malvezzi M, Bosetti C, Bertuccio P, Levi F, et al. Worldwide trends in gastric cancer mortality (1980–2011), with predictions to 2015, and incidence by subtype. Eur J Cancer. 2014;50(7):1330–44.
7. Fuccio L, Eusebi L, Bazzoli F. Gastric cancer, helicobacter pylori infection and other risk factors. World J Gastrointest Oncol. 2010;2(9):342.
8. Smalley SR, Benedetti JK, Haller DG, Hundahl SA, Estes NC, Ajani JA, et al. Updated Analysis of SWOG-Directed Intergroup Study 0116: A Phase III Trial of Adjuvant Radiochemotherapy Versus Observation After Curative Gastric Cancer Resection. J Clin Oncol. 2012;30(19):2327–33.
9. Cunningham D, Allum WH, Stenning SP, Thompson JN, Van de Velde CJ, Nicolson M, et al. Perioperative chemotherapy versus surgery alone for resectable gastroesophageal cancer. N Engl J Med. 2006;355(1):11–20.
10. Van Hagen P, Hulshof M, van Lanschot JJB, Steyerberg EW, van Berge Henegouwen M, Wijnhoven BPL, et al. Preoperative chemoradiotherapy for esophageal or junctional cancer. N Engl J Med. 2012;366(22):2074–84.
11. Noh SH, Park SR, Yang H-K, Chung HC, Chung I-J, Kim S-W, et al. Adjuvant capecitabine plus oxaliplatin for gastric cancer after D2 gastrectomy (CLASSIC): 5-year follow-up of an open-label, randomised phase 3 trial. Lancet Oncol. 2014;15(15):1389–96.

12. Perreira JM, Chin CR, Feeley EM, Brass AL. IFITMs restrict the replication of multiple pathogenic viruses. J Mol Biol. 2013;425(24):4937–55.

13. Popson SA, Ziegler ME, Chen X, Holderfield MT, Shaaban CI, Fong AH, et al. Interferon-Induced Transmembrane Protein 1 Regulates Endothelial Lumen Formation During Angiogenesis. Arterioscler Thromb Vasc Biol. 2014;34(5):1011–9.

14. Harris RA, Nagy-Szakal D, Mir SA, Frank E, Szigeti R, Kaplan JL, et al. DNA methylation-associated colonic mucosal immune and defense responses in treatment-naïve pediatric ulcerative colitis. Epigenetics. 2014;9(8):1131–7.

15. Kim B-S, Kim H-J, Kim JS, You Y-O, Zadeh H, Shin H-I, et al. IFITM1 increases osteogenesis through Runx2 in human alveolar-derived bone marrow stromal cells. Bone. 2012;51(3):506–14.

16. Andreu P, Colnot S, Godard C, Laurent-Puig P, Lamarque D, Kahn A, et al. Identification of the IFITM Family as a New Molecular Marker in Human Colorectal Tumors. Cancer Res. 2006;66(4):1949–55.

17. Balbous A, Cortes U, Guilloteau K, Villalva C, Flamant S, Gaillard A, et al. A mesenchymal glioma stem cell profile is related to clinical outcome. Oncogenesis. 2014;3(3):e91.

18. Yu F, Ng SSM, Chow BKC, Sze J, Lu G, Poon WS, et al. Knockdown of interferon-induced transmembrane protein 1 (IFITM1) inhibits proliferation, migration, and invasion of glioma cells. J Neurooncol. 2011;103(2):187–95.

19. Choi HJ, Lui A, Ogony J, Jan R, Sims PJ, Lewis-Wambi J. Targeting interferon response genes sensitizes aromatase inhibitor resistant breast cancer cells to estrogen-induced cell death. Breast Cancer Res. 2015;17(1):6.

20. Hatano H, Kudo Y, Ogawa I, Tsunematsu T, Kikuchi A, Abiko Y, et al. IFN-Induced Transmembrane Protein 1 Promotes Invasion at Early Stage of Head and Neck Cancer Progression. Clin Cancer Res. 2008;14(19):6097–105.

21. Kim N, Sung H, Choi E, Lyu D, Choi H, Ju W, et al. Aberrant DNA methylation in the IFITM1 promoter enhances the metastatic phenotype in an intraperitoneal xenograft model of human ovarian cancer. Oncol Rep. 2014;31(5):2139–46.

22. Chattopadhyay I, Phukan R, Singh A, Vasudevan M, Purkayastha J, Hewitt S, et al. Molecular profiling to identify molecular mechanism in esophageal cancer with familial clustering. Oncol Rep. 2009;21(5):1135–46.

23. Lee J, Goh S-H, Song N, Hwang J-A, Nam S, Choi IJ, et al. Overexpression of IFITM1 Has Clinicopathologic Effects on Gastric Cancer and Is Regulated by an Epigenetic Mechanism. Am J Pathol. 2012;181(1):43–52.

24. Pan Z, Chen S, Pan X, Wang Z, Han H, Zheng W, et al. Differential gene expression identified in Uigur women cervical squamous cell carcinoma by suppression subtractive hybridization. Neoplasma. 2010;57(2):123–8.

25. Yang G, Xu Y, Chen X, Hu G. IFITM1 plays an essential role in the antiproliferative action of interferon-γ. Oncogene. 2007;26(4):594–603.

26. Huang H, Colella S, Kurrer M, Yonekawa Y, Kleihues P, Ohgaki H. Gene expression profiling of low-grade diffuse astrocytomas by cDNA arrays. Cancer Res. 2000;60(24):6868–74.

27. Akyerli CB, Beksac M, Holko M, Frevel M, Dalva K, Özbek U, et al. Expression of IFITM1 in chronic myeloid leukemia patients. Leuk Res. 2005;29(3):283–6.

28. Fristedt R, Gaber A, Hedner C, Nodin B, Uhlén M, Eberhard J, et al. Expression and prognostic significance of the polymeric immunoglobulin receptor in esophageal and gastric adenocarcinoma. J Transl Med. 2014;12(1):83.

29. Jonsson L, Hedner C, Gaber A, Korkocic D, Nodin B, Uhlén M, et al. High expression of RNA-binding motif protein 3 in esophageal and gastric adenocarcinoma correlates with intestinal metaplasia-associated tumours and independently predicts a reduced risk of recurrence and death. Biomark Res. 2014;2:11.

30. Hedner C, Gaber A, Korkocic D, Nodin B, Uhlén M, Kuteeva E, et al. SATB1 is an independent prognostic factor in radically resected upper gastrointestinal tract adenocarcinoma. Virchows Arch. 2014;465(6):649–59.

31. Hedner C, Tran L, Borg D, Nodin B, Jirström K, Eberhard J. Discordant HER2 overexpression in primary and metastatic upper gastrointestinal adenocarcinoma signifies poor prognosis. Histopathology. 2016;68(2):230–40.

32. Hedner C, Borg D, Nodin B, Karnevi E, Jirström K, Eberhard J. Expression and Prognostic Significance of Human Epidermal Growth Factor Receptors 1 and 3 in Gastric and Esophageal Adenocarcinoma. PLoS One. 2016;11(2):e0148101.

33. The Human Protein Atlas [Internet]. Available from: http://www.proteinatlas.org/ENSG00000185885-IFITM1/antibody. Accessed 08 Feb 2016

34. Kitahara O, Furukawa Y, Tanaka T, Kihara C, Ono K, Yanagawa R, et al. Alterations of Gene Expression during Colorectal Carcinogenesis Revealed by cDNA Microarrays after Laser-Capture Microdissection of Tumor Tissues and Normal Epithelia. Cancer Res. 2001;61:3544–9.

35. Yang Y, Lee J-H, Yong Kim K, Keun Song H, Kwang Kim J, Ran Yoon S, et al. The interferon-inducible 9–27 gene modulates the susceptibility to natural killer cells and the invasiveness of gastric cancer cells. Cancer Lett. 2005; 221(2):191–200.

36. Pinheiro H, Carvalho J, Oliveira P, Ferreira D, Pinto MT, Osorio H, et al. Transcription initiation arising from E-cadherin/CDH1 intron2: a novel protein isoform that increases gastric cancer cell invasion and angiogenesis. Hum Mol Genet. 2012;21(19):4253–69.

37. Fumoto S, Shimokuni T, Tanimoto K, Hiyama K, Otani K, Ohtaki M, et al. Selection of a novel drug-response predictor in esophageal cancer: a novel screening method using microarray and identification of IFITM1 as a potent marker gene of CDDP response. Int J Oncol. 2008;32(2):413–23.

38. Lee H, No HK, Ryu CJ, Park H-J. Brahma-related gene 1-associated expression of 9–27 and IFI-27 is involved in acquired cisplatin resistance of gastric cancer cells. Mol Med Rep. 2013;8:747–50.

4

DNA methyltransferases and their roles in tumorigenesis

Wu Zhang and Jie Xu[*]

Abstract

DNA methylation plays an important role in gene expression, chromatin stability, and genetic imprinting. In mammals, DNA methylation patterns are written and regulated by DNA methyltransferases (DNMTs), including DNMT1, DNMT3A and DNMT3B. Recent emerging evidence shows that defects in DNMTs are involved in tumor transformation and progression, thus indicating that epigenetic disruptions caused by DNMT abnormalities are associated with tumorigenesis. Herein, we review the latest findings related to DNMT alterations in cancer cells and discuss the contributions of these effects to oncogenic phenotypes.

Keywords: DNA methyltransferases, Tumorigenesis, DNA methylation

Background

DNA methylation is one of the most important epigenetic modifications [1], playing key roles in the regulation of gene expression, genomic imprinting, X chromosome inactivation, and tumorigenesis [2, 3]. In mammals, DNMT1, DNMT3A and DNMT3B, the generally recognized three types of DNA methyltransferases (DNMTs), execute the genomic methylation process [4]. These proteins are highly conserved and have similar amino acid sequences. The N-terminus contains a regulatory domain, which allows DNMTs to anchor in the nucleus and recognize nucleic acids or nucleoproteins, and the C-terminus possesses a catalytic domain, which is responsible for the enzymatic activity [5]. DNMT1, DNMT3A and DNMT3B have different functions in the methylation process. DNMT1 is required for the maintenance of all methylation in the genome. During replication, DNMT1 restores the specific methylation pattern on the daughter strand in accordance with that of the parental DNA. DNMT3A and DNMT3B are referred to as *de novo* methyltransferases, which are responsible for establishing DNA methylation patterns during embryogenesis and setting up genomic imprints during germ cell development [6]. Although they are highly expressed in early mammalian embryos, DNMT3A and DNMT3B decrease in expression over the course of cell differentiation. These two proteins have distinct functions throughout embryonic development, showing both spatial and temporal differences. DNMT3A primarily methylates a set of genes and sequences at the late stage of embryonic development and especially after birth, whereas DNMT3B modifies a broader region of genomic sequences in early embryos [2, 6]. Very recently, one study identified a new *de novo* DNA methyltransferase DNMT3C in murine germ cells. DNMT3C exhibits high identity with DNMT3B, and is specialized at methylating the young retrotransposons [7]. Beside the above-mentioned enzymes, which are essential for the methylation of mammalian DNA, the DNMT family also includes two additional members, DNMT2 and DNMT3L. Although DNMT2 is not currently considered to be a DNA methylase, this enzyme methylates small transfer RNAs (tRNAs) [8]. DNMT3L, an important regulator without catalytic activity, operates in the form of DNMT3L-DNMT3A heterotetramers and facilitates the methylation of cytosine residues [2, 5, 6]. In animal models, Dnmt3a knockout mice have been found to exhibit postnatal growth retardation and dysplasia and to die by 4 weeks of age [9]. Mice deficient in either Dnmt1 or Dnmt3b exhibit embryonic lethality [9, 10]. Male mice without Dnmt3c are sterile [7]. Thus, these phenotypes demonstrate that the establishment and maintenance of global genomic methylation processes is the basis for cell proliferation and differentiation.

* Correspondence: nbxujie1011@163.com
State Key Laboratory for Medical Genomics, Shanghai Institute of Hematology, Rui-Jin Hospital affiliated to Shanghai Jiao-Tong University School of Medicine, 197 Rui Jin Er Road, 200025 Shanghai, China

In recent years, interest in the relationship between DNA methylation and human diseases has increased. Alterations in DNA methylation patterns have been implicated in tumorigenesis in several studies [11–13]. Owing to the revolutionary progress of next-generation sequencing technology, a variety of genomic landscapes of human tumor tissues have been described, and a number of defective genes associated with illnesses have been discovered [4, 13]. Sequencing studies on hematologic disorders achieve big success in identifying previously unrecognized mutated genes [14]. Among these mutated genes, many, such as *DNMT3A*, *TET2*, and *IDH1*, are involved in epigenetic processes [15–18] and are directly or indirectly related to DNA methylation. These discoveries bring new prospects for cancer diagnosis and treatment, enabling researchers to fully realize the enormous potential of genomic methylation abnormalities in tumorigenesis. The following content will describe the relationship between defective DNMTs and tumorigenesis, and finally will focus on the DNMT3A alteration that has been especially well studied.

Emerging evidence of DNMTs in malignant transformation

Tumor cells typically exhibit aberrant DNA methylation patterns during malignant transformation [3, 19]. Although this phenomenon is generally attributed to different mechanisms, alteration in the DNMT family of genes and the resulting dysregulation of genomic methylation is a primary causative factor [20, 21]. Numerous samples with lesions in the DNMT genes have been studied to identify methylation changes and to evaluate cancer development. These lesions can be classified into three categories: overexpression, mutation and deletion (Table 1).

Overexpression

Overexpression of DNMTs (DNMT1, DNMT3A, and DNMT3B) in a variety of tumors results in hypermethylation and oncogenic activation [11]. DNMT1 overexpression correlates well with aberrant DNA methylation in solid tumors, thus resulting in lymph node metastasis and poor prognosis in patients [22–24]. Similarly, highly expressed DNMT3A or DNMT3B has been found in a large number of patient specimens, and increased DNMT3A expression is involved in hepatocellular carcinogenesis [25]. Moreover, high expression levels of DNMT3B and CTCF are critical in the epigenetic inactivation of *BRCA1* in sporadic breast tumors [26]. Additional studies have suggested that DNMT3B is required for the outgrowth of colonic micro-adenomas [27, 28]. Several studies have provided explanations for the relationship between overexpressed DNMTs and tumorigenesis. Zhao et al. have shown that DNMT1 knockdown has an inhibitory effect on the cell cycle in esophageal squamous cell carcinoma, indicating that increased methylation levels promote cell mitosis [22]. Two groups have demonstrated that DNMT3B overexpression is closely related to CIMP-high in colon cancers [29, 30]. Additional studies performed on cultured primary prostate cells have shown that the overexpression of DNMT3B1 and DNMT3B2, the two subtypes of DNMT3B, leads to an increase in methylation [31].

Mutation

Somatic mutations in DNMTs are the prominent features of many tumors and substantially contribute to malignant transformation [32]. As shown in Table 1, DNMT1 mutations in colon tumors and DNMT3A mutations in hematological malignancies have been observed in the cancer genome. Kanai et al. have shown that DNMT1 inactivation due to mutational changes in colon cancers results in genome-wide alterations of the DNA methylation status [33]. Critical findings on DNMT3A variation have suggested that DNMT3A is frequently mutated in acute myeloid leukemia (AML), myelodysplastic syndrome (MDS) and adult early T-cell precursor acute lymphoblastic leukemia (ETP-ALL) and is associated with disease aggressiveness and treatment resistance [15, 16, 34–36]. Mice expressing the Dnmt3a Arg882 mutant protein developed chronic myelomonocytic leukemia with thrombocytosis [37]. Moreover, DNMT3A mutations, particularly those in the catalytic domain, substantially decrease enzymatic activity [16, 34]. In DNMT3A-mutated AML samples and relevant mouse models, such loss of function results in the hypomethylation of *HOX* family genes [16, 37]. Together, these studies suggest that mutated DNMTs disrupt genomic methylation and play significant roles in tumor formation.

Deletion

An in vivo mouse model with embryonically inactive DNMT3A and DNMT3B has shown that the deletion of *de novo* methyltransferases leads to lethal phenotypes [9]. Recently, the effects of *de novo* methyltransferase on hematopoiesis have been evaluated through conditional knockout technology. The deletion of Dnmt3a in adult mice induces the proliferation of hematopoietic progenitors [38]. On the basis of this abnormality, researchers then demonstrated that mutated NRAS- or FLT3-ITD-driven malignancy is accelerated by a lack of Dnmt3a [39–42]. Furthermore, the ectopic introduction of c-Kit variants into a Dnmt3a-deficient background produces acute leukemia [43]. Moreover, DNMT3A inactivation leads to the progression of peripheral T cell lymphoma (PTCL) and lung tumors, thus indicating that *DNMT3A* may act as a tumor-suppressor gene [44, 45]. Studies have also shown that DNMT3B acts as a tumor suppressor in Myc-induced lymphomas and MLL-AF9-driven AML [46]. A lack of maintenance methyltransferase

Table 1 Emerging evidence of DNMTs in malignant transformation

Tumor type	DNMT subtype	Model studied	Alteration	Reference
AML	DNMT3A	Patients	Mutation	[15, 16, 34]
	DNMT3A	Mouse tumor model	Mutation	[72]
	DNMT3A	Mouse tumor model	Deletion	[39–43]
	DNMT3B	Mouse tumor model	Deletion	[46]
	DNMTs	Patients	Overexpression	[74]
MDS	DNMT3A	Patients	Mutation	[35]
CMML	DNMT3A	Mouse model	Mutation	[37]
CML	DNMTs	Patients	Overexpression	[74]
ALL	DNMT3A	Patients	Mutation	[36]
Lymphoma	DNMT1	Mouse tumor model	Deletion	[47]
	DNMT3A	Mouse model	Deletion	[44]
	DNMT3B	Mouse tumor model	Deletion	[75]
Breast	DNMT1	Mouse tumor model	Deletion	[76]
	DNMT1	Patients	Overexpression	[77]
	DNMT3B	Patients	Overexpression	[26]
Lung	DNMT3A	Mouse tumor model	Deletion	[45]
Colon	DNMT1	Patients	Mutation	[33]
	DNMT3B	Patients	Overexpression	[29, 30]
	DNMT3B	Mouse tumor model	Overexpression	[27, 28]
Liver	DNMT1	Patients	Overexpression	[24]
	DNMT3A	Patients	Overexpression	[25]
Melanoma	DNMT3A	Mouse tumor model	Overexpression	[78]
Pancreas	DNMT1	Patients	Overexpression	[23]
Prostate	DNMT3B	Patients	Overexpression	[31]
Esophagus	DNMT1	Patients	Overexpression	[22]

activity is also related to carcinogenesis. Studies have shown that DNMT1 deletion leads to DNA demethylation and that DNMT1 is critical for T-cell lymphoma prevention and maintenance, contributing to aberrant methylation by *de novo* and maintenance methylation [47]. Therefore, deletion of genes encoding DNMTs also participates in tumor development.

Epigenetic disruptions involving DNMTs in tumorigenesis

Epigenetic disorders, which are commonly found in cancer, are attributed in part to DNMT dysfunction [3, 4]. Because of its catalytic role and inhibition of target gene transcription, DNMTs play a significant role in the maintenance of chromosomal homeostasis [6]. Defective DNMTs induce imbalances in DNA and/or histone modification, thus resulting in chromatin remodeling, genomic instability and gene inactivation. Unlike the genomes in normal tissue, the genomes of tumor cells generally display global hypomethylation throughout, with localized hypermethylation in particular regions [20]. Moreover, crosstalk between DNMTs and other chromatin regulators, such as histone methyltransferases and transcriptional co-suppressors, is highly important in epigenetic disruption [48–50]. These characteristics

may contribute to diagnosis and targeted therapy in clinical applications (Fig. 1).

Global hypomethylation

DNA hypomethylation of tumor cells is the first process characterized as an epigenetic abnormality [19]. The genome-wide hypomethylation of tumor cells results in a reduction of 5-mC, mainly in gene-coding regions and satellite repeats (Fig. 1). These changes cause mitotic recombination, copy number deletion and chromosomal rearrangement, and even genomic imprinting annihilation. Gaudet et al. have demonstrated that deletion or reduction of DNMT1 leads to substantial genome-wide hypomethylation and chromosomal instability [51]. Through methylated DNA immunoprecipitation (MeDIP)-chip analysis, hypomethylated CpG islands (CGIs) of the *HOXB* cluster have been found in AML samples with *DNMT3A* mutations [16]. Although the underlying mechanism governing the effects of genome-wide hypomethylation on the process of tumorigenesis is not fully understood, these limited data have provided alternative insight into a relationship between aberrant DNMTs and global hypomethylation, along with subsequent tumor occurrence [1].

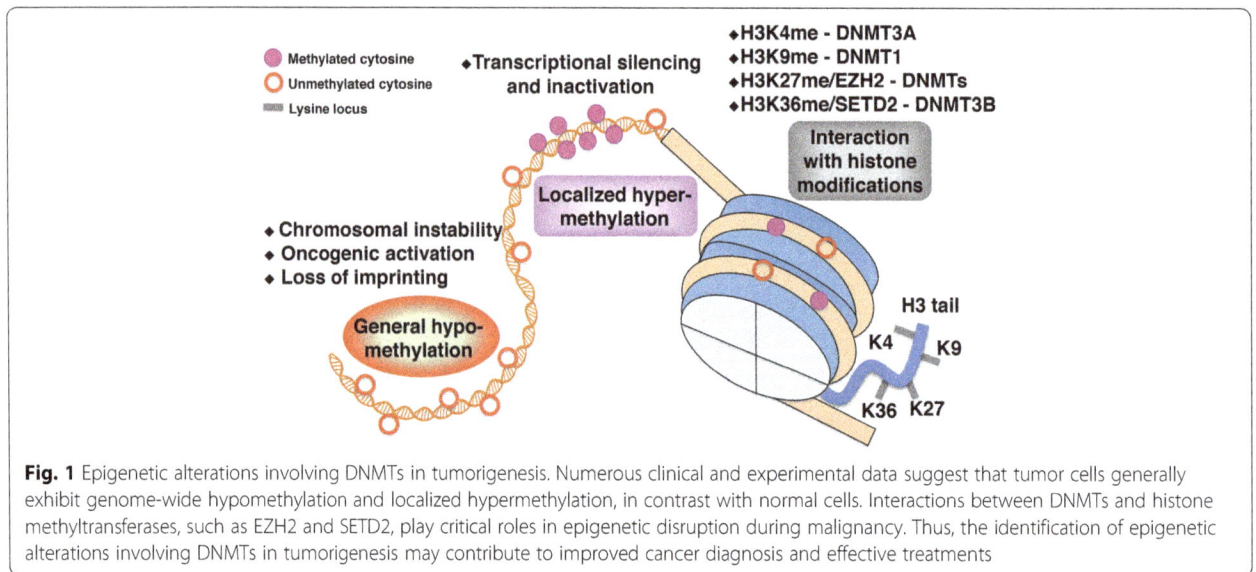

Fig. 1 Epigenetic alterations involving DNMTs in tumorigenesis. Numerous clinical and experimental data suggest that tumor cells generally exhibit genome-wide hypomethylation and localized hypermethylation, in contrast with normal cells. Interactions between DNMTs and histone methyltransferases, such as EZH2 and SETD2, play critical roles in epigenetic disruption during malignancy. Thus, the identification of epigenetic alterations involving DNMTs in tumorigenesis may contribute to improved cancer diagnosis and effective treatments

Localized hypermethylation

In normal somatic cells, DNA methylation occurs primarily in dinucleotides containing less CpG, whereas the CpG-enriched region is unmethylated [6, 50]. Throughout malignant transformation, the global methylation level of DNA changes, thus leading to non-CpG island hypomethylation and CGI hypermethylation. As a result, the number of genes that are hypermethylated on their promoters increases. In particular, hypermethylation induces the silencing of several key tumor-suppressor genes (TSGs), which play important roles in tumor progression (Fig. 1). Generally, abnormal CGI hypermethylation is an epigenetic characteristic of tumors, of which hypermethylated TSGs are the most common feature [1, 13].

A great deal of research has been performed to explore the mechanism of aberrant TSG methylation in tumor tissue. As expected, DNMTs have been included in the aforementioned studies. In leukemia, deletions or mutations in DNMTs often disrupt the distribution of 5-mC in the genome [52]. Butcher et al. have shown that in some sporadic breast tumors, hypermethylation of the BRCA1 promoter is partially due to DNMT3B overexpression [26]. Using a conditional Dnmt3a knockout mouse model, researchers have observed a general decrease in hypomethylation in the transcription factor-binding sites of cross-regions (Canyons) [53]. Additionally, canyon-associated genes, including HOX genes, are markedly enriched in DNMT3A mutant AMLs [53].

Tumor-associated DNA methylation generally occurs in the promoter regions of TSGs [13]. However, owing to rapid advancements in methylation sequencing, data increasingly indicate that a large number of non-TSGs are methylated at the early stage of tumor initiation, and methylation changes within the gene body have a

substantial effect on the process of transcription. The TCGA network has reported the integrated methylation profiles of AML samples with mutations in DNMT3A, as determined with Human Methylation 450 Bead Chip arrays [54]. This complete epigenomic landscape reveals a large amount of hypermethylated cytosine bases in the gene body and intergenic regions. Similarly, in a Dnmt3a mutant-transduced mouse model, hypermethylation is greater in the intergenic regions, and a cluster of suppressed genes related to lymphocyte development, such as Notch1 and Gata3, are hypermethylated in the gene body regions [37]. Furthermore, Yang et al. have suggested that DNMT3B-dependent gene body methylation enhances transcription and may be a potential therapeutic target in cancer [55].

Interaction with histone modifications

The entire epigenetic profile of the genome shows that active chromatin regions are generally characterized by acetylated histones and unmethylated DNA, whereas methylated histones associated with repressed chromatin and methylated DNA are enriched in suppressed regions [50]. Thus, the two chromatin markers interact in a highly orchestrated manner and are closely linked: DNA methylation helps guide histone modification, and histone modification directs DNA methylation (Fig. 1). For example, DNMT1 is required for the maintenance of H3K9 methylation in human cancer cells [56], and DNMT3A PWWP interacts with H3K36me3 and consequently enhances DNMT3A activity [57]. These effects can be regarded as the outcome of cooperation between histone methyltransferase (HMT) and DNMTs. Indeed, DNMTs form complexes with HMTs and consequently regulate transcription. Both the H3K36 methyltransferase

SETD2 and the PWWP domain of DNMT3B are required for the *de novo* methylation of transcribed genes [58]. Likewise, the ADD domain of DNMT3A recognizes un-modified H3, which is repressed by H3K4 methylation [59]. In undifferentiated human embryonic carcinoma cells, promoter-related DNMTs overlap with different histone modifications [60]. Two groups have demonstrated that DNMT1 improves genomic methylation through enhanced histone modification by EZH2. EZH2 polycomb group protein mediates H3K27 methylation and recruits and directly controls DNA methylation [61, 62]. Thus, the above-mentioned investigations confirm that abnormal DNA methylation in tumor cells is closely related to histone modification. The relationship between DNA methylation and histone modification should provide more comprehensive insights into epigenetic regulation in tumorigenesis.

DNMT3A alterations lead to epigenetic reprogramming in leukemia

In recent years, mutated genes encoding a group of epigenetic modification regulators have attracted attention because of their high frequency of variation in hematological diseases [63]. Epigenetic disruption due to genetic alterations is the root cause of malignant transformation, particularly in hematologic malignancies [64]. Most notably, through a variety of high-throughput techniques, somatic mutations involving the *DNMT3A* gene have been identified in AML at a mutation rate of ~20%, and the prognosis for mutant patients is relatively poor [65]. Currently, DNMT3A abnormalities are the most common subject in the field of epigenetic medical research, because of its significance in tumor pathogenesis and the potential for target medication. Herein, the organization characteristic of DNMT3A and critical implications of DNMT3A alterations in hematological cancers are highlighted.

DNMT3A structure and function

As a member of the DNMT family, DNMT3A possesses the characteristic peptide structure: its catalytic domain directly binds to S-adenosyl-L-methionine (SAM) and DNA strands, and the N-terminus regulation domain is primarily involved in nuclear localization and protein interactions, in which the PWWP domain interacts with methyl lysine histones, and the PHD domain recognizes unmethylated histones. These functions serve as a signal of the histone transfer effect, thus ensuring diverse epigenetic modification [5]. Specifically, DNMT3A forms a butterfly-shaped tetramer (DNMT3L-DNMT3A-DNMT3A-DNMT3L) in the C-terminus with DNMT3L, thus changing the conformation of DNMT3A and facilitating its catalytic activity. The N-terminus of DNMT3A also operates as a transcriptional repressor.

The regulatory domain recruits nucleoproteins into the complex and performs histone modifications, chromatin remodeling and gene transcription. A range of partners is known to interact with DNMT3A, including histone methyltransferases, histone deacetylases, and various transcription factors, even enzymes in the DNMT family [50]. DNMTs are bound to each other, and *de novo* methyltransferase said in coordination during methylation maintenance [66]. Studies have shown that H3K9 methyltransferases, such as SUV39H1 and SETDB1, can directly bind to the PHD domain of DNMT3A and improve each other's catalytic activity, thus indicating that different epigenetic modifications can enhance chromatin inhibition by cooperating together [67].

DNMT3A mutation in leukemia

Clinically, in patients with *DNMT3A* mutations, the number of leukocytes present at diagnosis is relatively higher, and survival is comparatively shorter [15, 16]. To date, numerous functional experiments have provided a better understanding of the effects of *DNMT3A* mutation on leukemia pathogenesis (Fig. 2). For instance, *DNMT3A* mutation is an early event in the initiation of hematopoietic disorders and is one of several causative factors for the establishment of founder clones and the transformation of hematopoietic stem cells (HSCs) to pre-leukemic stem cells (Pre-LSCs) [68]. In addition, DNMT3A mutants harbor dominant-negative effects, such as those exhibited by DNMT3A R882H (R878H in mouse) mutated protein against wild-type DNMT3A [69, 70]. DNMT3A mutations also disrupt hematopoiesis. Researchers have used a bone marrow transplantation mouse model to determine that the function of Dnmt3a mutants in blood cell production is aberrant [37]. Additional studies have shown that mutated DNMT3A disrupts normal hematopoiesis and promotes the transformation to malignant cells, in combination with other epigenetic regulators [71]. In Dnmt3a-mutated models, a double-hit is essential for clonal expansion. In vivo experiments suggest that the mutation or deletion of Dnmt3a induces the development of leukemia by cooperating with oncogenic factors, such as *RAS* mutation, *c-Kit* variation, or FLT3-ITD abnormalities [39–43, 72]. DNMT3A mutations may also play an important role in tumor metastasis. For example, DNMT3A mutant leukemia cells may undergo leukemic extramedullary infiltration in NOD/SCID mice, a result partially linked to high expression levels of TWIST1, an epithelial-mesenchymal transition (EMT) inducer [73]. In summary, *DNMT3A* mutation exerts a great influence in hematological malignancy. A variety of small molecule compounds targeting relevant epigenetic disruptions have been

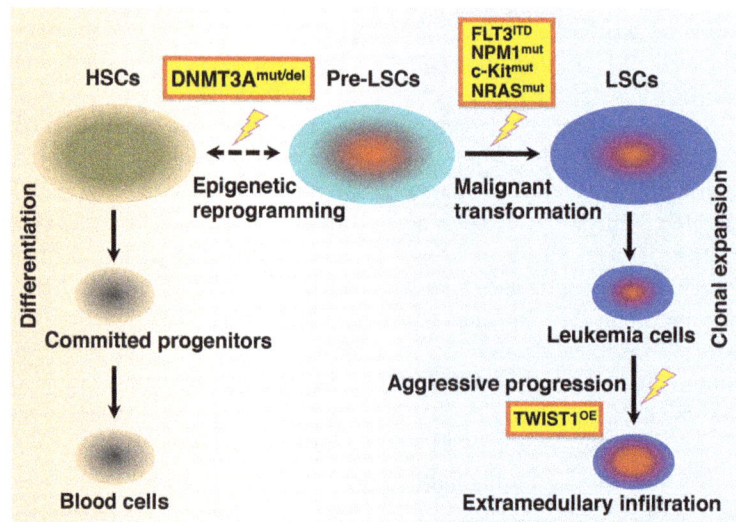

Fig. 2 DNMT3A alterations lead to epigenetic reprogramming in leukemia. Leukemia is a heterogeneous disease caused by cumulative multi-step disruption. In the initial stage of leukemogenesis, accumulated DNA lesions, emergent stimuli, and metabolic stress are observed in hematopoietic stem cells (HSCs). These conditions lead to gene alterations and link epigenetic reprogramming to leukemia development. Currently, DNMT3A gene lesions are considered to be critical epigenetic alterations in the occurrence of leukemia. In patient specimens and mouse models, the mutation or deletion of *DNMT3A* causes the apparent reversal of normal HSCs into pre-leukemia stem cells (Pre-LSCs). Frequently, Pre-LSCs are quiescent and stable in the early phases of leukemia. The accumulation of other transformative changes, such as a series of mutations (RAS^{mut}, $NPM1^{mut}$, $c-Kit^{mut}$) or oncogenic alterations ($FLT3^{ITD}$) causes Pre-LSCs to undergo malignant transformation into leukemia stem cells (LSCs), which finally enter the clonal expansion stage. Furthermore, during the aggressive progression of leukemia in a xenograft mouse model of OCI-AML3 with mutated DNMT3A, DNMT3A mutation promotes leukemic extramedullary infiltration by up-regulating the expression of the EMT inducer TWIST1. HSCs: hematopoietic stem cells; Pre-LSCs: pre-leukemia stem cells; LSCs: leukemia stem cells; mut: mutation; del: deletion; ITD: internal tandem duplication; OE: overexpression; EMT: epithelial-mesenchymal transition

developed and applied in the treatment of leukemia, which also provide a comprehensive innovation for the study of pathogenesis and targeted therapy of solid tumors.

Conclusions

Owing to advances in sequencing technologies, numerous gene alterations associated with epigenetics have been identified in cancer genomes. Furthermore, whole-epigenome approaches, including array-based methylation profiling and bisulfite sequencing, afford a comprehensive view of the tumor methylome, and potential mechanisms of epigenetic disruption caused by DNMT changes have been explored. However, the effects of DNMT aberrations in the promotion of tumorigenesis are not entirely clear, and novel strategies for relevant targeted therapies must be developed. Future work should focus on the elucidation of tumorigenic mechanisms induced by defective DNMTs and the production of effective therapeutic approaches.

Abbreviations
AML: Acute myeloid leukemia; BMT: Bone marrow transplantation; CGIs: CpG islands; CIMP: CpG island methylator phenotype; CTCF: CCCTC-binding factor; DNMTs: DNA methyltransferases; EMI: Extramedullary infiltration; EMT: Epithelial–mesenchymal transition; ETP-ALL: Early T-cell precursor acute lymphoblastic leukemia; HMTs: Histone methyltransferases; HSCs: Hematopoietic stem cells; LSCs: Leukemia stem cells; MDS: Myelodysplastic syndrome; MeDIP: Methylated DNA immunoprecipitation; Pre-LSCs: Pre-leukemia stem cells; SAM: S-adenosyl-L-methionine; TSGs: Tumor suppressor genes

Acknowledgements
We would like to thank Zhu Chen and Sai-Juan Chen for support and encouragement. We further acknowledge Jiang Zhu for selfless assistance in our research.

Funding
This work was supported by the National Natural Science Foundation of China (81400106), the Shanghai Young Doctor Training Program (2015), and the Doctoral Innovation Fund Projects from Shanghai Jiao Tong University School of Medicine (BXJ201407).

Authors' contributions
WZ and JX conceived the topic of this review, prepared the figures, and wrote the manuscript. Both authors read and approved the final manuscript.

Competing interest
The authors declare that they have no competing interests.

References

1. Baylin SB, Jones PA. Epigenetic Determinants of Cancer. Cold Spring Harb Perspect Biol. 2016;8:a019505.
2. Smith ZD, Meissner A. DNA methylation: roles in mammalian development. Nat Rev Genet. 2013;14:204–20.
3. Jones PA, Baylin SB. The epigenomics of cancer. Cell. 2007;128:683–92.
4. Hamidi T, Singh AK, Chen T. Genetic alterations of DNA methylation machinery in human diseases. Epigenomics. 2015;7:247–65.
5. Chen T, Li E. Structure and function of eukaryotic DNA methyltransferases. Curr Top Dev Biol. 2004;60:55–89.
6. Li E, Zhang Y. DNA methylation in mammals. Cold Spring Harb Perspect Biol. 2014;6:a019133.
7. Barau J, Teissandier A, Zamudio N, Roy S, Nalesso V, Herault Y, et al. The DNA methyltransferase DNMT3C protects male germ cells from transposon activity. Science. 2016;354:909–12.
8. Goll MG, Kirpekar F, Maggert KA, Yoder JA, Hsieh CL, Zhang X, et al. Methylation of tRNAAsp by the DNA methyltransferase homolog Dnmt2. Science. 2006;311:395–8.
9. Okano M, Bell DW, Haber DA, Li E. DNA methyltransferases Dnmt3a and Dnmt3b are essential for de novo methylation and mammalian development. Cell. 1999;99:247–57.
10. Li E, Bestor TH, Jaenisch R. Targeted mutation of the DNA methyltransferase gene results in embryonic lethality. Cell. 1992;69:915–26.
11. Esteller M. Epigenetics in cancer. N Engl J Med. 2008;358:1148–59.
12. Suva ML, Riggi N, Bernstein BE. Epigenetic reprogramming in cancer. Science. 2013;339:1567–70.
13. Feinberg AP, Koldobskiy MA, Gondor A. Epigenetic modulators, modifiers and mediators in cancer aetiology and progression. Nat Rev Genet. 2016;17:284–99.
14. Ntziachristos P, Abdel-Wahab O, Aifantis I. Emerging concepts of epigenetic dysregulation in hematological malignancies. Nat Immunol. 2016;17:1016–24.
15. Ley TJ, Ding L, Walter MJ, McLellan MD, Lamprecht T, Larson DE, et al. DNMT3A mutations in acute myeloid leukemia. N Engl J Med. 2010;363:2424–33.
16. Yan XJ, Xu J, Gu ZH, Pan CM, Lu G, Shen Y, et al. Exome sequencing identifies somatic mutations of DNA methyltransferase gene DNMT3A in acute monocytic leukemia. Nat Genet. 2011;43:309–15.
17. Mardis ER, Ding L, Dooling DJ, Larson DE, McLellan MD, Chen K, et al. Recurring mutations found by sequencing an acute myeloid leukemia genome. N Engl J Med. 2009;361:1058–66.
18. Delhommeau F, Dupont S, Della Valle V, James C, Trannoy S, Masse A, et al. Mutation in TET2 in myeloid cancers. N Engl J Med. 2009;360:2289–301.
19. Herman JG, Baylin SB. Gene silencing in cancer in association with promoter hypermethylation. N Engl J Med. 2003;349:2042–54.
20. Dawson MA, Kouzarides T. Cancer epigenetics: from mechanism to therapy. Cell. 2012;150:12–27.
21. Rodriguez-Paredes M, Esteller M. Cancer epigenetics reaches mainstream oncology. Nat Med. 2011;17:330–9.
22. Zhao SL, Zhu ST, Hao X, Li P, Zhang ST. Effects of DNA methyltransferase 1 inhibition on esophageal squamous cell carcinoma. Dis Esophagus. 2011;24:601–10.
23. Peng DF, Kanai Y, Sawada M, Ushijima S, Hiraoka N, Kitazawa S, et al. DNA methylation of multiple tumor-related genes in association with overexpression of DNA methyltransferase 1 (DNMT1) during multistage carcinogenesis of the pancreas. Carcinogenesis. 2006;27:1160–8.
24. Saito Y, Kanai Y, Nakagawa T, Sakamoto M, Saito H, Ishii H, et al. Increased protein expression of DNA methyltransferase (DNMT) 1 is significantly correlated with the malignant potential and poor prognosis of human hepatocellular carcinomas. Int J Cancer. 2003;105:527–32.
25. Zhao Z, Wu Q, Cheng J, Qiu X, Zhang J, Fan H. Depletion of DNMT3A suppressed cell proliferation and restored PTEN in hepatocellular carcinoma cell. J Biomed Biotechnol. 2010;2010:737535.
26. Butcher DT, Rodenhiser DI. Epigenetic inactivation of BRCA1 is associated with aberrant expression of CTCF and DNA methyltransferase (DNMT3B) in some sporadic breast tumours. Eur J Cancer. 2007;43:210–9.
27. Lin H, Yamada Y, Nguyen S, Linhart H, Jackson-Grusby L, Meissner A, et al. Suppression of intestinal neoplasia by deletion of Dnmt3b. Mol Cell Biol. 2006;26:2976–83.
28. Linhart HG, Lin H, Yamada Y, Moran E, Steine EJ, Gokhale S, et al. Dnmt3b promotes tumorigenesis in vivo by gene-specific de novo methylation and transcriptional silencing. Genes Dev. 2007;21:3110–22.
29. Ibrahim AE, Arends MJ, Silva AL, Wyllie AH, Greger L, Ito Y, et al. Sequential DNA methylation changes are associated with DNMT3B overexpression in colorectal neoplastic progression. Gut. 2011;60:499–508.
30. Nosho K, Shima K, Irahara N, Kure S, Baba Y, Kirkner GJ, et al. DNMT3B expression might contribute to CpG island methylator phenotype in colorectal cancer. Clin Cancer Res. 2009;15:3663–71.
31. Kobayashi Y, Absher DM, Gulzar ZG, Young SR, McKenney JK, Peehl DM, et al. DNA methylation profiling reveals novel biomarkers and important roles for DNA methyltransferases in prostate cancer. Genome Res. 2011;21:1017–27.
32. Baylin SB, Jones PA. A decade of exploring the cancer epigenome - biological and translational implications. Nat Rev Cancer. 2011;11:726–34.
33. Kanai Y, Ushijima S, Nakanishi Y, Sakamoto M, Hirohashi S. Mutation of the DNA methyltransferase (DNMT) 1 gene in human colorectal cancers. Cancer Lett. 2003;192:75–82.
34. Yamashita Y, Yuan J, Suetake I, Suzuki H, Ishikawa Y, Choi YL, et al. Array-based genomic resequencing of human leukemia. Oncogene. 2010;29:3723–31.
35. Walter MJ, Ding L, Shen D, Shao J, Grillot M, McLellan M, et al. Recurrent DNMT3A mutations in patients with myelodysplastic syndromes. Leukemia. 2011;25:1153–8.
36. Neumann M, Heesch S, Schlee C, Schwartz S, Gokbuget N, Hoelzer D, et al. Whole-exome sequencing in adult ETP-ALL reveals a high rate of DNMT3A mutations. Blood. 2013;121:4749–52.
37. Xu J, Wang YY, Dai YJ, Zhang W, Zhang WN, Xiong SM, et al. DNMT3A Arg882 mutation drives chronic myelomonocytic leukemia through disturbing gene expression/DNA methylation in hematopoietic cells. Proc Natl Acad Sci U S A. 2014;111:2620–5.
38. Challen GA, Sun D, Jeong M, Luo M, Jelinek J, Berg JS, et al. Dnmt3a is essential for hematopoietic stem cell differentiation. Nat Genet. 2011;44:23–31.
39. Yang L, Rodriguez B, Mayle A, Park HJ, Lin X, Luo M, et al. DNMT3A Loss Drives Enhancer Hypomethylation in FLT3-ITD-Associated Leukemias. Cancer Cell. 2016;29:922–34.
40. Mayle A, Yang L, Rodriguez B, Zhou T, Chang E, Curry CV, et al. Dnmt3a loss predisposes murine hematopoietic stem cells to malignant transformation. Blood. 2015;125:629–38.
41. Chang YI, You X, Kong G, Ranheim EA, Wang J, Du J, et al. Loss of Dnmt3a and endogenous Kras(G12D/+) cooperate to regulate hematopoietic stem and progenitor cell functions in leukemogenesis. Leukemia. 2015;29:1847–56.
42. Meyer SE, Qin T, Muench DE, Masuda K, Venkatasubramanian M, Orr E, et al. DNMT3A Haploinsufficiency Transforms FLT3ITD Myeloproliferative Disease into a Rapid, Spontaneous, and Fully Penetrant Acute Myeloid Leukemia. Cancer Discov. 2016;6:501–15.
43. Celik H, Mallaney C, Kothari A, Ostrander EL, Eultgen E, Martens A, et al. Enforced differentiation of Dnmt3a-null bone marrow leads to failure with c-Kit mutations driving leukemic transformation. Blood. 2015;125:619–28.
44. Haney SL, Upchurch GM, Opavska J, Klinkebiel D, Hlady RA, Roy S, et al. Dnmt3a Is a Haploinsufficient Tumor Suppressor in CD8+ Peripheral T Cell Lymphoma. PLoS Genet. 2016;12:e1006334.
45. Gao Q, Steine EJ, Barrasa MI, Hockemeyer D, Pawlak M, Fu D, et al. Deletion of the de novo DNA methyltransferase Dnmt3a promotes lung tumor progression. Proc Natl Acad Sci U S A. 2011;108:18061–6.
46. Zheng Y, Zhang H, Wang Y, Li X, Lu P, Dong F, et al. Loss of Dnmt3b accelerates MLL-AF9 leukemia progression. Leukemia. 2016;30:2373–84.
47. Peters SL, Hlady RA, Opavska J, Klinkebiel D, Novakova S, Smith LM, et al. Essential role for Dnmt1 in the prevention and maintenance of MYC-induced T-cell lymphomas. Mol Cell Biol. 2013;33:4321–33.
48. Esteller M. Cancer epigenomics: DNA methylomes and histone-modification maps. Nat Rev Genet. 2007;8:286–98.
49. Cedar H, Bergman Y. Linking DNA methylation and histone modification: patterns and paradigms. Nat Rev Genet. 2009;10:295–304.
50. Du J, Johnson LM, Jacobsen SE, Patel DJ. DNA methylation pathways and their crosstalk with histone methylation. Nat Rev Mol Cell Biol. 2015;16:519–32.
51. Gaudet F, Hodgson JG, Eden A, Jackson-Grusby L, Dausman J, Gray JW, et al. Induction of tumors in mice by genomic hypomethylation. Science. 2003;300:489–92.
52. Celik H, Kramer A, Challen GA. DNA methylation in normal and malignant hematopoiesis. Int J Hematol. 2016;103:617–26.

53. Jeong M, Sun D, Luo M, Huang Y, Challen GA, Rodriguez B, et al. Large conserved domains of low DNA methylation maintained by Dnmt3a. Nat Genet. 2014;46:17–23.

54. Cancer Genome Atlas Research N. Genomic and epigenomic landscapes of adult de novo acute myeloid leukemia. N Engl J Med. 2013;368:2059–74.

55. Yang X, Han H, De Carvalho DD, Lay FD, Jones PA, Liang G. Gene body methylation can alter gene expression and is a therapeutic target in cancer. Cancer Cell. 2014;26:577–90.

56. Espada J, Ballestar E, Fraga MF, Villar-Garea A, Juarranz A, Stockert JC, et al. Human DNA methyltransferase 1 is required for maintenance of the histone H3 modification pattern. J Biol Chem. 2004;279:37175–84.

57. Dhayalan A, Rajavelu A, Rathert P, Tamas R, Jurkowska RZ, Ragozin S, et al. The Dnmt3a PWWP domain reads histone 3 lysine 36 trimethylation and guides DNA methylation. J Biol Chem. 2010;285:26114–20.

58. Baubec T, Colombo DF, Wirbelauer C, Schmidt J, Burger L, Krebs AR, et al. Genomic profiling of DNA methyltransferases reveals a role for DNMT3B in genic methylation. Nature. 2015;520:243–7.

59. Guo X, Wang L, Li J, Ding Z, Xiao J, Yin X, et al. Structural insight into autoinhibition and histone H3-induced activation of DNMT3A. Nature. 2015;517:640–4.

60. Jin B, Ernst J, Tiedemann RL, Xu H, Sureshchandra S, Kellis M, et al. Linking DNA methyltransferases to epigenetic marks and nucleosome structure genome-wide in human tumor cells. Cell Rep. 2012;2:1411–24.

61. Vire E, Brenner C, Deplus R, Blanchon L, Fraga M, Didelot C, et al. The Polycomb group protein EZH2 directly controls DNA methylation. Nature. 2006;439:871–4.

62. Schlesinger Y, Straussman R, Keshet I, Farkash S, Hecht M, Zimmerman J, et al. Polycomb-mediated methylation on Lys27 of histone H3 pre-marks genes for de novo methylation in cancer. Nat Genet. 2007;39:232–6.

63. Shih AH, Abdel-Wahab O, Patel JP, Levine RL. The role of mutations in epigenetic regulators in myeloid malignancies. Nat Rev Cancer. 2012;12:599–612.

64. Welch JS, Ley TJ, Link DC, Miller CA, Larson DE, Koboldt DC, et al. The origin and evolution of mutations in acute myeloid leukemia. Cell. 2012;150:264–78.

65. Yang L, Rau R, Goodell MA. DNMT3A in haematological malignancies. Nat Rev Cancer. 2015;15:152–65.

66. Jia D, Jurkowska RZ, Zhang X, Jeltsch A, Cheng X. Structure of Dnmt3a bound to Dnmt3L suggests a model for de novo DNA methylation. Nature. 2007;449:248–51.

67. Matsui T, Leung D, Miyashita H, Maksakova IA, Miyachi H, Kimura H, et al. Proviral silencing in embryonic stem cells requires the histone methyltransferase ESET. Nature. 2010;464:927–31.

68. Shlush LI, Zandi S, Mitchell A, Chen WC, Brandwein JM, Gupta V, et al. Identification of pre-leukaemic haematopoietic stem cells in acute leukaemia. Nature. 2014;506:328–33.

69. Kim SJ, Zhao H, Hardikar S, Singh AK, Goodell MA, Chen T. A DNMT3A mutation common in AML exhibits dominant-negative effects in murine ES cells. Blood. 2013;122:4086–9.

70. Russler-Germain DA, Spencer DH, Young MA, Lamprecht TL, Miller CA, Fulton R, et al. The R882H DNMT3A mutation associated with AML dominantly inhibits wild-type DNMT3A by blocking its ability to form active tetramers. Cancer Cell. 2014;25:442–54.

71. Koya J, Kataoka K, Sato T, Bando M, Kato Y, Tsuruta-Kishino T, et al. DNMT3A R882 mutants interact with polycomb proteins to block haematopoietic stem and leukaemic cell differentiation. Nat Commun. 2016;7:10924.

72. Lu R, Wang P, Parton T, Zhou Y, Chrysovergis K, Rockowitz S, et al. Epigenetic Perturbations by Arg882-Mutated DNMT3A Potentiate Aberrant Stem Cell Gene-Expression Program and Acute Leukemia Development. Cancer Cell. 2016;30:92–107.

73. Xu J, Zhang W, Yan XJ, Lin XQ, Li W, Mi JQ, et al. DNMT3A mutation leads to leukemic extramedullary infiltration mediated by TWIST1. J Hematol Oncol. 2016;9:106.

74. Mizuno S, Chijiwa T, Okamura T, Akashi K, Fukumaki Y, Niho Y, et al. Expression of DNA methyltransferases DNMT1, 3A, and 3B in normal hematopoiesis and in acute and chronic myelogenous leukemia. Blood. 2001;97:1172–9.

75. Vasanthakumar A, Lepore JB, Zegarek MH, Kocherginsky M, Singh M, Davis EM, et al. Dnmt3b is a haploinsufficient tumor suppressor gene in Myc-induced lymphomagenesis. Blood. 2013;121:2059–63.

76. Pathania R, Ramachandran S, Elangovan S, Padia R, Yang P, Cinghu S, et al. DNMT1 is essential for mammary and cancer stem cell maintenance and tumorigenesis. Nat Commun. 2015;6:6910.

77. Agoston AT, Argani P, Yegnasubramanian S, De Marzo AM, Ansari-Lari MA, Hicks JL, et al. Increased protein stability causes DNA methyltransferase 1 dysregulation in breast cancer. J Biol Chem. 2005;280:18302–10.

78. Deng T, Kuang Y, Wang L, Li J, Wang Z, Fei J. An essential role for DNA methyltransferase 3a in melanoma tumorigenesis. Biochem Biophys Res Commun. 2009;387:611–6.

5

Metastatic biomarkers in synovial sarcoma

Rosalia de Necochea-Campion[1], Lee M. Zuckerman[2], Hamid R. Mirshahidi[3], Shahrzad Khosrowpour[4], Chien-Shing Chen[1,3] and Saied Mirshahidi[1*]

Abstract

Synovial sarcoma (SS) is an aggressive soft tissue sarcoma (STS) that typically occurs in the extremities near a joint. Metastatic disease is common and usually occurs in the lungs and lymph nodes. Surgical management is the mainstay of treatment with chemotherapy and radiation typically used as adjuvant treatment. Although chemotherapy has a positive impact on survival, the prognosis is poor if metastatic disease occurs. The biology of sarcoma invasion and metastasis remain poorly understood. Chromosomal translocation with fusion of the SYT and SSX genes has been described and is currently used as a diagnostic marker, although the full impact of the fusion is unknown. Multiple biomarkers have been found to be associated with SS and are currently under investigation regarding their pathways and mechanisms of action. Further research is needed in order to develop better diagnostic screening tools and understanding of tumor behavior. Development of targeted therapies that reduce metastatic events in SS, would dramatically improve patient prognosis.

Keywords: SYT-SSX, CDCA2, KIF14, IGFBP7, Secernin-1, E2H2, MMPs, NY-ESO-1, CXCR4

Background

Synovial sarcoma (SS) is the fourth most common type of soft tissue sarcoma (STS) and accounts for 5–10% of all soft tissue sarcomas [1]. SS was originally described by Simon in 1865, and given the name "synovial sarcoma" by Sabrazes et al. in 1934 based on a similar appearance to developing synovial tissue under light microscopy [2]. SS has a tendency to arise in the soft tissue surrounding larger joints, but it does not have a synovial cell origin [3]. While the exact cellular origin is an ongoing topic of investigation, it is likely to arise from undifferentiated mesenchymal stem cells [4]. Compared with other soft tissue sarcomas, SS occurs predominantly in younger adults with a median age of diagnosis of 35 years [5]. The most common tumor location is in the extremities, where approximately 70% of these tumors develop [6], and these patients have significantly better long term survival outcomes than those with non-extremity involvement [7]. In patients with localized disease, 10 year survival outcomes vary from 8 to 88% depending on tumor size and location [8]. Standard treatment for synovial sarcoma is tumor resection

frequently accompanied by radiotherapy and/or chemotherapy, although some data suggests that therapies in addition to surgery substantially increase long-term metastatic risks [7].

Metastasis negatively impacts patient prognosis and significantly reduces survival outcomes [9]. For patients who present with or develop metastatic tumors median survival outcomes vary from 7 to 37 months depending on lymph node involvement and metastatic location [10]. SS can evolve slowly and there is a high incidence of late metastasis which occurs in about 50% of all cases [7]. Most metastatic tumors develop in the lungs (80%), although bone (9.9%) and liver (4.5%) are the next most frequent locations [9]. Synovial sarcoma can metastasize through the lymph nodes with clinically detectable disease found in 15–20% of newly diagnosed patients [11]. Histologically, synovial sarcoma is classified into four subtypes consisting of a biphasic (BPSS), monophasic fibrous or monophasic epithelial (MPSS), and poorly differentiated (PDSS, round cell) tumor cells [1]. While these histological subtypes do not seem to be associated with metastatic events [7, 12], they have been linked to survival. A study of 3756 SS patients registered in the National Cancer Data Base from 1998 to 2010 showed a significant difference in average 5-year

---

* Correspondence: smirshahidi@llu.edu

[1]Biospecimen Laboratory, Loma Linda University Cancer Center, Loma Linda University School of Medicine, 11175 Campus Street, Chan Shun Pavilion 11017, Loma Linda, CA 92354, USA

Full list of author information is available at the end of the article

survival numbers among patients with biphasic (65%), monophasic (56%) and undifferentiated (52%) tumors [13].

While many factors that influence synovial sarcoma patient outcome have been identified, tumor behavior remains highly unpredictable [14]. An extremely high level of metastasis means that further studies are needed to characterize the mechanisms that influence tumor action. Ultimately, the identification of highly relevant molecular biomarkers associated with metastatic outcomes and patient prognosis establishes the foundation for development of better therapeutic strategies to target these oncogenic factors. Several metastatic biomarkers that have been described to date are described in the following sections and summarized in Fig. 1.

Significance of the syt-ssx fusion gene

The chromosomal translocation t(X;18)(p11.2;q11.2) fuses the SS18 (SYT) gene to the SSX gene (predominantly SSX1 or SSX2) and is regarded as a founding event in the oncogenic development of synovial sarcoma [15]. Yet, the exact transformative event of the chimeric SYT-SSX gene product has not been fully elucidated. It has

been shown that SYT-SSX can interfere with assembly of BAF (BRG-/BRM-associated factor) complexes affecting the integration of a tumor suppressor component and consequent SRY (sex-determining region Y)-box 2 (SOX2) activation which stimulates cell proliferation [16]. Over 95% of SS can be characterized by expression of the SYT-SSX gene and it is used as a routine diagnostic marker for this type of cancer [15]. Although both SYT and SSX proteins contain transcriptional regulation domains, they lack any DNA binding regions, so their regulatory effects are surmised to occur through interactions with other proteins [17]. Accordingly, the SYT-SSX fusion oncogene has been shown to interact with several major epigenetic regulators as well as other DNA binding proteins and exert both direct and indirect effects on transcript regulation [17, 18]. Of note, SYT-SSX has been shown to act as a scaffold linking two master transcription regulators TLE1 (transducin like enhancer of split 1) and ATF2 (activating transcription factor 2) such that TLE1 acts as a repressor of ATF2 target genes regulating cell cycle, apoptosis, and more, demonstrating that the SYT-SSX/TLE1/ATF2 complex is important not only to oncogenic transformation but also tumor cell survival

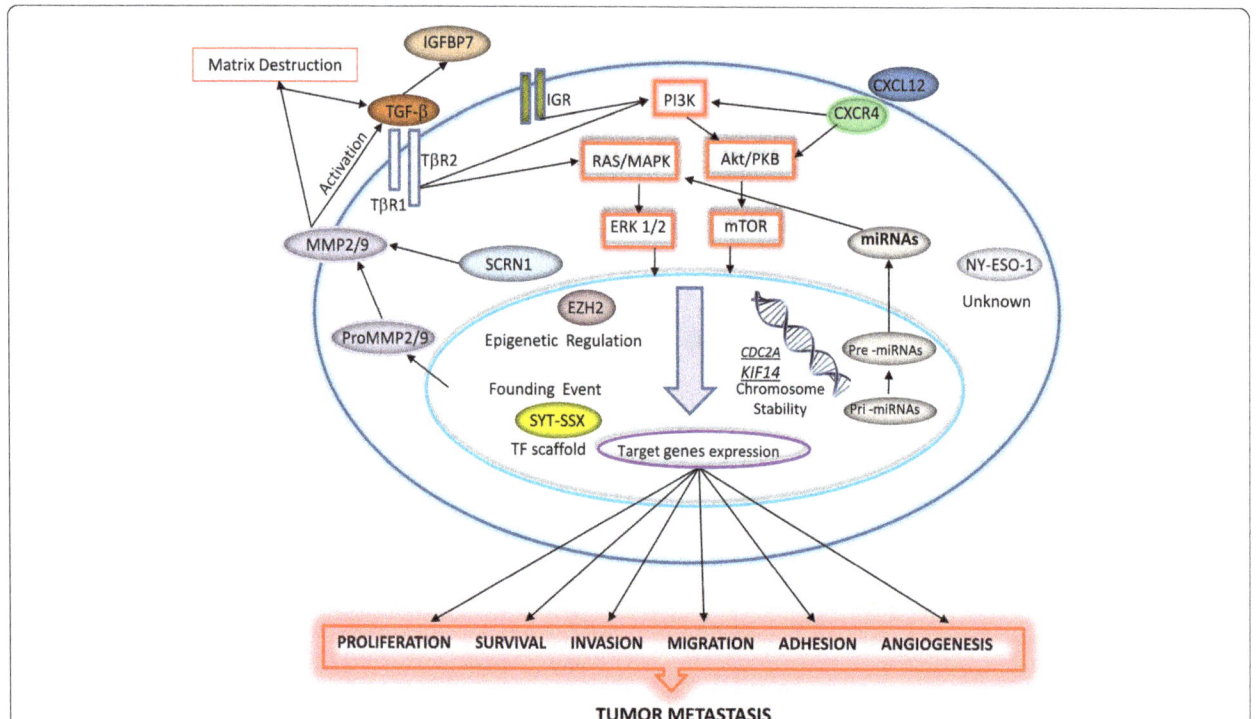

Fig. 1 Schematic diagram summarizing functional relevance of metastatic signals in synovial sarcoma. SYT-SSX fusion is a founding event in the development of this cancer which frequently results in the production of molecular signals that promote tumor metastasis. Abbreviations: Akt (Serine/threonine kinase); CDCA2 (Cell division cycle A2); CXCR (Chemokine receptor); ERK1/2 (Extracellular signal-regulated kinase 1/2); EZH2 (Enhancer of zeste homologue 2); IGFBP7 (Insulin-like growth factor-binding protein-7); IGR (Insulin like growth factor receptor); KIF14 (Kinesin family member 14); MAPK (Mitogen-activated protein kinases); MicroRNAs (miRNAs); MMPs (Matrix metalloproteinases); mTOR (Mammalian target of rapamycin); NY-ESO-1 (New York esophageal squamous cell carcinoma 1); PI3K (Phosphatidylinositol-3-kinase); pri-miRNA (primary microRNA); pre-miRNA (precursor microRNA); PKB (Protein kinase B); RAS (Ras GTPase); SCRN1 (Secernin-1); TGF-β (Transforming growth factor beta); TβR (TGF-beta receptor); TF (transcription factor)

[19]. TLE has emerged as a useful diagnostic marker of SS with robust expression detected in approximately 95% of these tumors however a low level of positive staining in non-SS tumors indicates that this antibody should only be used in a panel with other antibodies to confirm diagnosis [20]. Recently, a highly specific assay to detect the association of SYT-SSX and TLE in either localized or metastatic SS tumors was developed and shown to be useful in drug discovery assays seeking to disrupt this interaction [21].

A number of studies have investigated the association between SYT-SSX gene fusion type and metastatic risk. Some have reported that the SYT-SSX1 fusion approximately doubles the risk of metastatic tumor development compared with SYT-SSX2 [22, 23]. Intriguingly, a similar pattern was evident in a survival study demonstrating a median survival of 6.1 years for SS patients with an SYT-SSX1 fusion gene compared with 13.7 years for those with SYT-SSX2 [24]. In contrast, several other studies report no significant associations between SYT-SSX fusion type and metastasis or survival [7, 25]. These conflicting data appear to suggest that the influence of unspecified additional factors have a much larger role in determining metastatic outcomes. These clinicopathological characteristics must be better defined to understand in which context SYT-SSX has an important versus an inconsequential role.

Circulating biomarkers

Development of a diagnostic blood test to detect SS and assess metastatic risk would be a valuable tool for the management of this disease. A whole blood microRNA signature shows that SS patients demonstrate significant upregulation of seven microRNAs (miR-99a-5p, miR-146b-5p, miR-148b-3p, miR-195-5p, miR-223-3p, miR-500b-3p and miR-505-3p) compared with patients in remission and healthy controls [26]. Furthermore, expression levels of these seven microRNAs are significantly reduced by 5–50 fold increments after local tumor resection, but once again dramatically upregulated if a patient develops recurrent local or metastatic disease [26]. Thus, since a clearly defined microRNA expression panel can be used to distinguish SS from other malignancies as well as characterize metastatic and recurrent tumor status, this method could be useful in therapeutic monitoring of patients [26]. miRNAs have a critical role in activation of the Ras GTPase/Mitogen-activated protein kinases (Ras/MAPK) pathway necessary for tumor development [27], and miRNA suppression significantly inhibits SS cell proliferation in vitro [28].

Detection of a circulating SYT-SSX fusion gene product could be another important method for assessing metastatic risk in patients with SS. In culture, it has been shown that SS cells produce microvesicles containing the SYT-SSX fusion gene, yet this research group was unable to detect the biomarker in microvesicles or PBMCs (peripheral blood mononuclear cell) obtained from patient blood samples regardless of their metastatic status [29]. In contrast, the SYT-SSX gene was detected in peripheral blood in a case study of a single SS patient who developed multiple lung metastasis 2 months after local tumor resection from the thigh [30]. The presence of circulating tumor cells (CTC) could be indicative of a patient's metastatic risk given their potential to extravasate and form tumors in new locations [31], and CTC abundance may account for discrepancies in SYT-SSX detection abilities. CTCs can be readily isolated from patient blood by size exclusion, and CTC quantities vary considerably among different SS patients [32].

Cinsarc signature genes

Gene expression profiling of soft tissue sarcomas revealed a prognostic panel of 67 genes (CINSARC, complexity index in sarcomas) with functional roles in mitosis and chromosome management that are also highly predictive of metastatic risk [33]. While many CINSARC genes have been identified as molecular markers associated with metastasis in other types of cancers, they are usually ascribed a proliferative function, although they may actually have a greater role in chromosome instability [33]. When the CINSARC classification criteria were used to stratify SS tumor specimens into two prognostic groups, a highly significant difference was observed in metastatic outcomes among these patients [34]. However, since the CINSARC profile emerged from an analysis of multiple types of soft tissue sarcomas, these authors sought to determine if a better metastatic prognostic profile could be developed for SS [34]. Comparison of whole genome expression in 51 metastatic and 49 non-metastatic SS tumors revealed significant upregulation of 59 genes in metastatic specimens, 24% of which were common to the CINSARC classification panel [34]. Importantly, singular expression of the 2 most differentially regulated genes, CDCA2 (cell division cycle A2) and KIF14 (kinesin family member 14), could better predict metastatic outcomes than the overall CINSARC score in this patient cohort [34]. Functionally, both of these genes code for proteins that help to maintain chromosome integrity and are essential for the completion of cytokinesis. KIF14 is localizes to the central spindle during late phase mitosis and its inhibition in tumor cells results in cell cycle arrest and the formation of binucleated cells [35]. KIF14 was also found to regulate adhesive components on the tumor cell surface influencing migratory and invasive properties that promote cell motility during metastasis [36]. CDCA2 has critical catalytic and structural functions during late mitosis that help coordinate chromosome segregation and nuclear envelope reformation after division of nuclear contents [37].

IGFBP7

Insulin-like growth factor-binding protein-7 (IGFBP7,) also termed IGFBP-related protein-1 (IGFBP-rP1), is a secreted 31-kDa protein belonging to the IGFBP family [38]. In various cancer types including hepatocellular carcinoma [39], breast [40], brain [41], and colon [42], IGFBP7 can function as a tumor suppressor and have the ability to suppress proliferation, adhesion, angiogenesis, survival, or induce apoptosis and senescence [43–45]. Yet the role of this protein in tumor behavior is complex, as it undergoes extensive proteolytic processing that reverses its cellular function and influence over cell proliferation and adhesion activities [46]. In the tumor stroma microenvironment, IGFBP7 expression is closely related with the transforming growth factor beta (TGF-β secretion [47], which is a potent factor promoting tumor cell invasiveness and metastasis [48, 49]. TGF-β upregulates expression of IGFBP7 and angiogenic capacity of tumor cells [50]. Recently, it was shown that IGFBP7 expression in SS was higher that other types of STSs and significantly associated with metastatic events [51]. In addition, nuclear expression of another IGFBP family protein, insulin like growth factor 1 receptor (IGF1R),, was significantly related to poor survival in SS patients who did not receive adjuvant chemotherapy [52]. In sarcoma, IGF1R activation is known to activate the phosphatidylinositol-3-kinase/serine/threonine kinase Akt/Mammalian target of rapamycin (PI3K/Akt/ mTOR) pathway which promotes cancer progression and metastasis [53]. These studies, highlight the potential for proteins from the IGF family to be used as prognostic biomarkers to help guide treatment decisions in SS.

MMPs

The matrix metalloproteinases (MMPs), a family of zinc and calcium dependent proteolytic enzymes, are involved in the degradation extracellular matrix (ECM) components and play key roles in tumor cell invasion and metastasis [54]. Notably, the proteolytic activity of MMPs can help release inactive TGFB in the extracellular space so that it can bind to its receptors and activate downstream pathways such as PI3k/Akt and MAPK which are critical to the epithelial mesenchymal transition (EMT) process underlying metastasis [55]. Benassi et al. demonstrated that high levels of MMP2 and MMP9 in biopsied tissue from patients with SS, was significantly associated with metastasis ($P = 0.008$ and $P = 0.005$, respectively) [56]. In addition, lack of expression the tissue inhibitors of metalloproteinases (TIMP) was found to be a poor prognostic factor for disease-free

survival in synovial sarcoma ($P = 0.009$) [56]. The proteolytic activity of MMPs and their activation process can be inhibited by the TIMPs [57]. The presence of TIMPs can suppress metastasis by preserving ECM integrity [58]. It has been shown that a decrease in TIMP-1 correlated with a poor outcome in high-risk STS [59] and colorectal cancer patients [60]. Both MMPs and TIMPs can further be evaluated as biological markers for predicting progression, metastasis and prognosis of human SS.

Secernin-1

Secernin-1 (SCRN1), a 50-kDa cytosolic protein, is a member of the secernin gene family that regulates exocytosis in mast cells through a mechanism that has not been well defined [61]. Exocytosis is a process by which cells transport and release secretory products through the cytoplasm to the cell membrane and several studies have described that this promotes tumor growth, metastasis and invasion [62, 63]. In colon cancer, SCRN1 expression promoted exocytosis secretion of MMP2 and MMP, while silencing this gene reduced MMP2 secretion, inhibited cell proliferation and decreased invasion capability [63]. The poor prognostic significance of SCRN1 expression in colon cancer [63, 64], is contrary to that reported in synovial sarcoma [65]. A proteomics analysis of tumor specimens collected from 13 SS patients, identified SCRN1 as positive prognostic factor with significantly higher expression among patients who were alive and disease free for at least 5 years [65]. Further analysis of SCRN1 expression in 45 SS tumor specimens revealed a 5-year survival rate was 77.6 and 21.8% for patients with secernin-1 positive and negative primary tumors, respectively ($p = 0.0015$), and significantly associated with metastatic outcomes [65]. Metastasis-free survival was significantly higher (62.8% vs. 16.7%) in the SS patient group with SCRN1 positive tumors compared to that with SCRN1 negative tumors ($p = 0.0012$) [65].

EZH2

Enhancer of zeste homologue 2 (EZH2) is a member of the polycomb group (PcG) protein family, which is composed of epigenetic transcriptional regulators that participate in cell cycle regulation, DNA damage repair, cell differentiation, senescence, and apoptosis [66]. In cancer, EZH2 expression is associated with a worse prognosis and required for promotion of metastasis [67]. In SS, overexpression of EZH2 helps to distinguish PDSS, which is defined by high cellularity, high nuclear grade, high mitotic activity and an agresssive clinical course that tends to include early recurrence and metastasis, from the MPSS and BPSS histological subtypes [68]. EZH2 overexpression in SS is correlated with high

H3K27 trimethylation, which facilitates chromatin compaction and gene silencing [68]. Importantly, high expression of EZH2 is predictive of developing distant metastasis even in the better-differentiated MPSS and BPSS subtypes [68]. In a recent preclinical study, the anti-tumor effect of EZH2 inhibition was evidenced in human SS models in vitro, as well as xenograft and patient-derived xenograft (PDX) models in vivo [69]. Moreover, Ramagila et al. found high EZH2 expression to be correlated with metastatic disease in pediatric soft tissue sarcomas [70]. Low expression of EZH2 restricts cell proliferation and induces cell cycle arrest at the G2 phase, whereas the overexpression of EZH2 can shorten the G1 phase of the cell cycle and lead to cell accumulation in the S phase [71, 72]. Moore et al. showed that EZH2 knockdown is sufficient to reduce distant metastasis in vivo [73]. EZH2-specific inhibition is an active area of researcher, with several human phase 1 and 2 trials now underway, such as an ongoing phase II, multicenter study of the EZH2 inhibitor tazemetostat in adult subjects with INI1-negative tumors or relapsed/refractory SS (https://clinicaltrials.gov/ct2/show/NCT02601950).

NY-ESO-1

New York esophageal squamous cell carcinoma 1 (NY-ESO-1), encoded by the *CTAG1B* gene, is a 22 kD hydrophobic protein cancer-testis antigen [74]. NY-ESO-1 is expressed in many cancers, associated with poor prognosis, and elevated metastatic risk [75]. The function of NY-ESO-1 is still unknown, but is of particular interest to researchers because it is highly immunogenic eliciting both cellular and humoral responses, and a large number of major histocompatibility complex (MHC) class I- and class II-restricted NY-ESO-1 epitopes have been identified [76]. Furthermore, NY-ESO-1 protein expression is significantly higher in metastatic versus primary tumors [75, 77, 78]. NY-ESO-1 is an attractive target for SS treatment because chemotherapy has a limited durable efficacy in relapsed or metastatic SS demonstrating the need for novel more effective therapies. NY-ESO-1 is expressed in approximately 80% of patients with SS which could be useful for distinguishing this cancer from other types of mesenchymal tumors, and identifying patients who would benefit from NY-ESO-1 targeted therapies [79]. In a clinical trial using genetically engineered T cells reactive with NY-ESO-1 in patients with metastatic synovial cell sarcoma, tumor regression was achieved in 67% of the patients [80]. Several clinical trials employing NY-ESO-1 are currently under way in patients with SS (https://clinicaltrials.gov/ct2/show/NCT01343043, NCT02609984).

CXCR4

Chemokine receptor 4 (CXCR4), is a 352-amino acid seven-transmembrane G protein-coupled cell surface receptor with an important role in homing of hematopoietic stem cells and lymphocyte trafficking that has been found to promote cell migration, invasion and angiogenesis [52, 81]. The CXCR4 pathway has been shown to be associated with tumor progression and poor prognosis in many types of cancer including breast [82], lung [83], colon [84], melanoma [85] and soft tissue sarcomas [86]. CXCR4 promotes metastasis by activating activating extracellular signal-regulated kinase 1/2 (ERK1/2), Akt/PKB and Nuclear factor-κB (NF-κB), which increases the adhesion and invasive ability of cancer cells in part by the activity of MMP2 and MMP9 [87–89]. CXCR4 has a pivotal role in the migration of cancer cells between the primary and the metastatic site in synovial sarcoma [52, 90]. Tumor cells expressing CXCR4 that detach from the primary tumor and enter the circulatory system can migrate toward organs that express its ligand CXCL12 [91]. Lung, lymph node, bone marrow, and liver, the most frequent metastatic locations in SS [9], all express very high levels of CXCL12 [92]. A study of SS patients found that 5-year overall survival (OS) rates were 47% for those with positive CXCR4 staining, and 86% ($P = 0.0003$) for those with negative CXCR4 staining [52]. A second study, reported that 5 year survival outcomes for SS patients with positive CXCR4 staining was less than 30% [4]. Importantly, it was found that SS cultures contain a subpopulation of cells expressing high levels of CXCR4 that also express high levels stem cell markers (NANOG, OCT4, SOX2), and these cells have an increased tumor initiating capacity in xenographic mouse models [4]. Although no group has directly measured the metastatic risk of CXCRX4 expression in SS, perhaps due to limited patient numbers, expression of this marker appears to be a key factor both for cell migration and tumor propagation at a distal site. Perhaps the use of CXCR4 antagonists, many of which are already in various stages of clinical development [93], and shown to significantly reduce lung metastasis in mouse models of osteosarcoma [94], would be a beneficial treatment option for patients with metastatic SS, particularly in cases where tumors are unresectable.

Conclusions

SS is a rare, aggressive subtype of soft tissue sarcoma. It has a predilection for metastases to multiple organs, including the lungs, lymph nodes, and bone. The ability of this tumor to metastasize to multiple organs demonstrates that the tumor can interact and invade multiple environments. The overall prognosis is poor given the high rate of metastatic disease and lack of effective therapeutic agents. Nearly all mortality in patients with SS is caused by metastatic disease, yet the biological cause of these events has not been well characterized.

The full transformation that occurs with the X;18 chromosomal translocation has not been completely elucidated at this time. Several oncogenic biomarkers have been found to be elevated in SS. As summarized in Fig. 1, many of these biomarkers may be used to evaluate for recurrence and metastatic disease and also help determine prognosis. The lack of the full understanding of how the translocation and elevated biomarkers interact with the host is a significant limitation in our ability to effectively treat SS. Further research should be done to help develop a greater understanding of these interactions and the downstream effects that occur in SS, with an emphasis on preventing metastatic disease. This will not only enable patients to be monitored for progression of disease and allow for counseling regarding prognosis, but also be used to develop better treatments for this subtype of soft tissue sarcoma.

Abbreviations

Akt: Serine/threonine kinase; ATF2: Activating transcription factor 2; BAF: BRG-/BRM-associated factor; BPSS: Biphasic synovial sarcoma; CDCA2: Cell division cycle A2; CTC: Circulating tumor cells; C-X-C motif: Chemokine; CXCL12: ligand 12; CXCR4: Chemokine receptor 4; ECM: extracellular matrix; EMT: Epithelial mesenchymal transition; ERK1/2: extracellular signal-regulated kinase 1/2; EZH2: Enhancer of zeste homologue 2; IGF1R: Insulin like growth factor 1 receptor; IGFBP7: Insulin-like growth factor-binding protein-7; IGFBP-rP1: IGFBP-related protein-1; KIF14: Kinesin family member 14; MAPK: Mitogen-activated protein kinases; MMPs: Matrix metalloproteinases; MPSS: Monophasic synovial sarcoma; mTOR: Mammalian target of rapamycin; NF-κB: Nuclear factor-κB; NY-ESO-1: New York esophageal squamous cell carcinoma 1; PBMCs: Peripheral blood mononuclear cell; PcG: Polycomb group; PDSS: Poorly differentiated synovial sarcoma; PDX: Patient-derived xenograft; PI3K: Phosphatidylinositol-3-kinase; PKB: Protein kinase B; RAS: Ras GTPase; SCRN1: Secernin-1; SOX2: SRY (sex-determining region Y)-box 2; SS: Synovial sarcoma; STS: Soft tissue sarcoma; TGF-β: Transforming growth factor beta; TIMP: Tissue inhibitors of metalloproteinases; TLE1: Transducin like enhancer of split 1

Acknowledgements

We would like to thank Loma Linda University School of Medicine Dean's Office & Department of Orthopedic Surgery for the Grants to Promote Collaborative and Translational Research (GCAT 2016, #681163) for supporting synovial sarcoma research and providing professional materials relevant to this review topic.

Funding

All costs associated with the study design, collection, analysis, interpretation of data, and writing the manuscript were funded by the Loma Linda University Cancer Center.

Authors' contributions

RN prepared the manuscript draft, LZ contributed information and important written content, SK critically reviewed the literature, HRM and CSC provided important material and suggestions, SM designed the study, prepared the figure, and revised the manuscript. All authors read and approved the final manuscript draft.

Competing interests

The authors declare that they have no competing interests.

Author details

[1]Biospecimen Laboratory, Loma Linda University Cancer Center, Loma Linda University School of Medicine, 11175 Campus Street, Chan Shun Pavilion 11017, Loma Linda, CA 92354, USA. [2]Department of Orthopaedic Surgery, Loma Linda University Medical Center, 11406 Loma Linda Drive, Suite 218, Loma Linda, CA 92354, USA. [3]Division of Hematology/Oncology, Loma Linda University School of Medicine, 11175 Campus Street, Chan Shun Pavilion 11015, Loma Linda, CA 92354, USA. [4]Chapman University, One University Drive, Orange, CA 92866, USA.

References

1. Rajwanshi A, Srinivas R, Upasana G. Malignant small round cell tumors. J Cytol. 2009;26(1):1–10.
2. Rong R, et al. Metastatic poorly differentiated monophasic synovial sarcoma to lung with unknown primary: a molecular genetic analysis. Int J Clin Exp Pathol. 2009;3(2):217–21.
3. Thway K, Fisher C. Synovial sarcoma: defining features and diagnostic evolution. Ann Diagn Pathol. 2014;18(6):369–80.
4. Kimura T, et al. Identification and analysis of CXCR4-positive synovial sarcoma-initiating cells. Oncogene. 2016;35(30):3932–43.
5. Eilber FC, Dry SM. Diagnosis and management of synovial sarcoma. J Surg Oncol. 2008;97(4):314–20.
6. Sultan I, et al. Comparing children and adults with synovial sarcoma in the Surveillance, Epidemiology, and End Results program, 1983 to 2005: an analysis of 1268 patients. Cancer. 2009;115(15):3537–47.
7. Krieg AH, et al. Synovial sarcomas usually metastasize after >5 years: a multicenter retrospective analysis with minimum follow-up of 10 years for survivors. Ann Oncol. 2011;22(2):458–67.
8. Deshmukh R, Mankin HJ, Singer S. Synovial sarcoma: the importance of size and location for survival. Clin Orthop Relat Res. 2004;419:155–61.
9. Vlenterie M, et al. Outcome of chemotherapy in advanced synovial sarcoma patients: Review of 15 clinical trials from the European Organisation for Research and Treatment of Cancer Soft Tissue and Bone Sarcoma Group; setting a new landmark for studies in this entity. Eur J Cancer. 2016;58: 62–72.
10. Salah S, et al. Factors influencing survival in metastatic synovial sarcoma: importance of patterns of metastases and the first-line chemotherapy regimen. Med Oncol. 2013;30(3):639.
11. Amankwah EK, Conley AP, Reed DR. Epidemiology and therapies for metastatic sarcoma. Clin Epidemiol. 2013;5:147–62.
12. Spurrell EL, et al. Prognostic factors in advanced synovial sarcoma: an analysis of 104 patients treated at the Royal Marsden Hospital. Ann Oncol. 2005;16(3):437–44.
13. Corey RM, Swett K, Ward WG. Epidemiology and survivorship of soft tissue sarcomas in adults: a national cancer database report. Cancer Med. 2014; 3(5):1404–15.
14. Vlenterie M, Jones RL, van der Graaf WT. Synovial sarcoma diagnosis and management in the era of targeted therapies. Curr Opin Oncol. 2015;27(4): 316–22.
15. Kubo T, et al. Prognostic value of SS18-SSX fusion type in synovial sarcoma; systematic review and meta-analysis. Springerplus. 2015;4:375.
16. Kadoch C, Crabtree GR. Reversible disruption of mSWI/SNF (BAF) complexes by the SS18-SSX oncogenic fusion in synovial sarcoma. Cell. 2013;153(1): 71–85.
17. Przybyl J, et al. Downstream and intermediate interactions of synovial sarcoma-associated fusion oncoproteins and their implication for targeted therapy. Sarcoma. 2012;2012:249219.
18. Garcia CB, Shaffer CM, Eid JE. Genome-wide recruitment to Polycomb-modified chromatin and activity regulation of the synovial sarcoma oncogene SYT-SSX2. BMC Genomics. 2012;13:189.

19. Su L, et al. Deconstruction of the SS18-SSX fusion oncoprotein complex: insights into disease etiology and therapeutics. Cancer Cell. 2012;21(3): 333–47.

20. Rekhi B, et al. Immunohistochemical validation of TLE1, a novel marker, for synovial sarcomas. Indian J Med Res. 2012;136(5):766–75.

21. Laporte AN et al. Identification of cytotoxic agents disrupting synovial sarcoma oncoprotein interactions by proximity ligation assay. Oncotarget, 2016; 7(23):34384–94.

22. Panagopoulos I, et al. Clinical impact of molecular and cytogenetic findings in synovial sarcoma. Genes Chromosomes Cancer. 2001;31(4):362–72.

23. Sun Y, et al. Prognostic implication of SYT-SSX fusion type and clinicopathological parameters for tumor-related death, recurrence, and metastasis in synovial sarcoma. Cancer Sci. 2009;100(6):1018–25.

24. Ladanyi M, et al. Impact of SYT-SSX fusion type on the clinical behavior of synovial sarcoma: a multi-institutional retrospective study of 243 patients. Cancer Res. 2002;62(1):135–40.

25. Takenaka S, et al. Prognostic implication of SYT-SSX fusion type in synovial sarcoma: a multi-institutional retrospective analysis in Japan. Oncol Rep. 2008;19(2):467–76.

26. Fricke A, et al. Identification of a blood-borne miRNA signature of synovial sarcoma. Mol Cancer. 2015;14:151.

27. Masliah-Planchon J, Garinet S, Pasmant E. RAS-MAPK pathway epigenetic activation in cancer: miRNAs in action. Oncotarget. 2016;7(25):38892–907.

28. Hisaoka M, et al. Identification of altered MicroRNA expression patterns in synovial sarcoma. Genes Chromosomes Cancer. 2011;50(3):137–45.

29. Fricke A, et al. Synovial Sarcoma Microvesicles Harbor the SYT-SSX Fusion Gene Transcript: Comparison of Different Methods of Detection and Implications in Biomarker Research. Stem Cells Int. 2016;2016:6146047.

30. Hashimoto N, et al. Detection of SYT-SSX fusion gene in peripheral blood from a patient with synovial sarcoma. Am J Surg Pathol. 2001;25(3):406–10.

31. Chang L, et al. Circulating tumor cells in sarcomas: a brief review. Med Oncol. 2015;32(1):430.

32. Chinen LT, et al. Isolation, detection, and immunomorphological characterization of circulating tumor cells (CTCs) from patients with different types of sarcoma using isolation by size of tumor cells: a window on sarcoma-cell invasion. Onco Targets Ther. 2014;7:1609–17.

33. Chibon F, et al. Validated prediction of clinical outcome in sarcomas and multiple types of cancer on the basis of a gene expression signature related to genome complexity. Nat Med. 2010;16(7):781–7.

34. Lagarde P, et al. Chromosome instability accounts for reverse metastatic outcomes of pediatric and adult synovial sarcomas. J Clin Oncol. 2013;31(5): 608–15.

35. Gruneberg U, et al. KIF14 and citron kinase act together to promote efficient cytokinesis. J Cell Biol. 2006;172(3):363–72.

36. Ahmed SM, et al. KIF14 negatively regulates Rap1a-Radil signaling during breast cancer progression. J Cell Biol. 2012;199(6):951–67.

37. Vagnarelli P, et al. Repo-Man coordinates chromosomal reorganization with nuclear envelope reassembly during mitotic exit. Dev Cell. 2011;21(2):328–42.

38. Hwa V, Oh Y, Rosenfeld RG. The insulin-like growth factor-binding protein (IGFBP) superfamily. Endocr Rev. 1999;20(6):761–87.

39. Chen D, et al. Insulin-like growth factor-binding protein-7 functions as a potential tumor suppressor in hepatocellular carcinoma. Clin Cancer Res. 2011;17(21):6693–701.

40. Burger AM, et al. Essential roles of IGFBP-3 and IGFBP-rP1 in breast cancer. Eur J Cancer. 2005;41(11):1515–27.

41. Jiang W, et al. Insulin-like growth factor binding protein 7 mediates glioma cell growth and migration. Neoplasia. 2008;10(12):1335–42.

42. Shao L, et al. Detection of the differentially expressed gene IGF-binding protein-related protein-1 and analysis of its relationship to fasting glucose in Chinese colorectal cancer patients. Endocr Relat Cancer. 2004;11(1):141–8.

43. Gambaro K, et al. Low levels of IGFBP7 expression in high-grade serous ovarian carcinoma is associated with patient outcome. BMC Cancer. 2015;15:135.

44. Nousbeck J, et al. Insulin-like growth factor-binding protein 7 regulates keratinocyte proliferation, differentiation and apoptosis. J Invest Dermatol. 2010;130(2):378–87.

45. Wajapeyee N, et al. Oncogenic BRAF induces senescence and apoptosis through pathways mediated by the secreted protein IGFBP7. Cell. 2008; 132(3):363–74.

46. Ahmed S, et al. Proteolytic processing of IGFBP-related protein-1 (TAF/ angiomodulin/mac25) modulates its biological activity. Biochem Biophys Res Commun. 2003;310(2):612–8.

47. Rao C, et al. High expression of IGFBP7 in fibroblasts induced by colorectal cancer cells is co-regulated by TGF-beta and Wnt signaling in a Smad2/3-Dvl2/3-dependent manner. PLoS One. 2014;9(1):e85340.

48. Padua D, Massague J. Roles of TGFbeta in metastasis. Cell Res. 2009;19(1): 89–102.

49. Massague J. TGFbeta in Cancer. Cell. 2008;134(2):215–30.

50. Pen A, et al. Glioblastoma-secreted factors induce IGFBP7 and angiogenesis by modulating Smad-2-dependent TGF-beta signaling. Oncogene. 2008; 27(54):6834–44.

51. Benassi MS, et al. Tissue and serum IGFBP7 protein as biomarker in high-grade soft tissue sarcoma. Am J Cancer Res. 2015;5(11):3446–54.

52. Palmerini E, et al. Prognostic and predictive role of CXCR4, IGF-1R and Ezrin expression in localized synovial sarcoma: is chemotaxis important to tumor response? Orphanet J Rare Dis. 2015;10:6.

53. Wan X, Helman LJ. The biology behind mTOR inhibition in sarcoma. Oncologist. 2007;12(8):1007–18.

54. Roomi MW, et al. Modulation of u-PA, MMPs and their inhibitors by a novel nutrient mixture in adult human sarcoma cell lines. Int J Oncol. 2013;43(1): 39–49.

55. Willis BC, Borok Z. TGF-beta-induced EMT: mechanisms and implications for fibrotic lung disease. Am J Physiol Lung Cell Mol Physiol. 2007;293(3):L525–34.

56. Benassi MS, et al. Metalloproteinase expression and prognosis in soft tissue sarcomas. Ann Oncol. 2001;12(1):75–80.

57. Hidalgo M, Eckhardt SG. Development of matrix metalloproteinase inhibitors in cancer therapy. J Natl Cancer Inst. 2001;93(3):178–93.

58. Ferrari C, et al. Role of MMP-9 and its tissue inhibitor TIMP-1 in human osteosarcoma: findings in 42 patients followed for 1–16 years. Acta Orthop Scand. 2004;75(4):487–91.

59. Benassi MS, et al. Tissue and serum loss of metalloproteinase inhibitors in high grade soft tissue sarcomas. Histol Histopathol. 2003;18(4):1035–40.

60. Moran A, et al. Clinical relevance of MMP-9, MMP-2, TIMP-1 and TIMP-2 in colorectal cancer. Oncol Rep. 2005;13(1):115–20.

61. Way G, et al. Purification and identification of secernin, a novel cytosolic protein that regulates exocytosis in mast cells. Mol Biol Cell. 2002;13(9):3344–54.

62. Hendrix A, et al. The tumor ecosystem regulates the roads for invasion and metastasis. Clin Res Hepatol Gastroenterol. 2011;35(11):714–9.

63. Lin S, et al. Secernin-1 contributes to colon cancer progression through enhancing matrix metalloproteinase-2/9 exocytosis. Dis Markers. 2015;2015: 230703.

64. Miyoshi N, et al. SCRN1 is a novel marker for prognosis in colorectal cancer. J Surg Oncol. 2010;101(2):156–9.

65. Suehara Y, et al. Secernin-1 as a novel prognostic biomarker candidate of synovial sarcoma revealed by proteomics. J Proteomics. 2011;74(6):829–42.

66. Wang W, et al. Polycomb Group (PcG) Proteins and Human Cancers: Multifaceted Functions and Therapeutic Implications. Med Res Rev. 2015; 35(6):1220–67.

67. Volkel P, et al. Diverse involvement of EZH2 in cancer epigenetics. Am J Transl Res. 2015;7(2):175–93.

68. Changchien YC, et al. Poorly differentiated synovial sarcoma is associated with high expression of enhancer of zeste homologue 2 (EZH2). J Transl Med. 2012;10:216.

69. Kawano S, et al. Preclinical Evidence of Anti-Tumor Activity Induced by EZH2 Inhibition in Human Models of Synovial Sarcoma. PLoS One. 2016; 11(7):e0158888.

70. Ramaglia M, et al. High EZH2 expression is correlated to metastatic disease in pediatric soft tissue sarcomas. Cancer Cell Int. 2016;16:59.

71. Yamaguchi H, Hung MC. Regulation and Role of EZH2 in Cancer. Cancer Res Treat. 2014;46(3):209–22.

72. Fujii S, et al. Enhancer of zeste homologue 2 (EZH2) down-regulates RUNX3 by increasing histone H3 methylation. J Biol Chem. 2008;283(25):17324–32.

73. Moore HM, et al. EZH2 inhibition decreases p38 signaling and suppresses breast cancer motility and metastasis. Breast Cancer Res Treat. 2013;138(3): 741–52.

74. Schultz-Thater E, et al. NY-ESO-1 tumour associated antigen is a cytoplasmic protein detectable by specific monoclonal antibodies in cell lines and clinical specimens. Br J Cancer. 2000;83(2):204–8.

75. Park TS, et al. Expression of MAGE-A and NY-ESO-1 in Primary and Metastatic Cancers. J Immunother. 2016;39(1):1–7.

76. Li M, et al. Effective inhibition of melanoma tumorigenesis and growth via a new complex vaccine based on NY-ESO-1-alum-polysaccharide-HH2. Mol Cancer. 2014;13:179.

77. Giesen E, et al. NY-ESO-1 as a potential immunotherapeutic target in renal cell carcinoma. Oncotarget. 2014;5(14):5209–17.

78. Aung PP, et al. Expression of New York esophageal squamous cell carcinoma-1 in primary and metastatic melanoma. Hum Pathol. 2014;45(2): 259–67.

79. Lai JP, et al. NY-ESO-1 expression in sarcomas: A diagnostic marker and immunotherapy target. Oncoimmunol. 2012;1(8):1409–10.

80. Robbins PF, et al. Tumor regression in patients with metastatic synovial cell sarcoma and melanoma using genetically engineered lymphocytes reactive with NY-ESO-1. J Clin Oncol. 2011;29(7):917–24.

81. Xu C, et al. CXCR4 in breast cancer: oncogenic role and therapeutic targeting. Drug Des Devel Ther. 2015;9:4953–64.

82. Dewan MZ, et al. Stromal cell-derived factor-1 and CXCR4 receptor interaction in tumor growth and metastasis of breast cancer. Biomed Pharmacother. 2006;60(6):273–6.

83. Gangadhar T, Nandi S, Salgia R. The role of chemokine receptor CXCR4 in lung cancer. Cancer Biol Ther. 2010;9(6):409–16.

84. Lv S, et al. The association of CXCR4 expression with prognosis and clinicopathological indicators in colorectal carcinoma patients: a meta-analysis. Histopathology. 2014;64(5):701–12.

85. Scala S, et al. Expression of CXCR4 predicts poor prognosis in patients with malignant melanoma. Clin Cancer Res. 2005;11(5):1835–41.

86. Oda Y, et al. Chemokine receptor CXCR4 expression is correlated with VEGF expression and poor survival in soft-tissue sarcoma. Int J Cancer. 2009; 124(8):1852–9.

87. Yuecheng Y, Xiaoyan X. Stromal-cell derived factor-1 regulates epithelial ovarian cancer cell invasion by activating matrix metalloproteinase-9 and matrix metalloproteinase-2. Eur J Cancer Prev. 2007;16(5):430–5.

88. Uchida D, et al. Possible role of stromal-cell-derived factor-1/CXCR4 signaling on lymph node metastasis of oral squamous cell carcinoma. Exp Cell Res. 2003;290(2):289–302.

89. Guo F, et al. CXCL12/CXCR4: a symbiotic bridge linking cancer cells and their stromal neighbors in oncogenic communication networks. Oncogene. 2016;35(7):816–26.

90. Kim RH, Li BD, Chu QD. The role of chemokine receptor CXCR4 in the biologic behavior of human soft tissue sarcoma. Sarcoma. 2011;2011:593708.

91. Murphy PM. Chemokines and the molecular basis of cancer metastasis. N Engl J Med. 2001;345(11):833–5.

92. Muller A, et al. Involvement of chemokine receptors in breast cancer metastasis. Nature. 2001;410(6824):50–6.

93. Debnath B, et al. Small molecule inhibitors of CXCR4. Theranostics. 2013; 3(1):47–75.

94. Kim SY, et al. Inhibition of the CXCR4/CXCL12 chemokine pathway reduces the development of murine pulmonary metastases. Clin Exp Metastasis. 2008;25(3):201–11.

6

A meta-analysis of hypoxia inducible factor 1-alpha (HIF1A) gene polymorphisms: association with cancers

Md. T Anam[1], Alokta Ishika[2], Md. B Hossain[1] and Jesmin[2*]

Abstract

Background: Hypoxia inducible factor 1-alpha (HIF1A) is a transcription factor that plays important role in regulating cascade of reactions. In this study, the effect of rs11549465 (1772 C/T) and rs11549467 (1790 G/A) polymorphisms of HIF1A gene and its association with cancers were investigated through meta-analysis.

Methods: Meta-analysis of genome wide association studies of HIF1A 1772 C/T polymorphism were conducted on 22 case-control studies of sample size 19024 and for 1790 G/A polymorphism 19 case-control studies were included with sample size 10654. Genotype and allelic frequency compared between cases and controls together with further subgroup analyses were carried out by cancer type and ethnicity.

Results: Meta-analysis from this study indicated that HIF1A 1772 C/T polymorphism is significantly associated with overall cancer risk. T allele and genotype TT are significantly associated with increasing overall cancer risk; odds ratios (OR) dominant model [TT + CT vs. CC: OR 1.30, 95 % CI (1.06-1.59), p-value: 0.0115], and T allele vs. C allele: OR 1.32, 95 % CI (1.07-1.63), p-value: 0.0098. Also, HIF1A 1790 G/A polymorphism, analyses showed that A allele and genotype AA are significantly associated with increasing overall cancer risk; odds ratios (OR) homozygote comparison [AA vs. GG: OR 5.10, 95 % CI (3.12-8.33), p-value: <0.0001], heterozygote comparison [GA vs. GG: OR 1.74, 95 % CI (1.20-2.52), p-value: 0.0033], dominant model [AA + GA vs. GG: OR 1.82, 95 % CI (1.26-2.62), p-value: 0.0014], recessive model [AA vs. GA + GG: OR 3.79, 95 % CI (2.34-6.15), p-value: <0.0001] and A allele vs. G allele: OR 1.82, 95 % CI (1.31-2.52), p-value: 0.0003.

Conclusion: In detail meta-analysis indicated that both the polymorphisms 1772 C/T and 1790 G/A are significantly associated with overall cancer risk. The subgroup analyses showed that lung cancer is significantly associated with both polymorphisms. Although the 1772 C/T polymorphism is significantly associated with decreasing risk of renal cell carcinoma but the 1790 G/A polymorphism has shown to significantly increase the cancer risk in both Caucasian and Asian population. Thus, HIF1A could be a useful prognostic marker for cancers early predisposition.

Keywords: HIF1A, Genome wide association studies, Cancer, Meta-analysis

Background

Cancer is the second leading cause of morbidity and mortality worldwide [1]. One major feature of cancer is uncontrolled cell proliferation, which can then invade adjacent parts of the body and spread to other organs, the latter process is referred as metastases, which are the major cause of death from cancer [2]. The most common causes of cancer deaths are due to cancers of the: lung (1.59 million deaths), liver (745,000 deaths), stomach (723,000 deaths), colorectal (694,000 deaths), breast (521,000 deaths) and esophageal (400,000 deaths) [1, 2]. Alongside, metabolic alterations and tumor hypoxia have consistently been identified as classical features with aggressive malignancy [3, 4]. Hypoxia regulates tumor cell phenotype mainly by altering genes that are sensitive to oxygen pressure [5]. However, the exact mechanism of carcinogenesis is yet to be elucidated. In recent years, an increasing number of studies have focused on

* Correspondence: jesmin@du.ac.bd
[2]Department of Genetic Engineering & Biotechnology, University of Dhaka, Dhaka 1000, Bangladesh
Full list of author information is available at the end of the article

understanding the relationship between genetic factors and cancer risk [3, 4]. Through the years, it has become well accepted that single nucleotide polymorphisms (SNPs) are the most common and effective type of genetic variations studied in association with disease susceptibility and are the markers of many complex diseases [6].

Hypoxia inducible factor 1α (HIF1A), is a transcription factor that has major impacts in the process of development and progression of cancers [7]. HIF1A regulates the expression of over 100 genes that control the major cellular functions including apoptosis, cell proliferation, glucose metabolism, erythropoiesis, iron metabolism and angiogenesis. It is a master regulator of oxygen homeostasis [7]. In the scientific community, HIF1A has been a research focus and a number of SNPs within HIF1A gene have been identified in association with cancers, with the most widely studied polymorphisms are C1772T (rs11549465) and G1790A (rs11549467) polymorphisms [8–38]. These two SNPs are located within the same domain (ODD/ pVHL) in exon 12 of the HIF1A gene [8, 9]. Recently a meta-analysis has revealed that C1772T is not in substantial linkage disequilibrium (LD) with G1790A [38]. A number of studies have suggested that these two nonsynonymous mutations might alter the transcriptional activity of HIF1A gene by causing structural changes with varied stability, which in turn, might influence the downstream target genes expression and regulation [8, 9, 38]. In the recent years, a good number of studies have investigated the impact of HIF1A polymorphisms on cancer risk in different populations; however reported results varied across studies and remain inconclusive [10–38]. In this study, the effect of rs11549465 (1772 C/T) and rs11549467 (1790 G/A) polymorphisms of HIF1A gene and its association with cancers were investigated systematically through meta-analysis.

Methods

Search study and study selection
The PubMed, PubMed Central and Google Scholar databases were searched systematically to retrieve compatible and pertinent peer reviewed publications of empirical studies. Published articles of last 15 years (ended on December 2014), in English language were only considered for this study. The search terms included were (1) HIF1A, (2) GWAS, (3) SNPs, (4) polymorphisms, (5) C1772T/ P582S, (6) A1790G/ A588T, (7) case-control study, and (8) cancer.

Eligibility criteria
Two authors independently investigated titles and abstracts of all the articles. Irrelevant and incompatible studies were excluded primarily. For final review, criteria's for further study elimination were: if (1) the study population was not defined completely; (2) it is not a case-control study; (3) not a genome wide association study; (4) incomplete information of allele frequency; and (5) the year of study conducted was not specified. Also, reviews, editorials, meta-analysis and non-human researches were excluded. Only case-control studies, genome wide association study (GWAS) and human researches were considered for the final review. Further, the references of the selected studies were screened carefully for incorporation of additional relevant studies. Only English language articles were considered for this study. Discrepancies and difficulties were discussed with corresponding authors where necessary. Following information were extracted from each study: (1) authors name, (2) year of study, (3) ethnicity of the study subjects, (4) cancer type and (5) allelic frequency (Fig. 1).

Meta-analysis
For HIF1A 1772 C/T polymorphism 22 case-control studies were included of sample size 19024 and for 1790 G/A polymorphism 19 case-control studies were included with sample size 10654. The meta-analysis was prepared in accordance with PRISMA statement [39].

Statistical analysis
Meta-analysis of genome wide association studies (GWAS) of HIF1A were conducted for two polymorphisms, 1772 C/T and 1790 G/A using odds ratios (ORs). A slightly amended estimator of OR was used to avoid the computation of reciprocal of zeros among observed values in the calculation of the original OR [40]. Pooled ORs with 95 % CIs were calculated using random effects model (REM) incorporating the inverse variance weighted method [41]. Heterogeneity among studies was assessed using the Q statistic [42] and quantified using I^2 index [43]. Subgroup analyses were carried out by cancer type and ethnicity. The Hardy Weinberg Equilibrium (HWE) test was performed for the controls of each study. The studies with control not in HWE were supervised for sensitivity analysis. Publication bias was assessed visually by conventionally constructed funnel plot where the inverse of the standard error (1/se) of the effect estimates were plotted against the logarithm transformation of Odds Ratios [log(OR)] [44]. Furthermore, Egger's test was performed to provide quantitative evidence of publication bias [45]. "Gap: Genetic analysis package" was used to perform the Hardy Weinberg Equilibrium (HWE) test [46, 47]. All analyses were conducted using "meta" package in R environment [46].

Summary measures
Odds Ratios (OR) with a 95 % confidence interval (CI) were calculated to evaluate the genotype contrasts. The genotype contrasts for the HIF1A 1772 C/T polymorphisms were: homozygote comparison [TT versus CC],

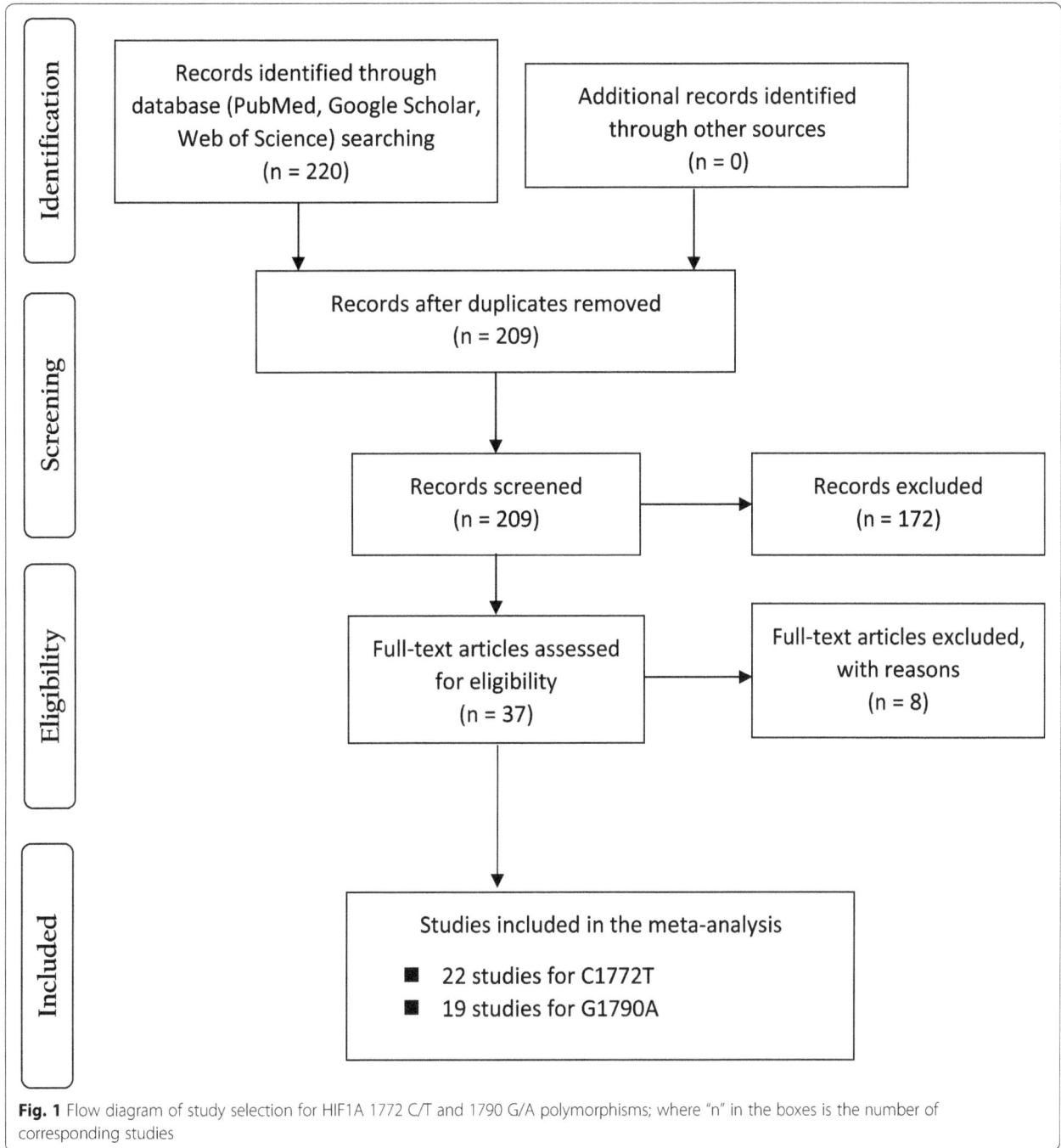

Fig. 1 Flow diagram of study selection for HIF1A 1772 C/T and 1790 G/A polymorphisms; where "n" in the boxes is the number of corresponding studies

heterozygote comparison [CT versus CC], and dominant model [TT + CT versus CC], recessive model [TT versus CT + CC] and T allele versus C allele. For HIF1A 1772 C/T polymorphism, three studies were found with genotype information of CC and CT + TT. These three studies were included only to evaluate genotype contrast of dominant model [TT + CT vs. CC]. The genotype contrasts for the HIF1A 1790 G/A polymorphism were: homozygote comparison [AA versus GG], heterozygote comparison [GA versus GG] and dominant model [AA + GA versus GG], recessive model [AA versus GA + GG] and [G versus A allele].

Results and discussion
Study characteristics
In the meta-analysis of the HIF1A 1772 C/T polymorphism, ten different types of cancers consisted of 22 studies with 8149 cancer cases and 10,875 controls were included.

The types of cancer included in these studies were prostate cancer, colorectal cancer, renal cell carcinoma, breast cancer, lung cancer, oral squamous cell carcinoma (OSCC), head-neck cancer, cervical cancer, bladder carcinoma and pancreatic cancer. For the following cancer types: head-neck, cervical, bladder and pancreatic only one study of each were found for the final review. So, these cancer types with single studies were incorporated in subgroup analysis as Other Cancers (Table 1).

For the meta-analysis of HIF1A 1790 G/A polymorphism, 19 studies with eleven different cancer types consisted of 4681 cancer cases and 5973 controls were included. The cancer types associated with this polymorphism were: renal cancer, prostate cancer, breast cancer, lung cancer, oral squamous cell carcinoma (OSCC), head-neck cancer, gastric cancer, hepatocellular carcinoma, lymph node metastasis, pancreatic cancer and colorectal cancer. For final review, only one study of each of the following cancer types was found: head-neck cancer, gastric cancer, hepatocellular carcinoma, lymph node metastasis, pancreatic cancer and colorectal cancer. These cancer types with single studies were incorporated in subgroup analysis as Other Cancers (Table 2).

Association of the HIF1A 1772 C/T polymorphism with cancer risk

The pooled ORs for overall cancer suggested that the HIF1A 1772 C/T polymorphism was significantly associated with increasing cancer risk for the dominant model [TT + CT vs. CC: OR 1.30, 95 % CI (1.06-1.59), p-value: 0.0115] and [T vs. C allele: OR 1.32, 95 % CI (1.07-1.63), p-value: 0.0098] (Fig. 2).

Subgroup analyses performed by cancer type

The subgroup analyses of prostate cancer, colorectal cancer, breast cancer and oral squamous-cell carcinoma suggested no significant association of the HIF1A 1772 C/T polymorphism. However, the subgroup analyses of renal cell carcinoma suggested that the HIF1A 1772 C/T polymorphism is significantly associated with lowering renal cell carcinoma risk in homozygote comparison [TT vs. CC: OR 0.27, 95 % CI (0.08-0.90), p-value:0.0335]. Interestingly, the results of subgroup analyses of lung cancer suggested that the HIF1A 1772 C/T polymorphism is highly associated with increasing lung cancer risk in homozygote comparison [TT vs. CC: OR 4.88, 95 % CI (2.42-9.84), p-value: <0.0001], recessive model [TT vs. CT + CC: OR 4.04, 95 % CI (2.02-8.08), p-value:<0.0001].

Table 1 Characteristic of eligible studies included in meta-analysis of HIF1A 1772 C/T polymorphism

Study	Year	Country	Ethnicity	Cancer	Case/Control	HWE
Clifford et al. [8]	2001	UK	Caucasian	Renal cell carcinoma	35/143	0.018 (N)
Tanimoto et al. [9]	2003	Japanese	Asian	Head-neck cancer	55/110	0.545 (Y)
Ollerenshawa et al. [10]	2004	European	Caucasian	Renal cell carcinoma	160/162	<0.001 (N)
Chau et al. [11]	2005	USA	Mixed	Prostate cancer	196/196	<0.001 (N)
Franse et al. [12]	2006	Swedish	Caucasian	Colorectal cancer	198/258	0.916 (Y)
Konac et al. [13]	2007	Turkish	Caucasian	Cervical cancer	32/107	0.229 (Y)
Li et al. [14]	2007	American	Mixed	Prostate cancer	1041/1234	0.159 (Y)
Lee et al. [15]	2008	Korean	Asian	Breast cancer	1332/1369	0.250 (Y)
Kim et al. [16]	2008	Korean	Asian	Breast cancer	90/102	0.641 (Y)
Nadaoka et al.[a] [17]	2008	Japanese	Asian	Transitional cell carcinoma of bladder	219/461	
Jacobs et al. [18]	2008	American	Mixed	Prostate cancer	1420/1450	0.041 (N)
Foley et al. [19]	2009	Ireland	Caucasian	Prostate cancer	95/188	0.623 (Y)
Morris et al. [20]	2009	Polish	Caucasian	Renal cell carcinoma	332/313	0.083 (Y)
Chen et al. [21]	2009	Taiwanese	Asian	Oral squamous cell carcinoma (OSCC)	174/347	0.722 (Y)
Shieh et al. [22]	2010	Taiwan	Asian	Oral squamous cell carcinoma (OSCC)	305/96	0.710 (Y)
Knechtel et al.[a] [23]	2010	Austria	Caucasian	Colorectal cancer	368/2156	
Kang et al.[a] [24]	2011	Korean	Asian	Colorectal cancer	50/50	
Putra et al. [25]	2011	Japanese	Asian	Lung cancer	83/110	0.545 (Y)
Wang et al. [26]	2011	Chinese	Asian	Pancreatic cancer	263/271	0.352 (Y)
Kuo et al. [27]	2012	Taiwanese	Asian	Lung cancer	285/300	0.132 (Y)
Li et al. [28]	2012	China	Asian	Prostate cancer	662/716	0.267 (Y)
Fraga et al. [29]	2014	Portuguese	Caucasian	Prostate cancer	754/736	0.400 (Y)

[a]Frequency of genotypes "CT + TT". *HWE* Hardy-Weinberg Equilibrium

Table 2 Characteristic of eligible studies included in meta-analysis of HIF1A 1790G/A polymorphism

Study	Year	Country	Ethnicity	Cancer	Case/Control	HWE
Clifford et al. [8]	2001	Caucasian	Caucasian	Renal cancer	48/144	0.866(Y)
Tanimoto et al. [9]	2003	Japan	Asian	Head neck squeamish cell carcinoma	55/110	0.655(Y)
Ollerenshaw et al. [10]	2004	Caucasian	Caucasian	Renal cancer	146/288	<0.001(N)
Fransen et al. [12]	2006	Sweden	Caucasian	Colorectal cancer	198/256	0.775(Y)
Orr-Urtreger et al. [30]	2007	Israel	Caucasian	Prostate cancer	200/300	0.954(Y)
Li et al. [14]	2007	USA	Mixed	Prostate cancer	1066/1264	0.810(Y)
Apaydin et al. [31]	2008	Turkey	Caucasian	Breast cancer	102/102	0.840(Y)
Kim et al. [16]	2008	Korea	Asian	Breast cancer	90/102	0.06(Y)
Muñoz et al. [32]	2009	Spain	Caucasian	Oral squamous cell carcinoma	64/139	0.693(Y)
Chen et al. [21]	2009	Taiwanese	Asian	Oral squamous cell carcinoma	174/347	0.701(Y)
Morris et al. [20]	2009	polish	Caucasian	Renal cancer	325/309	0.662(Y)
Li K et al. [33]	2009	Tibetan	Asian	Gastric cancer	87/106	0.764(Y)
Hsiao et al. [34]	2010	Taiwan	Asian	Hepatocellular carcinoma	102/347	0.701(Y)
Putra et al. [25]	2011	Japan	Asian	Lung cancer	83/110	0.655(Y)
Wang et al. [26]	2011	Japan	Asian	Pancreatic cancer	263/271	0.486(Y)
Kuo et al. [27]	2012	China	Asian	Lung cancer	285/300	0.154(Y)
Li et al. [28]	2012	China	Asian	Prostate cancer	662/716	0.554(Y)
Mera-Mene et al. [35]	2012	Spain	Caucasian	Lymph node metastasis	111/139	0.693(Y)
Qin et al. [36]	2012	Asian	Asian	Renal cancer	620/623	0.411(Y)

HWE Hardy-Weinberg Equilibrium

The subgroup analyses of Other Cancers suggested that the HIF1A 1772 C/T polymorphism is highly associated with increasing Other Cancer risk in homozygote comparison [TT vs. CC: OR 27.20, 95 % CI (5.04-146.78), *p*-value: 0.0001], heterozygote comparison [CT vs. CC: OR 2.16, 95 % CI (1.46-3.18), *p*-value: 0.0056], dominant model [TT + CT vs. CC: OR 1.92, 95 % CI (1.17-3.14), *p*-value: 0.0093], recessive model [TT vs. CT + CC: OR 17.5, 95 % CI (3.49-87.70), *p*-value: 0.0005] and [T vs. C allele: OR 2.42, 95 % CI (1.55-3.77), *p*-value: <0.0001] (Table 3).

Subgroup analyses by ethnicity group
The analyses data for the HIF1A 1772 C/T polymorphism suggested that there was no significant effect on the Caucasian population. However, the subgroup analyses of the Asian population suggested that the HIF1A 1772 C/T polymorphism was significantly associated with increasing cancer risk in homozygote comparison [TT vs. CC: OR 4.98, 95 % CI (2.66-9.31), *p*-value: <0.0001], heterozygote comparison [CT vs. CC: OR 1.30, 95 % CI (1.01-1.69), *p*-value: 0.0455], dominant model [TT + CT vs. CC: OR 1.41, 95 % CI (1.08-1.84), *p*-value: 0.0109], recessive model [TT vs. CT + CC: OR 4.28, 95 % CI (2.31-7.95), *p*-value:<0.0001] and [T vs. C allele: OR 1.43, 95 % CI (1.07-1.90), *p*-value: 0.0156] (Table 3). The subgroup analyses of mixed ethnic groups suggested that there were no significant association between HIF1A 1772 C/T polymorphism and cancer risk (Table 3).

Sources of heterogeneity
There were significant heterogeneity observed in the analyses of HIF1A 1772 C/T polymorphism for overall cancer heterozygote comparison [CT vs. CC: Q = 69.67, d.f = 18, *p*-value 0.0001, I^2 = 74.2 % (59.5 %-83.5 %)], dominant model [TT + CT vs. CC: Q = 90.25, d.f = 21, *p* <0.0001, I^2 = 76.7 % (65.1 %-84.5 %)], and [T vs. C allele: Q = 96.87, d.f = 18, *p* <0.0001, I^2 = 81.4 % (71.9 %-87.7 %). To detect the sources of heterogeneity subgroup analyses by cancer type and ethnicity group were performed. In the subgroup analyses by cancer type heterogeneity was significantly reduced. The results suggested that the studies in prostate cancer, renal cell carcinoma, lung cancer, Caucasian ethnicity and Asian ethnicity were the main sources of heterogeneity (Additional file 1).

Association of the HIF1A 1790 G/A polymorphism with cancer risk
The pooled ORs for overall cancer suggested that the HIF1A 1790 G/A polymorphism was significantly associated with increasing cancer risk for homozygote comparison [AA vs. GG: OR 5.10, 95 % CI (3.12-8.33), *p*-value: <0.0001, heterozygote comparison [GA vs. GG: OR 1.74, 95 % CI (1.20-2.52), *p*-value: 0.0033, dominant model [AA + GA vs. GG: OR 1.82, 95 % CI (1.26-2.62), *p*-value: 0.0014], recessive model [AA vs. GA + GG: OR 3.79, 95 % CI (2.34-6.15), *p*-value: <0.0001] and [A vs. G allele: OR 1.82, 95 % CI (1.31-2.52), *p*-value: 0.0003] (Fig. 3).

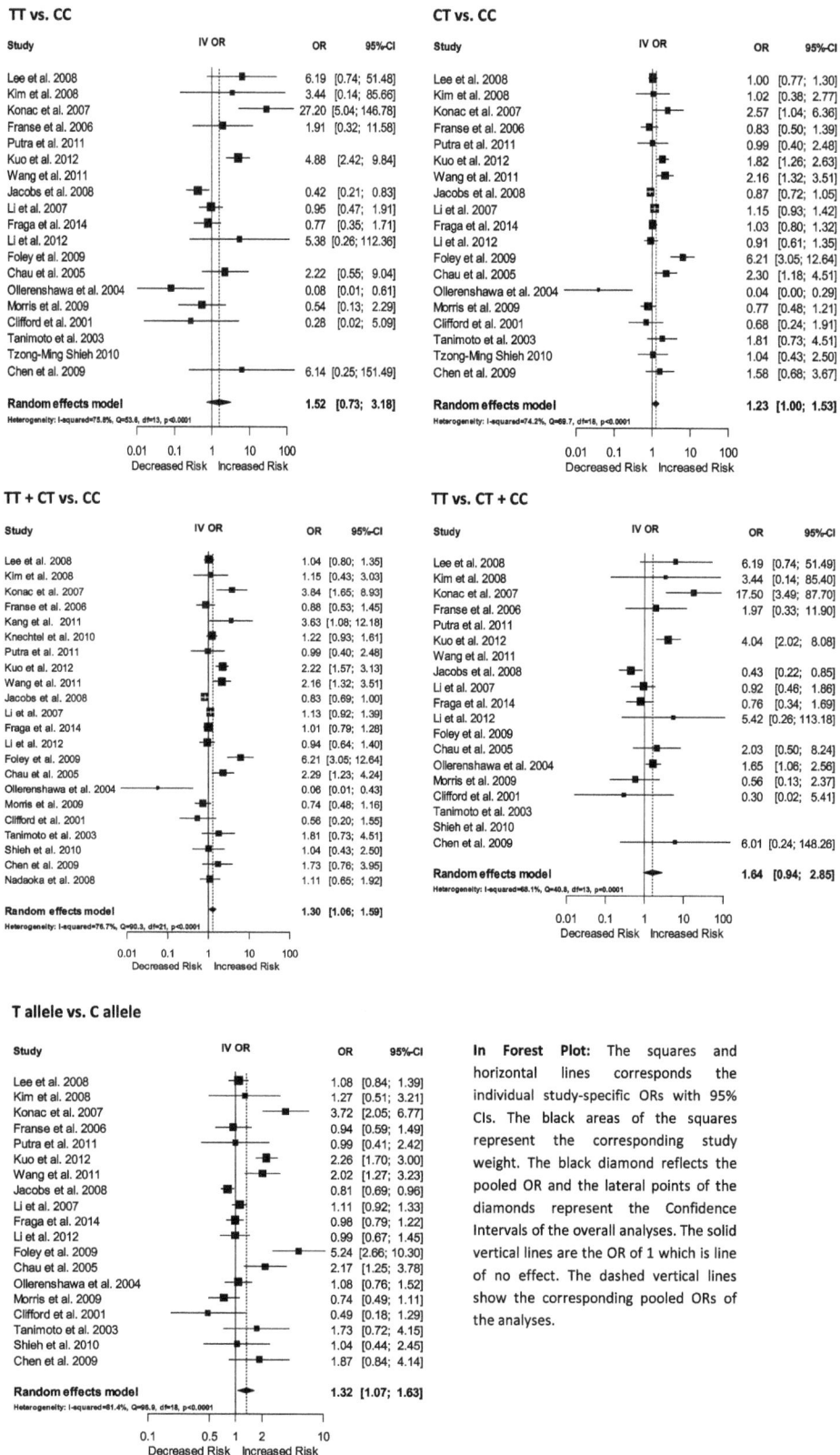

Fig. 2 Forest plot of HIF1A polymorphism 1772 C/T for overall cancer

Table 3 Meta-analysis of the HIF1A 1772 C/T polymorphism association with cancer

	Study number	Sample size	TT vs. CC OR (95 % CI)	p value	CT vs. CC OR (95 % CI)	p value	TT + CT vs. CC OR (95 % CI)	p value	TT vs. CT + CC OR (95 % CI)	p value	T vs. C OR (95 % CI)	p value
Overall cancer	22	19024	1.52 [0.73–3.18]	0.2648	1.23 [1.00–1.53]	0.0536	1.30 [1.06–1.59]	0.0115	1.64 [0.94–2.85]	0.0832	1.32 [1.07–1.63]	0.0098
Prostate cancer	6	8688	0.84 [0.47–1.49]	0.5449	1.34 [0.95–1.87]	0.0913	1.33 [0.95–1.87]	0.0982	0.81 [0.47–1.40]	0.4535	1.29 [0.94–1.76]	0.1178
Colorectal cancer	3	3080	1.91 [0.32–11.58]	0.4801	0.83 [0.50–1.39]	0.4817	1.24 [0.77–2.01]	0.3756	1.97 [0.33–11.90]	0.4603	0.94 [0.59–1.49]	0.7833
Renal cancer	3	1145	0.27 [0.08–0.90]	0.0335	0.40 [0.12–1.34]	0.1369	0.43 [0.15–1.20]	0.1082	1.08 [0.44–2.64]	0.8703	0.84 [0.58–1.22]	0.3548
Breast cancer	2	2893	5.18 [0.88–30.38]	0.0683	1.00 [0.77–1.29]	0.9964	1.05 [0.81–1.35]	0.7221	5.18 [0.88–30.36]	0.0684	1.09 [0.86–1.39]	0.4701
Lung cancer	2	778	4.88 [2.42–9.84]	< 0.0001	1.56 [0.94–2.61]	0.088	1.67 [0.79–3.54]	0.1832	4.04 [2.02–8.08]	< 0.0001	1.68 [0.77–3.64]	0.1908
OSCC	2	922	6.14 [0.25–151.49]	0.2673	1.29 [0.70–2.37]	0.4142	1.36 [0.75–2.49]	0.3127	6.01 [0.24–148.26]	0.2729	1.43 [0.79–2.56]	0.2348
Other cancers	4	1518	27.20 [5.04–146.78]	0.0001	2.16 [1.46–3.18]	0.0056	1.92 [1.17–3.14]	0.0093	17.5 [3.49 – 87.70]	0.0005	2.42 [1.55–3.77]	< 0.0001
Ethnicity												
Caucasian	8	6037	0.97 [0.24–3.93]	0.9654	1.09 [0.60–2.00]	0.7751	1.19 [0.75–1.89]	0.4528	1.48 [0.65–3.39]	0.352	1.31 [0.84–2.06]	0.237
Asian	11	7450	4.98 [2.66–9.31]	< 0.0001	1.30 [1.01–1.69]	0.0455	1.41 [1.08–1.84]	0.0109	4.28 [2.31–7.95]	< 0.0001	1.43 [1.07–1.90]	0.0156
Mixed	3	5537	0.82 [0.36–1.87]	0.6408	1.16 [1.00–1.65]	0.4178	1.16 [0.79–1.70]	0.4526	0.79 [0.37–1.71]	0.5544	1.14 [0.78–1.67]	0.505

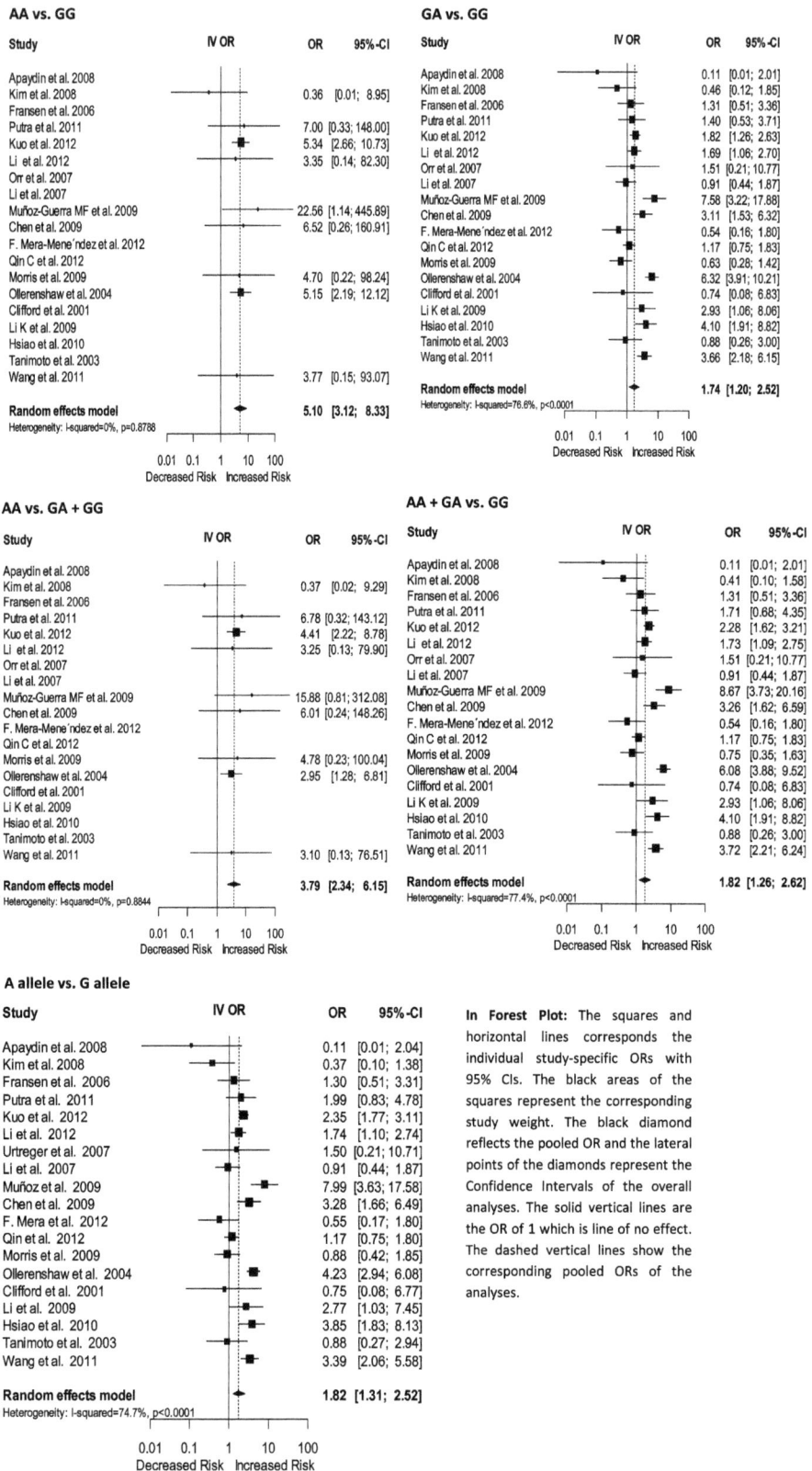

Fig. 3 Forest plot of the HIF1A polymorphism 1790 G/A for overall cancer

Subgroup analyses by cancer type

The analyzed data of prostate cancer suggested no significant association with the HIF1A 1790 G/A polymorphism. The subgroup analyses of renal cancer suggested that the HIF1A 1790 G/A polymorphism was significantly associated with increasing cancer risk for homozygote comparison [AA vs. GG: OR 5.11, 95 % CI (2.24-11.66), *p*-value: 0.0001], recessive model [AA vs. GA + GG: OR 3.05, 95 % CI (1.36-6.84), *p*-value: 0.0068] whereas the subgroup analyses of breast cancer showed that the HIF1A 1790 G/A polymorphism was significantly associated with decreasing cancer risk for [A vs. G allele: OR 0.30, 95 % CI (0.09-1.00), *p*-value: 0.0495]. The subgroup analyses of lung cancer suggested that the HIF1A 1790 G/A polymorphism was significantly associated with increasing cancer risk for homozygote comparison [AA vs. GG: OR 5.41, 95 % CI (2.74-10.69), *p*-value: <0.0001], heterozygote comparison [GA vs. GG: OR 1.76, 95 % CI (1.25-2.49), *p*-value: 0.0013], dominant model [AA + GA vs. GG: OR 2.20, 95 % CI (1.60-3.03), *p*-value:<0.0001], recessive model [AA vs. GA + GG: OR 4.51, 95 % CI (2.31-8.81), *p*-value:<0.0001] and [A vs. G allele: OR 2.31, 95 % CI (1.77-3.02), *p*-value: <0.0001]. Also, the subgroup analyses of oral squamous cell carcinoma (OSCC) suggested that the HIF1A 1790 G/A polymorphism was significantly associated with increasing cancer risk for homozygote comparison [AA vs. GG: OR 12.68, 95 % CI (1.43-112.64), *p*-value: 0.0227], heterozygote comparison [GA vs. GG: OR 4.69, 95 % CI (1.96-11.21), *p*-value: 0.0005], dominant model [AA + GA vs. GG: OR 5.17, 95 % CI (1.99-13.43), *p*-value: 0.0008], recessive model [AA vs. GA + GG: OR 10.12, 95 % CI (1.14-89.72), *p*-value: 0.0376] and [A vs. G allele: OR 5.00, 95 % CI (2.10-11.97), *p*-value: 0.0003] (Table 4). The subgroup analyses of Other Cancers suggested that the HIF1A 1790 G/A polymorphism is highly associated with increasing Other Cancer risk heterozygote comparison [GA vs. GG: OR 1.96, 95 % CI (1.05-3.65), *p*-value: 0.0336], dominant model [AA + GA vs. GG: OR 1.96, 95 % CI (1.05-3.67), *p*-value: 0.0341], and [A vs. G allele: OR 1.91, 95 % CI (1.06-3.44), *p*-value: 0.0306] (Table 4).

Subgroup analyses by ethnicity group

For Caucasian population, the analyzed data suggested that the HIF1A 1790 G/A polymorphism was highly associated with increasing cancer risk for homozygote comparison [AA vs. GG: OR 5.68, 95 % CI (2.57-12.58), *p*-value: <0.0001], recessive model [AA vs. GA + GG: OR 3.42, 95 % CI (1.57-7.45), *p*-value: 0.002]. For the Asian population, the subgroup analyses of ethnicity group suggested that the HIF1A 1790 G/A polymorphism was highly associated with increasing cancer risk for homozygote comparison [AA vs. GG: OR 4.76, 95 % CI (2.55-8.91), *p*-value: <0.0001], heterozygote comparison [GA vs.

GG: OR 1.94, 95 % CI (1.38-2.72), *p*-value: 0.0001], dominant model [AA + GA vs. GG: OR 2.04, 95 % CI (1.44-2.87), *p*-value: <0.0001], recessive model [AA vs. GA + GG: OR 4.05, 95 % CI (2.18-7.51), *p*-value: <0.0001] and [A vs. G allele: OR 2.03, 95 % CI (1.46-2.81), *p*-value: <0.0001] (Table 4).

Sources of heterogeneity

There were significant heterogeneity observed in the analyses of HIF1A 1790G/A polymorphism for overall cancer heterozygote comparison [GA vs. GG: Q = 77.05, d.f = 18, *p*-value: <0.0001, I^2 = 76.6 % (63.8 %-84.9 %), dominant model [AA + GA vs. GG: Q = 79.66, d.f = 18, *p*-value: <0.0001, I^2 = 77.4 % (65.1 %-85.4 %)], and [A vs. G allele: Q = 71.09, d.f = 18, *p*-value: <0.0001, I^2 = 74.7 % (60.4 %-83.8 %)]. To detect the sources of heterogeneity subgroup analyses by cancer type and ethnicity group were performed. The results suggested that the studies in renal cell carcinoma, oral squamous cell carcinoma (OSCC), Caucasian ethnicity and Asian ethnicity were the main sources of heterogeneity (Additional file 2).

Publication bias

To investigate the evidence of publication bias of the HIF1A 1772 C/T polymorphism for T versus C allele and HIF1A 1790 G/A polymorphism for G versus A allele funnel plot were used. The conventionally constructed funnel plot (log odds ratio [log(OR) vs 1/ standard error, 1/se) of HIF1A polymorphism 1772 C/T for T vs. C allele suggested that there was evidence of publication bias (Fig. 4). Also the funnel plot of HIF1A polymorphism 1790 G/A for A vs. G allele suggested that there was evidence of publication bias (Fig. 4). However, the Egger's linear regression analyses suggested no evidence of significant publication bias in [T vs C allele: t = 1.83, d.f = 17, *p*-value 0.0847] for HIF1A 1772 C/ T polymorphism. Also, for HIF1A 1790 G/A polymorphism results showed no significant evidence of publication bias in [A vs G allele: t = -1.87, d.f = 17, *p*-value 0.0787] (Additional file 3).

Sensitivity analysis

Studies which were not in HWE were excluded to evaluate the stability of the acquired results. The statistical significance of the results was not shifted after omitting the studies which were not in HWE which confirmed the obtained results of the meta-analysis were stable and robust.

Conclusion

Results generated from this meta-analysis indicated that both 1772 C/T and 1790 G/A polymorphisms are significantly associated with increasing overall cancer risk. The subgroup analyses by cancer type showed that both 1772 C/ T and 1790 G/A polymorphisms have significant association

Table 4 Meta-analysis of the HIF1A 1790 G/A polymorphism association with cancer

	Study number	Sample size	AA vs. GG		GA vs. GG		AA vs. GA + GG		AA + GA vs. GG		A vs. G	
			OR (95 % CI)	p value	OR (95 % CI)	p value	OR (95 % CI)	p value	OR (95 % CI)	p value	OR (95 % CI)	p value
Overall	19	10654	5.10 [3.12–8.33]	< 0.0001	1.74 [1.20–2.52]	0.0033	3.79 [2.34–6.15]	< 0.0001	1.82 [1.26–2.62]	0.0014	1.82 [1.31–2.52]	0.0003
Renal cancer	4	2503	5.11 [2.24–11.66]	0.0001	1.51 [0.45–5.05]	0.5038	3.05 [1.36–6.84]	0.0068	1.58 [0.49–5.03]	0.442	1.53 [0.60–3.92]	0.3747
Prostate cancer	3	4208	3.35 [0.14–82.30]	0.4597	1.41 [0.96–2.08]	0.0822	3.25 [0.13–79.90]	0.4707	1.41 [0.93–2.15]	0.1043	1.42 [0.93–2.17]	0.1093
Breast cancer	2	396	0.36 [0.01–8.95]	0.5332	0.35 [0.10–1.24]	0.1045	0.37 [0.02–9.29]	0.5484	0.32 [0.09–1.10]	0.0702	0.30 [0.09–1.00]	0.0495
Lung cancer	2	778	5.41 [2.74–10.69]	< 0.0001	1.76 [1.25–2.49]	0.0013	4.51 [2.31–8.81]	< 0.0001	2.20 [1.60–3.03]	< 0.0001	2.31 [1.77–3.02]	< 0.0001
OSCC	2	724	12.68 [1.43–112.64]	0.0227	4.69 [1.96–11.21]	0.0005	10.12 [1.14–89.72]	0.0376	5.17 [1.99–13.43]	0.0008	5.00 [2.10–11.97]	0.0003
Other cancers	6	2045	3.77 [0.15–93.07]	0.4171	1.96 [1.05–3.65]	0.0336	3.10 [0.13–76.51]	0.4887	1.96 [1.05–3.67]	0.0341	1.91 [1.06–3.44]	0.0306
Ethnicity												
Caucasian	8	2666	5.68 [2.57–12.58]	< 0.0001	1.43 [0.54–3.74]	0.4691	3.42 [1.57–7.45]	0.002	1.50 [0.58–3.85]	0.3987	1.52 [0.68–3.42]	0.3103
Asian	10	4914	4.76 [2.55–8.91]	< 0.0001	1.94 [1.38–2.72]	0.0001	4.05 [2.1 –7.51]	< 0.0001	2.04 [1.44–2.87]	< 0.0001	2.03 [1.46–2.81]	< 0.0001

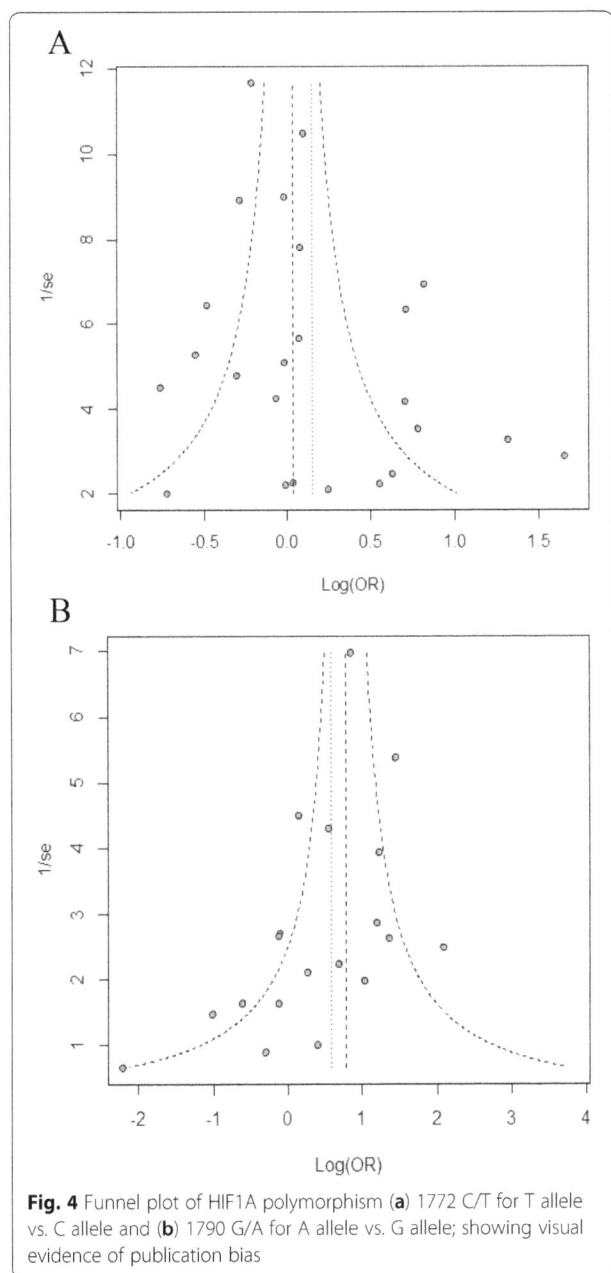

Fig. 4 Funnel plot of HIF1A polymorphism (**a**) 1772 C/T for T allele vs. C allele and (**b**) 1790 G/A for A allele vs. G allele; showing visual evidence of publication bias

Abbreviations

GWAS: Genome wide association studies; SNP: Single nucleotide polymorphism; REM: Random effects model; CI: Confidence interval; SE: Standard error; Log: Logarithm; HWE: Hardy-Weinberg Equilibrium; HIF1: Hypoxia- inducible factor -1; HIF1A: Hypoxia- inducible factor -1α; OR: Odds ratio; OSCC: Oral squamous cell carcinoma..

Competing interests

The authors declare that they have no competing interests.

Authors' contributions

Jesmin and MBH designed the research, MBH designed the experimental data analysis model and validate interpretation, MTA and AI collected, screened and analyzed the data. Jesmin, MBH and MTA analyzed and interpreted the result, drafted and revised the manuscript. All authors have read and approved the final manuscript.

Acknowledgements

This work was supported in part by NST Grant 39.012.002.01,03.021.2014-09/260 from the Ministry of Science & Technology (MOST), Government of the People's Republic of Bangladesh (to AI and Jesmin).

Author details

¹Department of Statistics, Biostatistics & Informatics, University of Dhaka, Dhaka 1000, Bangladesh. ²Department of Genetic Engineering & Biotechnology, University of Dhaka, Dhaka 1000, Bangladesh.

References

1. World Cancer Report. WHO|Cancer. 2014. (http://www.who.int/mediacentre/factsheets/fs297/en/).
2. Jemal A, Siegel R, Ward E, Hao Y, Xu J, Thun MJ. Cancer statistics, 2009, CA Cancer. J Clin. 2009;59:225–49. doi:10.3322/caac.20006.
3. Yanh X, Zhu HC, Zhang C, Qin Q, Liu J, Xu LP, et al. HIF1A 1771 C/T and 1790 G/A polymorphism are significantly associated with higher cancer risk: an updated Meta-analysis from 34 case-control studies. Plos one. 2013;8(11):e80396.
4. Hill RP, Marie-Egyptienne DT, Hedley DW. Cancer stem cells, hypoxia and metastasis. Semin Radient Oncol. 2009;19:106–11. doi:10.1016/j.semradonc.2008.12.002.
5. Huang Y, Lorenzo AD, Jiang W, Cantalupo A, Sessa WC, Giordano FJ. HIF-1α in vascular smooth muscle regulates blood pressure homeostasis through a PPARγ-angiotensin II receptor type 1 (ATR1) axis. Hypertension. 2013;62(3):634–40.
6. Shastry BS. SNP alleles in human disease and evolution. J Hum Genet. 2002;47:561–6.
7. Ke Q, Costa M. Hypoxia-inducible factor-1 (HIF-1). Mol Pharmacol. 2006;70:1469–80.
8. Clifford SC, Astuti D, Hooper L, Maxwell PH, Ratcliffe PJ, Maher ER. The pVHL-associated SCF ubiquitin ligase complex: molecular genetic analysis of elongin B and C, Rbx1 and HIF-1alpha in renal cell carcinoma. Oncogene. 2001;20(36):5067–74. PMID 11526493.
9. Tanimoto K, Yoshiga K, Eguchi H, Kaneyasu M, Ukon K, Kumazaki T, et al. Hypoxia-inducible factor-1alpha polymorphisms associated with enhanced transactivation capacity, implying clinical significance. Carcinogenesis. 2003;24(11):1779–8. PMID 12919954.
10. Ollerenshaw M, Page T, Hammonds J, Demaine A. Polymorphisms in the hypoxia inducible factor-1alpha gene (HIF1A) are associated with the renal cell carcinoma phenotype. Cancer Genet Cytoenet. 2004;153(2):122–6. PMID 15350301.

with lung cancer, whereas these two polymorphisms showed no significant association with prostate cancer. In oral squamous cell carcinoma (OSCC) subgroup analyses data showed that only 1790 G/A polymorphism has significant association whereas the HIF1A 1772 C/T polymorphism showed no significant association. However, the 1772 C/T polymorphism has indicated significantly decreased risk in renal cell carcinoma. Also, 1790 G/A polymorphism has increased the cancer risk significantly in both Caucasian and Asian ethnicity. Taken together all analyzed data, HIF1A could be a prognostic marker useful for early detection and diagnosis for cancers. In future, further experimental validations would be necessary to confirm the results.

11. Chau CH, Permenter MG, Steinberg SM, Retter AS, Dahut WL, Price DK, et al. Polymorphism in the hypoxia-inducible factor 1alpha gene may confer susceptibility to androgen-independent prostate cancer. Cancer Biol Ther. 2005;4(11):1222–5. PMID 16205110.

12. Fransén K, Fenech M, Fredrikson M, Dabrosin C, Söderkvist P. Association between ulcerative growth and hypoxia inducible factor-1alpha polymorphisms in colorectal cancer patients. Mol Carcinog. 2006;45(11):833–40. PMID 16865676.

13. Konac E, Onen HI, Metindir J, Alp E, Biri AA, Ekmekci A. An investigation of relationships between hypoxia-inducible factor-1 alpha gene polymorphisms and ovarian, cervical and endometrial cancers. Cancer Detect Prev. 2007;31(1):102–9. PMID 17418979.

14. Li H, Bubley GJ, Balk SP, Gaziano JM, Pollak M, Stampfer MJ. Hypoxia-inducible factor-1alpha (HIF-1alpha) gene polymorphisms, circulating insulin-like growth factor binding protein (IGFBP)-3 levels and prostate cancer. Prostate. 2007;67(12):1354–61. PMID 17624927.

15. Lee JY, Choi JY, Lee KM, Park SK, Han SH, Noh DY, et al. Rare variant of hypoxia-inducible factor-1alpha (HIF-1A) and breast cancer risk in Korean women. Clin Chim Acta. 2008;389(1-2):167–70. PMID 18160046.

16. Kim HO, Jo YH, Lee J, Lee SS, Yoon KS. The C1772T genetic polymorphism in human HIF-1alpha gene associates with expression of HIF-1alpha protein in breast cancer. Oncol Rep. 2008;20(5):1181–7. PMID 18949419.

17. Nadaoka J, Horikawa Y, Saito M, Kumazawa T, Inoue T, Narita S, et al. Prognostic significance of HIF-1 alpha polymorphisms in transitional cell carcinoma of the bladder. Int J Cancer. 2008;122(6):1297–302. PMID 18000826.

18. Jacobs EJ, Hsing AW, Bain EB, Stevens VL, Wang Y, Chen J, et al. Polymorphisms in angiogenesis-related genes and prostate cancer. Cancer Epidemiol Biomarkers Prev. 2008;17(4):972–7. PMID 18398039.

19. Foley R, Marignol L, Thomas AZ, Cullen IM, Perry AS, Tewari P, et al. The HIF-1alpha C1772T polymorphism may be associated with susceptibility to clinically localised prostate cancer but not with elevated expression of hypoxic biomarkers. Cancer Biol. 2009;8(2):118–24. PMID 19106642.

20. Morris MR, Hughes DJ, Tian YM, Ricketts CJ, Lau KW, Gentle D. Mutation analysis of hypoxia-inducible factors HIF1A and HIF2A in renal cell carcinoma. Anticancer Res. 2009;29(11):4337–43. PMID 20032376.

21. Chen MK, Chiou HL, Su SC, Chung TT, Tseng HC, Tsai HT, et al. The association between hypoxia inducible factor-1alpha gene polymorphisms and increased susceptibility to oral cancer. Oral Oncol. 2009;45(12):e222–6. PMID 19717330.

22. Shieh TM, Chang KW, Tu HF, Shih YH, Ko SY, Chen YC, et al. Association between the polymorphisms in exon 12 of hypoxia-inducible factor-1alpha and the clinic-pathological features of oral squamous cell carcinoma. Oral Oncol. 2010;46(9):e47–53. PMID 20656543.

23. Knechtel G, Szkandera J, Stotz M, Hofmann G, Langsenlehner U, Krippl P, et al. Single nucleotide polymorphisms in the hypoxia-inducible factor-1 gene and colorectal cancer risk. Mol Carcinog. 2010;49(9):805–9. PMID 20572162.

24. Kang MJ, Jung SA, Jung JM, Kim SE, Jung HK, Kim TH, et al. Associations between single nucleotide polymorphisms of MMP2, VEGF, and HIF1A genes and the risk of developing colorectal cancer. Anticancer Res. 2011;31(2):575–84. PMID 21378341.

25. Putra AC, Tanimoto K, Arifin M, Hiyama K. Hypoxia-inducible factor-1α polymorphisms are associated with genetic aberrations in lung cancer. Respirology. 2011;16(5):796–802. PMID 21435097.

26. Wang X, Liu Y, Ren H, Yuan Z, Li S, Sheng J, et al. Polymorphisms in the hypoxia-inducible factor-1α gene confer susceptibility to pancreatic cancer. Cancer Biol Ther. 2011;12(5):383–7. PMID 21709439.

27. Kuo WH, Shih CM, Lin CW, Cheng WE, Chen SC, Chen W, et al. Association of hypoxia inducible factor-1α polymorphisms with susceptibility to non-small-cell lung cancer. Transl Res. 2012;159(1):42–50. PMID 22153809.

28. Li P, Cao Q, Shao PF, Cai HZ, Zhou H, Chen JW, et al. Genetic polymorphisms in HIF1A are associated with prostate cancer risk in a Chinese population. PMID 23042446 Asian J Androl. 2012;14(6):864–9. PMID 23042446.

29. Fraga A, Ribeiro R, Príncipe P, Lobato C, Pina F, Maurício J, et al. The HIF1A functional genetic polymorphism at locus +1772 associates with progression to metastatic prostate cancer and refractoriness to hormonal castration. Eur J Cancer. 2014;50(2):359–65. PMID 24090974.

30. Orr-Urtreger A, Bar-Shira A, Matzkin H, Mabjeesh NJ. The homozygous P582S mutation in the oxygen-dependent degradation domain of HIF-1 alpha is associated with increased risk for prostate cancer. Prostate. 2007;67(1):8–13. PMID 16998808.

31. Apaydin I, Konac E, Onen HI, Akbaba M, Tekin E, Ekmekci A. Single nucleotide polymorphisms in the hypoxia-inducible factor-1alpha (HIF-1alpha) gene in human sporadic breast cancer. Arch Med Res. 2008;39(3):338–45. PMID 18279708.

32. Muñoz-Guerra MF, Fernández-Contreras ME, Moreno AL, Martín ID, Herráez B, Gamallo C. Polymorphisms in the hypoxia inducible factor 1-alpha and the impact on the prognosis of early stages of oral cancer. Ann Surg Oncol. 2009;16(8):2351–8. PMID 19449077.

33. Li K, Zhang Y, Dan Z, Wang Y, Ren ZC. Association of the hypoxia inducible factor-1-alpha gene polymorphisms with gastric cancer in Tibetans. Biochem Genet. 2009;47(9-10):625–34. PMID 19504235.

34. Hsiao PC, Chen MK, Su SC, Ueng KC, Chen YC, Hsieh YH, et al. Hypoxia inducible factor-1alpha gene polymorphism G1790A and its interaction with tobacco and alcohol consumptions increase susceptibility to hepatocellular carcinoma. J Surg Oncol. 2010;102(2):163–9. PMID 20648588.

35. Mera-Menéndez F, Hinojar-Gutiérrez A, Guijarro Rojas M, de Gregorio JG, Mera-Menéndez E, Sánchez JJ, et al. Polymorphisms in HIF-1alpha affect presence of lymph node metastasis and can influence tumor size in squamous-cell carcinoma of the glottic larynx. Clin Transl Oncol. 2013; 15(5):358–63. PMID 22914908.

36. Qin C, Cao Q, Ju X, Wang M, Meng X, Zhu J, et al. The polymorphisms in the VHL and HIF1A genes are associated with the prognosis but not the development of renal cell carcinoma. Ann Oncol. 2012;23(4):981–9. PMID 21778301.

37. Hu X, Fang Y, Zheng J, He Y, Zan X, Lin S, et al. The association between HIF-1α polymorphism and cancer risk: a systematic review and meta-analysis. Tumor Biol. 2014;35:903–16. PMID:24046090.

38. Yan Q, Chen P, Wang S, Liu N, Zhao P, Gu A. Association between HIF-1α C1772T/G1790A polymorphisms and cancer susceptibility: an updated systematic review and meta-analysis based on 40 case-control studies. BMC Cancer. 2014;14:950. PMID:25496056.

39. Liberati A, Altman DG, Tetzlaff J, Mulrow C, Gøtzsche PC, Ioannidis JP, et al. The PRISMA statement for reporting systemic reviews and meta-analyses of studies that evaluate health care interventions: explanation and elaboration. Ann Intern Med. 2009;151:W-65-94.

40. Liu IM, Agresti A. Mantel-Haenszel-type inference for cumulative odds ratios with a stratified ordinal response. Biometrics. 1996;52(4):1223–34.

41. Sutton AJ, Abrams KR, Jones DR, Sheldon TA, Song F. Methods for Meta-analysis in medical research. Chichester: John Wiley; 2000.

42. Cochran WG. The combination of estimates from different experiments. Biometrics. 1954;10:101–29.

43. Higgins JPT, Thompson SG. Quantifying heterogeneity in a meta-analysis. Stat Med. 2002;21:1539–58.

44. Light RJ, Pillemar DG. Summing Up: The science of Reviewing Research. Cambridge, MA: Harvard University Press; 1984.

45. Egger M, Smith GD, Schneider M, Minder C. Bias in meta-analysis detected by a simple, graphical test. BMJ. 1997;315(7109):629–4. doi:10.1136/bmj.315.7109.629.PMC2127453.

46. Zhao J. H. Gap: Genetic Analysis Package. R package version 1.1-12, 2014. http://cran.r-project.org/web/packages/gap/index.htmlFoundation for statistical computing (2008). R: a language and environment for statistical computing. Version 2.8.0. Vienna.

47. Zhao JH. Gap: genetic analysis package. J of Stat Software. 2007;23(8):1–18. http://www.jstatsoft.org/v23/i08.

7

Diagnosis and treatment of CD20 negative B cell lymphomas

Tasleem Katchi and Delong Liu[*]

Abstract

CD20 negative B cell non-Hodgkin lymphoma (NHL) is rare and accounts for approximately 1-2% of B cell lymphomas. CD20- negative NHL is frequently associated with extranodal involvement, atypical morphology, aggressive clinical behaviour, resistance to standard chemotherapy and poor prognosis. The most common types of these include plasmablastic lymphoma, primary effusion lymphoma, large B-cell lymphoma arising from HHV8-associated multicentric Castleman's disease, and ALK+ large B cell lymphoma. This review provides an overview of the diagnostic and treatment modalities for CD20 negative B cell NHL.

Background

CD20 is a glycosylated phosphoprotein expressed on the surface of all B cells (except early pro-B cells and plasma cells). Human CD20 molecule is encoded by the MS4A1 gene located on chromosome 11q12.2 [1, 2]. CD20 molecule is a tetra-transmembrane polypeptide with 297 amino acid residues. It plays a role in the differentiation, maturation and activation of B cells. CD20 is involved in the phosphorylation cascade of intracellular proteins by binding to Src family tyrosine kinases, such as Lyn, Fyn, and Lck. The CD20 molecule remains on the membrane of B cells without dissociation or internalization upon binding of CD20 antibody. CD20 expression varies in different lymphoma subtypes [3–5]. It is present from late pro-B cells through memory B cells, but not on early pro-B cells, plasmablasts and plasma cells. Plasma cell differentiation of B cells results in acquisition of plasma cell markers and loss of B cell antigens including the expression of CD20. CD20 was first defined by the murine monoclonal antibody (MoAb) tositumomab [6, 7]. Rituximab, a chimeric CD20 MoAb, was later developed and approved for treatment of human B cell malignancies. Rituximab destroys B lymphoid malignancies through complement-dependent cytotoxicity (CDC) and antibody-dependent cellular cytotoxicity (ADCC). The addition of rituximab, to cyclophosphamide, doxorubicin, vincristine, and prednisone (CHOP) has dramatically improved the survival of patients with diffuse large B cell lymphoma (DLBCL) [8, 9]. R-CHOP has since become the gold standard for the treatment of newly diagnosed DLBCL. In addition, rituximab has been found highly effective in a variety of B cell malignancies as well as relapsed and refractory lymphomas. Through recombinant DNA technology, second- and third- generation CD20 MoAbs were developed [2]. Among these, ofatumumab and obinutuzumab have been approved for clinical treatment of B cell malignancies, such as chronic lymphoid leukemia, and follicular lymphoma [10–15].

Genetic mutations of MS4A1 leading to conformational changes in the protein have been speculated to be a molecular mechanism of the CD20 negative phenotype [16]. The loss of CD20 expression is associated with extranodal involvement, a more aggressive clinical course, loss of responsiveness to rituximab and conventional chemotherapy, leading to poor prognosis. It poses a diagnostic and therapeutic dilemma and further studies need to be undertaken to establish the standard of care in this group of patients.

CD20 negative non-Hodgkin lymphomas

The pan-B lymphocyte markers include CD19, CD20, CD79a, and PAX-5 [2, 17–19]. Almost all B cell NHLs are positive for CD20. CD20- negative NHLs are rare with a rate of 1–2% of all B cell NHLs [20]. The most common types of these include plasmablastic lymphoma, primary effusion lymphoma, large B-cell lymphoma arising from

* Correspondence: DELONG_LIU@NYMC.EDU
Division of Hematology & Oncology, New York Medical College and Westchester Medical Center, Valhalla, NY 10595, USA

HHV8-associated multicentric Castleman's disease, and ALK+ large B cell lymphoma [20, 21].

Plasmablastic lymphoma (PBL) is the most common subtype of CD20 negative DLBCL, accounting for 75% of the cases with a median survival of 12 months [22, 23]. PBL is frequently associated with HIV and/or Epstein-Barr virus (EBV) co-infection. Immunoblastic lymphoma is frequently related and can be difficult to differentiate from PBL.

Primary effusion lymphoma (PEL), as the name suggests, presents as pleural, peritoneal and/or pericardial effusion. It is associated with HIV, EBV, and human herpesvirus 8 (HHV8) co-infection and has a median survival of 9 months [24].

Large B-cell lymphoma arising from HHV8-associated multicentric Castleman disease (MCD) usually presents in the setting of HIV infection. Unlike HHV-8 associated PEL, large B-cell lymphomas arising from MCD frequently has unmutated immunoglobulin IgM and lambda-chain restriction, suggesting an origin from HHV-8- positive plasmablasts [25].

Anaplastic lymphoma kinase (ALK) -positive DLBCL is a very rare type of DLBCL [26]. Unlike ALK+ anaplastic large cell lymphoma which harbors the ALK-NPM fusion gene from t(2;5) translocation with favorable prognosis, ALK+ DLBCL usually has t(2;17) (p23; q23) translocation which leads to a fusion gene of ALK-CLTC [27, 28]. Unlike the common DLBCL, ALK+ DLBCL is usually positive for CD38, CD138, and negative for CD20, CD30, and CD79a [28]. This type of lymphoma has a median survival of 20 months.

In addition to the above rare CD20 negative lymphomas, CD20 positive lymphoma can relapse as CD20 negative lymphoma after CD20 antibody therapy [29].

Diagnosis of CD20 negative NHL

DLBCL is identified by morphology and B cell biomarker analysis by immunohistochemistry and flow cytometry studies. However, CD20 negative DLBCL can pose a diagnostic dilemma. Immunohistochemical detection of CD19, CD79a and PAX-5 are the major biomarkers in establishing the diagnosis of CD20 negative B cell lymphoma. CD5 expression in DLBCL is mostly associated with Richter's transformation from a low-grade B-cell lymphoma, but has been seen in 5% of de novo DLBCL [30]. Similarly, CD10 expression is seen in both de novo DLBCL as well as in transformed follicular lymphomas [31]. Oct-2, Bob-1, and SOX11 are frequently examined and useful for differential diagnosis and accurate classification of lymphoma diagnosis [32, 33]. Flow cytometric analysis can reveal positivity for CD19, CD79a, CD5 and CD10 in cases of CD20 negative lymphoma.

Molecular analysis using cytogenetics or FISH (fluorescent in-situ hybridization) to detect rearrangements or translocations of Bcl-2, Bcl-6 and MYC is an important part of diagnosis. BCL-2 mutation was found frequently in human B cell lymphomas [34, 35]. Rearrangements or translocations of both BCL-2 and MYC are hallmarks of "double-hit" lymphomas which are typically more resistant to R-CHOP and portent poor prognosis. More intensive chemotherapy regimens and new agents like ibrutinib and lenalidomide appear to improve responses in these double-hit lymphomas [36].

Treatment strategies

There is still no standard of care for CD20 negative B cell lymphomas. Response to standard CHOP chemotherapy is inadequate. CODOX-M/IVAC (cyclophosphamide, vincristine, doxorubicin, methotrexate alternating with ifosfamide, etoposide, cytarabine) [37–44], dose-adjusted EPOCH (infusional etoposide, vincristine and doxorubicin along with bolus cyclophosphamide and prednisone) [45–47], and HyperCVAD (cyclophosphamide, vincristine, doxorubicin and dexamethasone alternating with high-dose methotrexate and cytarabine) [48–52], are the suggested therapies. Upregulation of the expression of CD20 in CD20-negative B cell acute lymphoblastic leukemia following treatment with 5-azacytidine has been reported [53]. In addition, good response to bortezomib in combination with infusional dose-adjusted EPOCH for the treatment of plasmablastic lymphoma has also been reported [54]. Upregulation of CD20 expression by epigenetic agents may be another option to re-sensitize B lymphoma to CD20 antibodies [55]. Plerixafor, a CXCR4 antagonist, has been shown to enhance rituximab-induced killing of lymphoma cells [56]. It would be interesting to examine whether plerixafor can have similar effect in CD20 negative lymphomas.

Conclusion

CD20 negative lymphoma is uncommon and has poor prognosis. It poses a diagnostic and therapeutic dilemma. Further studies need to be undertaken to establish the standard of care for this group of patients. Novel agents targeting B cell signalling pathways, such as, inhibitors of Bruton tyrosine kinase and phosphoinositol-3 kinase, may play important role in the therapy of this rare entity of B cell lymphomas [57–62]. PD-1 antibodies are active in lymphomas [63–65], it remains important to evaluate whether immune check point inhibitors have activity in CD20 negative lymphomas. Bcl-2 inhibitors may be another option for CD20 negative lymphomas and warrant further investigations [34, 66, 67].

Abbreviations
CHOP: cyclophosphamide, doxorubicin, vincristine, and prednisone; CODOX-M/IVAC: cyclophosphamide, vincristine, doxorubicin, methotrexate

alternating with ifosfamide, etoposide, cytarabine; EPOCH: etoposide, vincristine and doxorubicin along with bolus cyclophosphamide and prednisone; HyperCVAD: cyclophosphamide, vincristine, doxorubicin and dexamethasone alternating with high-dose methotrexate and cytarabine; MoAb: monoclonal antibody

Acknowledgement
We are indebted to our families for their unconditional support.

Funding
There was no funding involved in this study.

Author's contributions
DL designed the study. TK and DL drafted the manuscript. All authors involved in manuscript preparation and revisions. Both authors read and approved final manuscript.

Competing interests
The authors declare that they have no competing interests.

References
1. Tedder TF, Engel P. CD20: a regulator of cell-cycle progression of B lymphocytes. Immunol Today. 1994;15(9):450–4.
2. Cang S, Mukhi N, Wang K, Liu D. Novel CD20 monoclonal antibodies for lymphoma therapy. J Hematol Oncol. 2012;5:64.
3. Khandakar B, Wang W, Li S. Primary splenic red pulp diffuse large B-cell lymphoma with anaplastic features. Stem Cell Invest. 2016;3(4):9.
4. Liu Y, Zhang X, Zhong J-F. Current approaches and advance in mantle cell lymphoma treatment. Stem Cell Invest. 2015;2:18.
5. Mamorska-Dyga A, Ronny FMH, Puccio C, Islam H, Liu D. A rare case of the upper extremity diffuse large B-cell lymphoma mimicking soft tissue sarcoma in an elderly patient. Stem Cell Invest. 2016;3:25.
6. Alduaij W, Illidge TM. The future of anti-CD20 monoclonal antibodies: are we making progress? Blood. 2011;117(11):2993–3001.
7. Alduaij W, Ivanov A, Honeychurch J, Cheadle EJ, Potluri S, Lim SH, Shimada K, Chan CH, Tutt A, Beers SA, Glennie MJ, Cragg MS, Illidge TM. Novel type II anti-CD20 monoclonal antibody (GA101) evokes homotypic adhesion and actin-dependent, lysosome-mediated cell death in B-cell malignancies. Blood. 2011;117(17):4519–29.
8. Coiffier B. Rituximab in diffuse large B-cell lymphoma. Clin Adv Hematol Oncol. 2004;2(3):156–7.
9. Coiffier B, Lepage E, Briere J, Herbrecht R, Tilly H, Bouabdallah R, Morel P, Van Den Neste E, Salles G, Gaulard P, Reyes F, Lederlin P, Gisselbrecht C. CHOP chemotherapy plus rituximab compared with CHOP alone in elderly patients with diffuse large-B-cell lymphoma. N Engl J Med. 2002;346(4):235–42.
10. Mayes S, Brown N, Illidge TM. New antibody drug treatments for lymphoma. Expert Opin Biol Ther. 2011;11(5):623–40.
11. Tiwari A, Ayello J, Van de ven C, Cairo MS. Effect of obinutuzumab (GA101), a type II glycoengineered monoclonal antibody targeting CD20, against rituximab resistant and sensitive cell lines in B-cell non-Hodgkin lymphoma. ASCO Meet Abstr. 2012;30(15_suppl):e21150.
12. Umana P, Ekkehard M, Peter B, Gabriele K, Ursula P, Suter T, Grau R, Schmidt C, Herter S, Gerdes C, Nopora A, Patre M, Moser S, Sondermann P, Wheat L, Dyer MJS, Poppema S, Bauer S, Kubbies M, Strein P, Fertig G, Friess T, Dabbagh K, DalPorto J, Klein C. GA101, a novel humanized type II CD20 antibody with glycoengineered Fc and enhanced cell death induction, exhibits superior anti-tumor efficacy and superior tissue B cell depletion in vivo. ASH Annu Meet Abstr. 2007;110(11):2348.
13. van Meerten T, Hagenbeek A. CD20-targeted therapy: the next generation of antibodies. Semin Hematol. 2010;47(2):199–210.
14. Wierda WG, Kipps TJ, Mayer J, Stilgenbauer S, Williams CD, Hellmann A, Robak T, Furman RR, Hillmen P, Trneny M, Dyer MJS, Padmanabhan S, Piotrowska M, Kozak T, Chan G, Davis R, Losic N, Wilms J, Russell CA, Österberg A. Ofatumumab as single-agent CD20 immunotherapy in fludarabine-refractory chronic lymphocytic leukemia. J Clin Oncol. 2010;28(10):1749–55.
15. Wierda WG, Padmanabhan S, Chan GW, Gupta IV, Lisby S, Osterborg A, Hx CDSI. Ofatumumab is active in patients with fludarabine-refractory CLL irrespective of prior rituximab: results from the phase two international study. Blood. 2011;118(19):5126–9.
16. Gamonet C, Bole-Richard E, Delherme A, Aubin F, Toussirot E, Garnache-Ottou F, Godet Y, Ysebaert L, Tournilhac O, Dartigeas C, Larosa F, Deconinck E, Saas P, Borg C, Deschamps M, Ferrand C. New CD20 alternative splice variants: molecular identification and differential expression within hematological B cell malignancies. Exp Hematol Oncol. 2016;5(1):7.
17. Wang K, Wei G, Liu D. CD19: a biomarker for B cell development, lymphoma diagnosis and therapy. Exp Hematol Oncol. 2012;1(1):36.
18. Armitage JO. A clinical evaluation of the international lymphoma study group classification of non-Hodgkin's lymphoma. The Non-Hodgkin's lymphoma classification project. Blood. 1997;89(11):3909–18.
19. Dong HY, Browne P, Liu Z, Gangi M. PAX-5 is invariably expressed in B-cell lymphomas without plasma cell differentiation. Histopathology. 2008;53(3):278–87.
20. Castillo JJ, Chavez JC, Hernandez-Ilizaliturri FJ, Montes-Moreno S. CD20-negative diffuse large B-cell lymphomas: biology and emerging therapeutic options. Expert Rev Hematol. 2015;8(3):343–54.
21. Garg M, Lee BE, McGarry K, Mangray S, Castillo JJ. CD20-negative diffuse large B-cell lymphoma presenting with lactic acidosis. Am J Hematol. 2015;90(3):E49–50.
22. Castillo JJ, Furman M, Beltran BE, Bibas M, Bower M, Chen W, Diez-Martin JL, Liu JJ, Miranda RN, Montoto S, Nanaji NM, Navarro JT, Seegmiller AC, Vose JM. Human immunodeficiency virus-associated plasmablastic lymphoma: poor prognosis in the era of highly active antiretroviral therapy. Cancer. 2012;118(21):5270–7.
23. Gaur S, Padilla O, Nahleh Z. Clinical features and prognosis of CD20 negative aggressive B-cell Non-hodgkins lymphoma. Lymphoma. 2013;2013:290585.
24. Castillo JJ, Shum H, Lahijani M, Winer ES, Butera JN. Prognosis in primary effusion lymphoma is associated with the number of body cavities involved. Leuk Lymphoma. 2012;53(12):2378–82.
25. Du MQ, Bacon CM, Isaacson PG. Kaposi sarcoma-associated herpesvirus/human herpesvirus 8 and lymphoproliferative disorders. J Clin Pathol. 2007;60(12):1350–7.
26. Pan Z, Hu S, Li M, Zhou Y, Kim YS, Reddy V, Sanmann JN, Smith LM, Chen M, Gao Z, Wang HY, Yuan J. ALK-positive large B-cell lymphoma: a clinicopathologic study of 26 cases with review of additional 108 cases in the literature. Am J Surg Pathol. 2017;41(1):25–38.
27. De Paepe P, Baens M, van Krieken H, Verhasselt B, Stul M, Simons A, Poppe B, Laureys G, Brons P, Vandenberghe P, Speleman F, Praet M, De Wolf-Peeters C, Marynen P, Wlodarska I. ALK activation by the CLTC-ALK fusion is a recurrent event in large B-cell lymphoma. Blood. 2003;102(7):2638–41.
28. Chikatsu N, Kojima H, Suzukawa K, Shinagawa A, Nagasawa T, Ozawa H, Yamashita Y, Mori N. ALK+, CD30-, CD20- large B-cell lymphoma containing anaplastic lymphoma kinase (ALK) fused to clathrin heavy chain gene (CLTC). Mod Pathol. 2003;16(8):828–32.
29. Hiraga J, Tomita A, Sugimoto T, Shimada K, Ito M, Nakamura S, Kiyoi H, Kinoshita T, Naoe T. Down-regulation of CD20 expression in B-cell lymphoma cells after treatment with rituximab-containing combination chemotherapies: its prevalence and clinical significance. Blood. 2009;113(20):4885–93.
30. Matolcsy A, Chadburn A, Knowles DM. De novo CD5-positive and Richter's syndrome-associated diffuse large B cell lymphomas are genotypically distinct. Am J Pathol. 1995;147(1):207–16.
31. Lossos IS, Alizadeh AA, Diehn M, Warnke R, Thorstenson Y, Oefner PJ, Brown PO, Botstein D, Levy R. Transformation of follicular lymphoma to diffuse large-cell lymphoma: alternative patterns with increased or decreased expression of c-myc and its regulated genes. Proc Natl Acad Sci U S A. 2002;99(13):8886–91.
32. Browne P, Petrosyan K, Hernandez A, Chan JA. The B-cell transcription factors BSAP, Oct-2, and BOB.1 and the pan-B-cell markers CD20, CD22, and CD79a are useful in the differential diagnosis of classic Hodgkin lymphoma. Am J Clin Pathol. 2003;120(5):767–77.

33. Narurkar R, Alkayem M, Liu D. SOX11 is a biomarker for cyclin D1-negative mantle cell lymphoma. Biomark Res. 2016;4(1):6.

34. Cang S, Iragavarapu C, Savooji J, Song Y, Liu D. ABT-199 (venetoclax) and BCL-2 inhibitors in clinical development. J Hematol Oncol. 2015;8(1):129.

35. Cao Y, Yang G, Hunter ZR, Liu X, Xu L, Chen J, Tsakmaklis N, Hatjiharissi E, Kanan S, Davids MS, Castillo JJ, Treon SP. The BCL2 antagonist ABT-199 triggers apoptosis, and augments ibrutinib and idelalisib mediated cytotoxicity in CXCR4 wild-type and CXCR4 WHIM mutated waldenstrom macroglobulinaemia cells. Br J Haematol. 2015;170(1):134–8.

36. Younes A, Thieblemont C, Morschhauser F, Flinn I, Friedberg JW, Amorim S, Hivert B, Westin J, Vermeulen J, Bandyopadhyay N, de Vries R, Balasubramanian S, Hellemans P, Smit JW, Fourneau N, Oki Y. Combination of ibrutinib with rituximab, cyclophosphamide, doxorubicin, vincristine, and prednisone (R-CHOP) for treatment-naive patients with CD20-positive B-cell non-Hodgkin lymphoma: a non-randomised, phase 1b study. Lancet Oncol. 2014;15(9):1019–26.

37. Alwan F, He A, Montoto S, Kassam S, Mee M, Burns F, Edwards S, Wilson A, Tenant-Flowers M, Marcus R, Ardeshna KM, Bower M, Cwynarski K. Adding rituximab to CODOX-M/IVAC chemotherapy in the treatment of HIV-associated Burkitt lymphoma is safe when used with concurrent combination antiretroviral therapy. AIDS. 2015;29(8):903–10.

38. Sun H, Savage KJ, Karsan A, Slack GW, Gascoyne RD, Toze CL, Sehn LH, Abou Mourad Y, Barnett MJ, Broady RC, Connors JM, Forrest DL, Gerrie AS, Hogge DE, Narayanan S, Nevill TJ, Nantel SH, Power MM, Sutherland HJ, Villa D, Shepherd JD, Song KW. Outcome of patients with Non-Hodgkin lymphomas with concurrent MYC and BCL2 rearrangements treated with CODOX-M/IVAC with rituximab followed by hematopoietic stem cell transplantation. Clin Lymphoma Myeloma Leuk. 2015;15(6):341–8.

39. Evens AM, Carson KR, Kolesar J, Nabhan C, Helenowski I, Islam N, Jovanovic B, Barr PM, Caimi PF, Gregory SA, Gordon LI. A multicenter phase II study incorporating high-dose rituximab and liposomal doxorubicin into the CODOX-M/IVAC regimen for untreated Burkitt's lymphoma. Ann Oncol. 2013;24(12):3076–81.

40. Rodrigo JA, Hicks LK, Cheung MC, Song KW, Ezzat H, Leger CS, Boro J, Montaner JS, Harris M, Leitch HA. HIV-associated Burkitt lymphoma: good efficacy and tolerance of intensive chemotherapy including CODOX-M/IVAC with or without rituximab in the HAART Era. Adv Hematol. 2012;2012: 735392.

41. Corazzelli G, Frigeri F, Russo F, Frairia C, Arcamone M, Esposito G, De Chiara A, Morelli E, Capobianco G, Becchimanzi C, Volzone F, Saggese M, Marcacci G, De Filippi R, Vitolo U, Pinto A. RD-CODOX-M/IVAC with rituximab and intrathecal liposomal cytarabine in adult Burkitt lymphoma and 'unclassifiable' highly aggressive B-cell lymphoma. Br J Haematol. 2012; 156(2):234–44.

42. Barnes JA, Lacasce AS, Feng Y, Toomey CE, Neuberg D, Michaelson JS, Hochberg EP, Abramson JS. Evaluation of the addition of rituximab to CODOX-M/IVAC for Burkitt's lymphoma: a retrospective analysis. Ann Oncol. 2011;22(8):1859–64.

43. Mead GM, Barrans SL, Qian W, Walewski J, Radford JA, Wolf M, Clawson SM, Stenning SP, Yule CL, Jack AS, UKNCRILCS Group, Australasian L, Lymphoma G. A prospective clinicopathologic study of dose-modified CODOX-M/IVAC in patients with sporadic Burkitt lymphoma defined using cytogenetic and immunophenotypic criteria (MRC/NCRI LY10 trial). Blood. 2008;112(6):2248–60.

44. Davidson KL, Devaney MB, Tighe JE, Rogers SY, Dunlop DJ, Mackie MJ, Thomas RV, Johnson PR, Scotland and Newcastle Lymphoma Group Study. A pilot study of CODOX-M/IVAC in primary refractory or relapsed high-grade non-Hodgkin's lymphoma. A Scotland and Newcastle lymphoma group study. Haematologica. 2003;88(12):1366–71.

45. Dunleavy K, Pittaluga S, Shovlin M, Roschewski M, Lai C, Steinberg SM, Jaffe ES, Wilson WH. Phase II trial of dose-adjusted EPOCH in untreated systemic anaplastic large cell lymphoma. Haematologica. 2016;101(1):e27–29.

46. Purroy N, Bergua J, Gallur L, Prieto J, Lopez LA, Sancho JM, Garcia-Marco JA, Castellvi J, Montes-Moreno S, Batlle A, de Villambrosia SG, Carnicero F, Ferrando-Lamana L, Piris MA, Lopez A. Long-term follow-up of dose-adjusted EPOCH plus rituximab (DA-EPOCH-R) in untreated patients with poor prognosis large B-cell lymphoma. A phase II study conducted by the spanish PETHEMA group. Br J Haematol. 2015;169(2):188–98.

47. Dunleavy K, Pittaluga S, Maeda LS, Advani R, Chen CC, Hessler J, Steinberg SM, Grant C, Wright G, Varma G, Staudt LM, Jaffe ES, Wilson WH. Dose-adjusted EPOCH-rituximab therapy in primary mediastinal B-cell lymphoma. N Engl J Med. 2013;368(15):1408–16.

48. Linder K, Gandhiraj D, Hanmantgad M, Seiter K, Liu D. Complete remission after single agent blinatumomab in a patient with pre-B acute lymphoid leukemia relapsed and refractory to three prior regimens: hyperCVAD, high dose cytarabine mitoxantrone and CLAG. Exp Hematol Oncol. 2015;5:20.

49. Saste A, Arias-Stella J, Kuriakose P. Progression of a hepatosplenic gamma delta T-cell leukemia/lymphoma on hyperCVAD/MTX and ara-C: literature review and our institutional treatment approach. Clin Case Rep. 2016;4(1):67–71.

50. Daver N, Boumber Y, Kantarjian H, Ravandi F, Cortes J, Rytting ME, Kawedia JD, Basnett J, Culotta KS, Zeng Z, Lu H, Richie MA, Garris R, Xiao L, Liu W, Baggerly KA, Jabbour E, O'Brien S, Burger J, Bendall LJ, Thomas D, Konopleva M. A phase I/II study of the mTOR inhibitor everolimus in combination with HyperCVAD chemotherapy in patients with relapsed/refractory acute lymphoblastic leukemia. Clin Cancer Res. 2015;21(12):2704–14.

51. Romaguera JE, Fayad LE, Feng L, Hartig K, Weaver P, Rodriguez MA, Hagemeister FB, Pro B, McLaughlin P, Younes A, Samaniego F, Goy A, Cabanillas F, Kantarjian H, Kwak L, Wang M. Ten-year follow-up after intense chemoimmunotherapy with Rituximab-HyperCVAD alternating with Rituximab-high dose methotrexate/cytarabine (R-MA) and without stem cell transplantation in patients with untreated aggressive mantle cell lymphoma. Br J Haematol. 2010;150(2):200–8.

52. Dimopoulos MA, Weber D, Kantarjian H, Delasalle KB, Alexanian R. HyperCVAD for VAD-resistant multiple myeloma. Am J Hematol. 1996;52(2):77–81.

53. Rahme R, Benayoun E, Pautas C, Cordonnier C, Wagner-Ballon O, Maury S. Treatment with 5-azacytidin upregulates the expression of CD20 in CD20-negative B cell acute lymphoblastic leukemia: a case report. Exp Hematol. 2013;41(6):505–7.

54. Castillo JJ, Reagan JL, Sikov WM, Winer ES. Bortezomib in combination with infusional dose-adjusted EPOCH for the treatment of plasmablastic lymphoma. Br J Haematol. 2015;169(3):352–5.

55. Damm JK, Gordon S, Ehinger M, Jerkeman M, Gullberg U, Hultquist A, Drott K. Pharmacologically relevant doses of valproate upregulate CD20 expression in three diffuse large B-cell lymphoma patients in vivo. Exp Hematol Oncol. 2015;4(1):4.

56. Reinholdt L, Laursen MB, Schmitz A, Bødker JS, Jakobsen LH, Bøgsted M, Johnsen HE, Dybkær K. The CXCR4 antagonist plerixafor enhances the effect of rituximab in diffuse large B-cell lymphoma cell lines. Biomark Res. 2016;4(1):12.

57. Treon SP, Tripsas CK, Meid K, Warren D, Varma G, Green R, Argyropoulos KV, Yang G, Cao Y, Xu L, Patterson CJ, Rodig S, Zehnder JL, Aster JC, Harris NL, Kanan S, Ghobrial I, Castillo JJ, Laubach JP, Hunter ZR, Salman Z, Li J, Cheng M, Clow F, Graef T, Palomba ML, Advani RH. Ibrutinib in previously treated Waldenstrom's macroglobulinemia. N Engl J Med. 2015;372(15):1430–40.

58. Wu J, Liu C, Tsui ST, Liu D. Second-generation inhibitors of Bruton tyrosine kinase. J Hematol Oncol. 2016;9:80.

59. Wu J, Zhang M, Liu D. Acalabrutinib (ACP-196): a selective second-generation BTK inhibitor. J Hematol Oncol. 2016;9(1):21.

60. Wu J, Zhang M, Liu D. Bruton tyrosine kinase inhibitor ONO/GS-4059: from bench to bedside. Oncotarget. 2017;8:7201–7208.

61. Rai KR. Therapeutic potential of new B cell-targeted agents in the treatment of elderly and unfit patients with chronic lymphocytic leukemia. J Hematol Oncol. 2015;8:85.

62. Rai KR, Barrientos JC. Movement toward optimization of CLL therapy. N Engl J Med. 2014;370(12):1160–2.

63. Bi X-w, Wang H, Zhang W-w, Wang J-h, Liu W-j, Xia Z-j, Huang H-q, Jiang W-q, Zhang Y-j, Wang L. PD-L1 is upregulated by EBV-driven LMP1 through NF-κB pathway and correlates with poor prognosis in natural killer/T-cell lymphoma. J Hematol Oncol. 2016;9(1):109.

64. Shi L, Chen S, Yang L, Li Y. The role of PD-1 and PD-L1 in T-cell immune suppression in patients with hematological malignancies. J Hematol Oncol. 2013;6(1):74.

65. Ansell SM, Lesokhin AM, Borrello I, Halwani A, Scott EC, Gutierrez M, Schuster SJ, Millenson MM, Cattry D, Freeman GJ, Rodig SJ, Chapuy B, Ligon AH, Zhu L, Grosso JF, Kim SY, Timmerman JM, Shipp MA, Armand P. PD-1 blockade with nivolumab in relapsed or refractory Hodgkin's lymphoma. N Engl J Med. 2015;372(4):311–9.

66. Roberts AW, Davids MS, Pagel JM, Kahl BS, Puvvada SD, Gerecitano JF, Kipps TJ, Anderson MA, Brown JR, Gressick L, Wong S, Dunbar M, Zhu M, Desai

MB, Cerri E, Heitner Enschede S, Humerickhouse RA, Wierda WG, Seymour JF. Targeting BCL2 with venetoclax in relapsed chronic lymphocytic leukemia. N Engl J Med. 2016;374(4):311–22.

67. Souers AJ, Leverson JD, Boghaert ER, Ackler SL, Catron ND, Chen J, Dayton BD, Ding H, Enschede SH, Fairbrother WJ, Huang DC, Hymowitz SG, Jin S, Khaw SL, Kovar PJ, Lam LT, Lee J, Maecker HL, Marsh KC, Mason KD, Mitten MJ, Nimmer PM, Oleksijew A, Park CH, Park CM, Phillips DC, Roberts AW, Sampath D, Seymour JF, Smith ML, et al. ABT-199, a potent and selective BCL-2 inhibitor, achieves antitumor activity while sparing platelets. Nat Med. 2013;19(2):202–8.

8

Machine learning and systems genomics approaches for multi-omics data

Eugene Lin[1,2,3] and Hsien-Yuan Lane[1,4*]

Abstract

In light of recent advances in biomedical computing, big data science, and precision medicine, there is a mammoth demand for establishing algorithms in machine learning and systems genomics (MLSG), together with multi-omics data, to weigh probable phenotype-genotype relationships. Software frameworks in MLSG are extensively employed to analyze hundreds of thousands of multi-omics data by high-throughput technologies. In this study, we reviewed the MLSG software frameworks and future directions with respect to multi-omics data analysis and integration. Our review was targeted at researching recent approaches and technical solutions for the MLSG software frameworks using multi-omics platforms.

Keywords: Genomics, Pharmacogenomics, Single nucleotide polymorphisms, Machine learning, Multi-omics, Systems genomics

Background

Over the past few years, researchers and scientists have made remarkable progress in the interdisciplinary fields of precision medicine, data mining and predictive algorithms, bioinformatics, and computational medicine [1]. Machine learning and systems genomics (MLSG) approaches integrate multiple data types from multi-omics data by using data mining and predictive algorithms, pointing out that the MLSG approaches can support a more meaningful interpretation of phenotype-genotype relationships than an analysis using only a single data type. Therefore, there is an acute need for development of the MLSG software frameworks that can generate prediction of a given quantitative or categorical phenotype using next-generation multi-omic data [2].

Precision medicine, an emerging field of medicine, is becoming the cornerstone of medical practices with prospects of the customization of healthcare, which means medical decisions, practices, and treatments are tailored to individual patients [3]. The use of genomic biomarkers, such as multi-omics data, has played a major role in precision medicine in oncology and other chronic diseases such as asthma [4], mental disorders [5, 6], and diabetes [7–9]. More specifically, patients are divided into groups by genetic variability and other biomarkers so that medications may be tailored to individual patients with similar or related genetic characteristics [10, 11]. For example, accumulating evidence reveals that selected single nucleotide polymorphisms (SNPs) could be used as genetic markers to influence clinical treatment response and adverse drug reactions for antidepressants in patients with major depressive disorder [12–14]. With the advent of technology in multi-omics approaches such as genomics, proteomics, metabolomics, and epigenomics, we are able to employ materials or devices that can interact with biological systems at the molecular level and then target different molecules with high precision.

In big data science, machine learning methods are computer algorithms that can automatically learn to recognize complex patterns based on empirical data [15, 16]. The goal of an machine learning method is to enable an algorithm to learn from data of the past or present and use that knowledge to make predictions or decisions for unknown future events [17, 18]. In the general terms, the workflow for an machine learning method consists of three phases including build the model from example inputs, evaluate and tune the model, and then put the model into production in prediction-making. Some of the best-known algorithms in machine learning methods include

* Correspondence: hylane@gmail.com
[1]Graduate Institute of Biomedical Sciences, China Medical University, Taichung, Taiwan
[4]Department of Psychiatry, China Medical University Hospital, Taichung, Taiwan
Full list of author information is available at the end of the article

naive Bayes [19], C4.5 decision tree [20], artificial neural networks (ANNs) [21–23], support vector machine (SVM) [24], k-Means [25], k-nearest neighbors (kNN) [26], and regression [27, 28]. There were some key emerging diagnostics studies for various diseases and treatments of significance for public health with consideration of machine learning methods, including applications in mental health [29–33], cancer [34–38], and pharmacogenetics [39–41].

In this review, we surveyed the MLSG software frameworks that could enable definite assessment of the phenotype-genotype interplay status by using multi-omics platforms. The MLSG software frameworks encompass the model-based integration (MBI), concatenation-based integration (CBI), and transformation-based integration (TBI) approaches (Table 1). Furthermore, we investigated some potential data reduction and feature selection approaches that can be leveraged together with the MLSG software frameworks. Finally, we summarized the future perspectives with respect to the MLSG approaches.

Model-based integration approach

First, we explored the MBI approach, which generates multiple models using different data types as training sets, and then generates a final model from the multiple models created during the training phase (Fig. 1). One advantage of the MBI approach is that this approach can merge predictive models from different data types and each data type can be assembled from a different set of patients with same phenotype [42].

In order to identify interactions between different levels of genomic data associated with certain disease or phenotype (for example, survival in ovarian cancer), the MBI approach can integrate multi-omics data, including, but not limited to, miRNA, methylation, gene expression, and copy number variation data. The MBI approach can then conduct the final multi-dimensional model from a particular machine learning algorithm (for example, Bayesian networks) with variables from the best models of each individual genomic dataset. Next,

the MBI approach can compare the predictive power of the integration model with the one of the individual model from single level of genomic data to see whether the integration model can show the improvement. Finally, the MBI approach can obtain the best multi-dimensional model of all variables from multi-omics dimension as well as a balanced accuracy for the final model.

In the literature, the MBI approach encompasses the following computational frameworks for constructing a model: a majority voting approach [43], an ensemble classifier approach [44], and probabilistic causal networks [45]. In addition, we can employ the Analysis Tool for Heritable and Environmental Network Associations methodology, which is a suite of analysis tools for integrating multi-omics data [46].

Probabilistic causal network framework

In order to integrate highly dissimilar types of data, we can leverage Bayesian networks that are one type of probabilistic causal networks [47]. Bayesian networks are directed acyclic graphs where the edges of the graph are represented by conditional probabilities, which define the distribution of states of each node given the state of its parents [47]. In Bayesian networks, each node characterizes a quantitative trait that can be a genomic factor (such as variation in DNA, gene expression, methylation, metabolite, and protein). These conditional probabilities represent not only relationships between genomic factors, but also the stochastic nature of these relationships. By assuming the observed data as a function of our prior belief, the Bayes formula is used to determine the likelihood of a Bayesian network model. Because the number of potential network structures grows super-exponentially with the number of nodes, it is infeasible to find the best model by an exhaustive search of all possible structures. Therefore, we can utilize Monte Carlo Markov Chain simulation [48] to pinpoint probably a huge amount of different plausible Bayesian networks, which are then integrated to accomplish a consensus network model. In the beginning, there

Table 1 Summary, strength, and limitation of each method of machine learning and systems genomics (MLSG) software frameworks

Software framework	Summary	Strength	Limitation
Model-based integration (MBI)	Multiple predictive models are generated by using various multi-omics data types; then a final predictive model is generated by using the multiple models.	Predictive models can be consolidated from various multi-omics data types, and each data type can be gathered from a various set of patients with same phenotype.	It may be challenging to avoid overfitting.
Concatenation-based integration (CBI)	Multiple data matrices of different multi-omics data types are incorporated into a large input matrix; then a predictive model is generated by using the large input matrix.	It is fairly easy to leverage various machine learning methods for analyzing continuous or categorical data once a large input matrix is formed.	It may be challenging to combine a large input matrix.
Transformation-based integration (TBI)	Datasets for various multi-omics data types are first converted into intermediate forms, which are united into a large input matrix; then a predictive model is generated by using the large input matrix.	Unique variables such as patient identifiers can be used to link multi-omics data types and integrate a variety of continuous or categorical data values.	It may be challenging to transform into intermediate forms.

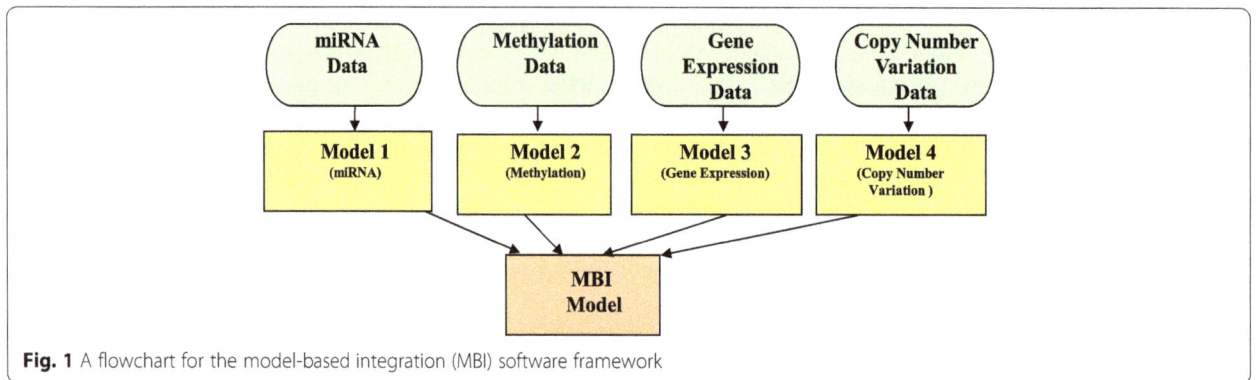

Fig. 1 A flowchart for the model-based integration (MBI) software framework

is a null network. Then, slight arbitrary changes are made to the network by flipping, adding, or deleting individual edges. Ultimately, accepting those changes will lead to an overall improvement by fitting the network to the data. In order to avoid over-fitting owing to the addition of new parameters, the Bayesian information criterion score [49] can be employed to assess whether a change improves the network model.

Ensemble classifier framework

In order to reduce the variance caused by the distinctiveness of a single genomic factor, Shen and Chou employed ensemble classifier models to integrate multiple classifiers, where each of those classifiers was based on individual genomic factor [50]. Thus, ensemble classifier models were able to obtain a more concrete concept in classification than a single classifier. The final output of the ensemble classifier model was the weighted fusion of the outputs generated by the individual basic classifiers. The weighted factor was assigned with the value of the success rate obtained by the individual basic classifier. Here, Shen and Chou adopted the optimized evidence-theoretic K-nearest-neighbors algorithm for the basic classifier [50].

Concatenation-based integration approach

Second, we investigated the CBI approach, which combines multiple data matrices for each dataset into one large input matrix before constructing a model (Fig. 2).

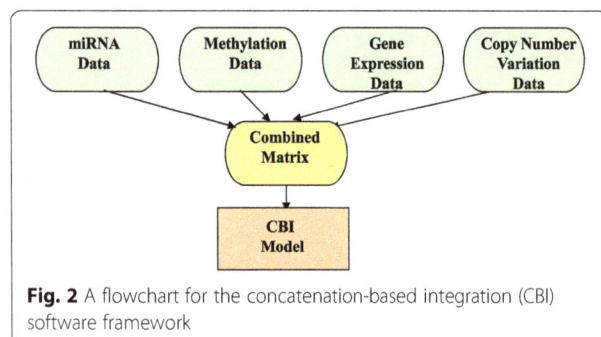

Fig. 2 A flowchart for the concatenation-based integration (CBI) software framework

One advantage of the CBI approach is that, after we determine how to combine all of the variables into one matrix, it is relatively simple to employ a variety of machine learning methods for analyzing continuous or categorical data [42].

In the literature, the CBI approach encompasses the following computational frameworks for constructing a model: Bayesian networks [51], multivariate Cox LASSO models [52], grammatical evolution neural networks [53], iCluster [54], Bayesian correlated clustering [55], and Bayesian consensus clustering [56]. In addition, We can consider some of the best-known machine learning algorithms including naive Bayes [19], C4.5 decision tree [20], ANNs [21–23], SVM [24], k-Means [25], kNN [26], and regression [27, 28]. Depending on the number of variables in the data matrix, we can also employ data reduction and feature selection methods as described below.

In order to assess response to cancer therapeutics such as gemcitabine, Fridley et al. employed a Bayesian integrative model, which combines the ideas of Bayesian pathway analysis with Bayesian variable selection using stochastic search variable selection [51]. They employed two various high-throughput multi-omics datasets, such as mRNA expression and SNPs data, which were integrated into one large input matrix [51]. Fridley et al. reported that the Bayesian integrative model had greater sensitivity to detect genomic effects in the drug gemcitabine, as compared to the traditional single data type analysis [51].

Furthermore, instead of a single data type, Shen et al. implemented the iCluster framework to carry out cancer subtype discovery in glioblastoma using three multi-omics data types such as copy number data, mRNA expression data, and methylation data [54]. The iCluster framework is a CBI method that can simultaneously accomplish both data integration and dimension reduction to combine multi-omics data into one large input matrix [54]. Shen et al. revealed three distinct integrated tumor subtypes by using iCluster and multi-omics data [54].

Transformation-based integration approach

Third, we assessed the TBI approach, which transforms each dataset into an intermediate form, such as a graph or a kernel matrix, and then merges multiple graphs or kernels into one before constructing a model (Fig. 3). One advantage of the TBI approach is that this approach can be employed to integrate a variety of continuous or categorical data values if the data contain unique variables such as patient identifiers for linking multi-omics data types [42].

In the literature, the TBI approach encompasses the following statistical frameworks for constructing a model: a kernel-based integration method [57] and a graph-based semi-supervised learning method [58]. The TBI approach investigates whether there is a relevant intermediate representation, such as a kernel or graph, for each multi-omics data type.

In order to find metabolic consequences underlying body weight change, Wahl et al. implemented a weighted correlation network approach [59], which was inferred using the Gaussian graphical model [60]. Instead of a single data type, they leveraged two different high-throughput multi-omics datasets, such as serum metabolomics and whole blood gene expression [59]. Wahl et al. first clustered multi-omics data into intermediate forms, namely modules of closely connected molecules, and then constructed a partial correlation network from the modules. Their analysis revealed that four metabolite and two gene expression modules were significantly associated with body weight change, indicating an association of long-term weight change with serum metabolite concentrations [59].

Data reduction and feature selection approach

Accounting for models is not a trivial task because even a relatively small set of factors results in the large number of possible models [61]. For example, if we study 10 factors, then these 10 factors yield 2^{10} possible models. The purpose of data reduction and feature selection approaches is to find a subset of factors that maximizes the performance of the prediction model, depending on how these methods incorporate the feature selection search with the classification algorithms. There are two data reduction and feature selection approaches including extrinsic approaches (which use information external to the data set itself) and intrinsic approaches (which use the data set and some analytical technique for filtering). The extrinsic approaches, such as Biofilter [62], employ prior knowledge that is accessible in the public domain. Additionally, the intrinsic approaches encompass factor analysis [63], ReliefF [64], chi-square statistics, principal component analysis [65], and genetic algorithms [66].

Furthermore, a hybrid approach, which combines the information-gain method and the chi-squared method, is designed to reduce bias introduced by each of the methods [67]. Each feature is measured and ranked according to its merit in both methods. The measurement of the merit for the two methods is defined as follows. The information-gain method measures the decrease in the entropy of a given feature provided by another feature, and the chi-squared method is based on Pearson chi-squared statistic to measure divergence from the expected distribution. Next, all features are sorted by their average rank across these two methods. After the features are ranked, the classifiers are utilized to add one feature at a time based on its individual ranking and then select the desired number of the top ranked features that provides the best predictive performance, respectively.

Moreover, in a wrapper-based feature selection approach, the feature selection algorithm acts as a wrapper around the classification algorithm. The wrapper-based feature selection approach conducts best-first search for a good subset using the classification algorithm itself as

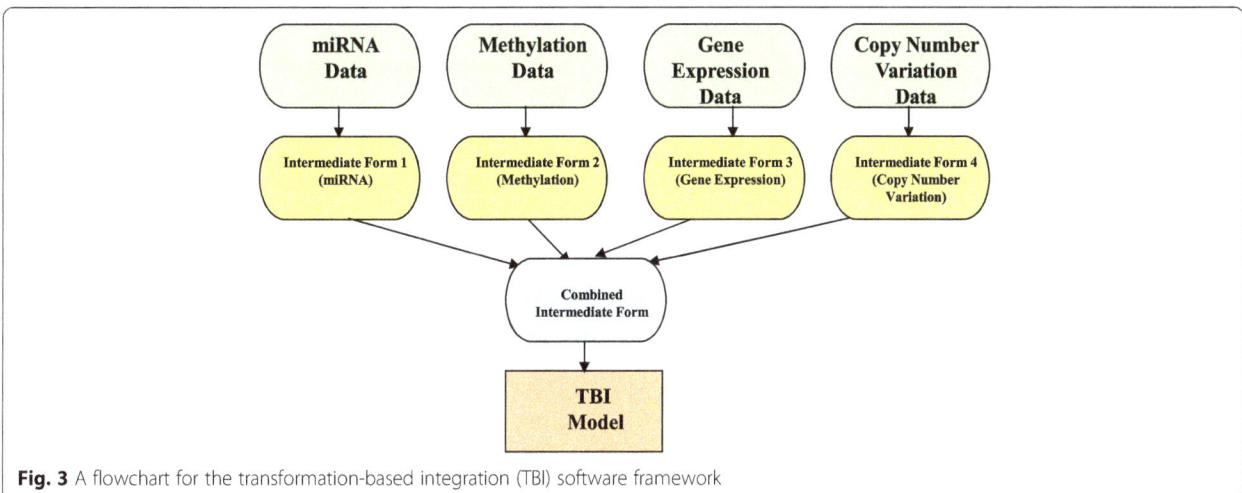

Fig. 3 A flowchart for the transformation-based integration (TBI) software framework

part of the function for evaluating feature subsets [68, 69]. Best first search starts with empty set of features and searches forward to select possible subsets of features by greedy hill-climbing augmented with a backtracking technique [18].

Future perspective

The MLSG modeling is essential to root out the false positive candidate genes discovered at the current association analyses by using meta-analysis, epistasis analysis, and pathway models [13]. Using multi-omics data not only could take care of missing information from any single data source, but also could help bridge the gap between phenotypes and more comprehensive biological regulation models [70]. In future research, models in MLSG will be established to predict the probability of drug efficacy to guide clinicians in choosing medications. In order to establish models for predicting drug efficacy, techniques in MLSG may provide a plausible way to predict drug efficacy in therapy. Finally, data analysis and integration in MLSG may play a key role in weighing gene–gene and gene–environment interactions.

Conclusions

In this study, we reviewed several recent findings and relevant studies in terms of the MLSG software frameworks. The work also underscores the importance of techniques in MLSG to track down a greater diversity of populations in the clinical settings of diseases and their treatments. In fact, facilitating the MLSG tools based on multi-omics data plays a pivotal role, economically and clinically, in predicting the possible outcomes of diseases and treatments. Future research using the MLSG approaches is needed in order to weigh the interplay among clinical factors and multi-omics data.

Abbreviations
ANNs: Artificial neural networks; CBI: Concatenation-based integration; kNN: k-nearest neighbors; MBI: Model-based integration; MLSG: Machine learning and systems genomics; SNPs: Single nucleotide polymorphisms; SVM: Support vector machine; TBI: Transformation-based integration

Acknowledgements
Not applicable.

Funding
This work was supported by the Ministry of Economic Affairs in Taiwan (SBIR Grant S099000280249-154), Taiwan Ministry of Health and Welfare Clinical Trial and Research Center of Excellence (MOHW105-TDU-B-212-133019), and China Medical University Hospital, Taiwan (DMR-101-091 and DMR-102-069). The funding supports had no role in study design, data collection and analysis, decision to publish, or preparation of the manuscript.

Authors' contributions
The present manuscript was drafted by EL and revised by EL and HYL. Both authors read and approved the final manuscript.

Competing interests
Both authors declare that they have no competing interests.

Author details
[1]Graduate Institute of Biomedical Sciences, China Medical University, Taichung, Taiwan. [2]Vita Genomics, Inc, Taipei, Taiwan. [3]TickleFish Systems Corporation, Seattle, WA, USA. [4]Department of Psychiatry, China Medical University Hospital, Taichung, Taiwan.

References
1. Katsanis SH, Javitt J, Hudson K. A case study of personalized medicine. Science. 2008;v320(4):53–4.
2. Snyderman R. Personalized health care: from theory to practice. Biotechnol J. 2012;v7:973–9.
3. Lin E. Novel drug therapies and diagnostics for personalized medicine and nanomedicine in genome science, nanoscience, and molecular engineering. Pharma Regul Aff. 2012;1:e116.
4. Lin E, Lin CG, Wang JY, Wu LS. Gene-gene interactions among genetic variants from seven candidate genes with pediatric asthma in a Taiwanese population. Curr Topics Genet. 2009;3:83–8.
5. Lin E, Hong CJ, Hwang JP, Liou YJ, Yang CH, Cheng D, et al. Gene-gene interactions of the brain-derived neurotrophic-factor and neurotrophic tyrosine kinase receptor 2 genes in geriatric depression. Rejuvenation Res. 2009;12(6):387–93.
6. Lin E, Tsai SJ. Gene-gene interactions in a context of individual variability in antipsychotic drug pharmacogenomics. Curr Pharmacogenomics Person Med. 2011;9:323–31.
7. Lin E, Pei D, Huang YJ, Hsieh CH, Wu LS. Gene-gene interactions among genetic variants from obesity candidate genes for nonobese and obese populations in type 2 diabetes. Genet Test Mol Biomarkers. 2009;13(4):485–93.
8. Wu LS, Hsieh CH, Pei D, Hung YJ, Kuo SW, Lin E. Association and interaction analyses of genetic variants in ADIPOQ, ENPP1, GHSR, PPARgamma and TCF7L2 genes for diabetic nephropathy in a Taiwanese population with type 2 diabetes. Nephrol Dial Transplant. 2009;24(11):3360–6.
9. Wang CH, Ke WS, Lin E. Evaluation of the ENPP1 and PLIN single nucleotide polymorphisms with type 2 diabetes in a Taiwanese population: evidence for replication and gene-gene interaction. J Investig Med. 2012;60(8):1169–73.
10. Lin E, Tsai SJ. Novel diagnostics R&D for public health and personalized medicine in Taiwan: current state, challenges and opportunities. Curr Pharmacogenomics Person Med. 2012;10:239–46.
11. Lin E, Hwang Y, Tzeng CM. A case study of the utility of the HapMap database for pharmacogenomic haplotype analysis in the Taiwanese population. Mol Diagn Ther. 2006;10:367–70.
12. Lin E, Chen PS. Pharmacogenomics with antidepressants in the STAR*D study. Pharmacogenomics. 2008;9:935–46.
13. Lin E, Lane HY. Genome-wide association studies in pharmacogenomics of antidepressants. Pharmacogenomics. 2015;16(5):555–66.
14. Lin E, Tsai SJ. Genome-wide microarray analysis of gene expression profiling in major depression and antidepressant therapy. Prog Neuropsychopharmacol Biol Psychiatry. 2016;64:334–40.
15. Kononenko I. Machine learning for medical diagnosis: history, state of the art and perspective. Artif Intell Med. 2001;23(1):89–109.
16. Lane HY, Tsai GE, Lin E. Assessing gene-gene interactions in pharmacogenomics. Mol Diagn Ther. 2012;16(1):15–27.
17. Landset S, Khoshgoftaar TM, Richter AN, Hasanin T. A survey of open source tools for machine learning with big data in the hadoop ecosystem. J Big Data. 2015;2:24.
18. Lin E, Tsai SJ. Machine learning and predictive algorithms for personalized medicine: from physiology to treatment. In: Turnbull A, editor. Personalized medicine. New York: Nova Science Publishers (in press).
19. Domingos P, Pazzani M. On the optimality of the simple Bayesian classifier under zero–one loss. Mach Learn. 1997;29:103–37.

20. Quinlan JR. C4.5: programs for machine learning. San Francisco: Morgan Kaufmann Publishers; 1993.

21. Kung SY, Hwang JN. Neural networks for intelligent multimedia processing. Proc IEEE. 1998;86:1244–72.

22. Bishop CM. Neural networks for pattern recognition. Oxford: Clarendon; 1995.

23. Rumelhart DE, Hinton GE, William RJ. Learning internal representation by error propagation. In: Parallel distributed processing: explorations in the microstructure of cognition. Cambridge: MIT Press; 1996. p. 318–62.

24. Vapnik V. The nature of statistical learning theory. New York: Springer; 1995.

25. Lloyd SP. Least squares quantization in PCM. IEEE Trans Inform Theory (Special Issue on Quantization). 1982;IT-28:129–37.

26. Altman NS. An introduction to kernel and nearest-neighbor nonparametric regression. Am Stat. 1992;46(3):175–85.

27. Friedman J, Hastie T, Tibshirani R. Regularization paths for generalized linear models via coordinate descent. J Stat Softw. 2010;33(1):1–22.

28. Zou H, Hastie T. Regularization and variable selection via the elastic net. J R Stat Soc Series B Stat Methodol. 2005;67(suppl):301–20.

29. Kessler RC, Warner CH, Ivany C, Petukhova MV, Rose S, Bromet EJ, et al. Predicting suicides after psychiatric hospitalization in US army soldiers. JAMA Psychiatry. 2015;72(1):49–57.

30. Huang LC, Hsu SY, Lin E. A comparison of classification methods for predicting chronic fatigue syndrome based on genetic data. J Transl Med. 2009;7:81.

31. Lin E, Chen PS, Yang YK, Lee IH, Yeh TL, Gean PW, et al. Modeling short-term antidepressant responsiveness with artificial neural networks. Open Access Bioinform. 2010;2:55–60.

32. Lin E, Tsai SJ. Genetics and suicide. In: Courtet P, editor. Understanding suicide - from diagnosis to personalized treatment. Switzerland: Springer; 2016.

33. Lin E, Hsu SY. Gender differences and pharmacogenomics with antidepressants in depression. In: Hernandez P, Alonso S, editors. Women and Depression. New York: Nova; 2009.

34. Kim W, Kim KS, Lee JE, Noh DY, Kim SW, Jung YS, et al. Development of novel breast cancer recurrence prediction model using support vector machine. J Breast Cancer. 2012;15(2):230–8.

35. Tseng CJ, Lu CJ, Chang CC, Chen GD. Application of machine learning to predict the recurrence-proneness for cervical cancer. Neural Comput & Applic. 2014;24(6):1311–6.

36. Chen YC, Ke WC, Chiu HW. Risk classification of cancer survival using ANN with gene expression data from multiple laboratories. Comput Biol Med. 2014;48:1–7.

37. Chang SW, Abdul-Kareem S, Merican AF, Zain RB. Oral cancer prognosis based on clinicopathologic and genomic markers using a hybrid of feature selection and machine learning methods. BMC Bioinformatics. 2013;14:170.

38. Rosado P, Lequerica-Fernández P, Villallaín L, Peña I, Sanchez-Lasheras F, de Vicente JC. Survival model in oral squamous cell carcinoma based on clinicopathological parameters, molecular markers and support vector machines. Expert Syst Appl. 2013;40(12):4770–6.

39. Lin E, Hwang Y, Wang SC, Gu ZJ, Chen EY. An artificial neural network approach to the drug efficacy of interferon treatments. Pharmacogenomics. 2006;7:1017–24.

40. Ke WS, Hwang Y, Lin E. Pharmacogenomics of drug efficacy in the interferon treatment of chronic hepatitis C using classification algorithms. Adv Appl Bioinform Chem. 2010;3:39–44.

41. Lin E, Hwang Y. A support vector machine approach to assess drug efficacy of interferon-alpha and ribavirin combination therapy. Mol Diagn Ther. 2008;12:219–23.

42. Ritchie MD, Holzinger ER, Li R, Pendergrass SA, Kim D. Methods of integrating data to uncover genotype-phenotype interactions. Nat Rev Genet. 2015;16(2):85–97.

43. Draghici S, Potter RB. Predicting HIV drug resistance with neural networks. Bioinformatics. 2003;19:98–107.

44. Akavia UD, Litvin O, Kim J, Sanchez-Garcia F, Kotliar D, Causton HC, et al. An integrated approach to uncover drivers of cancer. Cell. 2010;143:1005–17.

45. Zhu J, Sova P, Xu Q, Dombek KM, Xu EY, Vu H, et al. Stitching together multiple data dimensions reveals interacting metabolomic and transcriptomic networks that modulate cell regulation. PLoS Biol. 2012;10:e1001301.

46. Kim D, Li R, Dudek SM, Ritchie MD. ATHENA: identifying interactions between different levels of genomic data associated with cancer clinical outcomes using grammatical evolution neural network. BioData Min. 2013;6:23.

47. Pearl J. Probabilistic reasoning in intelligent systems: networks of plausible inference. San Mateo: Morgan Kaufmann Publishers; 1988.

48. Madigan D, York J. Bayesian graphical models for discrete data. Int Stat Rev. 1995;63:215–32.

49. Schwarz G. Estimating the dimension of a model. Ann Stat. 1978;6:461–4.

50. Shen HB, Chou KC. Ensemble classifier for protein fold pattern recognition. Bioinformatics. 2006;22(14):1717–22.

51. Fridley BL, Lund S, Jenkins GD, Wang LA. Bayesian integrative genomic model for pathway analysis of complex traits. Genet Epidemiol. 2012;36:352–9.

52. Mankoo PK, Shen R, Schultz N, Levine DA, Sander C. Time to recurrence and survival in serous ovarian tumors predicted from integrated genomic profiles. PLoS ONE. 2011;6:e24709.

53. Holzinger ER, Dudek SM, Frase AT, Pendergrass SA, Ritchie MD. ATHENA: the analysis tool for heritable and environmental network associations. Bioinformatics. 2014;30:698–705.

54. Shen R, Mo Q, Schultz N, Seshan VE, Olshen AB, Huse J, et al. Integrative subtype discovery in glioblastoma using iCluster. PLoS ONE. 2012;7:e35236.

55. Kirk P, Griffin JE, Savage RS, Ghahramani Z, Wild DL. Bayesian correlated clustering to integrate multiple datasets. Bioinformatics. 2012;28:3290–7.

56. Lock EF, Dunson DB. Bayesian consensus clustering. Bioinformatics. 2013;29:2610–6.

57. Lanckriet GRG, De Bie T, Cristianini N, Jordan MI, Noble WS. A statistical framework for genomic data fusion. Bioinformatics. 2004;20:2626–35.

58. Shin H, Lisewski AM, Lichtarge O. Graph sharpening plus graph integration: a synergy that improves protein functional classification. Bioinformatics. 2007;23:3217–24.

59. Wahl S, Vogt S, Stückler F, Krumsiek J, Bartel J, Kacprowski T, et al. Multi-omic signature of body weight change: results from a population-based cohort study. BMC Med. 2015;13:48.

60. Krumsiek J, Suhre K, Illig T, Adamski J, Theis FJ. Gaussian graphical modeling reconstructs pathway reactions from high-throughput metabolomics data. BMC Syst Biol. 2011;5:21.

61. Lin E, Huang LC. Identification of significant genes in genomics using Bayesian variable selection methods. Adv Appl Bioinform Chem. 2008;1:13–8.

62. Bush WS, Dudek SM, Ritchie MD. Biofilter: a knowledge-integration system for the multi-locus analysis of genome-wide association studies. Pac Symp Biocomput. 2009;368–379.

63. Hastie T, Tibshirani R, Friedman J. The elements of statistical learning: data mining, inference, and prediction. New York: Springer; 2001.

64. Greene CS, Penrod NM, Kiralis J, Moore JH. Spatially uniform ReliefF (SURF) for computationally efficient filtering of gene–gene interactions. BioData Min. 2009;2:5.

65. Zou H, Hastie T, Tibshirani R. Sparse principal component analysis. J Comput Graph Stat. 2006;15:265–86.

66. Holland JH. Genetic algorithms. Sci Am. 1992;267:66–72.

67. Saeys Y, Inza I, Larrañaga P. A review of feature selection techniques in bioinformatics. Bioinformatics. 2007;23:2507–17.

68. Kohavi R, John GH. Wrappers for feature subset selection. Artif Intell. 1997;97:273–324.

69. Lin E, Hwang Y, Liang KH, Chen EY. Pattern-recognition techniques with haplotype analysis in pharmacogenomics. Pharmacogenomics. 2007;8(1):75–83.

70. Leung MKK, Delong A, Alipanahi B, Frey BJ. Machine learning in genomic medicine: a review of computational problems and data sets. Proc IEEE. 2016;104(1):176–97.

9

Identification of potential serum biomarkers for breast cancer using a functional proteomics technology

David L. Wang[1], Chuanguang Xiao[2], Guofeng Fu[3], Xing Wang[3*] ⓘ and Liang Li[2*]

Abstract

Background: Cancer is a genetic disease; its development and metastasis depend on the function of many proteins. Human serum contains thousands of proteins; it is a window for the homeostasis of individual's health. Many of the proteins found in the human serum could be potential biomarkers for cancer early detection and drug efficacy evaluation.

Methods: In this study, a functional proteomics technology was used to systematically monitor metabolic enzyme and protease activities from resolved serum proteins produced by a modified 2-D gel separation and subsequent Protein Elution Plate, a method collectively called PEP. All the experiments were repeated at least twice to ensure the validity of the findings.

Results: For the first time, significant differences were found between breast cancer patient serum and normal serum in two families of enzymes known to be involved in cancer development and metastasis: metabolic enzymes and proteases. Multiple enzyme species were identified in the serum assayed directly or after enrichment. Both qualitative and quantitative differences in the metabolic enzyme and protease activity were detected between breast cancer patient and control group, providing excellent biomarker candidates for breast cancer diagnosis and drug development.

Conclusions: This study identified several potential functional protein biomarkers from breast cancer patient serum. It also demonstrated that the functional proteomics technology, PEP, can be applied to the analysis of any functional proteins in human serum which contains thousands of proteins. The study indicated that the functional domain of the human serum could be unlocked with the PEP technology, pointing to a novel alternative for the development of diagnosis biomarkers for breast cancer and other diseases.

Keywords: Biomarkers, Diagnostic kits, Breast cancer, Functional proteomics, Enzyme activity, Hexokinases, Proteases, Protein Elution Plate

Background

Human breast cancer is a major cause of morbidity and mortality in women. Data from the International Agency for Research on Cancer (IARC) showed that the incidence of cancer has increased all over the world. Regarding breast cancer, the highest incidence rates were found in the United States and Western Europe with 101 and 85 new cases per 100.000 women, respectively [1]. The American Cancer Society estimates that each year more than 230,000 Americans women will be diagnosed with this neoplasia and that more than 40,000 will die of the disease in the United States. Presymptomatic screening to detect early-stage cancer while it is still resectable with potential for cure can significantly reduce breast cancer-related mortality. Unfortunately, only about half of the breast cancers diagnosed are before the metastatic stage [2]. One reason that contributes to the poor prognosis of patients diagnosed with breast cancer is the fact that the diagnosis is often delayed due to limitations in mammography. Screen-film mammography (SFM) is considered

* Correspondence: xing.wang@arraybridge.com; liliangzb@sina.com
[3]Array Bridge Inc., 4320 Forest Park Ave, Suite 303, St. Louis, MO 63108, USA
[2]Zibo Central Hospital, Zibo, China
Full list of author information is available at the end of the article

the gold standard for breast cancer screening and detection. However, its optimal performance is only observed among women over 50 years old. Also, SFM has other limitations such as high rates of false-negative (between 4 and 34%). In addition, there is a high rate of false-positives that lead to unnecessary biopsy procedures [1].

In the last decade, many new technologies have been utilized for biomarker discovery with significant progress. Each of these technologies has focused on a different type of biological entity such as circulating tumor cells (CTC), extracellular vesicles, micro-RNAs and cancer-derived cell-free DNA or circulating tumor-derived DNA (ctDNA) [3–12]. However, several fundamental issues such as tumor heterogeneity, plasticity and diversity of cancer stem cells (CSC) make biomarker discovery and development a challenging endeavor. The variation introduced during sample collection and storage and the lack of robust validation approach once biomarker leads are identified further complicate biomarker development. As a result of these hurdles, there are currently no United States FDA-approved serum tests for early detection of the disease [1]. Given the considerable public health importance of breast cancer, it is crucial to quickly identify new biomarkers with the potential to enhance early diagnosis and to predict patient prognosis, drug resistance development and treatment choice.

Blood based biomarkers have great potential in cancer screening and their role could extend further from general population risk assessment to treatment response evaluation and recurrence monitoring. The rich content of diverse cellular and molecular elements in blood, which provide information about the health status of an individual, make it an ideal compartment to develop noninvasive diagnostics for cancer [13]. However, despite a large literature collection related to biomarkers for common cancers, blood based diagnostic tests that inform about the presence of cancer at an early stage and predict treatment response have been difficult to develop [11, 14–16].

For the past decade, proteomics has been used for the discovery of potential biomarkers from human fluids including serum [4, 6, 17, 18]. So far, most efforts in proteomics has been focused on the identification and sequence annotation of the proteome by mass spectrometry analyses of peptides derived through proteolytic processing of the parent proteome [19]. In such a manner, thousands of proteins have been identified from human serum (www.serumproteome.org). However, no validated protein biomarker currently exists for use in routine clinical practice for breast cancer early detection, prognosis and the prediction of treatment response. It is generally recognized that sequence annotation alone cannot capture this vital information, so new strategies are necessary.

Two-Dimensional (2-D) Gel Electrophoresis is a powerful tool used to separate complex protein samples because more than 10,000 protein spots can be detected with information on their relative abundance and post-translational modifications. Recently, a modified 2-D Gel Electrophoresis process was integrated with a special protein elution and refolding process to achieve high resolution of protein species from a proteome called PEP [20]. Many of the fractions recovered by the PEP technology with enzyme activity appear to contain just one or two major proteins, making the positive identification of the protein of interest relatively easy.

It is hypothesized that the levels and distributions of certain enzyme functions in serum could produce proteomic features and collective profiles which reflect physiological changes of an individual and can serve as possible biomarkers or diagnostic parameters. Our earlier studies using lung cancer patient serum and normal serum have identified many fractions with metabolic enzyme activity and the enzymes identified could serve as potential functional biomarkers for the diagnostic of lung cancer [21]. In the current study, we used both enriched serum samples as well as original serum pools from breast cancer patients and normal people for the systematic analysis of metabolic enzyme and protease activities with the PEP technology. In both type of samples, a large number of fractions with metabolic enzymes and proteases were identified with significant differences between breast cancer and normal serum. We believe that the further identification and validation of those functional proteins could lead to the development of biomarkers for breast diagnosis.

Methods

Materials

All the chemicals were purchased from MilliporeSigma (St. Louis, MO). Isoelectric Focusing (IEF) unit that is capable of running IEF at different length is from Bio-Rad (PROTEAN IEF Cell). Spectrophotometer Plate Reader capable of reading 384-well plates with a wide wavelength selection and fluorescence reading is the SPECTRAMax Plus from Molecular Devices (Sunnydale, CA). Semi-Blot unit for protein transfer such as Bio-Rad's Trans-Blot SD Semi-Dry Transfer Cell. AlbuVoid™ serum protein enrichment beads was from Biotech Support Group (Monmouth Junction, NJ). Protein Elution Plate (PEP) is a product of Array Bridge (St. Louis, MO).

AlbuVoid™ treatment for low abundance serum protein enrichment

200 mg of AlbuVoid™ beads were used to process 0.8 ml of human serum (contains about 40 mg total serum protein). The breast cancer patient serum and the matching normal people serum were collected at Zibo Central Hospital in China after the approval from the Hospital Ethics Committee with reference number of 20140102. Serum samples from normal people or breast cancer

patient were pooled with equal volume (100 μl each) respectively and either used directly in the analysis or enriched for low abundance serum proteins with Albu-Void™ according to the manufacturer's instruction before loading to the IEF. The enriched low abundance serum proteins were eluted with 0.8 ml elution solution containing 8 M urea, 2% CHAPS in 25 mM phosphate buffer, pH 8.0. The protein concentration was determined by BCA before 2-D gel electrophoresis.

Isoelectric focusing (IEF) and 2-D gel electrophoresis

To prepare for the IEF separation, Bio-Lyte Ampholyte (Bio-Rad #1631112) was added to the serum solution directly or AlbuVoid™ elute above with a final concentration of 0.5%. Rehydration was using 0.4 ml sample solution with nonlinear pH 3–10 11 cm IPG strip (Bio-Rad Ready-Strip #1632016) overnight with a total loading of 1 mg protein/IPG strip. In the experiments without AlbuVoid™ enrichment, 1 mg of serum protein from the pooled breast cancer patient or unaffected individual was used directly following the same sample preparation as described above. All the enriched and unenriched serum proteins were separated in the same IEF run. The proteins were separated using the following setting: 0–7000 linear gradient voltage for 4 h hold at 7000 voltages overnight until running termination at room temperature. After IEF, the IPG strips were taken off the running unit, mineral oil from the IPG strip was absorbed with a paper towel and the IPG strip was transferred to a 12-lane refolding tray (Bio-Rad #1654025). 4 ml refolding solution was added to each lane with the IPG strip and incubated for 10 min., which allows the urea to diffuse out of the IPG strip and permits the refolding of the protein., This was followed by incubation in electrophoresis transfer buffer (Tris-glycine with 0.1% SDS), which allows for the further diffusion of urea from the IPG strip and the binding of SDS to the protein so that all the proteins were negatively charged. For protein refolding, a proprietary protein refolding solution was used; the solution contains multiple metal elements to replace the possible loss of metal ions as enzyme cofactors. A redox system to mimic the cell cytoplasm was used to assist the protein refolding process. After protein refolding, the IPG strip was laid down to a precast 2-D gel (Bio-Rad 10–20% Criterion Gel #3450107) with the acidic end of the IPG on the left side of the 2-D gel when facing the gel apparatus. The gel was operated at 80 V for 15 min. followed by running at 120 voltages until the dye front of the gel was 0.5 cm from the bottom edge of the gel.

Electroelution and protein recovery from the Protein Elution Plate (PEP)

After second dimension gel electrophoresis, the gel was taken out from the cassette, and laid on top of the PEP plate which was filled with elution solution. The proteins

were transferred from the gel to the PEP plate for 60 min. at 20 V using a Semi-Blot apparatus from Bio-Rad (#1703940.). After protein transfer, the gel was carefully lifted from the PEP plate, and a multi-channel pipette transferred the eluted proteins from the PEP plate to a master plate which contained 50 μl PBS in each well. About 40–45 μl of solution could be transferred from the PEP plate to the Master Plate for a total volume of 90–95 μl in each well. In this analysis, 25 μl solutions was taken from each well in the Master Plate and transferred to an enzyme assay plate to perform the enzyme assay.

Hexokinase activity assay

Hexokinase activity can be monitored by a cascade reaction as follows:

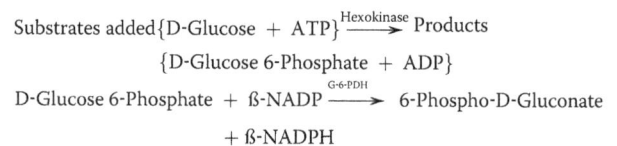

$$\text{Substrates added} \{\text{D-Glucose} + \text{ATP}\} \xrightarrow{\text{Hexokinase}} \text{Products}$$
$$\{\text{D-Glucose 6-Phosphate} + \text{ADP}\}$$
$$\text{D-Glucose 6-Phosphate} + \text{ß-NADP} \xrightarrow{\text{G-6-PDH}} \text{6-Phospho-D-Gluconate}$$
$$+ \text{ß-NADPH}$$

In the final assay solution, glucose was at 216 mM; $MgCl_2$ at 7.8 mM, ATP at 0.74 mM and NADP at 1.1 mM. 25 μl of this enzyme assay solution was mixed with 25 μl of sample from the Master Plate (described above) and the enzyme activity was monitored by the 340 nm absorbance from the reduction of NADP to NADPH. The readings at 0, 1 h., 2 h. was recorded for both the normal serum and breast cancer patient serum sample. However, in lieu of purified G-6-PDH, 0.25 mg/ml beef liver protein was used as the source of Glucose-6-Phosphate Dehydrogenase (G-6-PDH). The assay thus reports the additive contributions of the endogenous hexokinase activity present in the beef liver extract, and any exogenous activity from the presence of test sera protein in the PEP plate, which may influence the reduction of NAD or NADP (the reporting signal). In light of the ambiguities that may arise from such a reporting system, the primary goal of this investigation was to generate sufficient signal intensities and activity features which could monitored and compared between the two samples types within an 'omics' context. Therefore, this broader spectrum assay was chosen that could potentially detect the activities of downstream glycolytic and other cross-regulating proteins from the test sera.

Protease activity

FITC-labeled casein was used as general protease substrate at 0.5 mg/mL final concentration.

25 μl each of the PEP plate sample and substrate were incubated at room temperature overnight in the dark, after protease digestion, the casein was precipitated with 10% TCA (trichloroacetic acid) and the supernatant was

neutralized with Tris base and used for the fluorescence measurement.

Proteases Assay:

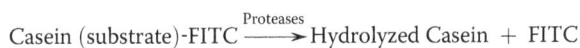

$$\text{Casein (substrate)-FITC} \xrightarrow{\text{Proteases}} \text{Hydrolyzed Casein} + \text{FITC}$$

Enzyme activity display

Two Microsoft Excel formats were used to display the enzyme activities. One is to use the 3-D column display and the other is to use the heat map.

Results

Comparison of hexokinase activity from normal serum and breast cancer patient serum

Previous effort in proteomics has identified thousands of proteins from human serum, a high percentage of the proteins identified are enzymes with significant numbers belongs to metabolic enzymes and proteases (www.serumproteome.org). There have been many reports of single or multiple protein panels as potential biomarkers for breast cancer diagnosis, however so far there are no routinely used serum-based biomarkers approved for breast cancer [1]. As a successful diagnostic biomarker, it will need to achieve a high level of sensitivity and specificity in its detection to minimize false negatives and false positives respectively because a high proportion of those false results have significant consequences both economically and also emotionally. During the development of serum biomarkers, one of the challenges is the wide range of physiological variations among the general population which causes potential biomarkers to overlap between the normal and patient group. In retrospective studies, a panel of serum biomarkers are often identified with excellent separation between the normal and disease group but failed during the validation process using collected clinical samples. In the current study, two aspects were unique: 1. the search for possible biomarkers is from a new domain of the serum proteome, i.e. the functional domain. It is hoped that this new dimension of information can provide a distinct signature for breast cancer when compared with normal serum. 2. When selecting the biomarker candidates, the effort was started with pooled serum instead of individuals. In this approach, the individual physiological variations of serum proteins from the normal or cancer patients were averaged, which will partially reduce the variations from the individuals and help identify those proteins that showed significant differences between the normal and disease groups. Once the potential biomarker(s) are identified, their discriminating power for the normal and disease individuals will be tested during the validation stage. 3. Only those fractions with qualitative differences (the detected active fraction is totally missing from a group) or 10-fold differences will be further investigated.

This will increase the possibility of eventual validation of the biomarker candida(s) in a large clinical sample collection. To demonstrate that hexokinase activity can be monitored from the PEP fractions, the reduction of NADP was measured at different time points. As can be seen in Figs. 1 and 2, many fractions from the normal serum have time-dependent hexokinase activities. Similarly, measurements on the serum from breast cancer patients also showed many fractions with hexokinase activities, and more interestingly, there are both qualitative and quantitative differences between the normal serum and cancer patient serum. For example, in the normal serum, F2 and G2 have significant levels of hexokinase activity whereas the corresponding fractions in the breast cancer patient serum are at baseline levels; the same is true for fractions P1 and P2. Conversely, from the breast cancer patient serum, fractions K3, I7, J7 and H8 each have significant hexokinase activities while the enzyme activity from the corresponding fractions in the normal group only showed baseline levels of activity (Fig. 2). As expected, those fractions with enzyme activity showed a time-dependent activity increase (Figs. 1 and 2). Another area that showed a significant difference in hexokinase activity was the high molecular weight region with pI between 7 and 8 (see the boxed area in Fig. 2). Interestingly, the fractions with hexokinase activity were detected across a wide range of molecular size and isoelectric points, suggesting that: 1.) there are many serum proteins that could directly or indirectly impact hexokinase activities within this assay system, and 2.) there could be protein variants that show different hexokinase activity among the fractions.

Comparison of protease activity from normal serum and breast cancer patient serum

Previous studies have shown that a large number of proteases exist in the human serum. (www.serumproteome.org) However, only a limited number of proteases were shown to have enzymatic activities [22]. In this study, protease activities were monitored systematically from the human serum directly using the PEP technology. Multiple fractions with protease activities were identified that showed significant different between normal and breast cancer patient serum (Fig. 3). The majority of the fractions with protease activities were detected in the acidic protein region (pI from 3 to 7) whereas very little activity was observed in the basic protein region. For protease activity detection, protein enrichment with AlbuVoid™ will make a significant difference, the principle of AlbuVoid™ is to use a chemically synthesized material to absorb serum proteins except albumin, by allowing albumin to be specifically wash off from the AlbuVoid™ column, the other low abundance serum proteins are enriched on the column and eluted with an elution solution ; details of the protease

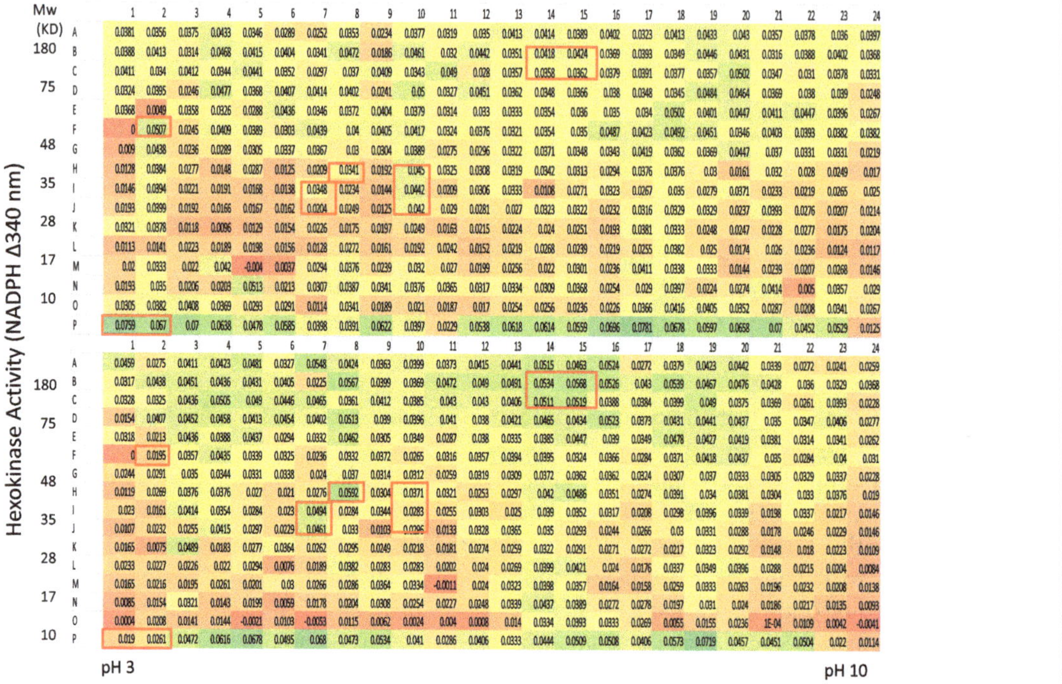

Fig. 1 Direct measurement of hexokinase activity from normal and breast cancer serum after PEP protein separation and elution (60 min). After elution of proteins from the 2-D gel into the 384-well PEP plate, the eluted proteins were further transferred into a 384-well Master Plate with 50 µl refolding solution. 25 µl of the solution from the Master Plate was further transferred into a 384-well Enzyme Assay plate, 25 µl of hexokinase assay components were was added to each well, the increase of OD 340 nm by NADP reduction was measured in a spectrophotometer, the OD readings were taken at 0 and 60 min. the OD340 nm increase from 60 min. was calculated by subtracting the value from the 0 min. reading. Boxed fractions indicated samples of interest

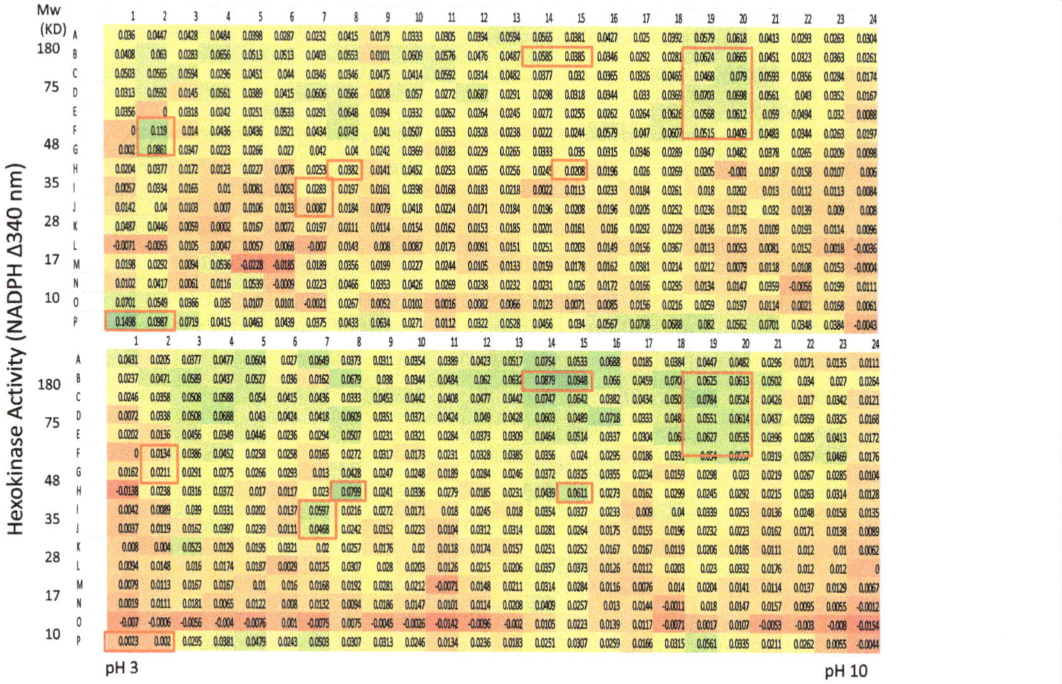

Fig. 2 Direct measurement of hexokinase activity from normal and breast cancer serum after PEP protein separation and elution (120 min). The conditions were the same as in Fig. 1, the OD readings were taken at 0 and 120 min. the OD340 nm increase from 120 min. was calculated by subtracting the value from the 0 min. reading. Boxed fractions indicated samples of interest

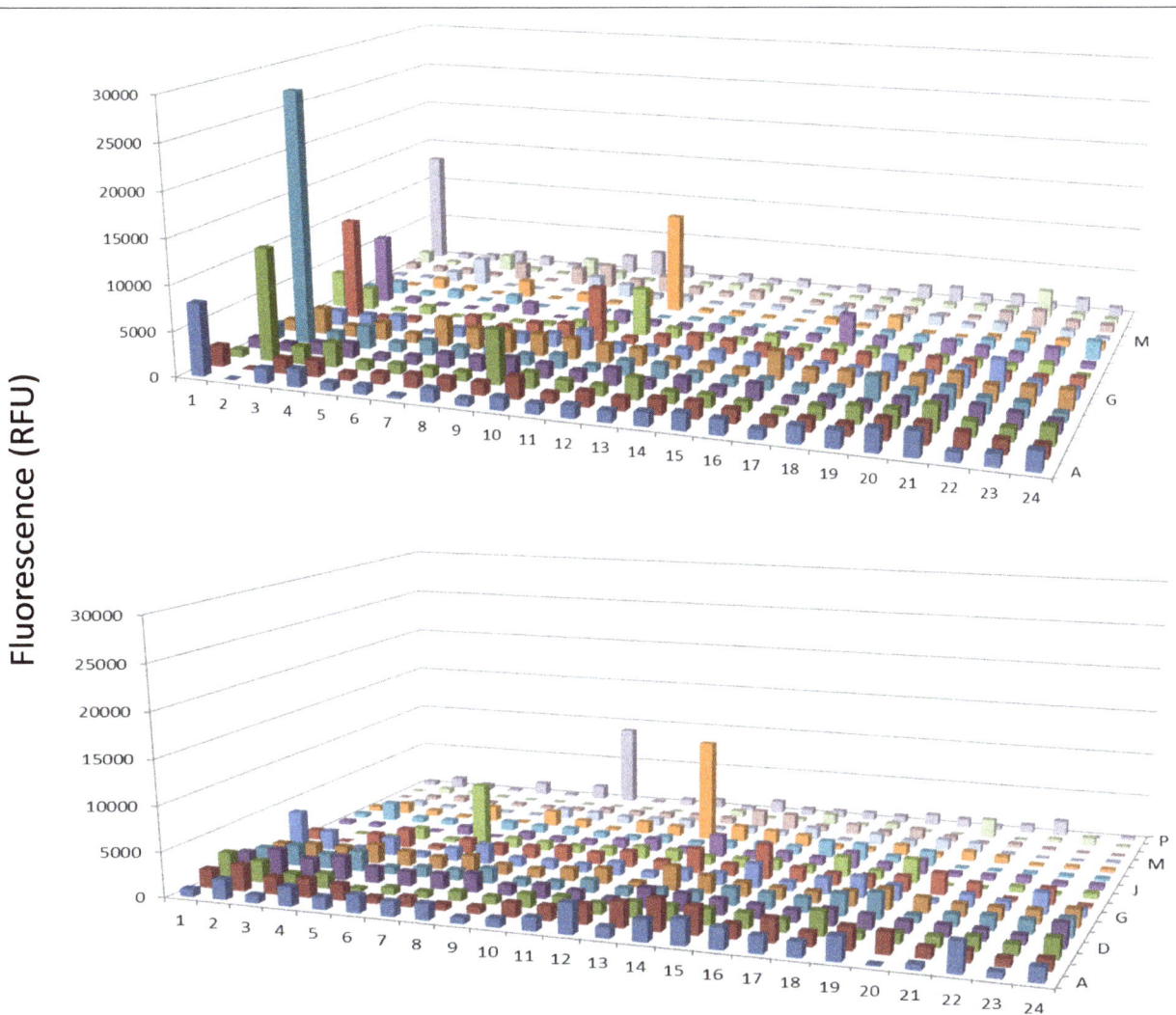

Fig. 3 Direct measurement of protease activity from normal and breast cancer serum after PEP protein separation and elution. The conditions were the same as in Fig. 1 except protease substrate was added to the assay plate. The assay was carried out at room temperature overnight, for more details please refer to the material and method. Boxed fractions indicated samples of interest

activity analysis will be discussed in the later part of this section.

Comparison of hexokinase activity from enriched normal serum and breast cancer patient serum

Previous work in using AlbuVoid™ has demonstrated that the profile of serum proteins and enzymatic activities will be changed significantly during the enrichment [21, 23]. (In this study, it was shown that the depletion of albumin can significantly enrich hexokinase activities (Figs. 4 and 5). Compared with the direct serum assay (Figs. 1 and 2), more fractions with hexokinase activities were detected across a wide range of molecular weight and isoelectric points (see Fig. 5 boxed). In the comparison of normal and breast cancer patient serum, many fractions with both qualitative and quantitative hexokinase activity differences were detected (see the boxed fractions

in Fig. 5 for details). This demonstrated that AlbuVoid™ is a very effective tool for the enrichment of low abundancy proteins with enzyme activity. As a result of this enrichment, there are more candidate fractions to choose from for further biological validation as potential biomarkers.

Comparison of protease activity from enriched normal serum and breast cancer patient serum

The most dramatic difference for enzyme activity detection in using the AlbuVoid™ for serum protein enrichment was demonstrated in the case of protease activity analysis. Figure 6 indicated that a large number of fractions were shown to have protease activities after serum protein enrichment. Compared with the direct serum proteinase measurement (Fig. 3), both the levels and species of proteases were increased significantly in the enriched serum sample. The fact that very few fractions were detected

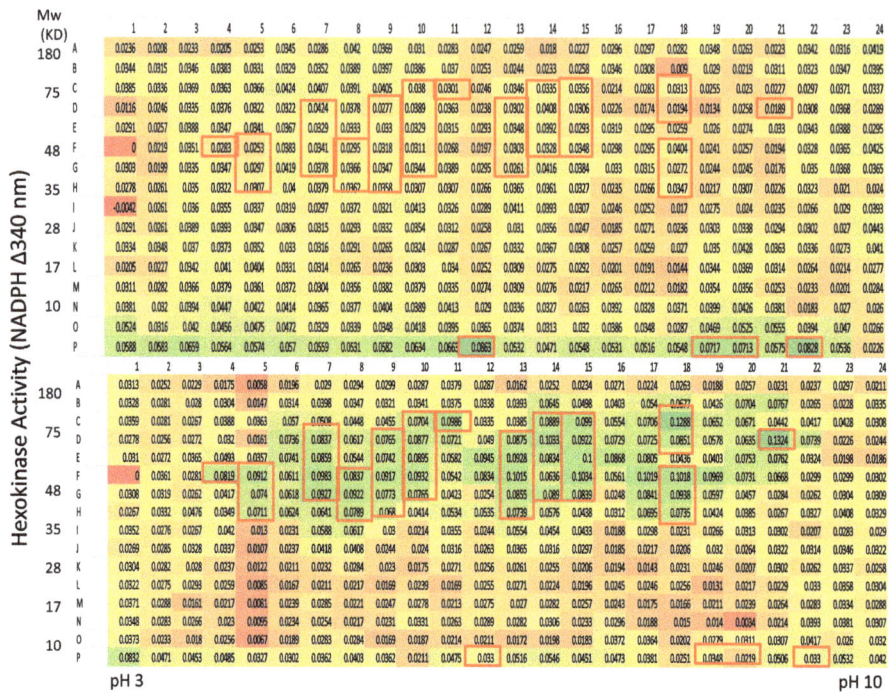

Fig. 4 Measurement of hexokinase activity from normal and breast cancer serum after AlbuVoid™ enrichment and PEP protein separation and elution (60 min). 800 μg AlbuVoid-enriched serum proteins from normal group was loaded onto an IPG strip and separated by IEF. After further separation by SDS-PAGE, the proteins were eluted into the PEP plate and hexokinase activities were analyzed from each of the 384 wells. Hexokinase activity was measured by NADP reduction at 340 nm at 0 and 60 min, the OD340 nm increase from 60 min. was calculated by subtracting the value from the 0 min. reading. Boxed fractions indicated samples of interest

with protease activity in the direct serum analysis suggested that the protease levels in the serum were below the detection threshold of protease activity method used in this study, and it is necessary to use AlbuVoid™ to enrich these low level proteases to bring them to a high enough level to be detected.

Discussion

In US, breast cancer is the most commonly diagnosed malignancies and the leading cause of cancer mortality among women. Approximately 40,000 deaths from the disease occur annually in the US. Worldwide, more than 450,000 deaths occur each year with 1,300,000 diagnosed [24]. The main factor that contributes to breast cancer mortality is the presence of metastasis. Of those diagnosed with breast cancer, 30 to 85% of the patients already have bone metastases and the median survival rate after diagnosis is 25 to 72 months. Human serum is one of the bodily health windows from which the homeostasis of the body can be monitored [13].

In human serum, more than 10,000 proteins have been detected and thousands of them have been identified by mass spectrometry. However, there is a bottleneck in the further use of those serum proteins as potential biomarkers: the clinical validation of the biomarker candidates that meet the requirements of both sensitivity and

specificity. Given the cost of developing useful assays such as monoclonal antibody-based immunoassays, it is not practical to test the hypothesis on thousands of serum proteins in a clinical setting. Therefore, different or more efficient approaches should be considered in the efforts for breast cancer biomarker discovery. Significant progress has been made in the field of breast cancer biomarker discovery in the past decade; however, the early accurate detection of the disease remains a challenge [1, 2, 9, 10, 12, 25, 26]. In a recent review of potential biomarkers for breast cancer, fifteen biomarkers with demonstrated promise in initial studies were reported two of them are for diagnosis and the rest are for prognosis [1]. In addition to protein based biomarker candidates, miRNA and other nucleic acid-based breast cancer biomarkers were also reported recently but no validated biomarker currently exists for use in routine clinical practice

It has long been recognized that cancer has significantly different metabolic behavior when compared with normal cells. Otto Warburg was the first to report the increased metabolic glucose activity in cancer tissue [27, 28], and there has been many reports linking increased metabolic activities with cancer development in the past few years [29–36]. As a result of extensive studies on cancer metabolism, many compounds targeting various metabolic enzymes are in different stages of clinical trials with some

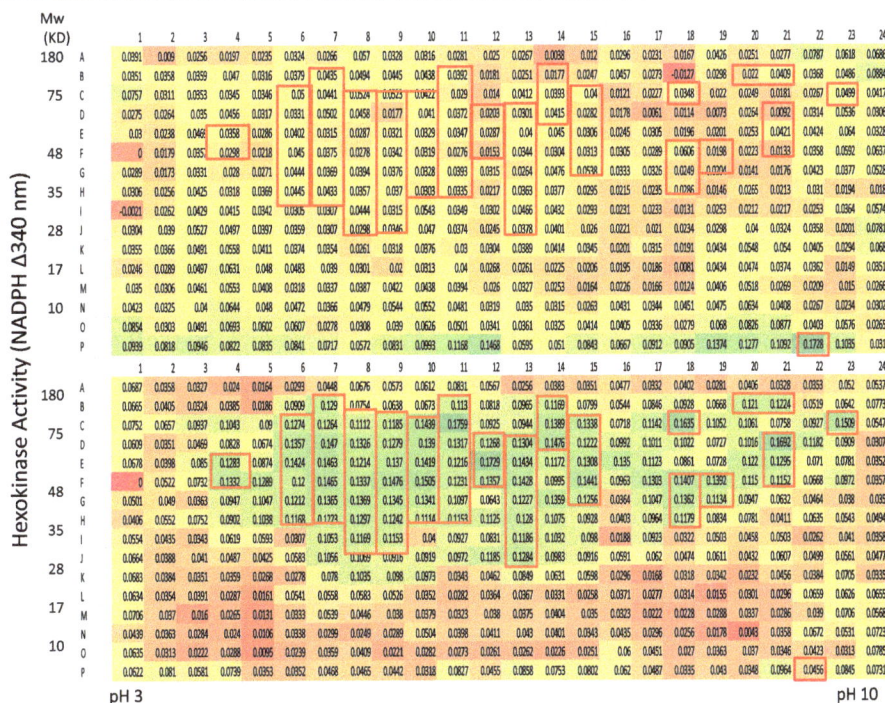

Fig. 5 Measurement of hexokinase activity from normal and breast cancer serum after AlbuVoid™ enrichment and PEP protein separation and elution (120 min). The conditions were the same as in Fig. 4, hexokinase activity was measured by NADP reduction at 340 nm at 0 and 120 min, the OD340 nm increase from 120 min. was calculated by subtracting the value from the 0 min. reading. Boxed fractions indicated samples of interest

encouraging efficacy. Up to now, most of the efforts in serum breast cancer biomarker discovery has been focused on the level of proteins or protein post-translational modifications [3–5, 13, 15, 37]. The goal is to find a protein-based signature for the disease has only been met with limited success. Since the human serum reflects the homeostasis of the body, we hypothesized that among the thousands of proteins identified, metabolic enzymes and other functional proteins may provide a unique window to look into the breast cancer status. Recently, a functional proteomics technology was developed that can analyze the function of serum proteins systematically after 2-D gel electrophoresis [20]. Using this technology, it was demonstrated that the activities of many metabolic enzymes could be monitored from mouse cochleae tissue after drug treatment, and that proteins with differential regulation could be identified directly by mass spectrometry because each fraction recovered in the PEP technology contained just one or a few proteins, In a further study with human lung cancer serum, it was shown that many fractions with metabolic enzyme activities could be detected from lung cancer patient serum [21]. In this further study, it was demonstrated that many fractions with metabolic enzyme activities or protease activities could be detected from normal and breast cancer patient serum with or without AlbuVoidTM protein enrichment. Comparison between the direct serum analysis and the enriched serum analysis

showed that the number of active fractions and levels of enzymatic activities were significantly increased after protein enrichment. This is not surprising given the high protein concentration of the serum protein and the earlier finding that human albumin is associated with many species of serum proteins. First of all, since the principle of AlbuVoid™ serum low abundance protein enrichment is through avoiding the binding of albumin to the column whereas proteins other than albumin will bind any proteins with similar biochemical properties as albumin could be in the flow-through fraction. Secondly, as mentioned above, since human albumin was found to be associated with large amount of low abundance proteins, the avoidance of albumin would also exclude those proteins that bind to albumin. In spite of the impact on the serum protein composition, the AlbuVoid™ enrichment is still a very effective method to enrich low abundance proteins from human serum [23]. This is especially important for certain functional enzymes because the detection and quantitation of enzyme activity is proportional to the quantity of the enzyme present and many enzymes may be below the detection threshold of the assay limit. This was the case in the protease activity assay as more and different enzyme fractions were detected with the protein enrichment (Figs. 3 and 6). It should be pointed out that in the current study, the hexokinase assay system was designed to detect any rate-limiting enzymes in the glycolytic pathway

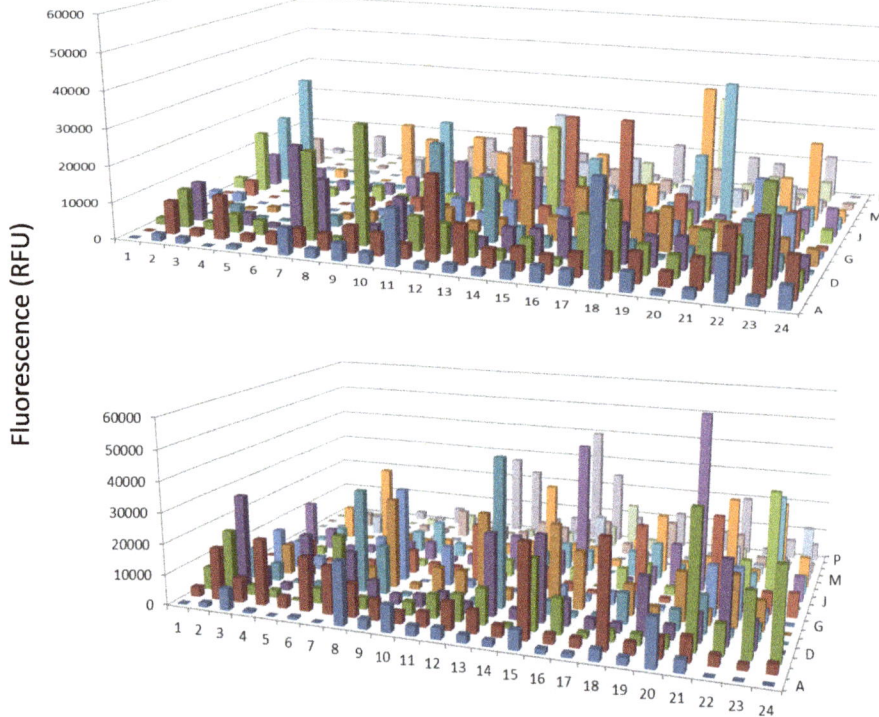

Fig. 6 Protease activity from normal and breast cancer serum after AlbuVoid™ enrichment and PEP protein separation and elution. The conditions were the same as in Fig. 3 except the testing sample is from AlbuVoid™ enrichment. The assay was carried out at room temperature overnight, for more details please refer to the material and method. Boxed fractions indicated samples of interest

because the first enzyme activity in the pathway, hexokinase, was selected and beef liver extract was used as the source of supporting enzymes for the assay. This design was intended to detect as many active metabolic enzymes from the serum as possible. Therefore, any glycolytic enzymes downstream of hexokinase could potentially enhance hexokinase activity by removing downstream products from the system. Because of this assay design, any downstream enzymes in the metabolic pathway could contribute to the detected activity. Previous studies have identified a large number of proteases from human serum through mass spectrometry and a few proteases have been shown to possess catalytic activity (www.serumproteome.org). In this study, a large number of fractions with protease activity were detected from human serum, and many differences were identified between normal and cancer patient serum (Figs. 3 and 6). As expected, there are more species of proteases being detected in the enriched serum samples as compared with the direct serum assay and the enzyme activity levels for many fractions were also significantly higher in the enriched samples. This suggested that for the protease activity assay used in the study, many of the serum proteases were below the detection or quantitation threshold, and the use of an effective serum protein

method is critical to reveal the important information in the functional aspects of proteins in the serum. In the earlier studies, several other enzymes have been tested in the PEP platform for serum proteins including protein kinases, alkaline phosphatases, NADH or NADPH-dependent oxidases and GAPDH [23]. In all the enzymes analyzed, multiple fractions were detected with enzymatic activities. Given the fact that most of the cellular proteins have variants because of post-translational modifications, it is possible that only one or a few protein variants released by the cancer cells and survived in the serum could retain a high correlation with human diseases.

Conclusions

In this study, multiple functional fractions with biomarker candidates were identified for the first time from breast cancer serum using the PEP technology. It is hoped that the combination of methods for serum protein enrichment and PEP technology, which allows functional proteins to be molecularly profiled and compared, can help discover new breast cancer biomarkers. Furthermore, these same technologies can easily be extended for the development of biomarkers, drug targets or diagnostic kits for other types of cancer or diseases.

Abbreviation
PEP: Protein Elution Plate

Acknowledgement
The authors would like to thank Array Bridge Inc. and Biotech Support Group for the supply of PEP and AlbuVoid™ reagents respectively to carry out this study.

Funding
No external funding was used.

Authors' contributions
DLW performed part of the experiments and wrote part of the manuscript; CX performed part of the experiments; GF performed part of the experiments; XW designed the study and wrote part of the manuscript. LL designed the study and wrote part of the manuscript. All authors read and approved the final manuscript.

Competing interests
The authors declare that they have no competing interests.

Author details
[1]Department of Biology, Vanderbilt University, Nashville, TN, USA. [2]Zibo Central Hospital, Zibo, China. [3]Array Bridge Inc., 4320 Forest Park Ave, Suite 303, St. Louis, MO 63108, USA.

References
1. Dos Anjos Pultz D, et al. Far beyond the usual biomarkers in breast cancer: a review. J Cancer. 2014;5(7):13.
2. Li J, et al. Proteomics and bioinformatics approaches for identification of serum biomarkers to detect breast cancer. Clin Chem. 2002;48(8):9.
3. Chan MK, Cooper JD, Bahn S. Commercialisation of biomarker tests for mental illnesses: advances and obstacles. Trends Biotechnol. 2015;33(12):12.
4. Chung L, et al. Novel serum protein biomarker panel revealed by mass spectrometry and its prognostic value in breast cancer. BioMed Central Breast Cancer Res. 2014;16(3):R63. doi:10.1186/bcr3676.
5. Henderson MC, et al. Integration of serum protein biomarker and tumor associated autoantibody expression data increases the ability of a blood-based proteomic assay to identify breast cancer. PLoS ONE. 2016;11(8): e0157692. doi:10.1371/journal.pone.0157692.
6. Ingvarsson J, et al. Design of recombinant antibody microarrays for serum protein profiling: targeting of complement proteins. J Proteome Res. 2007;6:10.
7. Lee JS, Magbanua MJ, Park JW. Circulating tumor cells in breast cancer: applications in personalized medicine. Breast Cancer Res Treat. 2016;160(3): 411-24. Epub 2016 Oct 19.
8. Mehan MR, et al. Validation of a blood protein signature for non-small cell lung cancer. BMC Clin Proteomics. 2014;11(32):12.
9. Ross JS, et al. Breast cancer biomarkers and molecular medicine. Expert Rev Mol Diagn. 2003;3(5):13.
10. Ross JS, et al. Breast cancer biomarkers and molecular medicine: part II. Expert Rev Mol Diagn. 2004;4(2):20.
11. Surinova S, et al. Prediction of colorectal cancer diagnosis based on circulating plasma proteins. EMBO Mol Med. 2015;7(9):13.
12. Yezhelyev MV, et al. In situ molecular profiling of breast cancer biomarkers with multicolor quantum dots. Adv Mater. 2007;19:6.
13. Kirmiz C, et al. A serum glycomics approach to breast cancer biomarkers. Mol Cell Proteomics. 2007;6:13.
14. Harsha HC, et al. A compendium of potential biomarkers of pancreatic cancer. PLoS Med. 2009;6(6):6.
15. Kaskas NM, et al. Serum biomarkers in head and neck squamous cell cancer. JAMA. 2014;140(1):7.
16. Wang C-H, et al. Current trends and recent advances in diagnosis, therapy and prevention of hepatocellular carcinoma. Asian Pac J Cancer Prev. 2015;16(9):10.
17. Alexander H, et al. Proteomic analysis to identify breast cancer biomarkers in nipple aspirate fluid. Clin Cancer Res. 2004;10:11.
18. Ma S, et al. Multiplexed serum biomarkers for the detection of lung cancer. EBio Med. 2016;11:9.
19. Evens MJ, Cravatt BF. Mechanism-based profiling of enzyme families. Chem Rev. 2006;106(8):3279–301.
20. Wang DL, et al. Identification of multiple metabolic enzymes from mice cochleae tissue using a novel functional proteomics technology. PLoS ONE. 2015;10(3):e0121826. doi:10.1371/journal.pone.0121826.
21. Sun Z, et al. Identification of functional metabolic biomarkers from lung cancer patient serum using PEP technology. BioMed Central Biomark Res. 2016;4(11). doi:10.1186/s40364-016-0065-4.
22. Sun Z, Yang P. Role of imbalance between neutrophil elastase and α1-antitrypsin in cancer development and progression. Lancet Oncol. 2004;5:9.
23. Wang X, et al. Bead based proteome enrichment enhances features of the protein elution plate (PEP) for functional proteomic profiling. Proteomes. 2015;3:13.
24. Amorim M, et al. Decoding the usefulness of non-coding RNAs as breast cancer markers. J Transl Med. 2016;14:15.
25. Mabert K, et al. Cancer biomarker discovery: current status and future perspectives. Int J Radiat Biol. 2014;90(8):18.
26. Surinova S, et al. Non-invasive prognostic protein biomarker signatures associated with colorectal cancer. EMBO Mol Med. 2015;7:13.
27. Orla T, et al. Metabolic signatures of malignant progression in prostate epithelial cells. Int J Biochem Cell Biol. 2011;43:8.
28. Teicher BA, Marston WL, Helman LJ. Targeting cancer metabolism. Clin Cancer Res. 2013;18(20):9.
29. Araujo EP, Carvalheira AB, Velloso LA. Disruption of metabolic parhways - perspectives for the treatment of cancer. Curr Cancer Drug Targets. 2006;6:77–87.
30. Bryksin AV, Laktionov PP. Role of glyceraldehyde-3-phosphate dehydrogenase in vesicular transport from golgi apparatus to endoplasmic reticulum. Biochemistry. 2008;73:7.
31. Cairns RA, Harris IS, Mak TW. Regulation of cancer cell metabolism. Nat Rev Cancer. 2011;11:11.
32. Chaneton B, Gottlieb E. Rocking cell metabolism: revised functions of the key glycolytic regulator PKM2 in cancer. Trends Biochem Sci. 2012;37(8):7.
33. Chang C-H, et al. Metabolic competition in the tumor microenvironment is a driver of cancer progression. Cell. 2015;162:13.
34. Chiaradonna FR, et al. From cancer metabolism to new biomarker and drug targets. Biotechnol Adv. 2012;30:30–51.
35. Favaro E, et al. Glucose utilization via glycogen phosphorylase sustains proliferation and prevents premature senescence in cancer cells. Cell Metab. 2012;16:14.
36. Ledford H. Metabolic quirks yield tumour hope. Nature. 2014;508:2.
37. Anderson NL, Anderson NG. The human plasma proteome: history, character, and diagnostic prospects. Mol Cell Proteomics. 2002;1:23.

10

Advance in microRNA as a potential biomarker for early detection of pancreatic cancer

Jing Huang[1], Jianzhou Liu[1], Kevin Chen-Xiao[2], Xuemei Zhang[2], W. N. Paul Lee[2], Vay Liang W. Go[2] and Gary Guishan Xiao[1,2,3]*

Abstract

Pancreatic cancer is characterized as a disease with low survival and high mortality because of no effective diagnostic and therapeutic strategies available in clinic. Conventional clinical diagnostic methods including serum markers and radiological imaging (CT, MRI, EUS, etc.) often fail to detect precancerous or early stage lesions. Development of effective biomarkers is unmet for reduction of mortality of pancreatic cancer. MicroRNAs (miRNAs) are a group of small non-protein-coding RNAs playing roles in regulation of cell physiology including tumorigenesis, apoptotic escape, proliferation, invasion, epithelial-mesenchymal transition (EMT), metastasis and chemoresistance. Various altered signaling pathways involving in molecular pathogenesis of pancreatic cancer are mediated by miRNAs as a role of either oncogenes or tumor suppressors. Among biomarkers developed including protein, metabolites, DNA, RNA, epigenetic mutation, miRNAs are superior because of its unique chemical property. Recent study suggests that miRNAs may be promising biomarkers used for early detection of pancreatic cancer. This review will update the progression made in early detection of pancreatic cancer.

Keywords: Early detection, Pancreatic cancer, Cancer stem cells, microRNAs, Signal transduction, Biomarker

Background

Pancreatic cancer has an exceptionally low 5-year survival rate (<5 %) and high mortality rate, making it the fourth leading cause of cancer mortality in developed countries [1]. As it is particularly located in an inaccessible position of the abdomen leading the common clinical presentation, greater than 80 % of the affected patients were diagnosed when occurring locally advancing or metastasis [2]. Thus the early diagnosis of pancreatic cancer is the key for successful treatment of the disease, though it is rendered uneasy to accomplish resulted from the deficiency of early warning signs. Although much more research into biomarkers has been investigated, few biomarkers are proven to be effective used for early diagnosis of the disease [3]. Therefore, seeking novel biomarkers with higher sensitivity or specificity is still a challenge.

miRNAs are small non-protein-coding RNAs consisting of 18–24 nucleotides in length involving in regulating multiple gene expression by degrading target mRNAs or inhibiting translation at the post-transcriptional level, thereby regulating various neoplastic processes including cell proliferation, migration, invasion, survival, and metastasis [4]. Disregulation of miRNA plays an important role in the pathogenesis, diagnosis and therapy of pancreatic cancer [3]. Here, we update progression made in miRNA as early diagnostic/prognostic biomarkers for pancreatic cancer.

Cancer diagnosis by imaging and biomarkers

Imaging technology has been widely applied as routine methods in diagnosis, therapy and prognosis of varied tumor types including pancreatic cancer. Although common imaging modalities consisting of computed tomography (CT), magnetic resonance imaging (MRI), endoscopic ultrasound (EUS), endoscopic retrograde

* Correspondence: gxiao@dlut.edu.cn
[1]School of Pharmaceutical Science and Technology, Dalian University of Technology, Dalian 116024, China
[2]Harbor-University of California Los Angeles Research and Education Institute, UCLA School of Medicine, Torrance, CA 90502, USA
Full list of author information is available at the end of the article

cholangiopancreatography (ERCP) have been remarkably improved in their detection of pancreatic tumor as by positron emission tomography (PET) or their combination, sensitivity and specificity of detection of pancreatic cancer at its early stage remains challenge [5, 6].

As for CA 19-9, widely used biomarker, fails to distinguish pancreatic cancer from benign pancreatic diseases and multiple carcinoma, which limits clinical utility because of its inadequate sensitivity and specificity [7]. Similarly, several other serum and tissue-based biomarkers (Table 1) suffering the same limitation as CA 19-9, thus none of them have good clinical utility for early diagnosis of pancreatic cancer [7]. Effective biomarkers thus coupled with imaging would provide an ideal approach for early detection of cancer [5].

MicroRNAs as effective biomarkers

Currently, a large sum of studies have identified the potential role of miRNAs in tumorigenesis and metastasis, suggesting that it may be developed as biomarkers used for diagnosis, prognosis and prediction of pancreatic cancer [8]. Given that miRNA-mediated transcriptional regulation is involved in every cellular process, abnormal alterations in miRNA expression are commonly associated with all the carcinogenic process of pancreatic ductal adenocarcinoma (PDAC), including apoptosis escape, proliferation, invasion, epithelial-mesenchymal transition (EMT), metastasis and chemoresistance [8, 9]. Based on their expression, a handful of miRNAs up-regulated in tumor cells are classified as potent oncogenes,

while some others are classified as tumor suppressors since they are conversely down-regulated during the tumorigenesis [10]. MiR-21, for instance, is classified as an oncogene because whose over-expression is associated with the increased proliferation, invasion, and chemoresistance of pancreatic cancer cells to Gemcitabine. Like miR-21, several other miRNAs, which clearly presented their over-expression in cancer tissues, include miR-155, miR-106a, miR-27a, miR-221/222, miR-224, miR-486, miR-194, miR-200b/c, miR-429, miR-10a/b, miR-367, miR-196a/b, miR-210, miR-375, and miR-301a [9, 10]. Meanwhile, another group of miRNAs showed inhibitory effects on cell proliferation, invasion and metastasis, thus functioned as tumor suppressors, including miR-34a/b, Let-7, miR-96, miR-124, miR-615-5p, miR-200a/b/c, miR-219-1-3p, miR-203, miR-146a, and miR-17-92 [9, 10]. An interesting study showed that miR-17-92 cluster is down-regulated in pancreatic cancer stem cells (CSCs), which showed highly resistant to chemotherapy by activating NODAL/ACTIVIN/TGF-β1 signaling pathways, thus, suppression of these pathways may enhance the sensitivity of pancreatic CSCs to chemotherapy [11].

miRNAs regulate key biological processes of tumor cells by altering signaling pathways involved in molecular pathogenesis of PDAC, including *K-ras*, p53, SMAD4, E-cad, PTEN, ADAM9, Bcl-2, STAT3, Cyclin D1, EGFR, TGF-β, JNK, Hedgehog, Notch, NF-κB, and Akt-2 [2]. RAS associated signaling pathways are derived from the most frequently mutated *KRAS* in 90 % of pancreatic cancer, whose translation was found to be

Table 1 Assay parameters of imaging modalities and classical biomarkers used in detection of pancreatic cancer

Item	AUC	Sensitivity (%)	Specificity (%)	PPV (%)	NPV (%)	Accuracy (%)	Reference
CT	0.832	92	-	80	67	-	[19]
MRI	0.92	100	-	90	100	-	[19]
EUS-FNA	-	82.1	100	100	79.2	89.4	[20]
MRCP	-	-	-	85	-	80	[21]
ERCP	-	-	-	88	-	85	[21]
MRI+ERCP	-	-	-	91	-	88	[21]
^{18}F-FDGPE/CT	0.759	67.50	72.73	94.74	23.53	68.13	[22]
CA19-9	0.857	75.00	81.82	96.77	31.03	75.82	[22]
^{18}F-FDGPE/CT + CA19-9	0.940	96.25	63.64	95.06	70.00	92.31	[22]
CA125	0.810	78.68	71.05	79.63	51.92	-	[23]
CEA	0.670	63.24	63.16	75.44	48.98	-	
CA50	0.630	52.21	78.95	81.61	48.00	-	
CA724	0.670	65.44	68.42	78.76	52.53	-	
CA242	0.640	64.71	60.53	74.58	48.94	-	
AFP	0.490	43.38	61.84	67.05	37.90	-	

The assay parameters are for diagnosis of differentiation between adenocarcinoma and nonadenocarcinoma. Small liver metastases (0.5 – 1 cm in diameter) were missed on CT and MRI. Adequate specimens were obtained by EUS-FNAB from 47 of the 50 pancreatic lesions (94.0 %). CA125, CEA, CA50, CA50, CA724, CA242 and AFP are for patients with unresectable pancreatic cancer misjudged as resectable tumor by CT scan. *AUC* area under the curve, *NPV* negative predictive value, *PPV* positive predictive value, – No data was available in these instances

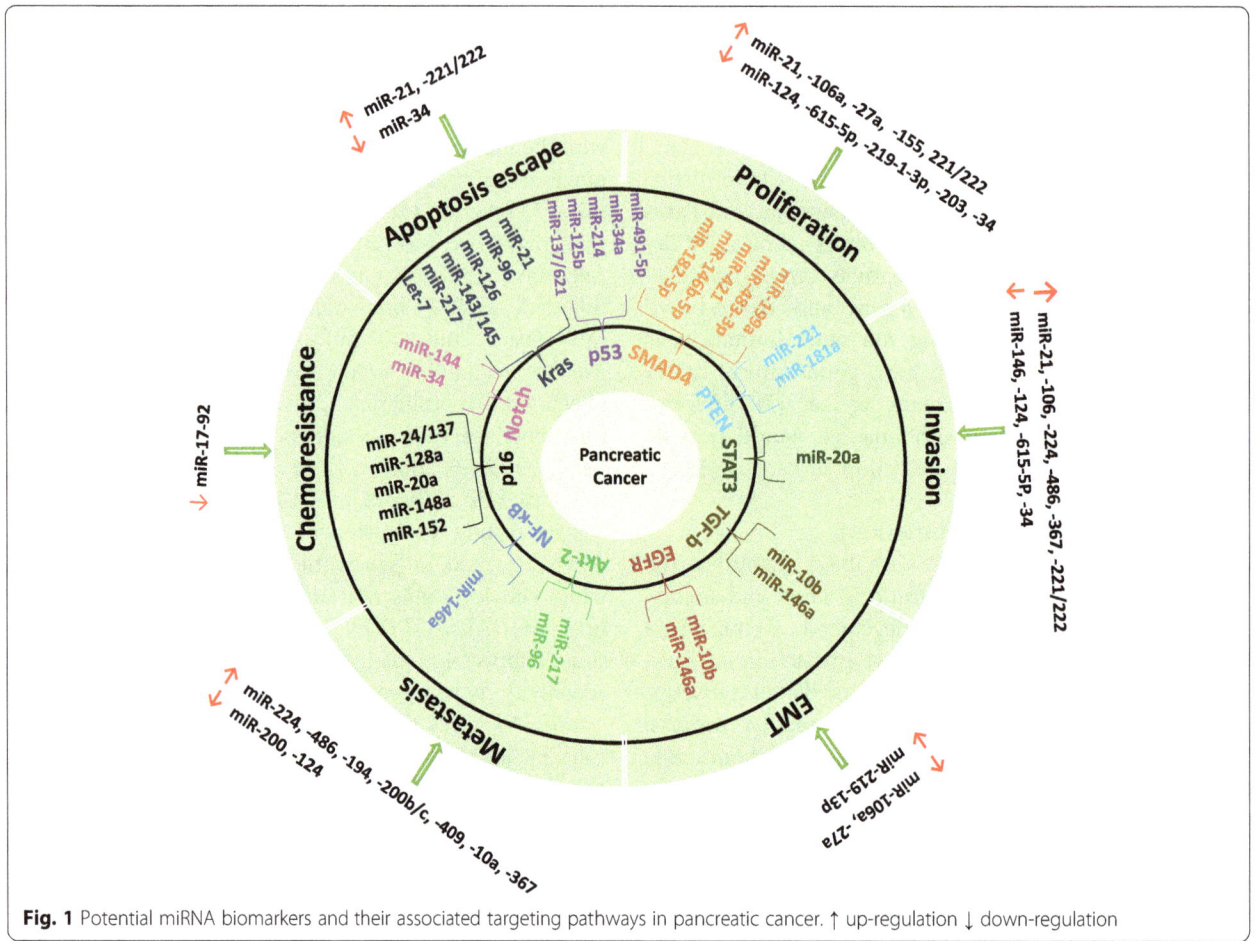

Fig. 1 Potential miRNA biomarkers and their associated targeting pathways in pancreatic cancer. ↑ up-regulation ↓ down-regulation

Table 2 The AUC, sensitivity and specificity of miRNA-based biomarkers for detection of pancreatic cancer

Item	Drived from	AUC		Sensitivity (%)		Specificity (%)		Reference
		PCa vs. Normal	PCa vs. CP	PCa vs. Normal	PCa vs. CP	PCa vs. Normal	PCa vs. CP	
miR-20a, 21, 24, 25, 99a, 185, 191	Serum	0.992		89		100		[13]
miR-10b, 155, 106b, 30c, 212	Plasma	>0.90		95		100		[14]
	Bile			96		100		
miR-21, 210, 155, 196a	Plasma	0.82		64		89		[15]
CA19-9	Serum	0.903	0.897	81.2	81.2	100.0	89.0	[17]
miR-16, 196a,	Plasma	0.895	0.790	87.0	75.4	73.5	66.4	
miR-16+miR-196a+CA19-9	-	0.979	0.956	92.0	88.4	95.6	96.3	
PaCIC marker	Serum	-		0.96		0.86		[18]
miR-1246, 4644, 3976, 4306	Serum	-		0.81		0.94		
PaCIC marker + miR-1246, 4644, 3976, 4306	Serum	-		1.00		0.80		

Serum miR-20a, 21, 24, 25, 99a, 185 and 191 were derived from 197 PCa cases and 158 age- and sex-matched cancer-free controls. MiR-10b, 155, 106b, 30c and 212 were derived from patients (*n* = 215) with treatment-naive PDAC (*n* = 77), CP with bile/pancreatic duct pathology (*n* = 67), and controls (*n* = 71). The plasma levels of miR-21, 210, 155, 196a were interrogated in 49 PCa and 36 normal healthy individuals. Plasma miR-16, 196a and CA19-9 were extracted from 140 PCa patients, 111 CP patients and 68 normal controls. PaCIC marker and miR-1246, 4644, 3976, 4306 were collected from 20 healthy donors, 131 PCa, 25 CP, 22 benign pancreatic tumors, 12 nonPCa. *PCa* pancreatic cancer, *CP* chronic pancreatitis, *AUC* area under the curve, – No data was available in the instances

mediated by miR-96, miR-126, miR-143/145, miR-217 and Let-7 [3]. Recently p53 has been shown to mediate regulation of miR-34 family (miR-34a/b/c). miRNAs such as miR-21, miR-143, miR-155, miR-130a/301a/454, miR-224, miR-146a, miR-483-3p, miR-494, miR-494, and miR-421 are involved in pancreatic cancer progression by regulating TGF-β/SMAD-4 signaling either directly or indirectly [3]. Moreover, miR-137 targets KDM4A mRNA during Ras-induced senescence, and activates both p53 and retinoblastoma (pRb) [12]. More information about miRNAs as biomarkers and their targeting pathways are summarized in Fig. 1.

As aberrant expression of miRNA occurs in molecular pathogenesis of pancreatic cancer, identification of miRNA signatures differentially expressed in different pathological stages of the disease may distinguish pancreatic cancer from pancreatic benign diseases with excellent sensitivity or specificity. A recent study in serum from patients with pancreatic cancer demonstrated that seven serum miRNAs, including miR-20a, miR-21, miR-24, miR-25, miR-99a, miR-185, miR-191, differentially expressed in pancreatic cancer compared to cancer-free subjects, suggesting this miRNA profile may be developed as an effective biomarker used for early detection of the disease with high sensitivity and specificity [13]. More study identified a panel of five miRNAs including miR-10b, −155, −106b, −30c, and −212 in plasma and bile had excellent accuracy, sensitivity, and specificity for detection of PDAC over the control(patients with choledocholithiasis but normal pancreata) [14]. Similarly, miR-21, miR-210, miR-155, and miR-196a showed significant difference in cancer versus healthy control, further study on miR-21 suggests that this miRNA can be developed as an independent prognostic biomarker distinguishing invasive from non-invasive macroscopic intraductal papillary mucinous neoplasms (IPMN), which is one of the precursor lesions of PDAC [15, 16]. It is worth noting that miRNA biomarkers can play a supplementary role with several protein markers in early identification of pancreatic cancer. The combination of a panel of miRNAs, especially miR-16 and miR-196a with CA19-9, for instance, showed effective at identification of tumors in Stage 1 [17]. Pancreatic cancer -initiating cell (PaCIC) markers, such as CD44v6, Tspan8, EpCAM, MET and CD104, combined with miRNA serum-exosome biomarkers including miR-1246, miR-4644, miR-3976 and miR-4306, improved sensitivity significantly with a specificity of 80 % for pancreatic cancer compared to all others groups [18]. Table 2 lists the sensitivity and the specificity of the miRNAs mentioned above.

Future perspective

Although more data suggest that miRNAs offers great potential as biomarkers for early detection of pancreatic cancer, there are limited prospective validation studies to prove their efficacy. Most studies thus far have been in the case-control stage, its application in clinic for prediction and diagnosis of pancreatic cancer at its early stages remained challenge. This may be due to lack of effective standard operational procedures (SOPs) used in standardized clinical assays. Secondarily, no consensus is agreed about the mechanisms underlying miRNA deregulation in tumor cells, hence understanding better the role of miRNAs in tumorigensis may eradicate the field of both molecular diagnosis and effective therapy of pancreatic cancer.

Conclusions

As gene regulators, miRNAs can regulate cell growth, differentiation and apoptosis in many cases of human tumor. Abnormal expression of miRNAs in pancreatic cancer is the early events of pancreatic cancer development, which makes it can be used as a new biological marker for early detection of pancreatic cancer. Evaluation of single miRNA plays an important role in biomarker research, however, a single biomarker is often limitaed in sensitivity and specificity. A miRNA profile consists of a panel of up-regulated or down-regulated miRNAs, thus it can reflect the tumor progression with high sensitivity and specificity. Although there have been a large number of literatures which stated the potetial role of miRNAs as biomarker in pancreatic cnacer early detection, the application in clinical is still remains to explore.

Abbreviations
CSCs: Cancer stem cells; CT: Computed tomography; EMT: Epithelial-mesenchymal transition; ERCP: Endoscopic retrograde cholangiopancreatography; EUS-FNA: Endoscopic ultrasound-Fine needle aspiration; IPMN: Intraductal papillary mucinous neoplasms; MRI: Magnetic resonance imaging; PaCIC: Pancreatic cancer-initiating cell; PDAC: Pancreatic ductal adenocarcinoma; PET: Positron emission tomography; pRb: p53 and retinoblastoma; SOPs: Standard operational procedures

Acknowledgements
Thank you to the DUT International Center for Metabolomics.

Funding
This work was supported by the DUT International Center for Metabolomics in the School of Pharmaceutical Science and Technology, Dalian University of Technology.

Authors' contributions
All authors read and approved the final manuscript.

Competing interests
The authors declare that they have no competing interests.

Author details

[1]School of Pharmaceutical Science and Technology, Dalian University of Technology, Dalian 116024, China. [2]Harbor-University of California Los Angeles Research and Education Institute, UCLA School of Medicine, Torrance, CA 90502, USA. [3]Genomics and Functional Proteomics Laboratories, Creighton University Medical Center, Omaha, NE 68131, USA.

References

1. Li A, Yu J, Kim H, Wolfgang CL, Canto MI, Hruban RH, et al. MicroRNA array analysis finds elevated serum mir-1290 accurately distinguishes patients with low-stage pancreatic cancer from healthy and disease controls. Clin Cancer Res. 2013;19(13):3600–10.

2. Chitkara D, Mittal A, Mahato RI. miRNAs in pancreatic cancer: therapeutic potential, delivery challenges and strategies. Adv Drug Deliv Rev. 2015;81:34–52.

3. Rachagani S, Macha MA, Heimann N, Seshacharyulu P, Haridas D, Chugh S, et al. Clinical implications of miRNAs in the pathogenesis, diagnosis and therapy of pancreatic cancer. Adv Drug Deliv Rev. 2015;81:16–33.

4. Munding JB, Adai AT, Maghnouj A, Urbanik A, Zöllner H, Liffers ST, et al. Global microRNA expression profiling of microdissected tissues identifies miR-135b as a novel biomarker for pancreatic ductal adenocarcinoma. Int J Cancer. 2012;131(2):E86–95.

5. Oberg K, Modlin IM, Herder WD, Pavel M, Klimstra D. Consensus on biomarkers for neuroendocrine tumour disease. Lancet Oncol. 2015;16: e435–46.

6. Miura F, Takada T, Amano H, Yoshida M, Furui S, Takeshita K. Diagnosis of pancreatic cancer. HPB. 2006;8(5):337–42.

7. Duffy MJ, Sturgeon C, Lamerz R, Haglund C, Holubec VL, Klapdor R, et al. Tumor markers in pancreatic cancer: a European Group on Tumor Markers (EGTM) status report. Ann Oncol. 2010;21(3):441–7.

8. Karius T, Schnekenburger M, Dicato M, Diederich M. MicroRNAs in cancer management and their modulation by dietary agents. Biochem Pharmacol. 2012;83(12):1591–601.

9. Brunetti O, Russo A, Scarpa A, Santini D, Reni M, Bittoni A, et al. MicroRNA in pancreatic adenocarcinoma: predictive/prognostic biomarkers or therapeutic targets? Oncotarget. 2015;6(27):23323–41.

10. Khan S, Ansarullah DK, Jaggi M, Chauhan SC. Targeting microRNAs in pancreatic cancer: microplayers in the big game. Cancer Res. 2013;73(22):6541–7.

11. Cioffi M, Trabulo SM, Sanchez-Ripoll Y, Miranda-Lorenzo I, Lonardo E, Dorado J, et al. The miR-17-92 cluster counteracts quiescence and chemoresistance in a distinct subpopulation of pancreatic cancer stem cells. Gut. 2015;64(12):1936–48.

12. Neault M, Mallette FA, Richard S. miR-137 modulates a tumor suppressor network-inducing senescence in pancreatic cancer cells. Cell Rep. 2016;14(8):1966–78.

13. Liu R, Chen X, Du Y, Yao W, Shen L, Wang C, et al. Serum MicroRNA expression profile as a biomarker in the diagnosis and prognosis of pancreatic cancer. Clin Chem. 2012;58(3):610–8.

14. Cote GA, Jesse Gore A, McElyea SD, Heathers LE, Xu H, Sherman S, et al. A pilot study to develop a diagnostic test for pancreatic ductal adenocarcinoma based on differential expression of select miRNA in plasma and bile. Am J Gastroenterol. 2014;109:1942–52.

15. Wang J, Chen J, Chang P, Leblanc A, Li D, Abbruzzesse JL, et al. MicroRNAs in plasma of pancreatic ductal adenocarcinoma patients as novel blood-based biomarkers of disease. Cancer Prev Res. 2009;2(9):807–13.

16. Caponi S, Funel N, Frampton AE, Mosca F, Santarpia L, Van der Velde AG, et al. The good, the bad and the ugly: a tale of miR-101, miR-21 and miR-155 in pancreatic intraductal papillary mucinous neoplasms. Ann Oncol. 2013;24(3):734–41.

17. Liu J, Gao J, Du Y, Li Z, Ren Y, Gu J, et al. Combination of plasma microRNAs with serum CA19-9 for early detection of pancreatic cancer. Int J Cancer. 2012;131(3):683–91.

18. Madhavan B, Yue S, Galli U, Rana S, Gross W, Müller M, et al. Combined evaluation of a panel of protein and miRNA serum-exosome biomarkers for pancreatic cancer diagnosis increases sensitivity and specificity. Int J Cancer. 2015;136(11):2616–27.

19. Schima W, Függer R, Schober E, Oettl C, Wamser P, Grabenwöger F, et al. Diagnosis and staging of pancreatic cancer: comparison of Mangafodipir Trisodium–enhanced MR imaging and contrast-enhanced helical hydro-CT. Am J Roentgenol. 2002;179:717–24.

20. Ryozawa S, Kitoh H, Gondo T, Urayama N, Yamashita H, Ozawa H, et al. Usefulness of endoscopic ultrasound-guided fine-needle aspiration biopsy for the diagnosis of pancreatic cancer. J Gastroenterol. 2005;40(9):907–11.

21. Diehl SJ, Lehmann KJ, Gaa J, Meier-Willersen HJ, Wendl K, Georgi M. Pancreatic cancer: value of MRI including MR cholangio-pancreatography (MRCP) compared to endoscopic retrograde cholangiopancreatography (ERCP). ROFO-FORTSCHRITTE AUF DEM GEBIET DER RONTGENSTRAHLEN UND DER BILDGEBENDEN VERFAHREN. 1999;170(5):463–9.

22. Sun Y, Duan Q, Wang S, Yuecan Zeng WR. Diagnosis of pancreatic cancer using 18 F-FDG PET/CT and CA19-9 with SUVmax association to clinical characteristics. JBUON. 2015;20(2):452–9.

23. Luo G, Xiao Z, Long J, Liu Z, Liu L, Liu C, et al. CA125 is Superior to CA19-9 in predicting the resectability of pancreatic cancer. J Gastrointest Surg. 2013;17(12):2092–8.

11

Prognostic models for alcoholic hepatitis

Erik Rahimi* and Jen-Jung Pan

Abstract

Alcoholic hepatitis (AH) is caused by acute inflammation of the liver in patients that consume excessive amounts of alcohol, usually in a background of cirrhosis. AH can range from mild to severe, life threatening disease with a high rate of short and long-term mortality. Prognostic models have been used to estimate mortality in order to identify those that may benefit from corticosteroids or pentoxifylline. This review focuses on the different prognostic models proposed. While limitations of the prognostic models exist, combining models may be beneficial in order to identify responders to therapy versus non-responders.

Keywords: Alcoholic hepatitis, Prognostic score, Mortality, Risk

Introduction

Alcoholic hepatitis (AH) is a syndrome due to acute inflammation of the liver in patients that consume excessive amounts of alcohol [1]. Rapid onset of jaundice due to parenchymal injury ranging from mild to severe, life-threatening disease usually in the background of concomitant cirrhosis is the hallmark presentation of AH [2]. Along with jaundice, varying symptoms and signs consist of fever, encephalopathy, abdominal distress, ascites, varices, anemia, leukocytosis, coagulopathy, and a ratio of serum aspartate aminotransferase (AST) to alanine aminotransferase (ALT) greater than 2, which rarely exceeds 300 IU per liter, are seen [3–5]. Although it is a treatable form of alcoholic liver disease, there is a high rate of short and long-term mortality. The overall inpatient mortality was 6.6 %–6.8 % for acute AH and 13.6 % for chronic AH in population-based studies [1,6]. In a Danish study, the 28-day mortality was 15 %, 84-day mortality was 24 %, and 5-year mortality was 56 % with a further increase of mortality in cirrhotic patients [7]. Another study from the United Kingdom estimated a 5-year survival of 31.8 % after index hospitalization with severe AH. Abstinence from alcohol was the only independent predictor of long-term survival [8].

While mild AH usually enjoys a good prognosis with alcohol abstinence only, severe AH is associated with high mortality rates and requires additional treatment. Corticosteroids and pentoxifylline are the main pharmacological treatment options that have shown to improve short-term survival, although the overall outcomes are still poor and can cause potential adverse events [9]. Estimating prognosis and identifying those who will need treatment is therefore extremely important. Prognostic models are developed by combining two or more items of patient data into a statistical model to potentially predict clinical outcomes [10]. Non-invasive scoring systems are important for prognosis as more invasive testing such as liver biopsies can lead to increased morbidity [11]. In this article, we review several scoring systems that are available to assess severity and prognosis of AH.

Maddrey discriminant function

The American Association for the Study of Liver Diseases (AASLD) practice guidelines recommend that patients suspected of having AH should have their outcome risk stratified using the discriminant function (DF), along with other available clinical data [2]. In a placebo-controlled study assessing benefits of prednisolone in AH, Maddrey et al. in 1978 first yielded the DF based on prothrombin time (PT) and serum bilirubin concentration that identified patients with a significant risk for early mortality [12]. This was later modified in 1989 to the modified DF (or mDF) = 4.6 (patient's PT in seconds- control PT in seconds) + total bilirubin (mg/dL) that is used today. Those patients with mDF >32 were considered to have severe AH. Patients with an elevated mDF and/or with encephalopathy that received corticosteroid therapy, showed a 28-day mortality of 6 % in the treatment group compared to 35 % in

* Correspondence: Erik.f.rahimi@uth.tmc.edu
Division of Gastroenterology, Hepatology and Nutrition, University of Texas Medical School at Houston, 6431 Fannin Street, MSB 4.234, Houston, TX 77030, USA

the placebo group [13]. On retrospective analysis, DF is a valid index of severity of disease identifying those at 50 % risk of death within 2 months [14]. DF has an inadequate specificity of <40 %–62 % and a sensitivity of 67 %–100 % for short-term (30 day) mortality [15,16]. The inaccuracy in using DF may be accounted for the cut-off point of 32, and had been the basis of debate on differing effectiveness of corticosteroid treatment. Higher cut-off values have been proposed such as cut-offs of 33, 37, 41, 42, or 44 to increase the specificity [15–18]. However, DF scores less than 32 have also been shown to be associated with a relatively high 28-day mortality of 16.7 %. DF was shown to have a poor diagnostic performance since it can only predict mortality or survival 66.6 % of the time [15]. A drawback of using DF is the variable results of PT across different laboratories. The PT test relies on thromboplastin, a variable reagent, making inter-laboratory results vary greatly [19]. Due to the aforementioned limitations of DF, several other prognostic models as listed below have therefore been developed.

Model for end-stage liver disease (MELD) score

The MELD score is calculated using bilirubin, creatinine and international normalized ratio (INR) levels. The objective parameters were originally used to predict early death following elective transjugular intrahepatic portosystemic shunts (TIPS) [20]. The use of objective and reproducible data was subsequently shown to be a reliable measure of short-term mortality risk in patients with end-stage liver disease independent of complications of portal hypertension, and is used as a disease severity index to determine organ allocation priorities [21]. Several studies have used the MELD score to assess disease severity in AH. In a study by Sheth et al [18], the MELD score had a similar performance as the DF in predicting mortality at 30 days. The sensitivity and specificity in predicting 30-day mortality was 86 % and 82 %, respectively, for MELD scores >11 compared to 86 % and 48 %, respectively, when DF was greater than 32. The utility of predicting mortality using MELD score represented as area under the curve (AUC) was 0.82 (95 % confidence intervals (CI): 0.65–0.98), and AUC of DF was 0.86 (95 % CI: 0.70–1.00). Sheth et al. therefore suggested that treatment for AH should be considered when MELD score is greater than 11.

Other studies have suggested higher cut-offs for MELD scores for predicting mortality. In a retrospective study, Srikureja et al [22] reported that MELD score is better than DF in predicting in-hospital mortality. An admission MELD score ≥18 showed a sensitivity and specificity of 85 % and 84 %, respectively, for predicting in-hospital mortality. First week MELD score ≥20 had a 91 % sensitivity and 85 % specificity, and first week change of MELD score ≥2 points had a 80 % sensitivity and 75 % specificity for predicting in-hospital mortality.

Dunn et al. [17], in a retrospective review of 73 patients showed that MELD score was the only independent predictor of mortality in patients with AH. MELD was shown to be comparable to DF in predicting 30-day and 90-day mortality. A MELD score of 21 in the study was shown to have a sensitivity of 75 % and a specificity of 75 % to predict mortality with an estimated 90-day mortality of 20 % in AH. Another study reported a 30-day and 90-day mortality rates of 5.9 % and 14.7 %, respectively in patients with AH. MELD score >30.5 had an excellent performance in predicting 30-day mortality with a sensitivity of 100 % and specificity 94 % (AUC 0.969). Furthermore, MELD score >19 only had a fair performance in predicting 90-day mortality with a sensitivity of 60 % and a specificity of 60 % (AUC 0.762) [23].

In a retrospective study of 26 patients, Vaa et al [24] compared MELD and MELD-Na in predicting 180-day mortality in patients with AH. MELD-Na is a modified MELD score that includes serum sodium (Na) which has been shown to improve prediction of death in cirrhotic patients. In the study, MELD-Na was a better predictor of 180-day mortality than MELD in patients with ascites. A MELD score of 27 and a MELD-Na score of 28 in patients without ascites had a sensitivity/specificity of 76.5 %/64.9 % and 87.5 %/52.5 %, respectively. After adjustment for MELD in AH patients without ascites, serum Na, specifically hyponatremia, was not a significant predictor of mortality ($p = 0.83$). However, in patients with ascites a MELD score of 29 and a MELD-Na score of 34 had sensitivity/specificity of 85.7 %/31.0 % and 83.3 %/16.7 %, respectively. In AH patients with ascites, MELD-Na had better predictability of 180-day mortality compared to MELD (odds ratio (OR), 2.27 for every 1-point increase in MELD-Na; 95 % CI: 1.22–36.68; $p = 0.008$ versus OR, 1.37 for every 1-point increase in MELD; 95 % CI: 1.07–2.12; $p = 0.006$).

Overall MELD score is a good predictor for mortality in patients with AH. According to therapeutic algorithms, an initial MELD score ≥18 and increasing serial MELD scores over time are considered high risk for mortality and should be used in guiding initiation of therapeutic intervention [2].

Glasgow alcoholic hepatitis score (GAHS)

In 2005, Forrest et al. [25] used 5 variables including age, blood urea, peripheral blood leukocyte count, serum bilirubin, and PT, expressed as a ratio of the control value to develop a new prognostic scoring system for AH. Values obtained ranged from 5 to 12, separated into those with value <9 or ≥9 points. Day 28 survival in patients with a day 1 GAHS score of <9 was 87 % compared to 46 % in those with GAHS ≥9. Based on the validation dataset, accuracy of GAHS day 1 and 7 data had a better prediction of 28 day and 84 day outcome than mDF. Accuracy of GAHS day 1 and 7 in predicting

28-day mortality was 67 % and 75 %, versus mDF accuracy of 48 % and 56 %; $p = 0.0016$ and $p = 0.0038$, respectively. Accuracy of GAHS day 1 and 7 in predicting 84-day mortality was 71 % and 75 %, versus mDF accuracy of 57 % and 62 %; $p = 0.0179$ and $p = 0.0477$, respectively. In a subsequent study in 2007 by Forrest et al. [26], patients with a mDF ≥32 and a GAHS <9 did not benefit from treatment with corticosteroids. However corticosteroids therapy was associated with better survival in those with both GAHS ≥9 and mDF ≥32 compared to no treatment (28-day survival 78 % vs. 52 %, $p = 0.002$). Day 84 survival was 59 % and 38 % ($p = 0.02$) in those treated and not treated with steroids, respectively. In a recent study, Lafferty et al. [27] showed that patients receiving corticosteroids with a GAHS ≥9, irrespective of mDF, had a 90-day survival of 58 % compared to 30 % in those not receiving treatment. The sensitivity and specificity of 90-day outcome for GAHS assessment on admission was 67 % and 78 %, respectively.

Age, serum bilirubin, INR, and serum creatinine (ABIC) score

In 2008, Dominguez et al. [28] built a predictive score from multivariate analysis of variables identified during admission. The resulting score: Age, serum Bilirubin, INR, and serum Creatinine (ABIC) score = (age × 0.1) + (serum bilirubin × 0.08) + (serum creatinine × 0.3) + (INR × 0.8) was validated in an independent prospective cohort. Using a cutoff value of 6.71 and 9 the score identified patients with AH that have a low (100 % survival), intermediate (70 % survival), and high risk (25 % survival) of death at 90 days. The sensitivity and specificity was 100 % and 50 % for the cut-off of 6.71, respectively, and 70 % and 33 %, respectively, for a cut-off of 9. In a retrospective study evaluating 9 different scoring systems, the sensitivity and specificity of the ABIC score for 30-day mortality were 100 % and 20 %, respectively, for a cut-off of 6.71, and 60 % and 80 %, respectively, for a cut-off of 9. A higher ABIC cut-off of 9.5 compared to original cut-off of 9 resulted in an increased specificity of 90 % vs. 80 % and 95 % vs. 84 % for a 30- and 90-day outcome respectively [16]. When comparing the 90-day mortality predictive accuracy of the ABIC score with MELD, mDF, and GAHS, the ABIC score was the best independent predictor of 90-day mortality (hazard ratio (HR) 2.78, 95 % CI 1.90–4.09, $p = 0.0001$). The ABIC score was also assessed to determine 1-year mortality, which could be used for liver transplantation assignment. The ABIC score was the only independent predictor of 1-year mortality (HR: 2.49, 95 % CI 1.77–3.52, $p = 0.0001$), when compared to other prognostic models. Analysis of the subgroup of patients treated with steroids showed that the greatest response was in the group with intermediate ABIC score (between 6.71–8.99) compared to those with either low ABIC

(<6.71) or high ABIC scores (>9). In patients treated with steroids, the ABIC score at 7 days has a better accuracy than the Lille model in predicting mortality at 6 months [28].

Lille model

In 2007, Louvet et al. [29] generated a prognostic model, the Lille model, to identify "non-responders" to corticosteroid therapy in patients with severe AH. The model combined six objective variables (age, renal insufficiency, albumin, PT, bilirubin, and evolution of bilirubin at day 7) which were highly predictive of death at 6 months in patients treated with corticosteroids (p < 0.000001). The Lille formula is available online at http://www.lillemodel.com or see formula in Table 1. A cut-off value of 0.45 was determined to be the best identifier of patients at high risk of death, with a sensitivity and specificity of 81 % and 76 %, respectively in the validation cohort, and 76 % and 85 %, respectively on overall patients. Patients with a Lille score ≥0.45 had a significant decrease in 6-month survival compared to patients with a Lille score <0.45 (25 % versus 85 %; p < 0.0001). Thus, 40 % of patients receiving steroids can be identified to have a poor prognosis using the Lille model. Patients receiving corticosteroids after 7 days with a score ≥0.45 may be futile and alternative treatments should be considered. In a prospective study regarding infection in AH patients, only the Lille model (OR, 11.14; 95 % CI: 3.2–39.2, p = 0.0002) independently predicted infection upon steroids use in multivariate analysis. Responders (Lille model <0.45) to steroids that developed infection had lower survival compared to responders that did not develop infection: 51 % vs 94 %, respectively (p = 0.000001). Non-responders (Lille model ≥0.45) that developed infection had similar survival to non-responders that did not develop infection: 42 % vs 52 %, respectively (p = 0.5). Thus adjuvant antibiotic therapy to corticosteroids in the setting of severe AH may improve survival mainly in responders [30].

Beclere model

The Beclere model was initially formulated by Poynard et al. [31] in 1994 to determine survival in alcoholic cirrhosis. The final model has four variables: age, encephalopathy, serum bilirubin, and serum albumin to obtain a risk score (R) for each patient using the formula R = (0.0484 × [Age in Years] + 0.469 × [encephalopathy] + 0.537 × Log$_e$ [Bilirubin in µmol/L] - 0.052 × [Albumin in g/L]. This model was then used by Mathurin et al. [32] as a simulated prognostic model for a control group in a study aimed to examine prognostic factors and long-term survival in AH patients receiving corticosteroids. There was no difference in 1 and 2 year survival in the observed placebo-randomized group and the simulated control group using the Beclere model. In a multivariate analysis,

Table 1 Prognostic scoring formulas to determine severity of acute alcoholic hepatitis

Scoring system	Formula			Severe Disease	
mDF	4.6 (patient's PT in seconds- control PT in seconds) + total bilirubin (mg/dL)			≥32	
CTP	1	2	3		
Bilirubin	<2 mg/dL	2–3 mg/dL	>3 mg/dL	Class A	5–6 points
Albumin	>3.5 g/dL	2.8–3.5 g/dL	<2.8 g/dL	Class B	7–9 points
INR	<1.7	1.7–2.2	>2.2	Class C	10–15 points
Ascites	None	Mild	Severe		
Encephalopathy	None	Grade I-II	Grade III-IV		
MELD	MELD Score = 0.957 x Loge (creatinine mg/dL) + 0.378 x Loge (bilirubin mg/dL) + 1.120 x Loge (INR) 0.6431* 10 (if hemodialysis, value for Creatinine is automatically set to 4.0)			MELD ≥ 21	
	MELD score = 3.8*loge (total bilirubin, mg/dL) + 11.2*loge (INR) + 9.6*loge (creatinine, mg/dL)				
	MELD score = 9.57 x loge (Cr mg/dL) + 3.78 x loge (bili mg/dL) + 11.20 x loge (INR) + 6.43				
MELD-Na	MELD-Na score = MELD Score - Na - 0.025*MELD* (140-Na) + 140				
GAHS	1	2	3	≥9	
Age	<50	≥50	-		
WBC (109/l)	<15	≥15	-		
Urea (mmol/l)	<5	≥5	-		
PT ratio	<1.5	1.5–2.0	>2.0		
Bilirubin (µmol/l)	<125	125 - 250	>250		
Lille Score	Lille Score = 3.19–0.101 * (age in years) + 0.147 * (albumin day 0 in g/L) + 0.0165 * (evolution in bilirubin level in µM) - (0.206 * renal insufficiency) - 0.0065 * (bilirubin day 0 in µM) - 0.0096 * (INR or prothrombin time in seconds).			≥0.45	
ABIC score	ABIC score = (age × 0.1) + (serum bilirubin × 0.08) + (serum creatinine × 0.3) + (INR × 0.8)			>9.0	
AHHS		Points			
	Stage of fibrosis			Mild (0–3)	
	No fibrosis or portal fibrosis	0		Moderate (4–5)	
	Expansive fibrosis	0		Severe (6–9)	
	Bridging fibrosis or cirrhosis	3			
	Bilirubinostasis				
	No	0			
	Hepatocellular only	0			
	Canalicular or ductular	1			
	Canalicular or ductular plus hepatocellular	2			
	PMN infiltration				
	No/ Mild	2			
	Severe	0			
	Megamitochondria				
	No Megamitochondria	2			
	Megamitochondria	0			

mDF modified Discriminant Function, *CTP* Child Turcotte Pugh, *MELD* Model for End-stage Liver Disease, *GAHS* Glasgow Alcoholic Hepatitis Score, *ABIC* Age serum Bilirubin INR and serum Creatinine, *AHHS* Alcoholic Hepatitis Histologic Score

the corticosteroid effect (p < 0.02) and the Beclere model risk score ($p = 0.0003$) had independent prognostic value for survival. Survival was significantly better in the treated groups compared to the non-treated groups. The prednisolone - randomized group had 69 % survival (95 % CI: 57 %–81 %) and 71 % (95 % CI: 55 %–87 %) in the prednisolone-open group, compared to 41 % (95 % CI: 23 %–59 %; $p = 0.01$) in the placebo-randomized group and 50 % (95 % CI: 37 %–63 %; $p = 0.05$) in the simulated control group. However, subsequent studies in AH patients did not further use this model for prognostic scoring.

Alcoholic hepatitis histologic score (AHHS)

The need for liver biopsy is controversial in diagnosing alcoholic hepatitis patients as the presence of ascites and coagulopathy may require a transjugular approach, which may not be readily available [33]. Altamirano et al. [34] developed a histologic scoring system based on liver biopsy findings to predict short-term (90-day) mortality in AH patients. The AHHS was initially developed from 121 patients admitted to a single center in Spain, and subsequently tested and validated in another set of 205 patients from 5 academic centers in the United States and Europe. After multivariate analysis, four independent histologic features were combined in the final score: fibrosis stage (0–3) which was separated as bridging fibrosis or cirrhosis giving a score of +3 versus a score of 0 for absence of these features; bilirubinostasis (0–2) was divided into a score of 0 for absence or hepatocellular only, +1 for canalicular or ductular, and +2 for canalicular or ductular plus hepatocellular; polymorphonuclear (PMN) infiltration (0–2) was described as "mild" PMN (score +2) when usually <15 PMN per focus were found around a hepatocyte and "marked" PMNs were easily recognized at low magnification and many PMNs found around damaged hepatocytes (with ballooning or Mallory–Denk bodies); and megamitochondria (0–2) where none seen was +2, and seen was 0, for a total of 9 points. Marked PMN infiltration and megamitochondria were independently associated with a favorable outcome. AHHS cut-off score categorized patients as low 0–3 (97 % survival), intermediate 4–5 (81 % survival), and high risk 6–9 (49 % survival) of death. When combing the AHHS with analytical scoring systems, the AHHS was able to refine the prognostic stratification of those with a MELD score <21 (low risk group). In patients with a MELD score <21 (low risk group) the AHHS was able to define 2 subgroups with different 90-day survival using a cut-off of 5 points (94 % vs 72 %; $p = 0.001$). The differences in the MELD with an AHHS <5 points and those with an AHHS ≥5 points (16 ± 8 vs 23 ± 9 points of MELD, respectively; $p < 0.0001$) suggest that analytic parameters in the MELD score, such as bilirubin, are reflected in severity of histologic abnormalities. This would, therefore, modify stratification of severity from a low to high risk group, and change treatment management in these patients.

Child–Turcotte–Pugh (CTP) score

The CTP is based on 5 variables including ascites, encephalopathy, serum bilirubin, albumin and PT, which the latter was modified in 1973 by Pugh et al. from the original use of nutritional status in the Child-Turcotte criteria. Each variable has a score of 1 to 3, and patients are classified as class A (best), B (moderate), or C (worse) to determine prognosis, originally for cirrhotic patients undergoing surgery [35,36]. The limitations to the scoring system include subjectivity in ascites and encephalopathy grading, variable PT results, and a "ceiling" and "floor" effect for arbitrary cut-off points with bilirubin and albumin, respectively [37]. The use of CTP score in AH is not widely used. In 2004, Said et al [38] reported that CTP compared to the MELD score had similar predictive abilities for 3- and 6-month mortality in AH patients, with a c-statistics of 0.85 (0.75–0.95) and 0.81 (0.70–0.92), respectively. Srikureja et al. [22] retrospectively compared MELD, CTP, and DF scores as predictive models to assess in-hospital mortality in AH patients. CTP score was independently associated with mortality on admission with an AUC of 0.87 (95 % CI: 0.81–0.94). However, this was lost with the first week change in CTP score (AUC 0.57; 95 % CI: 0.43–0.70) compared to first week change in MELD score (AUC 0.85; 95 % CI: 0.76–0.94; $p = 0.0004$).

TMA and pentane (TAP) score

A recent study by Hanouneh et al. [39] identified novel breath biomarkers in patients with AH. Six compounds including 2-propanol, acetaldehyde, acetone, ethanol, pentane, and trimethylamine (TMA) were initially shown to be increased in patients with liver disease compared with healthy control subjects. TMA, acetone and pentane were significantly higher in AH compared to those with acute decompensation or control subjects (for all, p < 0.001). After accounting for MELD score only the associations between TMA and pentane (TAP) to AH remained significant (TMA, p < 0.001; pentane, $p = 0.004$). Combining pentane and TMA levels in the breath was found to have an excellent prediction accuracy to diagnose AH (AUC 0.92). A model, named the TAP score, was then developed using the logistic regression (lr) function of the two variables (lr = –3.71 + [0.34*TMA] - [0.087*pentane]), and the following derived formula, TAP score = 100 × (exp [lr]/ 1 + exp [lr] was used. TAP scores of ≥36 identified patients with AH with 90 % sensitivity and 80 % specificity. There correlation of the so called breathprint and severity of liver disease was only moderate as presented by MELD score (r = 0.38; 95 % CI, 0.07–0.69; $p = 0.18$). Larger studies are needed to further validate these results, as only a small group of 40 patients with AH were assessed.

Combining static and dynamic models

Louvet et al. [40] evaluated the prognostic value of combining static models for AH, such as mDF, MELD score, and ABIC score with dynamic models, such as the Lille score. This joint effect model was able to predict outcome of survival after 2 and 6 months significantly better than either the static or dynamic models alone (p < 0.01). The MELD + Lille combination model predicted survival better than the mDF + Lille or ABIC + Lille models. Using the joint effect model of MELD + Lille score, a hypothetical patient with a MELD score of 21 and Lille score at 0.45 had a 15.3 % and 23.7 % mortality rate at 2 and 6 months, respectively. The overall predicted mortality at 6 months in the MELD + Lille model with a MELD score of 15–45 was between 8.5 %–49.7 % in a complete responder (Lille score, 0.16), and from 16.4 %–75.2 % in a non-responder (Lille score, 0.45). The use of the joint effect models has a better prediction of mortality in AH patients. This models can also identify high risk of death in patients previously classified as responders, and intermediate risk of death in previous classified non-responders.

Further indicators of prognosis in alcoholic hepatitis
Acute kidney Injury (AKI)
AKI, as per the AKIN (Acute Kidney Injury Network) criteria, is defined as an abrupt reduction (within 48 h) in kidney function that results in an absolute increase of at least 0.3 mg/dL (or a 50 % increase) in serum levels of creatinine from baseline [41]. In a retrospective study by Altamirano et al [42], AKI was shown to markedly influence 90 day mortality in patients with AH versus without AH (65 % vs. 7 %, p < 0.0001). The most accurate predictors of AKI were the presence of systemic inflammatory response syndrome, serum bilirubin (especially >16 mg/dL), and elevated INR >1.7 in patients with AH.

Change in bilirubin
Similar to the Lille score, early change in bilirubin levels (ECBL), defined as bilirubin level at 7 days lower than bilirubin level on the first day of treatment of steroids was shown to be an important prognostic factor in AH patients. Mathurin et al [43] reported that 95 % of patients with ECBL continued to have improved liver function during treatment. Six-month survival in patients with ECBL was 82.8 ± 3.3 % versus 23 ± 5.8 % (p < 0.0001) in the non-ECBL group. Another study by Morris and Forrest [44] identified steroid responders, defined as a 25 % fall in serum bilirubin after 6–9 days of treatment had a better survival than non-responders. Non-responders were found to have 28-day and 56-day mortality of 36.8 % and 57.9 %, respectively, versus responders with 0 % (*p* = 0.0148) and 11.1 % (*p* = 0.0084), respectively. The above studies, therefore, suggest stopping steroids in non-responders.

Gastrointestinal (GI) bleed
In a recent study, Rudler et al. [45] compared the mortality risk in AH patients who had concomitant GI bleeding (AH-GIB+) with AH patients without GI bleeding (AH-GIB-). There was no difference in 1, 3, and 6-month probability of survival in AH-GIB+ versus AH-GIB- groups (87.9 ± 4 % vs 84.1 ± 5 %, *p* = 0.56; 79.2 ± 5 % vs 71.1 ± 7 %, *p* = 0.24; and 73.9 ± 6 % vs 69.9 ± 7 %, *p* = 0.49, respectively). There was also no difference in response to therapy between the two groups as well.

Protein-Calorie malnutrition
Malnutrition, to some degree is found in every AH patient whether they do or do not have concomitant cirrhosis [46]. Mendenhall et al. [47] found that the severity of protein energy malnutrition (PEM) correlated with prognosis of AH patients. A moderate PEM of 60 %–79 % of normal was associated with a 29 % 6-month mortality, and severe malnutrition (PEM score <60 %) correlated with a 45 % mortality in 6 months. Patients with moderate malnutrition and adequate caloric intake (>2,500 kcal/day) that were given oxandrolone (an anabolic steroid) had a reduced 6-month mortality of 4 % versus 28 % in the placebo group (*p* = 0.002). These findings were not seen in cases of severe malnutrition [48]. In a randomized control trial, AH patients received either prednisone or total enteral nutrition (TEN) of 2,000 kcal/day for 28 days [49]. Short term (28-day period) mortality was 25 % and 31 % in the steroid group and TEN group, respectively. One-year survival probability was 39 % with steroids and 62 % with TEN. Thus there may be a synergistic effect in using steroid and TEN in AH treatment. In a meta-analysis, Antar et al. [50] pooled 7 randomized control trials that compared nutritional supplementation plus a normal hospital diet versus diet alone. There was no statistical difference in mortality between the two groups (OR, 0.80; 95 % CI: 0.42–1.52), although there was a trend toward survival benefit with supplemental nutrition and significant improvement in encephalopathy (OR, 0.24; 95 % CI: 0.06–0.93). Thus nutritional supplement is still regarded as beneficial.

Conclusion
The available scoring systems are useful in both prognostic stratification and selection of candidates for appropriate therapy. Limitations of the scoring systems include differing cut-offs to meet the best accuracy, clinical and laboratory parameters that may differ, and that one scoring system may be insufficient to determine some patients with severe AH. Combining more than one scoring system, e.g. DF and Lille score, MELD and AHHS, or static and dynamic models may better define severe AH with greater accuracy. Furthermore, determining responders versus non-responders to therapy is important to avoid untoward adverse events associated with treatment.

Abbreviations

AH: Alcoholic hepatitis; AST: Serum aspartate aminotransferase; ALT: Alanine aminotransferase; AASLD: American Association for the Study of Liver Diseases; DF: Discriminant function; PT: Prothrombin time; mDF: Modified DF; MELD: Model for End-Stage Liver Disease; INR: International normalized ratio; TIPS: Transjugular intrahepatic portosystemic shunts; AUC: Area under the curve; CI: Confidence intervals; OR: Odds ratio; GAHS: Glasgow Alcoholic Hepatitis Score; ABIC: Age serum Bilirubin INR and serum Creatinine; HR: Hazard ratio; AHHS: Alcoholic Hepatitis Histologic Score; PMN: Polymorphonuclear; CTP: Child–Turcotte–Pugh; AKI: Acute Kidney Injury; AKIN: Acute Kidney Injury Network; ECBL: Early change in bilirubin levels; GI: Gastrointestinal; PEM: Protein energy malnutrition; TEN: Total enteral nutrition.

Competing interests

All authors disclose no conflicts and no competing interests.

Authors' contributions

ER: Drafting of the manuscript; critical revision of the manuscript for important intellectual content. J-JP: Drafting of the manuscript; critical revision of the manuscript for important intellectual content. Both authors read and approved the final manuscript.

References

1. Liangpunsakul S. Clinical characteristics and mortality of hospitalized alcoholic hepatitis patients in the United States. J Clin Gastroenterol. 2011;45(8):714–9.
2. O'Shea RS, Dasarathy S, McCullough AJ. Diseases PGCotAAftSoL, Gastroenterology PPCotACo. Alcoholic liver disease. Hepatology. 2010;51(1):307–28.
3. Lucey MR, Mathurin P, Morgan TR. Alcoholic hepatitis. N Engl J Med. 2009;360(26):2758–69.
4. Ishak KG, Zimmerman HJ, Ray MB. Alcoholic liver disease: pathologic, pathogenetic and clinical aspects. Alcohol Clin Exp Res. 1991;15(1):45–66.
5. Cohen JA, Kaplan MM. The SGOT/SGPT ratio–an indicator of alcoholic liver disease. Dig Dis Sci. 1979;24(11):835–8.
6. Yang AL, Vadhavkar S, Singh G, Omary MB. Epidemiology of alcohol-related liver and pancreatic disease in the United States. Arch Intern Med. 2008;168(6):649–56.
7. Sandahl TD, Jepsen P, Thomsen KL, Vilstrup H. Incidence and mortality of alcoholic hepatitis in Denmark 1999–2008: a nationwide population based cohort study. J Hepatol. 2011;54(4):760–4.
8. Potts JR, Goubet S, Heneghan MA, Verma S. Determinants of long-term outcome in severe alcoholic hepatitis. Aliment Pharmacol Ther. 2013;38(6):584–95.
9. Chayanupatkul M, Liangpunsakul S. Alcoholic hepatitis: a comprehensive review of pathogenesis and treatment. World J Gastroenterol. 2014;20(20):6279–86.
10. Perel P, Edwards P, Wentz R, Roberts I. Systematic review of prognostic models in traumatic brain injury. BMC Med Inform Decis Mak. 2006;6:38.
11. Liver EAftSo. EASL clinical practical guidelines: management of alcoholic liver disease. J Hepatol. 2012;57(2):399–420.
12. Maddrey WC, Boitnott JK, Bedine MS, Weber FL, Mezey E, White RI. Corticosteroid therapy of alcoholic hepatitis. Gastroenterology. 1978;75(2):193–9.
13. Carithers RL, Herlong HF, Diehl AM, Shaw EW, Combes B, Fallon HJ, et al. Methylprednisolone therapy in patients with severe alcoholic hepatitis. A randomized multicenter trial. Ann Intern Med. 1989;110(9):685–90.
14. Ramond MJ, Poynard T, Rueff B, Mathurin P, Théodore C, Chaput JC, et al. A randomized trial of prednisolone in patients with severe alcoholic hepatitis. N Engl J Med. 1992;326(8):507–12.
15. Kulkarni K, Tran T, Medrano M, Yoffe B, Goodgame R. The role of the discriminant factor in the assessment and treatment of alcoholic hepatitis. J Clin Gastroenterol. 2004;38(5):453–9.
16. Papastergiou V, Tsochatzis EA, Pieri G, Thalassinos E, Dhar A, Bruno S, et al. Nine scoring models for short-term mortality in alcoholic hepatitis: cross-validation in a biopsy-proven cohort. Aliment Pharmacol Ther. 2014;39(7):721–32.
17. Dunn W, Jamil LH, Brown LS, Wiesner RH, Kim WR, Menon KV, et al. MELD accurately predicts mortality in patients with alcoholic hepatitis. Hepatology. 2005;41(2):353–8.
18. Sheth M, Riggs M, Patel T. Utility of the Mayo End-Stage Liver Disease (MELD) score in assessing prognosis of patients with alcoholic hepatitis. BMC Gastroenterol. 2002;2:2.
19. Robert A, Chazouillères O. Prothrombin time in liver failure: time, ratio, activity percentage, or international normalized ratio? Hepatology. 1996;24(6):1392–4.
20. Malinchoc M, Kamath PS, Gordon FD, Peine CJ, Rank J, ter Borg PC. A model to predict poor survival in patients undergoing transjugular intrahepatic portosystemic shunts. Hepatology. 2000;31(4):864–71.
21. Kamath PS, Wiesner RH, Malinchoc M, Kremers W, Therneau TM, Kosberg CL, et al. A model to predict survival in patients with end-stage liver disease. Hepatology. 2001;33(2):464–70.
22. Srikureja W, Kyulo NL, Runyon BA, Hu KQ. MELD score is a better prognostic model than Child-Turcotte-Pugh score or Discriminant Function score in patients with alcoholic hepatitis. J Hepatol. 2005;42(5):700–6.
23. Soultati AS, Dourakis SP, Alexopoulou A, Deutsch M, Vasilieva L, Archimandritis AJ. Predicting utility of a model for end stage liver disease in alcoholic liver disease. World J Gastroenterol. 2006;12(25):4020–5.
24. Vaa BE, Asrani SK, Dunn W, Kamath PS, Shah VH. Influence of serum sodium on MELD-based survival prediction in alcoholic hepatitis. Mayo Clin Proc. 2011;86(1):37–42.
25. Forrest EH, Evans CD, Stewart S, Phillips M, Oo YH, McAvoy NC, et al. Analysis of factors predictive of mortality in alcoholic hepatitis and derivation and validation of the Glasgow alcoholic hepatitis score. Gut. 2005;54(8):1174–9.
26. Forrest EH, Morris AJ, Stewart S, Phillips M, Oo YH, Fisher NC, et al. The Glasgow alcoholic hepatitis score identifies patients who may benefit from corticosteroids. Gut. 2007;56(12):1743–6.
27. Lafferty H, Stanley AJ, Forrest EH. The management of alcoholic hepatitis: a prospective comparison of scoring systems. Aliment Pharmacol Ther. 2013;38(6):603–10.
28. Dominguez M, Rincón D, Abraldes JG, Miquel R, Colmenero J, Bellot P, et al. A new scoring system for prognostic stratification of patients with alcoholic hepatitis. Am J Gastroenterol. 2008;103(11):2747–56.
29. Louvet A, Naveau S, Abdelnour M, Ramond MJ, Diaz E, Fartoux L, et al. The Lille model: a new tool for therapeutic strategy in patients with severe alcoholic hepatitis treated with steroids. Hepatology. 2007;45(6):1348–54.
30. Louvet A, Wartel F, Castel H, Dharancy S, Hollebecque A, Canva-Delcambre V, et al. Infection in patients with severe alcoholic hepatitis treated with steroids: early response to therapy is the key factor. Gastroenterology. 2009;137(2):541–8.
31. Poynard T, Barthelemy P, Fratte S, Boudjema K, Doffoel M, Vanlemmens C, et al. Evaluation of efficacy of liver transplantation in alcoholic cirrhosis by a case–control study and simulated controls. Lancet. 1994;344(8921):502–7.
32. Mathurin P, Duchatelle V, Ramond MJ, Degott C, Bedossa P, Erlinger S, et al. Survival and prognostic factors in patients with severe alcoholic hepatitis treated with prednisolone. Gastroenterology. 1996;110(6):1847–53.
33. Liangpunsakul S, Kleiner DE. The alcoholic hepatitis histologic score: structured prognostic biopsy evaluation comes to alcoholic hepatitis. Gastroenterology. 2014;146(5):1156–8.
34. Altamirano J, Miquel R, Katoonizadeh A, Abraldes JG, Duarte-Rojo A, Louvet A, et al. A histologic scoring system for prognosis of patients with alcoholic hepatitis. Gastroenterology. 2014;146(5):1231–1239.e1231-1236.
35. Child CG, Turcotte JG. Surgery and portal hypertension. Major Probl Clin Surg. 1964;1:1–85.
36. Pugh RN, Murray-Lyon IM, Dawson JL, Pietroni MC, Williams R. Transection of the oesophagus for bleeding oesophageal varices. Br J Surg. 1973;60(8):646–9.
37. Cholongitas E, Papatheodoridis GV, Vangeli M, Terreni N, Patch D, Burroughs AK. Systematic review: The model for end-stage liver disease–should it replace Child-Pugh's classification for assessing prognosis in cirrhosis? Aliment Pharmacol Ther. 2005;22(11–12):1079–89.
38. Said A, Williams J, Holden J, Remington P, Gangnon R, Musat A, et al. Model for end stage liver disease score predicts mortality across a broad spectrum of liver disease. J Hepatol. 2004;40(6):897–903.
39. Hanouneh IA, Zein NN, Cikach F, Dababneh L, Grove D, Alkhouri N, et al. The breathprints in patients with liver disease identify novel breath biomarkers in alcoholic hepatitis. Clin Gastroenterol Hepatol. 2014;12(3):516–23.
40. Louvet A, Labreuche J, Artru F, Boursier J, Kim DJ, O'Grady J, et al. Combining Data From Liver Disease Scoring Systems Better Predicts Outcomes of Patients With Alcoholic Hepatitis. Gastroenterology 2015. In Press.

41. Mehta RL, Kellum JA, Shah SV, Molitoris BA, Ronco C, Warnock DG, et al. Acute Kidney Injury Network: report of an initiative to improve outcomes in acute kidney injury. Crit Care. 2007;11(2):R31.

42. Altamirano J, Fagundes C, Dominguez M, García E, Michelena J, Cárdenas A, et al. Acute kidney injury is an early predictor of mortality for patients with alcoholic hepatitis. Clin Gastroenterol Hepatol. 2012;10(1):65–71.e63.

43. Mathurin P, Abdelnour M, Ramond MJ, Carbonell N, Fartoux L, Serfaty L, et al. Early change in bilirubin levels is an important prognostic factor in severe alcoholic hepatitis treated with prednisolone. Hepatology. 2003;38(6):1363–9.

44. Morris JM, Forrest EH. Bilirubin response to corticosteroids in severe alcoholic hepatitis. Eur J Gastroenterol Hepatol. 2005;17(7):759–62.

45. Rudler M, Mouri S, Charlotte F, Lebray P, Capocci R, Benosman H, et al. Prognosis of treated severe alcoholic hepatitis in patients with gastrointestinal bleeding. J Hepatol. 2015;62(4):816–21.

46. Mendenhall CL, Anderson S, Weesner RE, Goldberg SJ, Crolic KA. Protein-calorie malnutrition associated with alcoholic hepatitis. Veterans Administration Cooperative Study Group on Alcoholic Hepatitis. Am J Med. 1984;76(2):211–22.

47. Mendenhall CL, Moritz TE, Roselle GA, Morgan TR, Nemchausky BA, Tamburro CH, et al. A study of oral nutritional support with oxandrolone in malnourished patients with alcoholic hepatitis: results of a Department of Veterans Affairs cooperative study. Hepatology. 1993;17(4):564–76.

48. Mendenhall CL, Moritz TE, Roselle GA, Morgan TR, Nemchausky BA, Tamburro CH, et al. Protein energy malnutrition in severe alcoholic hepatitis: diagnosis and response to treatment. The VA Cooperative Study Group #275. JPEN J Parenter Enteral Nutr. 1995;19(4):258–65.

49. Cabré E, Rodríguez-Iglesias P, Caballería J, Quer JC, Sánchez-Lombraña JL, Parés A, et al. Short- and long-term outcome of severe alcohol-induced hepatitis treated with steroids or enteral nutrition: a multicenter randomized trial. Hepatology. 2000;32(1):36–42.

50. Antar R, Wong P, Ghali P. A meta-analysis of nutritional supplementation for management of hospitalized alcoholic hepatitis. Can J Gastroenterol. 2012;26(7):463–7.

12

Utility of PD-L1 immunohistochemistry assays for predicting PD-1/PD-L1 inhibitor response

Laurence P. Diggs and Eddy C. Hsueh[*]

Abstract

We have seen a notable increase in the application of PD-1/PD-L1 inhibitors for the treatment of several solid and hematogenous malignancies including metastatic melanoma, non-small-cell lung cancer and lymphoma to name a few. The need for biomarkers for identification of a suitable patient population for this type of therapy is now pressing. While specific biomarker assays have been developed for these checkpoint inhibitors based on their respective epitopes, the available studies suggested the clinical utility of these biomarker assays is for response stratification and not patient selection. Further improvement in assay development is needed to utilize this type of assay in identification of ideal patient population for this therapy.

Keywords: Metastatic melanoma, Non-Small-Cell Lung Cancer, PD-1/PD-L1 inhibitors, PD-L1 immunohistochemistry assays

Introduction

Immune modulation therapies have seen an impressive growth over the last decade [1]. Recently, inhibitors of programmed cell-death receptor (PD-1) and its associated ligand (PD-L1) have gained significant attention from the oncology community. PD-L1, typically expressed on the surface of healthy cells, binds PD-1 on primed cytotoxic T cells thereby inhibiting cell-mediated attack [1–3]. Multiple studies reported worse outcomes in tumors expressing PD-L1 [2, 3]. Purportedly, the expression of this ligand on tumor cells confers protection against immune-mediated attacks on tumor cells and may account for their particularly malignant potential. Anti-PD-L1 (or anti-PD-1) monoclonal antibodies inhibit PD-L1 binding to PD-1 and allow T cell activity at this immune checkpoint. Several clinical trials using these antibodies for the treatment of malignancies such as melanoma, non-small-cell lung cancer (NSCLC), head and neck cancer, renal cell cancer, urothelial cancer and lymphoma have shown great promise in prolonging survival [4–10].

However, not all patients respond to PD-1/PD-L1 inhibitors. Thus, predicting the likelihood of response to treatment would aid in appropriate patient selection for these drugs. Immunohistochemistry (IHC) biomarker assays for respective PD-1/PD-L1 inhibitors were designed to screen for the presence of specific PD-1/PD-L1 epitopes as well as to estimate the percentage of T cells or tumor cells expressing this receptor or ligand. At this time, 4 FDA-approved IHC biomarker assays have been designed [10]. Their ability to consistently and reproducibly quantify proportion of cells expressing PD-L1 has been evaluated in prospective trials. Given the inherent heterogeneity of gene expression between individual tumors and among tumor cells within the same tumor nodules, there are concerns that any single assay using a fixed percentage of PD-L1 positive tumor cells could accurately determine the appropriate patients for treatment [11, 12]. This is reflected in the finding that PD-1/PD-L1 inhibitors appear to have activity in a subset of individuals who do not meet the IHC bioassay cutoff. Furthermore, recent studies suggested that several additional factors could be involved in the response to anti-PD-1/PD-L1 antibodies.

Current PD-1 & PD-L1 inhibitors

Among the first generation of these drugs, Pembrolizumab (an anti PD-1 antibody) was approved for treatment

* Correspondence: hsuehec@slu.edu
Division of General Surgery, Department of Surgery, Saint Louis University, 3635 Vista at Grand Blvd., St. Louis, MO 63110, USA

of NSCLC [13–16] and melanoma [17–20] in 2014. Pembrolizumab has also recently been approved for use in advanced head and neck squamous cell carcinoma (HNSCC) [21, 22]. Nivolumab (an anti PD-1 antibody) was approved for melanoma in 2014 [23–28] NSCLC in 2015 [29–32] and renal cell carcinoma in 2015 [33, 34]. Pembrolizumab and Nivolumab have been demonstrated to improve overall and progression free survival in the above-mentioned tumors. Atezolizumab (an anti PD-L1 antibody) has received FDA designated breakthrough drug status for two malignancies. Clinical trials are currently underway for both metastatic NSCLC [35–37] and for urothelial carcinoma [38]. Durvalumab (an anti-PD-L1 antibody) is also being evaluated in clinical trials for the treatment of NSCLC (phase III) [39] and bladder cancer (phase III) [40, 41]. Pidilizumab (an anti PD-1 antibody) is currently being tested in the treatment of large B cell lymphoma (Phase II completed) [42]. Finally, Avelumab (an anti PD-L1 antibody) is currently being tested in patients with Merkel cell carcinoma (Phase II) [43] and NSCLC (Phase III) [44].

Current PD-1/PD-L1 bioassays

Several studies examining the usefulness of PD-L1 IHC assays have demonstrated a direct correlation of response rate to PD-L1 expression level. The distinction between a companion assay and a complementary assay should be underlined here. A companion assay is one that is considered to be essential to the use of its corresponding drug. Pembrolizumab is FDA approved only when used in conjunction with the Dako 22C3. Conversely, the other bioassays are considered complementary in that their use is recommended in order to optimize appropriate patient selection but is not considered mandatory for the use of its associated drug [45]. The cutoff values for these assays vary from as low as 1% to as high as 50%. To allow for comparison, sensitivity (SENS) and specificity (SPEC) of the bioassay for a given malignancy were calculated based on the reported objective response rate in individuals who were considered to have PD-L1 positive tumors (ORR+) and that of the individuals who were considered to have PD-L1 negative tumors (ORR-). Sensitivity was calculated as a ratio of true positives (ORR+) to the sum of true positives (ORR+) and False Negatives (ORR-). Specificity was calculated as a ratio of true negatives (1-ORR-) to the sum of true negatives (1-ORR-) and false positives (1-ORR+).

Pembrolizumab is currently approved for the treatment of NSCLC, advanced HNSCC and advanced melanoma. Its companion IHC biomarker assay, Dako 22C3, is used to detect PD-L1 in all three types of malignancies. It is the only assay that has FDA companion status [45]. This exceptional status is due to the assays reliability when testing for PD-L1 positivity making it an essential tool when assessing which candidates are appropriate for treatment with Pembrolizumab. The Dako 22C3 PD-L1 positivity cutoff is 1% for melanoma. The average ORR+ is 39% for PD-L1 positive tumors and the average ORR- is 10% for PD-L1 negative tumors. These estimates are based on the findings from Daud et al. [19] who graded PD-L1 positivity and negativity based on the MEL score. Using a 1% expression as a cutoff, MEL scores of 0 and 1 were considered negative whereas MEL scores of 2,3,4 and 5 were considered positive. The ORR- and ORR+ were weighted averages of MEL 0 and 1 and MEL 2–5 respectively. The associated SENS and SPEC for this bioassay are 80 and 60%, respectively. The cutoff for HNSCC PD-L1 positivity is also 1%. The ORR+ and ORR- are 22% and 4%, respectively [21, 22]. SENS is 85% and SPEC is 55%. For NSCLC, the Dako 22C3 PD-L1 positivity cutoff is 50%. ORR+ and ORR- are 41 and 13%, respectively [13–15]. The SENS is 76% and the SPEC is 60% (Table 1).

Nivolumab is currently approved for the treatment of squamous and non-squamous NSCLC, advanced RCC and advanced melanoma. Its companion PD-L1 IHC biomarker assay, Dako 28–8, is only used in tumor tissue from NSCLC and melanoma [46]. In the case of RCC, the PD-L1 expression detected on Dako 28–8 was not predictive of response to Nivolumab [33, 34]. Nivolumab is considered second line therapy for RCC regardless of PD-L1 status. For melanoma, the Dako 28–8 PD-L1 positivity cutoff is 5%. The ORR+ was 57% and the ORR- was 41% and the associated SENS and SPEC are 58 and 49%. An interesting set of findings was brought about when Nivolumab was combined with Ipilimumab, an anti- CTLA4 antibody. The ORR+ and ORR- are 72 and 55%, respectively and the associated SENS and SPEC for this bioassay are 57 and 54%, respectively [25, 27, 28]. The Dako 28–8 cutoff for NSCLC is 1%. For non-squamous NSCLC, the ORR+ and ORR- are 19 and 9%, respectively [32]. SENS is 68% and SPEC is 53%. For squamous NSCLC, there was no significant difference between ORR+ and ORR- which could be estimated at approximately 20% [30, 31]. The SENS and SPEC could therefore not be calculated (Table 1).

Durvalumab is currently approved for the treatment of NSCLC and bladder cancer. Its companion IHC biomarker assay is Roche Ventana SP263 [47]. The SP263 PD-L1 positivity cutoff is 25% for NSCLC. The ORR is 27% for PD-L1 positive tumors and 5% for PD-L1 negative tumors [39]. The associated SENS and SPEC are 84 and 78%, respectively. A recent study compared Durvalumab alone to combination therapy with Durvalumab and Tremelimumab (an anti CTLA-4 antibody). The ORR+ and ORR- were 22.5 and 29% respectively indicated that the ORR appeared to be negatively affected by higher PD-L1 expression. The SENS and SPEC were 36 and 48%. The SP263 cutoff for bladder cancer is also

Table 1 Biomarker assays for anti-PD-1/PD-L1 drugs and associated outcomes

Bioassay	Drug	Disease Target	Cut Off[b]	ORR+[c]	ORR-[d]	SENS[e]	SPEC[f]
Roche Ventana SP263	Durvalumab	NSCLC[a]	25%	27%	5%	84%	78%
Roche Ventana SP263	Durvalumab + Tremelimumab	NSCLC	25%	22.5%	29%	36%	48%
Roche Ventana SP263	Durvalumab	Bladder Cancer	25%	46%	0%	100%	65%
Roche Ventana SP142	Atezolizumab	Metastatic NSCLC	50%	45%	14%	76%	61%
Roche Ventana SP142	Atezolizumab	Urothelial Carcinoma	1%	27%	13%	NA	NA
Dako 22C3	Pembrolizumab	NSCLC	50%	41%	13%	76%	60%
Dako 22C3	Pembrolizumab	HNSCC	1%	22%	4%	85%	55%
Dako 22C3[g]	Pembrolizumab	Melanoma	1%	39%	10%	80%	60%
Dako 28-8	Nivolumab	Non-Squamous NSCLC	1%	19%	9%	68%	53%
Dako 28-8	Nivolumab	Squamous NSCLC	5%	20%	20%	NA	NA
Dako 28-8	Nivolumab	Melanoma	5%	57%	41%	58%	49%
Dako 28-8	Nivolumab + Ibilimumab	Melanoma	5%	72%	55%	57%	54%

[a]NSCLC: Non-Small-Cell Lung Cancer – [b]Cut Off: Proportion of tumor cells expressing PD-L1 below which tumor is considered PD-L1 negative. – [c]ORR+ Objective Response Rate in PD-L1 positive tumors. – [d]ORR-: Objective Response Rate in PD-L1 negative tumors. – [e]Sensitivity of bioassay for predicting response to PD-L1 blockade based on established cut off. [f]Specificity of bioassay for predicting response to PD-L1 blockade based on established cut off. – [g]ORR+ and ORR- based on weighted average of corresponding MEL scores

25%. The ORR+ and ORR- are 46 and 0%, respectively [40, 41] with an associated SENS of 100% and SPEC of 65% (Table 1).

Atezolizumab is currently approved for treatment of metastatic NSCLC and urothelial cancer [35]. Its companion IHC biomarker assay is Roche Ventana SP142. The SP142 PD-L1 positivity cutoff is 50% for NSCLC. ORR+ is 45% and ORR- is 14% [36, 37]. The associated SENS and SPEC are 76 and 61%, respectively. The cutoff for urothelial cancer is 1%. The ORR+ and ORR- are 27% and 15%, respectively [38]. However, in this study, the ORR- included both patients with IHC staining <1% and patients with IHC staining between 1 and 5%. Therefore, the SENS and SPEC for SP142 in urothelial cancer could not be calculated (Table 1).

In general, the average specificity for these assays is 58%. Thus, approximately 42% of patients who are not likely to respond to treatment are considered PD-L1+. Furthermore, the average overall sensitivity of these assays with their respective cutoff levels is 72%; suggesting an average of 28% of patients who are considered PD-L1 negative may benefit from this type of treatment. The estimates are based on the figures seen in table.

Factors influencing PD-L1 expression

The mechanism of PD-L1 expression is complex. Several factors appear to influence both PD-L1 expression and response to treatment [48–52]. BRAF and MEK mutations contribute to dysfunction of the Ras-Raf-MEK-ERK Map kinase mutations that are present in greater than 90% of melanomas. Specific BRAF mutations when pretreated with Dabrafenib have been associated with reduced response to PD-1/PD-L1 inhibition in melanoma [53–55]. However, when Dabrafenib was combined with MEK suppressor Tremelimumab, an improved response to PD-L1 inhibition was noted [55, 56]. Similarly, blockade of mutated BRAF and MEK was associated with improved response to PD-1/PD-L1 inhibition in NSCLC. Another interesting relationship is the one between mutations in EGFR and EML4-ALK and the expression of PD-L1. Recent studies indicate that EGFR mutations and rearrangements in EML4-ALK are associated with up regulation of PD-L1 synthesis and expression in NSCLC [57–59]. This was further established when patients with these mutations were treated with tyrosine kinase inhibitors and exhibited in lower overall response to PD-L1 blockade [60]. The presence of KRAS in the tumor also appears to be associated with increased expression of PD-L1 [60]. In a case report, KRAS pretreatment is reported to have increased response to Nivolumab in a patient who had not responded to several other treatment courses [61]. In addition, PD-L1 expression can increase due to local pro-inflammatory factors. Cigarette smoking in patients with NSCLC appears to increase the number of lymphocytes present as well as the overall proportion of PD-L1 present [62]. Platinum based chemotherapy [63] also appears to affect the tumor environment in a similar way to cigarette smoke. Additional studies have attributed tumor resistance to immunotherapies to immunosuppressive events occurring in the tumor microenvironment. Several of the mechanisms have been studied in clinical samples and validated in mouse models. The most important may be extrinsic suppression of CD8+ effector cells by CD4 + CD25 + FoxP3+ regulatory T cells (Tregs) [64, 65]. The metabolic deregulation via tryptophan catabolism by indoleamine-2,3-dioxygenase (IDO) may also play a role [66]. With multiple intrinsic and extrinsic factors influencing PD-L1 expression, PD-L1 expression may vary over time. Since tumor cells can exert an adaptive immune response over time, tumor tissue may express little PD-L1 at the moment of tissue sampling for IHC staining but expression may increase considerably at later time point in the disease course [52, 67, 68].

Conclusion

Modification of specific checkpoints in anti-tumor immune response has resulted in significant improvement for the treatment of various malignancies. The relationship between tumor expression of PD-L1 and patient outcome has been established. However, the currently available IHC biomarker assays could not provide clinically meaningful identification of responders and nonresponders [11, 12, 67, 68]. The sensitivity and specificity of the IHC assays are generally poor. The stringent application of the results of these assays would exclude up to 28% of individuals who may benefit from treatment and include up to 42% of patients who may not benefit.

Several tumor and patient characteristics appear to influence response to PD-1/PD-L1 inhibitor and should be considered when selecting patients for this treatment. Providing several tissue samples and obtaining tissue samples at different time intervals may allow for more accurate determination of appropriate patient for treatment.

A direct comparison of the clinical utility of these diagnostic assays for lung cancer was recently completed. In the Blueprint PD-L1 IHC Assay Comparison Project, the Pathology Committee of the International Association for the Study of Lung Cancer joined efforts with 6 of the commercial stakeholders (Astra Zeneca, Bristol Myers Squibb, Dako, Merck Sharpe Dohme, Roche/Genentech Pharmaceuticals, and Roche Ventana Diagnostics) to compare these tests. 3 of the 4 assays showed similar results but the SP142 demonstrated significantly less expression [72]. The interchangeability of the current assays is likely to be a challenge [69–71]. One promising strategy is the study of mRNA via in situ hybridization aimed at providing useful data for predicting success of these drugs on their targets [73].

Acknowledgements
Not applicable.

Funding
ECH receives research support from Saint Louis University Cancer Center.

Authors' contributions
LPD prepared the majority of the manuscript. ECH performed the final revision and was a major contributor in preparation of the manuscript. All authors read and approved the final manuscript.

Competing interests
ECH is on the Speaker Bureau of Amgen, Inc, and receives honoria for speaking engagement.

References
1. Tumeh PC, Harview CL, Yearley JH, Shintaku IP, Taylor EJ, Robert L, et al. PD-1 blockade induces responses by inhibiting adaptive immune resistance. Nature. 2014;515(7528):568–71. doi:10.1038/nature13954.
2. Gatalica Z, Snyder C, Maney T, Ghazalpour A, Holterman DA, Xiao N, et al. Programmed cell death 1 (PD-1) and its ligand (PD-L1) in common cancers and their correlation with molecular cancer type. Cancer Epidemiol Biomarkers Prev. 2014;23(12):2965–70.
3. Patel SP, Kurzrock R. PD-L1 expression as a predictive biomarker in cancer immunotherapy. Mol Cancer Ther. 2015;14(4):847–56.
4. Massi D, Brusa D, Merelli B, Ciano M, Audrito V, Serra S, et al. PD-L1 marks a subset of melanomas with a shorter overall survival and distinct genetic and morphological characteristics. Ann Oncol. 2014;25(12):2433–42.
5. Wang W, Lau R, Yu D, Zhu W, Korman A, Weber J. PD1 blockade reverses the suppression of melanoma antigen-specific CTL by CD4+ CD25(Hi) regulatory T cells. Int Immunol. 2009;21(9):1065–77.
6. Daud AI, Loo K, Pauli ML, Sanchez-Rodriguez R, Sandoval PM, Taravati K, et al. Tumor immune profiling predicts response to anti-PD-1 therapy in human melanoma. J Clin Invest. 2016;126(9):3447–52. doi:10.1172/JCI87324.
7. Callea M, Albiges L, Gupta M, Cheng SC, Genega EM, Fay AP, et al. PD-L1 expression in primary clear cell renal cell carcinoma (ccRCCs) and their metastases. J Clin Oncol. 2014;32:5s.
8. Brahmer JR. Harnessing the immune system for the treatment of non-small-cell lung cancer. J Clin Oncol. 2013;31(8):1021–8.
9. Cancer Genome Atlas Network. Comprehensive genomic characterization of head and neck squamous cell carcinomas. Nature. 2015;517(7536):576–82.
10. Ma W, Gilligan BM, Yuan J, Li T. Current status and perspectives in translational biomarker research for PD-1/PD-L1 immune checkpoint blockade therapy. J Hematol Oncol. 2016;9:47. doi:10.1186/s13045-016-0277-y.
11. Kerr KM, Hirsch FR. Programmed death ligand-1 immunohistochemistry friend or foe? Arch Pathol Lab Med. 2016;140:326–31.
12. Kerr KM, Tsao MS, Nicholson AG, Yatabe Y, Wistuba II, Hirsch FR, et al. Programmed death-ligand 1 immunohistochemistry in lung cancer: in what state is this art? J Thorac Oncol. 2015;10(7):985–9.
13. Reck M, Rodríguez-Abreu D, Robinson AG, Hui R, Csőszi T, Fülöp A, et al. Pembrolizumab versus chemotherapy for PD-L1-positive non-small-cell lung cancer. N Engl J Med. 2016;375:1823–33. doi:10.1056/NEJMoa1606774. November 10, 2016.
14. Garon EB, Rizvi NA, Hui R, Leighl N, Balmanoukian AS, Eder JP, et al. Pembrolizumab for the treatment of non-small-cell lung cancer. N Engl J Med. 2015;372(21):2018–28.
15. Herbst RS, Baas P, Kim DW, Felip E, Pérez-Gracia JL, Han JY, et al. Pembrolizumab versus docetaxel for previously treated, PD-L1-positive, advanced non-small-cell lung cancer (KEYNOTE-010): a randomised controlled trial. The Lancet. 2015;387(10027):1540–50.
16. Garon EB, Gandhi L, Rizvi N, Hui R, Balmanoukian AS, Patnaik A, et al. Antitumor activity of pembrolizumab (pembro; mk-3475) and correlation with programmed death ligand 1 (pd-l1) expression in a pooled analysis of patients (pts) with advanced non-small cell lung carcinoma (NSCLC). Ann Oncol. 2014;25 suppl 4:LBA43.
17. Ribas A, et al. Association of pembrolizumab with tumor response and survival among patients with advanced melanoma. JAMA. 2016;315:1600.
18. Robert C, Schachter J, Long GV, Arance A, Grob JJ, Mortier L. Pembrolizumab versus ipilimumab in advanced melanoma. N Engl J Med. 2015;372:2521–32.

19. Daud AI, Wolchok JD, Robert C, Hwu WJ, Weber JS, Ribas A, et al. Programmed death-ligand 1 expression and response to the anti-programmed death 1 antibody pembrolizumab in melanoma. J Clin Oncol. 2016;34(34):4102–9. Epub 2016 Oct 31.

20. Ribas A, Puzanov I, Dummer R, Schadendorf D, Hamid O, Robert C, et al. Pembrolizumab versus investigator-choice chemotherapy for ipilimumab-refractory melanoma (KEYNOTE-002): a randomised, controlled, phase 2 trial. Lancet Oncol. 2015;16(8):908–18.

21. Chow LQ, Haddad R, Gupta S, Mahipal A, Mehra R, Tahara M, et al. Antitumor activity of pembrolizumab in biomarker-unselected patients with recurrent and/or metastatic head and neck squamous cell carcinoma: results from the phase Ib KEYNOTE-012 expansion. Cohort J Clin Oncol. 2016;32:3838–45.

22. Seiwert TY, Burtness B, Mehra R, Weiss J, Berger R, Eder JP, et al. Safety and clinical activity of pembrolizumab for treatment of recurrent or metastatic squamous cell carcinoma of the head and neck (KEYNOTE-012): an open-label, multicentre, phase 1b trial. Lancet Oncol. 2016;17(7):956–65.

23. Topalian S, Sznol M, McDermott, Kluger HM, Carvajal RD, Sharfman WH, et al. Survival, durable tumor remission, and longterm safety in patients with advanced melanoma receiving nivolumab. J Clin Oncol. 2014;32(10):1020–30.

24. Weber JS, D'Angelo SP, Minor D, Hodi FS, Gutzmer R, Neyns B, et al. Nivolumab versus chemotherapy in patients with advanced melanoma who progressed after anti-CTLA-4 treatment (CheckMate 037): a randomised, controlled, open-label, phase 3 trial. Lancet Oncol. 2015;16(4):375–84.

25. Larkin J, Hodi FS, Wolchok JD. Combined Nivolumab and Ipilimumab or Monotherapy in Untreated Melanoma. N Engl J Med. 2015;373:23–34.

26. Robert C, Long GV, Brady B, Dutriaux C, Maio M, Mortier L, et al. Nivolumab in previously untreated melanoma without BRAF mutation. N Engl J Med. 2015;372(4):320–30.

27. Postow MA, Chesney J, Pavlick AC, Robert C, Grossmann K, McDermott D, et al. Nivolumab and ipilimumab versus ipilimumab in untreated melanoma. N Engl J Med. 2015;372:2006–17.

28. Hodi FS, Chesney J, Pavlick AC, Robert C, Grossmann KF, McDermott DF, et al. Combined nivolumab and ipilimumab versus ipilimumab alone in patients with advanced melanoma: 2-year overall survival outcomes in a multicentre, randomised, controlled, phase 2 trial. Lancet Oncol. 2016;17(11):1558–68.

29. Gettinger SN, Horn L, Gandhi L, Spigel DR, Antonia SJ, Rizvi NA, et al. Overall survival and long-term safety of nivolumab (anti-programmed death 1 antibody, BMS-936558, ONO-4538) in patients with previously treated advanced non-small-cell lung cancer. J Clin Oncol. 2015;33(18):2004–12.

30. Brahmer J, Reckamp KL, Baas P, Crinò L, Eberhardt WE, Poddubskaya E, et al. Nivolumab versus docetaxel in advanced squamous-cell non-small-cell lung cancer. N Engl J Med. 2015;373(2):123–35.

31. Rizvi NA, Mazières J, Planchard D, Stinchcombe TE, Dy GK, Antonia SJ, et al. Activity and safety of nivolumab, an anti-PD-1 immune checkpoint inhibitor, for patients with advanced, refractory squamous non-small-cell lung cancer (CheckMate 063): a phase 2, single-arm trial. Lancet Oncol. 2015;16(3):257–65.

32. Borghaei H, Paz-Ares L, Horn L, Spigel DR, Steins M, Ready NE, et al. Nivolumab versus docetaxel in advanced non-squamous non-small-cell lung cancer. N Engl J Med. 2015;373(17):1627–39.

33. McDermott DF, Drake CG, Sznol M, Choueiri TK, Powderly JD, Smith DC, et al. Survival, durable response, and long-term safety in patients with previously treated advanced renal cell carcinoma receiving nivolumab. J Clin Oncol. 2015;33(18):2013–20.

34. Nivolumab combined with ipilimumab versus sunitinib in previously untreated advanced or metastatic renal cell carcinoma (CheckMate 214). ClinicalTrials.gov Identifier: NCT02231749.

35. Herbst RS, Soria JC, Kowanetz M, Fine GD, Hamid O, Gordon MS, et al. Predictive correlates of response to the anti-PD-L1 antibody MPDL3280A in cancer patients. Nature. 2014;515(7528):563–7.

36. Fehrenbacher L, Spira A, Ballinger M, Kowanetz M, Vansteenkiste J, Mazieres J, et al. Atezolizumab versus docetaxel for patients with previously treated non-small-cell lung cancer (POPLAR): a multicentre, open-label, phase 2 randomised controlled trial. Lancet. 2016;387(10030):1837–46.

37. Herbst RS, De Marinis F, Jassem J, Lam S, Mocci S, Sandler A, et al. PS01.56: IMpower110: phase III trial comparing 1 L atezolizumab with chemotherapy in PD-L1–selected chemotherapy-naive NSCLC patients. J Thorac Oncol. 2016;11(11):S304–5.

38. Rosenberg JE, Hoffman-Censits J, Powles T, van der Heijden MS, Balar AV, Necchi A, et al. Atezolizumab in patients with locally advanced and

metastatic urothelial carcinoma who have progressed following treatment with platinum-based chemotherapy: a single-arm, multicentre, phase 2 trial. Lancet. 2016;387:1909–20.

39. Planchard D, Yokoi T, McCleod MJ, Fischer JR, Kim YC, Ballas M, et al. A phase III study of durvalumab (MEDI4736) with or without tremelimumab for previously treated patients with advanced NSCLC: rationale and protocol design of the ARCTIC study. Clin Lung Cancer. 2016;17(3):232.

40. Brower V. Anti-PD-L1 inhibitor Durvalumab in bladder cancer. Lancet Oncol. 2016;17(7):e275.

41. Massard C, Gordon MS, Sharma S, Rafii S, Wainberg ZA, Luke J, et al. Safety and efficacy of durvalumab (MEDI4736), an anti-programmed cell death ligand-1 immune checkpoint inhibitor, in patients with advanced urothelial bladder cancer. J Clin Oncol. 2016;34:26. 3119–3125.

42. Bryan LJ, Gordon LI. Pidilizumab in the treatment of diffuse large B-cell lymphoma. Expert Opin Biol Ther. 2014;14(9):1361–8.

43. Sidaway P. Skin cancer: Avelumab effective against Merkel-cell carcinoma. Nat Rev Clin Oncol. 2016;13(11):652.

44. A Phase III, Open-label, Multicenter Trial of Avelumab (MSB0010718C) Versus Platinum-based Doublet as a First-line Treatment of Recurrent or Stage IV PD-L1+ Non-small Cell Lung Cancer. ClinicalTrials.gov. Identifier: NCT02576574

45. Roach C, Zhang N, Corigliano E, Jansson M, Toland G, Ponto G, et al. Development of a companion diagnostic PD-L1 immunohistochemistry assay for pembrolizumab therapy in Non–small-cell lung cancer. Appl Immunohistochem Mol Morphol. 2016;24:392–7.

46. Phillips T, Simmons P, Inzunza HD, Cogswell J, Novotny Jr J, Taylor C, et al. Development of an automated PD-L1 immunohistochemistry (IHC) assay for non-small cell lung cancer. Appl Immunohistochem Mol Morphol. 2015;23(8):541–9.

47. Rebelatto MC, Midha A, Mistry A, Sabalos C, Schechter N, Li X, et al. Development of a programmed cell death ligand-1 immunohistochemical assay validated for analysis of non-small cell lung cancer and head and neck squamous cell carcinoma. Diagn Pathol. 2016;11:95.

48. McLaughlin J, Han G, Schalper KA, Carvajal-Hausdorf D, Pelekanou V, Rehman J, et al. Quantitative assessment of the heterogeneity of PD-L1 expression in non-small-cell lung cancer. JAMA Oncol. 2016;1:46–54.

49. Rizvi NA, Hellmann MD, Snyder A, Kvistborg P, Makarov V, Havel JJ, et al. Cancer immunology: mutational landscape determines sensitivity to PD-1 blockade in non-small cell lung cancer. Science. 2015;348(6230):124–8.

50. Taube JM, Klein A, Brahmer JR, Xu H, Pan X, Kim JH, et al. Association of PD-1, PD-L1 ligands, and other features of the tumor immune micro-environment with response to anti-PD-1 therapy. Clin Cancer Res. 2014;20(19):5064–74.

51. Zaretsky JM, Garcia-Diaz A, Shin DS, Escuin-Ordinas H, Hugo W, Hu-Lieskovan S, et al. Mutations associated with acquired resistance to PD-1 blockade in melanoma. N Engl J Med. 2016;375(9):819–29.

52. Kowanetz M, Koeppen H, Boe M, Chaft JE, Rudin CM, Zou W, et al. Spatiotemporal effects on programmed death ligand 1 (PD-L1) expression and immunophenotype of non-small cell lung cancer (NSCLC). J Thorac Oncol. 2015;10:9.

53. Johnson DB, Pectasides E, Feld E, Ye F, Zhao S, Johnpulle R, et al. Sequencing treatment in BRAFV600 mutant melanoma: anti-PD-1 before and after BRAF inhibition. J Immunother. 2017;40(1):31–5 [ABSTRACT].

54. Massi D, Brusa D, Merelli B, Falcone C, Xue G, Carobbio A, et al. The status of PD-L1 and tumor-infiltrating immune cells predict resistance and poor prognosis in BRAFi-treated melanoma patients harboring mutant BRAFV600. Ann Oncol. 2015;26(9):1980–7.

55. Rivalland G, Mitchell P. Combined BRAF and MEK inhibition in BRAF-mutant NSCLC. Lancet Oncol. 2016;17(7):860–2. doi:10.1016/S1470-2045(16)30203-0. Epub 2016 Jun 6.

56. Roskoski R. Allosteric MEK1/2 inhibitors including cobimetanib and trametinib in the treatment of cutaneous melanomas. Pharmacol Res. 2017;117:20–31.

57. Ota K, Azuma K, Kawahara A, Hattori S, Iwama E, Tanizaki J, et al. Induction of PD-L1 expression by the EML4-ALK oncoprotein and downstream signaling pathways in non-small cell lung cancer. Clin Cancer Res. 2015;21:4014–21.

58. Chen N, Fang W, Zhan J, Hong S, Tang Y, Kang S, et al. Upregulation of PD-L1 by EGFR activation mediates the immune escape of EGFR-Driven NSCLC: implications of optional immune targeted therapy for NSCLC patients with EGFR mutation. J Thorac Oncol. 2015;10:910–23.

59. Tang Y, Fang W, Zhang Y, Hong S, Kang S, Yan Y, et al. The association between PD-L1 and EGFR status and the prognostic value of PD-L1 in

advanced non-small cell lung cancer patients treated with EGFR-TKIs. Oncotoarget. 2015;6:14209–19.

60. Lin C, Chen X, Li M, Liu J, Qi X, Yang W, et al. Programmed death-ligand 1 expression predicts tyrosine kinase inhibitor response and better prognosis in a cohort of patients with epidermal growth factor receptor mutation-positive lung adenocarcinoma. Clin Lung Cancer. 2015;16:e25–35.

61. Calles A, Liao X, Sholl LM, Rodig SJ, Freeman GJ, Butaney M, et al. Expression of PD-1 and its ligands, PD-L1 and PD-L2, in smokers and never smokers with KRAS mutant lung cancer. J Thorac Oncol. 2015;10:1726–35.

62. Barsoum IB, Smallwood CA, Siemens DR, Graham CH. A mechanism of hypoxia-mediated escape from adaptive immunity in cancer cells. Cancer Res. 2014;74:665–74.

63. Hato SV, Khong A, De Vires IJ, Lesterhius WJ. Molecular Pathways: the immunogenic effects of platinum–based chemotherapeutics. Clin Cancer Res. 2014;20:2831–7.

64. Gajewski TF, Meng Y, Harlin H. Immune suppression in the tumor microenvironment. J Immunother. 2006;29:233–40.

65. Kline J, Brown IE, Zha YY, Blank C, Strickler J, Wouters H, Zhang L, Gajewski TF. Homeo-static proliferation plus regulatory T-cell depletion promotes potent rejection of B16 melanoma. Clin Cancer Res. 2008;14:3156–67.

66. Uyttenhove C, Pilotte L, Théate I, Stroobant V, Colau D, Parmentier N, Boon T, Van den Eynde BJ. Evidence for a tumoral immune resistance mechanism based on tryptophan degradation by indoleamine 2,3-dioxygenase. Nat Med. 2003;9:1269–74.

67. Chen Y-b, Chuan-Yong M, Huang J-A. Clinical significance of programmed death-1 ligand-1 expression in patients with non-small cell lung cancer: a 5-year-follow-up study. Tumori. 2012;2012(6):751–5.

68. Illie M, Long-Mira E, Bence C, Butori C, Lassalle S, Bouhlel L, et al. Comparative study of the PD-L1 status between surgically resected specimens and matched biopsies of NSCLC patients reveal major discordances: a potential issue for anti-PD-L1 therapeutic strategies. Ann Oncol. 2016;27:147–53.

69. Food US, Administration D. Public workshop—complexities in personalized medicine: harmonizing companion diagnostics across a class of targeted therapies. March. 2015;24.

70. Fitzgibbons PL, Bradley LA, Fatheree LA, Alsabeh R, Fulton RS, Goldsmith JD, et al. Principles of analytic validation of immunohistochemical assays: guideline from the College of American Pathologists Pathology and Laboratory Quality Center. Arch Pathol Lab Med. 2014;138(11):1432–43.

71. Carvajal-Hausdorf DE, Schalper KA, Neumeister VM, Rimm DL. Quantitative measurement of cancer tissue biomarkers in the lab and in the clinic. Lab Invest. 2015;95(4):385–96.

72. Hirsch FR, McElhinny A, Stanforth D, Ranger-Moore J, Jansson M, Kulangara K. PD-L1 immunohistochemistry assays for lung cancer: results from phase 1 of the blueprint PD-L1 IHC assay comparison project. J Thorac Oncol. 2017;12(2):208–22. doi:10.1016/j.jtho.2016.11.2228. Epub 2016 Nov 29.

73. Higgs BW, Robbins PB, Blake-Haskins JA, Zhu W, Morehouse C, Brohawn PZ, et al. High tumoral IFN mRNA, PD-L1 protein, and combined IFNg mRNA/PD-L1 protein expression associates with response to durvalumab (anti-PD-L1) monotherapy in NSCLC patients. Eur J Cancer. 2015;51 suppl 3:S717, 15LBA.

13

Mechanically produced schistosomula as a higher-throughput tools for phenotypic pre-screening in drug sensitivity assays: current research and future trends

Emmanuel Mouafo Tekwu[1,2]*, William Kofi Anyan[1], Daniel Boamah[3], Kofi Owusu Baffour-Awuah[1], Stephanie Keyetat Tekwu[4], Veronique Penlap Beng[2], Alexander Kwadwo Nyarko[5] and Kwabena Mante Bosompem[1]

Abstract

It is crucial to develop new antischistosomal drugs since there is no vaccine and the whole world is relying on only a single drug for the treatment of schistosomiasis. One of the obstacles to the development of drugs is the absence of the high throughput objective screening methods to assess drug compounds efficacy. Thus for identification of new drug compounds candidates, fast and accurate in vitro assays are unavoidable and more research efforts in the field of drug discovery can target schistosomula. This review presents a substantial overview of the present state of in vitro drug sensitivity assays developed so far for the determination of anti-schistosomula activity of drug compounds, natural products and derivatives using newly transformed schistosomula (NTS). It highlights some of the challenges involved in in vitro compound screening using NTS and the way forward.

Keywords: Schistosomiasis, Newly Transformed Schistosomula, Mechanical transformation, In vitro drug sensitivity, Drug discovery

Background

Hundreds of millions of people are living at risk of schistosomiasis infection [1]. More than 207 million people are infected worldwide with 85% living in Africa. This makes schistosomiasis one of the most devastating tropical diseases in the world and remains a major source of morbidity and mortality for developing countries, especially in Sub-Saharan Africa [1]. Also known as "snail fever", schistosomiasis is a water-borne trematodiasis carried by fresh water snails infected with one of the five varieties of the parasite *Schistosoma*. But three principal varieties are mainly the causative agents for human schistosomiasis: *Schistosoma mansoni*, *Schistosoma haematobium* and *Schistosoma japonicum*. The pathophysiology associated with schistosomiasis, is mainly due to immune response to the schistosome eggs that are trapped in tissues and organs. The liver, intestines and bladder usually trap eggs on their way out of the host. The spleen, as a lymphoid organ, becomes enlarged (splenomegaly) and together with the enlargement of the liver result in hepatosplenomegaly. Schistosomiasis has both an acute and a chronic phase. Acute schistosomiasis are generally short-term and mild and can develop a few weeks after the schistosome parasite first penetrates into the skin of the host. But if left untreated, schistosomiasis cause by any of the three species listed above may become a chronic inflammation which develops slowly into swelling, fibrosis and necrosis of the affected tissues such as intestinal organs, the liver and the bladder, as well as a wide range of other symptoms which gradually damage the host physiologically and even cognitively [2, 3].

Mass drug administration (MDA) in endemic areas using praziquantel (PZQ) remains a major cornerstone of schistosomiasis control programs [4]. Praziquantel

* Correspondence: ETekwu@noguchi.ug.edu.gh; etekwu@yahoo.fr
[1]Noguchi Memorial Institute for Medical Research (NMIMR), College of Health Sciences, University of Ghana, PO Box LG581 Legon, Accra, Ghana
[2]Laboratory for Tuberculosis Research and Pharmacology, Biotechnology Centre, Nkolbisson, University of Yaoundé 1, Yaoundé, Cameroon
Full list of author information is available at the end of the article

was discovered in the year 1970's and brought to the market in 1988 under the name Biltricide [5, 6]. It is so far the only drug available and recommended by World Health Organization (WHO) for the treatment of schistosomiasis. This single drug PZQ, is used for the treatment of millions of people annually and as stated in the recent publications, its coverage is projected to reach 235 million people by 2018, which raises concerns of increasing drug pressure [7, 8]. Furthermore, although there are several advantages of this drug, in particular its high efficacy on the adult worms of all the medically important *Schistosoma* species and its excellent tolerability, PZQ has some disadvantages, mostly its inefficiency against younger stage of schistosomes [9]. This mean that treatment does not rule out all the worms in those who are infected and necessitates the repeat of the treatment. Again, reliance on a single drug as the sole treatment, while positively reducing morbidity has led to big concerns over development of potential drug resistance [10]. These facts emphasize the imperative to search for the next generation of antischistosomal drugs. Therefore, a number of studies have recommended repeatedly the need for novel drugs, since the drug discovery and development pipeline is virtually dry [11]. Only a few candidates compounds have been studied in preclinical phases [12] and none of them have reached the clinical trials phase. For instance, the target product profile for a new antischistosomal drug [12] was not met by mefloquine and artemisinins [13, 14].

Formerly, procedures established at TDR-designated compound screening centers relied on adult worms incubated with the candidate drugs for 72 h [15]. Following the incubation period, the parasite viability was assessed microscopically [15]. This approach of in vitro drug screening based on the phenotype of the whole adult worm organism usually requires the intensive use of laboratory animals (hamster, rats, mice) since there is no existing in vitro life cycles for *Schistosoma*. This approach is also time consuming and low-throughput and relied on a small number of research groups experts that are able to handle the complex life cycle of *Schistosoma* and work with both high recovery of adult parasite from mammalian host and long screen timelines. The latter is the consequence of the long period that *Schistosoma* infection requires to become obvious since in the mouse model, it may take not less than 30 days for *S. mansoni* infections to become patent [16] and even more than 30 days for others specie such as *S. haematobium*.

Not long ago, the screening method using Newly Transformed Schistosomula (NTS) has been popularised as a higher-throughput [17–20]. Here, we have provided an overview for the alternative approach to phenotypic screening younger parasites that can be easily obtained from the intermediary host snails and in greater numbers

than adult worms. This review presents the current state of in vitro drug sensitivity assays developed so far for the determination of anti-schistosomula activity of drug compounds, natural products and derivatives using NTS and highlights some of the challenges involved in in vitro compound screening using NTS.

In which stage of the *Schistosoma* life cycle is schistosomula found?

Schistosomes have a complex life cycle (Fig. 1). The transmission of schistosomiasis occurs when people harboring the parasite contaminate freshwater sources (lakes, ponds, rivers and dams) inhabited by snails with their urine (for urogenital Schistosomiasis) or faeces (for intestinal schistosomiasis) containing parasite eggs. Under optimal conditions the fertilized eggs hatch in water and miracidia are released. Once released from the eggs, miracidia swim in the fresh water and penetrate specific intermediate snail hosts. In the snail host, the miracidiae multiply by asexual division of 2 generations of sporocysts (primary and then secondary sporocysts) and produce cercariae from 4 to 6 weeks [21, 22]. Upon release from the snail, the infective cercariae can remain infective in freshwater for 1 to 3 days [22]. They swim in the water in search of the definitive host. Upon contact with the host, cercariae penetrate the skin of the host, and lose their bifurcated tail to become schistosomulae [22]. It takes several days for the schistomules to move from the skin into the venous circulation then into the lungs [22]. This path generally takes within 5 to 7 days after penetration. The schistosomulae takes at least 15 days to travel through the circulatory system to the hepatoportal circulation where they grow and mature into adult worms and pair up. In humans, adult worms are found to reside in either the perivesicular or mesenteric venules in various locations. This seems to be specific for each species. Specifically, *S. japonicum* occurs frequently in the superior mesenteric veins draining the small intestine while *S. mansoni* is frequently found in the superior mesenteric veins draining the large intestine. Nevertheless, *S. japonicum* and *S. mansoni* can occupy either location, and they are capable of moving between both sites, therefore it is impossible to state unequivocally that one species is specifically found in one location. Generally, *S. haematobium* is found in the venous plexus of the bladder, but can sometime be found in the rectal venules. The females start laying eggs from 4 to 6 weeks after infection in their final infection site which is either the bladder or the intestine. This usually continues for 3 to 5 years equivalent to the lifespan of the worm [22]. Eggs are laid in the small venules of the portal and perivesical systems. For *S. mansoni* and *S. japonicum*, eggs gradually move towards the lumen of the intestine and of the bladder and ureters

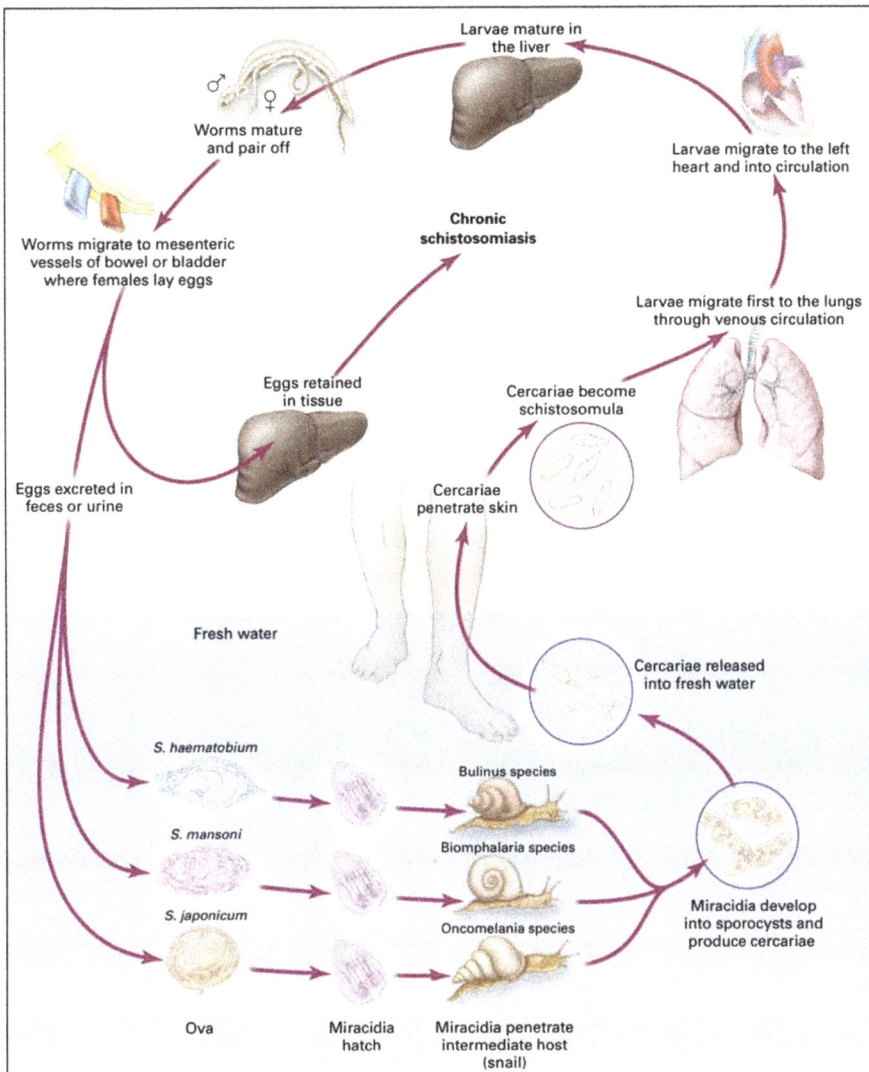

Fig. 1 Life cycle of *Schistosoma* (Source: [22])

for *S. haematobium*, and are excreted from the body through feces or urine, respectively [22]. The intermediate host snails are primary for transmission, and human contact with fresh water that harbors the infective larval form of the parasite known as cercariae is thus necessary for Schistosome infection [22].

Importance of in vitro drug screening using Newly Transformed Schistosomula (NTS)

The in vitro culture techniques were developed for parasites after the successful establishment of the life cycle of *S. mansoni* in the laboratory [15]. The process relied on adult worms incubated with the candidate drugs for 72 h after which the viability of the parasite is microscopically assessed [15]. This approach of phenotypic screening using whole worm organism requires the intensive use of laboratory animals such as hamster, rats and mice since currently there is no existing in vitro procedure to generate adult worms. Moreover, this method is time consuming and low-throughput. It is no wonder that, in the recent years, researchers are using the Newly Transformed Schistosomula (NTS) as a tools for higher-throughput screening for drug sensitivity assay in the field of antischistosomals drug discovrey [12, 17–20, 23–27].

The era of working with schistosomula began with the recovery of mature schistosmulae from the lungs of infected laboratory animals. This was associated with the inconvenience of recovering only limited worm [19]. The transformation of cercariae into schistosomula using simple techniques as centrifugation, repeated aspiration through a syringe needle or chemical stimulation was an important discovery in the field of schistosome cultivation. Nowadays, researchers use cercariae as the starting material for in vitro studies of schistosomes as large numbers of schistosomula can be easily obtained in a manner which is advantageous in economical point of view [18, 19]. Furthermore and most importantly, the use of mechanically transformed schistosomulae limits and replaces the use of live animals in accordance with the 3Rs (reduce, replace, refine) principles of animal protection. Using an artificially produced schistosomula in in vitro drug sensitivity assays might serve as pre-screen tools.

Changes associated with cercariae/ schistosomulum transformation

Schistosoma infection occurs when people get in contact with free-swimming larval forms of the parasite (cercariae) released by freshwater snails. Cercariae, with the aid of its tail swim in the water until they penetrate the skin of the definitive host during contact with the contaminated water. From its intermediate snail host to the definitive host (human), the cercariae undergoes a series of adaptive changes. All these changes are known as transformation. During the transformation process, the tail of cercariae is lost and the secretory glands release two substances: a mucus which promotes attachment to the skin and enzymes which degrade the skin [28]. Moreover, on the surface of schistosomula, appears the transient microvilli and a double unit membrane is formed on the tegument [29]. Concurrently, some of the glycocalyx is lost [29]. McLaren and Hockley reported that in vivo, microvilli are developed on the surface of schistosomula obtained throughout penetration of the host skin. This also occurs on schistosomula which have penetrated a mouse skin prepared in vitro and on artificial schistosomula prepared by mechanical separation of the tail from the head of the cercariae [30]. From their investigation, they reported that microvilli occur at approximately the same time, have about the same lifespan and show identical morphological characteristics in each of the three types of schistosomula [30].

Schistosomules rapidly undergo marked physiological and ultrastructural changes in the body of the definitive host in order to adapt to the host's internal environment [31]. Some of these changes are loss of the glycocalyx, conversion of trilaminate to heptalaminate tegumental membrane [29], sensitivity of schistosomula to water (loss of water tolerance) [28], and evacuation of secretory glands. All these changes result in the schistosomulum stage. Transformation is complete within about 2–3 h [30, 32]. Brink et al. published in 1977 a study conducted to compare schistosomula produced artificially and schistosomula recovered after cercariae had penetrated isolated skin [33]. They concluded that the schistosomula prepared by mechanical separation of the

tail from the head of the cercariae fulfill the main criteria of transformation from cercarial to schistosomulum. This is justified by the fact that, the surface membrane of all type of schistosomula (those mechanically obtained and those recovered after cercarial penetration of the isolated skin) had changed from trilaminate to heptalaminate structures and had loss their cercarial glycocalyx within 2 h of transformation [33]. They also reported that in vitro, the development of mechanical transformed schistosomules is similar to schistosomula obtained after cercarial had penetrated isolated skin although only 25–50% of mechanically transformed schistosomules reached the 'gut-closed' stage by day 12, while 50–70% of skin transformed schistosomules reached this stage [33]. Thus, 2 mains criteria were generated by the authors to help decide whether transformation from cercariae to schistosomula has been effective. The 2 criteria were, the NTS must have developed heptalaminate surface membranes and they must be capable to growth and develop in vitro, at least to the 'gut-closed' stage [33].

Requirement for in vitro drug screening using NTS

Drugs and chemicals

Praziquantel, mefloquine, auranofin, artesunate, metrifonate, oxamniquine, artemisinins, arthemeter are drugs used as antischistosomal compounds. These drugs are usually dissolved in dimethylsulphoxide (DMSO) to obtain drug stock solutions of 10 mg/ml or 10 mM and then diluted into culture media to serve as positive control [12, 20, 23, 25, 26, 34]. The highest concentration of DMSO used as drug solvent should not exceed 1% [15, 18, 24, 34].

Antifungal drug (Amphotericin B) and antibiotic drugs (penicillin 100 to 300 U/ml and streptomycin 100 to 300 µg/ml) are used to supplement the medium in order to avoid fungal and bacteria contamination during schistosomula culture [12, 17, 23, 25–27, 34].

Media

Different type of media such as Basch Medium 169 [18–20, 26, 27, 35, 36], Earles'Minimum Essential Medium [32, 33], Dulbecco's Modified Eagle's Medium (DMEM) [17, 19, 26, 31, 35, 37], Minimum Essential Medium (MEM) [19, 27, 35], Roswell Park Memorial Institute (RPMI 1640) [18, 31, 32, 38] and Medium 199 [12, 19, 23–26, 34, 35] have been used in different studies. Other investigations were developed to compare and obtain optimal culture conditions for the NTS. For the optimal culture condition for schistosomula, several studies have shown that the supplemented medium is appropriate. Different concentrations of heat inactivated fetal calf serum (iFCS) 1% [24], 5% [12, 20, 23, 25–27, 34, 38], 10%

[17, 37], or heat inactivated fetal bovine serum (FBS) 5% [38], 10% [36] have been used.

The supplemented medium 199 turned out to be the most suitable medium for the incubation of schistosomula and thus has been widely used for in vitro screening of others compounds with known activities against *Schistosoma* newly transformed schistosomula [12, 23–25, 34]. Thus 5 to 10% heat inactivated calf serum is the commonly used supplement by several researchers.

Snails and cercariae

The snails might be of the genus *Bulinus* which serves as the intermediate hosts of *S. haematobium* as well as of *S. intercalatum* or the genus *Biomphalaria* or *Oncomelania* for *S. mansoni* and *S. japonicum* respectively. Snails are individually infected with an average of 10 miracidia per snail [26]. In our laboratory, an average of 5 can be used to successfully infect snails. Usually, snails are kept in aquarium with dechlorinated water in a humid room simulating a 12 h day and night cycle. Intermediate host snails start shedding cercariae from 4 to 6 weeks post-infection with miracidia. According to the circadian rhythm, each snail species are then collected and placed individually into 24 or 48 well plates or in a test tube (1 ml of distilled or dechlorinated tap water/well or per tube). Each test tube or well plate can be exposed to artificial light for 30 min [39], 1 h [17], or 2 h [40–43]. The cercarial suspension is then collected, cleaned and concentrated by allowing to stand on ice for 30 to 60 min. During this time, cercariae form into a mass, settle and adhere to the bottom of the tube. The supernatant is poured off and replaced with ice-cold distilled water. This suspension is used for the preparation of schistosomula. There are several techniques for transforming cercariae into schistosomula and maintaining them [18, 33, 44–46]. Some of these techniques are performed in vivo and others in vitro. In vivo transformation occurs after host skin penetration [33] and in vitro transformation can be obtained when parasites penetrate excised skin [33, 47] or when cercariae tails are removed mechanically [12, 18–20, 23–25, 27, 33, 34, 45] or chemically [26] and cercariae bodies are incubated in physiological media (Fig. 2).

Newly transformed schistosomula (NTS)
In vitro transformation of Schistosome cercariae to schistosomula and maintenance

As the schistosomulum stage is becoming attractive for search of new antischistosomal drugs, this requires the development of efficient, reproducible and rapid means to generate large and suitable quantities of the biological material. The artificial transformation of cercariae into schistosomula can be induced by various effectors for instance the cell growth media at 37 °C [48, 49] or low osmolarity phosphate buffer saline solution [50] that seem to be able to start off the transformation of cercariae into schistosomula. In vitro, schistosomula can be obtained through excised skin preparation or by mechanical separation of the tail from the body of the cercariae [30]

Non-mechanical transformation

Excised skin preparation of schistosomula Schistosomula can be prepared from cercariae of schistosome by allowing them to penetrate excised rat [51] or mouse [52] skins into Hanks' Balanced Salt Solution (HBSS). The possibility of contamination by host material and the low yield of produced schistosomula as reported by Brink et al. [33] make the excised skin penetration technique inappropriate.

Chemical transformation using glucose The cercarial transformation can be performed using glucose. This is known as chemical transformation which is carried out based on protocol previously described [45]. Briefly, the cercariae suspension is cooled on ice for 30 min to reduce parasite motility. Afterwards, the cercariae suspension is centrifuged for 2 min at 2000 rpm, then resuspended in 5% glucose and incubated for 10 min at 30 °C [26]. The tails are removed from the bodies using the ice purification method as described below.

Mechanical preparation of schistosomula

The mechanical transformation protocol is the most popular method for obtaining artificially transformed schistosomula. This method is applied to freshly shed cercariae and includes centrifugation, passages through an emulsifying needle, or shaking. The separation of cercariae body from tails is usually done by centrifugation in a density gradient followed by incubation of the cercariae heads in culture media at 37 °C. In order to detach the tails from the body, these methods usually incorporate an initial step consisting of agitating the organisms sufficiently. Schistosomules prepared in vitro and incubated at 37 °C gradually undergo morphological and physiological changes [31]. Tucker in 2001 [31] reported that mechanically transformed schistsmula by 24 h in culture, resemble in most respects cercariae that have penetrated and resided in the skin for about 1 h. Thus, parasites obtained following this protocol is morphologically or biochemically closed enough to those recovered from natural infections [33, 48]. This makes the mechanical transformation the best alternative method for large production of schistosomula for high-throughput studies such as gene expression, identification of drug targets and identification of effective drugs against schistosmes [37].

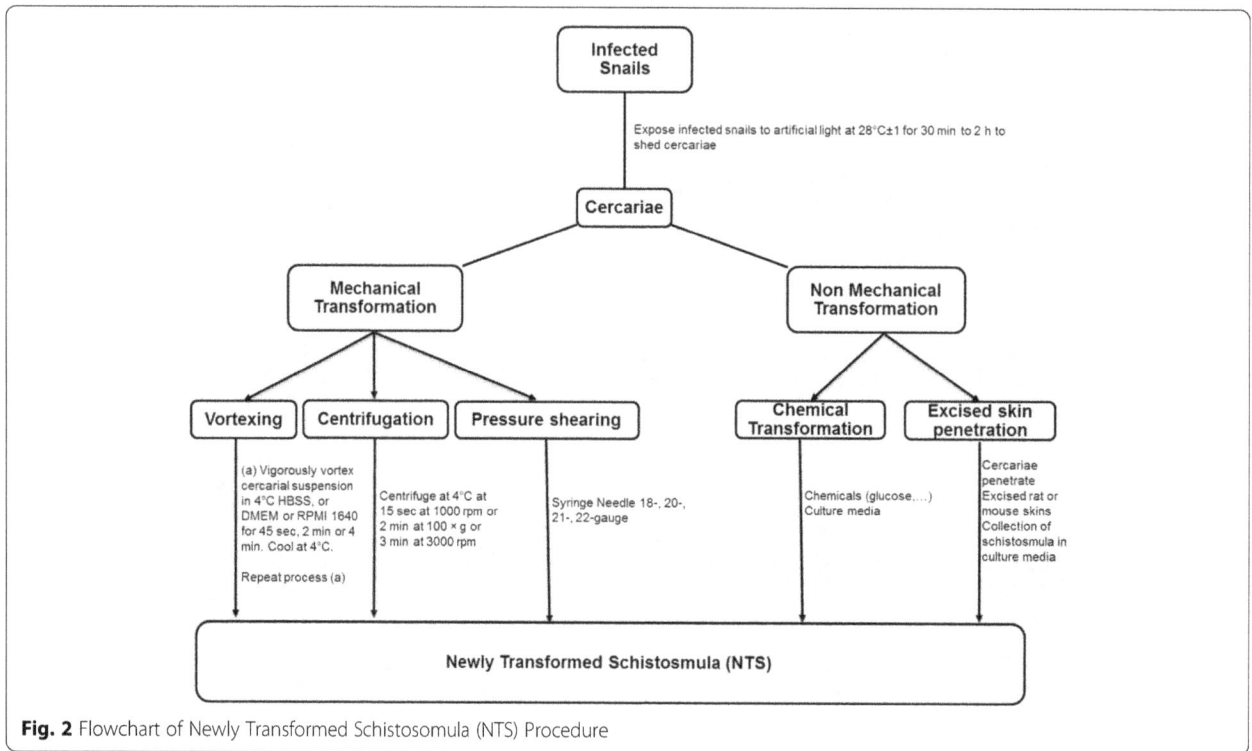

Fig. 2 Flowchart of Newly Transformed Schistosomula (NTS) Procedure

In this paper, we will describe the two of the three mechanical methods that have been employed for the acquisition of schistosomules. These include centrifugation, vortexing, or pressure shearing, such as using the 18-, 20-, 21-, 22-gauge–needle method [31, 37, 43–45]. The double-ended–needle method that presumably was developed recently, from the normal needle process seems to be the most widely used for cercariae transformation in vitro [31, 35, 37, 38, 43, 44].

In vitro transformation of cercariae to schistosomula by vortexing The transformation of cercariae to schistosomula by vortexing is performed based on a protocol of Ramalho-Pinto [45]. Many laboratories used a slightly adapted Ramalho-Pinto method [19, 26]. Briefly, cercarial suspension is cooled on ice for 10 min [33], 30–40 min [26, 31] in order to reduce parasite motility. Then cercariae are further concentrated by centrifuging for 15 s at 1000 rpm [33], 2 min at $100 \times g$ [31], 3 min at 3000 rpm [26], 4 °C. The supernatant is discarded and the cercarial pellet is resuspended in cold Hanks` Balanced Salt Solution (HBSS) containing or not penicillin-streptomycin and amphotericin B [18, 26], or in 4 °C DMEM or RPMI 1640 [31]. The suspension is vigorously vortexed for 2 min [27], 4 min [26], or 45 s twice separated by ice cooling for 3 min [31] in order to start off tail loss. This step is repeated after an incubation of the mixed tail-schistosomula suspension for 20 min at 37 °C [26]. Tucker [31]

recommended addition of antibiotics if incubation following the transformation will be longer than 8 to 12 h.

In vitro transformation of cercariae to schistosomula by needle and syringe Using a needle and syringe to separate the tails from the head of cercariae is an equally valid method for the initial phase of preparing schistosomula. In this case, cercarial suspension is placed into a plastic centrifuge tube and a syringe with 18-, 20-, 21-, or 22-gauge–needle is filled. The cercarial suspension is repeatedly passed through the needle (10–20 times back and forth) [31, 38, 43–45].

For the double-ended–needle method, an 18-, 20-, 21-, or 22- gauge double-hub, emulsifying needle with a stabilizing bar is fitted to a sterile 10 ml syringe [43]. Cercariae are drawn up using a second 10 ml syringe which is fitted to the open end of the emulsifying needle. The cercariae tails are sheared by approximately 10–20 passes back and forth through the needle [31, 37, 38]. This procedure involves manipulation of thousands of cercariae which is an obvious biohazard. Therefore mandate the use of protective clothing and gloves, including protection for the face and the eyes. Afterwards, the schistosomule bodies are isolated from the sheared tails by Percoll gradient centrifugation [53] or another purification method as described below. Table 1 compare the different schistosomula preparation procedure with advantages and disadvantages.

Table 1 Advantages and disadvantages of different ways for preparing schistosomula

	Advantages	Disadvantages
Mechanical methods (Centrifugation, Syringe needle method, Vortexing)	Relatively easy and Inexpensive	Increased parasite damage
	Manipulation of thousands of cercariae	Increased risk of infection to researchers (Potential biohazard to the researcher)
	Replaces the use of live animals	
	Help to obtain large number of schistosomula	
	Morphological characteristics identical to schistosmula obtained naturally	Only 25–50% of transformed schistosomula reach the 'gut-closed' stage by day 12
Non-mechanical methods (Chemical transformation & Excised skin penetration)	Ideal alternative to obtaining high numbers of viable schistosomula	Significantly less cercariae heads separated from the tails by chemical method
	Simpler Less damaging to the parasites	Low schistosomula yield and the possibility of contamination by host material
	50–70% of skin transformed schistosomula reach the 'gut-closed' stage by day 12	Require use of live animals (rat, mice, hamster, …) and skilled technician
	Schistosmula are obtained naturally	Less appropriate technique for high throughput

Purification of newly transformed schistosomula (NTS)

The schistosomule bodies can be isolated from the sheared tails by three purification methods which are Percoll, ice and swirling method.

The Percoll method is based on the method of Lazdins et al. [53]. The separation of the bodies from the tails is done on a 70% Percoll gradient (polyvinylpyrolidone-coated colloidal silica particles) by centrifuging for 15 min at 500 × g, 4 °C [31]. After centrifugation, the sample is collected from the bottom of the tube and the collected fraction is then diluted to the culture medium (RPMI 1640, DMEM, Medium 199, 169, MEM, etc...) and centrifuged [31, 37, 38]. The schistomula pellet is resuspended in fresh, warm supplemented medium.

Another purification method of schistosomula is a swirling technique which is a simple and easy. This method was described previously [31, 38]. In this case, schistosomula suspension is poured into a Petri dish with a sufficient warm medium such as 199 [26], 37 °C RPMI 1640 complete media [38] or incomplete medium 169 [18]. By swirling the dish gently, all the bodies are settled in the centre and the lighter tails can be aspirated and the bodies are left accumulated in the centre. The bodies (schistosomulae) will be further transferred into 15 or 50 ml centrifuge tubes. This step (swirling and collecting) is repeated until schistosomula are no longer present in the center of the dish. This objective can be reached approximately after 4 to 5 times [26] or 10 times [38].

For the ice method, 7 ml of cold HBSS is added to the schistosomula suspension and cooled on ice for 7 min. The supernatant is decanted, and the pellet resuspended again in 7 ml of cold HBSS. This step is repeated three times. The pellet that contained the recovered schistosomula is then resuspended in pre-warmed (37 °C) supplemented Medium 199 [26] or Basch medium [27].

The obtained purified schistosomula are kept in the schistosmula culture medium and incubate at an atmosphere of 37 °C of 5% CO_2 for further experiments.

After the purification, the transformation rate and the purification factor can be estimated. The rate of transformation is estimated by counting the total number of cercariae in the HBSS suspension before transformation, and placing them in relation to the total number of schistosomulae obtained after purification [26]. Marxer et al. [26] reported a transformation mean rate of 69% for five identically performed mechanical transformations by vortexing and 34% for the chemical transformation.

To estimate the purification factor, the total number of bodies and tails are counted in a sample of 50 μl after the experiment. The ratio is expressed as purification factor. Marxer et al. [26] after performing the three purification methods, they calculated the mean purification factor for each of the methods. The best purification method according to their analysis is Percoll with purification factor of 24.4 ± 11.4 [26]. This method was followed by the swirling method with a purification factor of 11.7 ± 3.2 [26]. The ice method presenting a very weak mean purification factor of 3 ± 1.7 [26].

Schistosomula culture and culture media

Techniques required to cultivate parasites in vitro is a major area of concern among present day researchers. Aside the dynamic study and understanding the physiology, behavior and metabolism of parasites, the nature of the antigenic molecules found in their excretory and secretory products need to be vigorously pursued and analyzed upon a successful establishment of the in vitro culture of the parasite. However, this is a difficult task since parasites have complex life-cycles comprising different stages and host species requirements. A good mention is in the case of parasitic helminths. Techniques involved in parasites culture requires knowledge of all types of microbiological cultures as different parasites demands particular culturing conditions such as nutrients, temperature and even incubation conditions.

Cultivation of parasites has immense usefulness in the production of vaccines, testing efficacy of vaccine, and production of antigens for obtaining serological reagents, detection of drug-resistance, screening of potential therapeutic agents and conducting epidemiological studies. Parasite cultivation is always a challenge. In the case of *schistosoma*, transformed schistosomula can be grown and maintained in vitro in a complex medium [35]. The growing rate of schistosomules cultured in vitro is not the same as those in a permissive host, nor will they become patent adults. Using good and appropriate methods, about 50% of the cultured parasites will mature with fully formed guts, and 10% will develop into sexually distinct male and female worms [31]. Starting with good number of parasites, a good amount of worms can be easily maintained and provide a vast quantity of parasite material for assay. There is also a possibility to increase the percentage of schistosomules forming guts and growing properly (50% versus 20%). This can be achieved by supplementing the growth media with conditioned media during the first week of culture [31]. Using the method described by Tucker et al. [31] with supplemented DMEM or RPMI1640 media, *Schistosoma spp.* schistosomules can be grown in culture media for at least two months. Abdulla et al. [18] noted that the Basch Medium 169 is chosen over RPMI for schistosomula culture since worms survive more in the Bash Medium with 10% mortality for up to 4 weeks whereas in RPMI medium, an average of 40 to 60% of the parasites die within 3 days with continued mortality up to two weeks . Keiser in 2010 reported that schistosmula can survive for at least 96 h in different culture media such as MEM, DMEM, Basch, or TC 199 [19]. Marxer et al. [26] showed that supplemented Medium 199 is most suitable for the incubation of schistosomula obtained by transformation in supplemented HBSS. After undertaken comparison study on three culture media (DMEM, Medium 199, Basch medium), they reported that in the supplemented Medium 199, the parasites were still alive after 120 h with an average viability value of 2.5 while all schistosomula died by 72 h in Basch medium and by 144 h in DMEM on the other hand as shown in Fig. 3 [26]. Schistosomules are cultured at 37 °C in a 5% CO_2 incubator [12, 17, 20, 23, 25–27, 31, 34, 37, 43, 45, 54]. It was also shown that over the course of one week's incubation, parasites in Basch Medium 169 appear robust and uniform in shape and appearance. The effects of culture media on the growth of schistosomula are summarized in Table 2.

Although the more suitable medium vary from one study to another, we can observe that studies initiated to screen compound FDA library [25], Medicines for Malaria Venture (MMV) box compounds [12], Mefloquine-related Arylmethanols [34] made used of supplemented Medium 199. Thus the supplemented medium 199 seems to be the most suitable medium for the cultivation of schistosomula and might justify why it has been widely used for in vitro screening of other compounds with known activities against *Schistosoma* newly transformed schistosomula [12, 23–25, 34].

The biggest obstacle to a successful schistosomules culture is contamination by fungal and bacterial, which is mainly due to the fact that the parasites originate from non-sterile snails. Therefore, the use of antibiotics (Penicillin and Streptomycin) is useful to prevent bacteria growth and amphotericin B, a fungizone that prevent fungal growth. Different concentration as indicated above are used.

In vitro drug sensitivity assays with newly transformed schistosomula
Schistosomula screening
Schistosoma NTS in vitro Assay is obtained using one of the transformation methods already described in this review. The NTS suspension adjusted to a concentration of 100 NTS per 50 μL [12, 25, 26, 34] is then incubated in culture medium at 37 °C, 5% CO_2 in ambient air for a minimum of 12 to 24 h to allow maturation or in order to achieve complete transformation into schistosomula before being further processed [12, 17, 20, 23–25, 34]. Other authors incubated NTS suspension just for 1 to 3 h before being used in subsequent experiments [18, 27]. The transformed schistosomula in schistosomula culture medium are then incubated with the test drugs in a 96-well flat bottom plate in duplicate or in triplicate and at least 2 to 3 time at a number of 100 NTS/well [12, 20, 25, 26, 34]. Since drug stock solution is prepared in DMSO, the highest concentration of DMSO diluted in Schistosomula culture medium is used to serve as control. Thereafter, drug effects are assessed microscopically under an inverted microscope.

Determination of schistosomula viability in response to test compound
Based on microscope readouts, phenotypic changes of NTS is recorded at 3 different time points (24 h, 48 h, 72 h post-drug exposure). The changes are recorded with regard to death of worms, changes in motility, viability and morphological alterations [12, 25, 34]. This makes use of a viability scale from 0 to 3 (3 = motile, no changes to morphology; 2 = reduced motility and/or some damage to tegument noted; 1 = severe reduction to

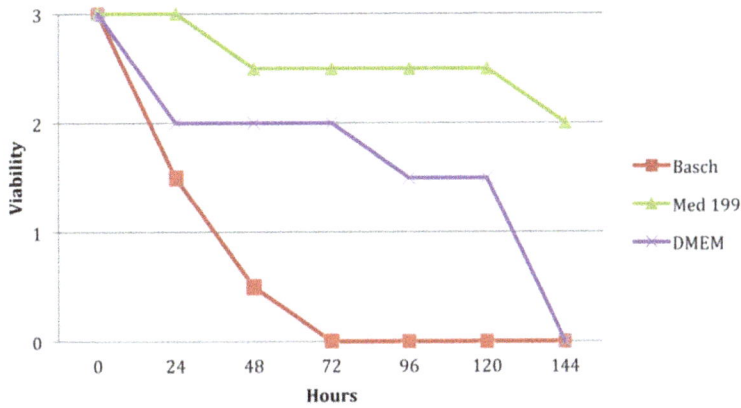

Fig. 3 Survival time of *S. haematobium* NTS in different culture media (Source: [26])

motility and/or damage to tegument observed; 0 = dead) [12, 13, 25–27, 34]. The 50% (IC50) and/or 99% (IC99) inhibitory concentration are determine for active compounds [12, 23–26, 34].

Inconvenience of microscopic read-out and development of automated technologies

Current methods utilized to assess schistosomula viability encompass microscopic techniques. In this case, the experimenter manipulates the parasite in vitro and assesses the effect of such manipulation by bright field examination of morphology. This procedure has been used in several drug screening protocols [18, 25–27] and general manipulations of parasite development [55]. Schistosome viability has been assessed in various research work using different criteria. Some of the criteria are intracellular granularity, schistosomula movement, schistosomula shape alterations. Nevertheless, evaluating

parasite viability through microscopic read-out are itself potential deterrents to the development of high throughput since these methods are slow and subjective and therefore represent a bottleneck for high-throughput screening. More often, high throughput methods are dependent upon assay miniaturisation, objectivity and very demanding in term of quantification. Several complementary techniques initially developed for single cell eukaryotes viability measurement have been adapted to multicellular schistosomes parasites. Among the existing viability assays that have been developed for use with single cell eukaryotes, it is amazing to find that only a limited range of techniques have successfully been translated to studies with schistosomes. This may be explained by the multicellular nature of schistosomes which size more than 1 cm with complex tissue and also its external tegument bound by a heptalaminate membrane [56]. The heptalaminate is thought to be

Table 2 Effects of different culture media on the growth of schistosomula

Culture Media	Shape and appearance of NTS	Motility of NTS	Duration/Viability of NTS
Basch Medium 169	Parasites (NTS) appear robust and uniform	High dynamic motility	Keeps parasites alive up to one week's incubation. Worms survive more with 10% mortality for up to 4 weeks
DMEM	Parasites (NTS) appear distorted including rounding and darkening	Slowed and less dynamic motility	Keeps parasites alive up to 144 h When the culture media is appropriately supplemented schistosomula can be grown for at least two months
Medium 199	Generate different degrees of distorted parasites (NTS) including rounding and darkening	Slowed and less dynamic motility	Supplemented Medium 199 keeps the parasites alive up to 120 h with an average viability value of about 2.5
RPMI 1640	Parasites (NTS) rounding	Slowed and less dynamic motility	Parasites degeneration and average death of 40 to 60% within 3 days with continued mortality up to two weeks When the culture media is appropriately supplemented schistosomula can be grown for at least two months

NTS newly transformed schistosomula, *DMEM* Dulbecco's modified eagle's medium, *RPMI* Roswell Park Memorial Institute

selectively permeable to macromolecules, simple compounds and water [57]. Nonetheless, there is a challenges due to parasite biology, there is also evidence that some techniques developed for single cell viability can successfully be adapted to schistosomes.

The size and complexity of schistosomes can partly be considered as useful attributes for determining viability. One of the valuable trait in assessing schistosome (both schistosomula and adult worm schistosome) viability in vitro is their regular movement, although lack of movement is thought to be not infallible indicator of death. Motility together with other microscopic characteristics such as morphology changes, granularity and tegument damaging [12, 25, 34] are currently the most common indicators for assessing schistosome viability and represent the "gold standard" for assessing drug screening protocols within the schistosomiasis research community [12, 18, 20, 25, 34].

Despite the wide application of bright-field, light microscopic assessment of schistosome viability, this technique presents several problems. Firstly, the personnel should be well trained to acquire sufficient knowledge on diverse schistosome phenotypes. Secondly, the bright-field, light microscopic detection of schistosome viability will always be subjective due to lack of immunological and molecular evidence that death has actually occurred when a schistosome is immobile. Even when the personnel has acquire the proficiency at identifying schistosome phenotypes, this technique is still slow and tedious. For instance a recent study performed the screening of only 640 potential antischistosomula compounds per month [18]. Finally, replication of results obtained by bright-field microscopic means is not always possible, because of the absence of uniformity between laboratories. With recent advancements in automated technologies, a number of alternatives read-out assay have been attempted with varying degrees of success in order to avoid the subjective nature of quantifying viability of schistosome from microscopic observation of phenotype alone [58]. For example, methylene blue has shown to stain differentially dead schistosomula and therefore was considered as a reliable dye for dead schistosomula [55] and has been used to assess the viability of mechanically transformed schistosomula [59]. Regardless, it was thought that vital dyes can be successfully translated from single cell viability markers to multicellular schistosomes.

Some fluorescent compounds such as DNA intercalating dyes, ethidium bromide (EB) and Propidium Iodide (PI) [60, 61], carboxyfluorescein [61] as well as resazurin have also been used to quantify schistosome viability in low-throughput, microscopic read-out methods. In more detail, resazurin, the active ingredient of Alamar Blue (AB), a non-toxic and cell permeable compound, is blue in color and virtually non-fluorescent. But when resazurin enters the cells, it is converted to resorufin which is red in color and highly fluorescent. Resazurin is continuously reduced to resorufin by viable cells. This staining technique was used to discriminate between live and dead schistosomula after 48 and 72 h of incubation with standard selected drug compounds of known antischistosomal activity [26]. Unfortunately this technique cannot be used for earlier time-points and to measure dose response drug effects [23].

Ethidium bromide has been used to differentiate dead schistosomula from live ones during microscopic examination [61], while PI has successfully been used for the same reason (as a differential stain of dead schistosomula) for both microscopic examination and flow cytometry [60]. Carboxyfluorescein in contrast to ethidium bromide and propidium iodide, has been tested as live staining for schistosomula. However, it was difficult to clearly differentiate live schistosomula to dead ones since the latter developed some fluorescence [61].

By promoting the use of single dye staining, a dual fluorescent viability assay has been developed for schistosomula [17]. In this case, authors combined the use of PI with fluorescein diacetate (FDA) to easily assess the percentage of viable schistosomula present in a sample. By using a microtiter plate reader, this fluorescent bioassay was developed for 96 or 384 well microtiter blacksided, flat-bottom plate optically clear. Ninety-six (96) well plate were designed for medium throughput and 384 for high throughput applications [17]. The use of the fluorescent bioassay has the added advantages that it could increase by 10-fold the number of compounds screened per month over existing microscope methodologies and also, it does not require extensive training of personnel in parasite morphology [58]. Therefore fluorescent bioassay has been shown to be entirely objective [58] and has been validated with schistosomula. Currently, there are indications that fluorescent bioassay can be adapted for use with adult worm schistosomes as well as other life stages. Although the combined use of PI and FDA, can objectively and rapidly quantify schistosome viability in a high-throughput format, the ability of PI and FDA to provide significant phenotypic data is slightly limited [58]. Therefore, there is still a need for the complementary technologies to the fluorescent bioassay and methodologies that allow the automated assessment of phenotype that could be seen as a great discovery in the field of novel antischistosomal drugs discovery.

Smout et al. [62] developed a motility assay that was thought to be one of the technological advance to offer a solution to this helminth phenotype quantification challenge, until high content screening as an affordable reality. This assay, which uses the xCELLigence system was a new application or device to monitoring cells in a

Table 3 In vitro drug sensitivity assays developed for the determination of anti-schistosomula activity of drug compounds

Methods	Principles	Advantages	Disadvantages
Microscope readouts without staining	Parasites are manipulated in vitro and the effect is assessed by bright field examination of morphology. Schistosomula viability is assessed using different criteria: - intracellular granularity - schistosomula movement - schistosomula shape alterations This makes use of a viability scale from 0 to 3	- Used to discriminate between live and dead schistosomula after incubation	- The personnel should be well trained to distinguish diverse schistosomula phenotypes - The bright-field, light microscopic detection of schistosomula viability is subjective due to lack of immunological and molecular evidence that death has actually occurred when a schistosomula is immobile - The technique is slow (time consuming) and tedious - Replication of results is not always possible, because of the absence of uniformity between laboratories
Microscope readouts with Staining using a single fluorescent dye	Parasites are manipulated in vitro and the effect is assessed by bright field examination of viable or dead cells	- Used to discriminate between live and dead schistosomula after incubation - Does not require extensive training of personnel in parasite morphology - The fluorescent bioassay is objective - Fluorescent bioassay can be adapted for use with adult worm schistosomes as well as other life stages	- Cannot be used for earlier time-points - Cannot be used to measure dose response drug effects - It is sometime difficult to clearly differentiate live schistosomula from dead ones
Microscope readouts with Staining using dual fluorescent viability assay	Combination of the use of DNA intercalating dyes (ethidium bromide (EB), Propidium Iodide (PI)) with Carboxyfluorescein (fluorescein diacetate), Resazurin to easily assess the percentage of viable schistosomula present in a sample	- This bioassay was developed for 96 or 384 well microtiter plate optically clear - Designed for medium throughput (96 well) and high throughput (384 well) applications - Increase by 10-fold the number of compounds screened per month over existing microscopy methodologies - Does not require extensive training of personnel in parasite morphology - The fluorescent bioassay objectively and rapidly quantify schistosomula viability in a high-throughput format - Fluorescent bioassay can be adapted for use with adult worm schistosomes as well as other life stages	- The ability of the dual fluorescent dye to provide significant phenotypic data is slightly limited
Motility assay	The assay uses the xCELLigence system for monitoring cells in a real-time manner. This technique is based on the detection of changing electrical currents running through mini gold electrodes incorporated into the bottom of tissue culture plates	- Simply and objectively assess anthelmintic effects by measuring parasite motility in real time in a fully automated high-throughput fashion - Help remove subjectivity in helminth phenotype characterization - Results can be compared directly from different laboratories	- The xCELLigence equipment used in this technology is costly and may restrict its applicability

Table 3 In vitro drug sensitivity assays developed for the determination of anti-schistosomula activity of drug compounds (*Continued*)

Fluorometric L-lactate assay	Consist of the measurement of lactate levels that reflect clearly the viability of schistosomula and this also correlate with schistosomula numbers	- Can be used as simple surrogate marker - Promising new approach to assess the viability of schistosomula in drug sensitivity assays	- This technique requires that the supernatant must be removed from the drug assay without aspirating the schistosomula and the drug assay should be diluted to an acceptable fluorescence range as needed. These make the fluorometric L-lactate assay less than high-throughput
CellTiterGlo® (Commercial luminescence-based cell viability kit)	Detection of schistosomula viability through quantitation of ATP	- Suitable for a Medium-Throughput Assay semi-automated for drug screening - Fast, highly reliable, sensitive and automation friendly	- Require a precise multi-drop dispenser to ensure an exact number of NTS present in each well

Table 4 Summary of the published studies

Objective	Media used	NTS procedure	Outcome	Reference
Mansour et al. (2016) screened almost 300,000 compounds using an assay based on motility of worm, larvae and image analysis of assay plates	M169 supplemented with 100 U/ml Penicillin, 300 µg/ml Streptomycin, 0.25 µg/ml Fungizone (Amphotericin B) and 5 % fetal calf serum (FCS)	Mechanical transformation using the Syringe needle Method	A number of compounds were identified as promising leads for further chemical optimization	[54]
Panic et al. (2015a) investigate a panel of fluorescence/luminescence dyes for their applicability as viability markers in drug sensitivity assays for Schistosoma mansoni schistosomula	Medium 199 supplemented with 5 % heat iFCS and 1 % penicillin-streptomycin mixture	Mechanical in vitro transformation (vortexing)	Of the 11 markers selected for testing, resazurin, Vybrant® and CellTiter-Glo® correlated best with NTS viability, produced signals ≥ 3-fold stronger than background noise and revealed a significant signal-to-NTS concentration relationship	[23]
Panic et al. (2015b) expands the knowledge of antischistosomal properties of already approved 1600 FDA compounds from a very diverse set of indications against Schistosoma mansoni	Medium 199 supplemented with 5 % heat iFCS and 1 % penicillin/streptomycin	Mechanical in vitro transformation (vortexing)	Of the 1600 compounds screened against schistosomula, 121 were identified as active and 36 of these were active on the adult worms after Screening. The two in vivo- moderately active drugs identified in this study, doramectin and clofazimine present as novel drug classes as starting points for further investigation	[25]
Lalli et al. (2015) describes the development and validation of a luminescence based, medium-throughput assay for the detection of schistosomula viability through quantitation of ATP	DMEM complete tissue culture medium	Mechanical in vitro transformation (vortexing)	Schistosomula viability luminescence based assay is successful and suitable for the identification of novel compounds potentially exploitable in future schistosomiasis therapies. Thus representing a valid alternative to fluorescence-based microscopy assays	[63]
Howe et al. (2015) assessed lactate as a surrogate marker for viability in Schistosoma drug screening assays by testing compounds with reported potencies	Phenol-red free medium 199 Supplemented with 5.5 mM D-glucose, 200 U/ml penicillin, 200 µg/ml streptomycin, 1 % heat iFCS	Mechanically transformed by vortexing	Lactate levels clearly reflected the viability of schistosomula and correlated with schistosomulum numbers. Lactate is a sensitive and simple surrogate marker to be measured to determine Schistosoma viability in compound screening assays	[24]
Ingram-Sieber et al.(2014) investigated the Medicines for Malaria Venture malaria box containing 200 diverse drug-like and 200 probe-like compounds with known antimalarial activity against larval stage of S. mansoni, followed by testing against adult worms in vitro and by in vivo studies of lead candidates	Supplemented Medium 199 with 5 % heat iFCS, penicillin (100 U/ml), and streptomycin (100 µg/ml)	Mechanically transformation by vortexing	Underlined the potential of compounds with an antimalarial background on schistosomes. Two entirely new chemical scaffolds with antischistosomal in vitro activity in the sub micromolar range and moderate in vivo activity identified	[12]
Protasio et al. (2013) analyzed differences in gene expression patterns between Mechanical and Skin Transformed Schistosoma mansoni Schistosomula and provide enough data to resolve a long-lasting controversy	Supplemented DMEM, 10 % FCS, 1 % Hepes buffer with 100 U/L penicillin, 0.1 mg/L streptomycin and 10 mM L-glutamine	- Mechanical transformation using the 21G Syringe needle method - Excised skin from mice	This work contributes to the validation of gene expression studies that have used Mechanical transformed schistosomula and provides further evidence that the MT is a good proxy for natural skin transformation	[37]
Coultas et al. (2012) compared a current and widely used double-ended-needle mechanical transformation method to a culture medium based on a nonmechanical method	RPMI 1640 medium enriched with L-glutamine; 150 units/ml penicillin, 100 µg/ml streptomycin and 5 % heat inactivated fetal bovine serum (iFBS)	Mechanical transformation using the 22-gauge double-ended, luer lok emulsifying needle	The mechanical and nonmechanical cercariae transformation methods both yielded significantly large and similar quantities of viable schistosomula	[49]

Table 4 Summary of the published studies (*Continued*)

Study	Medium	Transformation method	Findings	Ref
de Moraes et al. (2012) report the in vitro antischistosomal activity of piplartine on S. mansoni schistosomula of different ages	Basch 169 medium containing antibiotics and supplemented with 10 % fetal bovine serum (FBS)	Mechanical transformation, using a Vortex mixer	This report provides the first evidence that piplartine is able to kill schistosomula of different ages and reinforce that piplartine is a promising compound that could be used for the development of new schistosomicidal agent	[36]
Marxer et al. (2012) developed an in vitro drug screening assay for S. haematobium newly transformed schistosomula (NTS). The cercarial emergence rhythms of the intermediate hosts of S. mansoni and S. haematobium, Biomphalaria glabrata and Bulinus truncatus were studied, two artificial transformation methods for the production of the schistosomula were compared and the best purification method and optimal culture conditions were established by testing three different methods and several different media	Basch Medium 169, DMEM and Medium 199. All supplemented with 5 % heat iFCS and 200 U/ml penicillin and 200 µg/ml streptomycin	Mechanical transformation, using a Vortex mixer and chemical transformation using glucose	A circadian rhythm existed in both snail species. The highest transformation rate of S. haematobium cercariae into NTS was obtained with the vortex transformation and the highest purification factor was observed using Percoll. The fluorimetric readout based on resazurin was very precise in detecting dead schistosomula	[26]
Ingram et al. (2012) tested mefloquine-related compounds belonging to the three major groups of arylmethanols in order to elucidate their potential as antischistosomal lead candidates. The selected arylmethanols were tested against S. mansoni schistosomula and adults worms in vitro	Medium 199 supplemented with 5 % heat iFCS, penicillin (100 U/ml), and streptomycin (100 µg/ml)	Mechanically transformation by vortexing	The study confirmed the high antischistosomal activity of compounds with a mefloquine scaffold. Four candidates, WR7930, its two derivatives, and enpiroline, that are characterized by high antischistosomal properties in vivo were identified	[34]
Milligan et al. (2011) provide a visual description of cercarial transformation and in vitro culturing of schistosomules	RPMI 1640 supplemented with 5 % FBS, 1X Penicillin/Streptomycin	Mechanical transformation using the 22-gauge double-ended, luer lok emulsifying needle	This study developed a visual protocols for in vitro cercarial transformation and schistosomules culture techniques	[38]
Smout et al. (2010) describe a novel application for a real-time cell monitoring device (xCELLigence) that can simply and objectively assess anthelmintic effects by measuring parasite motility in real time in a fully automated high-throughput fashion	RPMI 1640, 1 % antibiotic/antimycotic and 10 mM Hepes	-	The study reported that the technique can be suitable for discovery and development of new anthelmintic drugs as well as for detection of phenotypic resistance to existing drugs for the majority of helminths and other pathogens where motility is a measure of pathogen viability	[62]
Mansour et al.(2010) report the development and validation of the Alamar Blue assay compared with morphology-based (microscopic) assessment of compound activity	M169 supplemented with 100 U/ml Penicillin, 100 mg/ml Streptomycin and 5 % FCS	Mechanical transformation using the Syringe Method	The Alamar Blue assay is readily able to detect compounds causing death or severe damage to the larvae but is less reliable than microscopy for more subtle morphological changes. It is concluded that an automated high throughput screen would benefit from integrated use of both alamar blue and automatic image-based morphology assays	[20]
Manneck et al.(2010) studied the temporal effect of this Mefloquine in vitro and in vivo, and examined alterations on the tegumental surface of schistosomula and adults of S. mansoni by means of scanning electron microscopy (SEM)	Basch medium 169 supplemented with 5 % heat iFCS and 100 U/ml penicillin and 100 mg/ml streptomycin	Mechanically transformation by vortexing	Mefloquine induces extensive morphological and tegumental alterations on both S. mansoni schistosomula and adults in vitro and in vivo	[27]

Table 4 Summary of the published studies *(Continued)*

Peak et al. (2010) presented a microtiter plate-based method for reproducibly detecting schistosomula viability that takes advantage of the differential uptake of fluorophores (propidium iodide and fluorescein diacetate) by living organisms	DMEM lacking phenol red, containing 4500 mg/l glucose, supplemented with 10 % FCS, 2 mM L-glutamine, 200 U/ml penicillin, 200 mg/ml streptomycin	Mechanically transformation by vortexing	The study showed that developed method is sensitive (200 schistosomula/well can be assayed), relevant to industrial (384-well microtiter plate compatibility) and academic (96-well microtiter plate compatibility) settings, translatable to functional genomics screens and drug assays	[17]
Abdulla et al. (2009) presented a partially automated, three component phenotypic screen workflow that utilizes at its apex the schistosomula stage of the parasite adapted to a 96-well plate format. Hits that arise are subsequently screened in vitro against adult parasites and finally for efficacy in a murine model of disease	Basch Medium 169	Mechanical transformation using the 22-gauge double-ended, luer lok emulsifying needle	The study has identified various compounds and drugs as hits in vitro and leads, with the prescribed oral efficacy, in vivo	[18]

NTS newly transformed schistosomula, *DMEM* Dulbecco's modified eagle's medium, *RPMI* Roswell Park Memorial Institute, *iFCS* heat inactivated fetal calf serum, *SEM* scanning electron microscopy

real-time manner. This was known to simply and object-ively assess anthelmintic effects by measuring parasite motility in real time in a fully automated high-throughput fashion. In principle, this technique is based on the detection of changing electrical currents running through mini gold electrodes incorporated into the bot-tom of tissue culture plates. When schistosomes in the immature and mature stages are quite dense, they usu-ally sediment during in vitro culturing and this make contact with the gold electrodes. It is known that, changes to the culturing conditions that may impact a worm's physiology will probably modifiy its behavior or phenotype. This result to a measurable fluctuation in current across the electrodes [58]. Since many anti-schistosomal drug compounds act by affecting the motil-ity of the target parasite, the importance of these meas-urable current fluctuations can be considered as an indicator of potential therapeutic activity. This biophys-ical characteristic to assess anthelmintic activity of com-pounds in real time in a high-throughput fashion was demonstrated by Smout et al. [62]. This technology was applied to adult schistosomes to illustrate that by in-creasing the doses of PZQ, the signal decreased from adult worm schistosomes, and this allowed to generate a dose dependent curve. Can this technology be applied to larval schistosome life stages? Although the answer to this question is currently unknown, it appears feasible. It is believed that this assay may provide an advanced methodology to microscopy that will help remove sub-jectivity in helminth phenotype characterization as well as making available a technology to compare results dir-ectly from different laboratories [58]. But the original cost of the xCELLigence equipment may restrict its widespread use.

Howe et al. [24] investigated a fluorometric L-lactate assay for viability in *schistosoma* drug screening assays. Lactate is a by-product of glycolysis. It is secreted via aquaglyceroporins from NTS and adult worm schisto-somes [23]. Authors fully investigated parameters of lac-tate measurement and performed drug sensitivity assays by applying schistosomulae and adult worms to establish a proof of concept. They showed that lactate levels re-flect clearly the viability of schistosomula and this was also correlated with schistosomulae numbers. They tested compounds with described potencies, and com-pared activities of fluorometric L-lactate assay with mi-croscopy. Howe et al. [24] concluded that lactate can be used as simple surrogate marker since its measurement can be a promising new approach to assess the viability of schistosomulae in drug sensitivity assays. However, this technique requires two things. Firstly, the super-natant must be removing from the drug assay without aspirating the Schistosomula and secondly, the drug assay should be diluted to an acceptable fluorescence

range as needed. These two aspects make the fluoromet-ric L-lactate assay less than high-throughput [23].

More recently, the commercial luminescence-based cell viability kit known as CellTiterGlo® was validated by Lalli et al. [63] for the in vitro assay using *S. mansoni* NTS and adult worms schistosomes. In this procedure unfortunately, a precise multi-drop dispenser is required to ensure an exact number of NTS present in each well. Although the investigation of marker-dye based assays has been a popular activity, we can simply note that, the aim of a simple, inexpensive and accurate dye that does not require much additional equipment or analysis has not so far been entirely met [23]. Table 3 summarizes different in vitro drug sensitivity assays developed so far for the determination of anti-schistosomula activity of drug compounds. The summary of publications cited in this review are contained in Table 4.

Conclusion

One of the great deal of new drug discovery against schistosomes is dependent on in vitro whole parasite screens. Access to adequate quantities and a substantial source of whole parasite organisms is a constant source of concern. Thus mechanically transformed schistoso-mula may be used as alternative for the purpose of high-throughput tools in the field of antischistosomal drugs discovery. This may help for the rapid discovery of ur-gently needed new drugs that will be useful in the con-trol of schistosmiasis which represent one of the major devastating parasitic infections. Although it is clear from recent publications that subjective measures of NTS via-bility, motility and phenotype are still the gold standard, none of the automated assessment of phenotype have so far been validated.

Abbreviations
AB: Alamar blue; DMEM: Dulbecco's modified eagle's medium; DMSO: Dimethyl sulfoxide; EB: Ethidium bromide; FBS: Fetal bovine serum; FDA: Fluorescein diacetate; HBSS: Hanks` balanced salt solution; IC: Inhibition concentration; iFCS: Inactivated fetal calf serum; MDA: Mass drug administration; MEM: Minimum essential medium; MMV: Medicines for malaria venture; NTS: Newly transformed schistosomula; PI: Propidium iodide; PZQ: Praziquantel; RPMI: Roswell Park Memorial Institute; TDR: Research and training in tropical diseases

Acknowledgement
Emmanuel Mouafo Tekwu is very grateful to the Bill and Melinda Gates Foundation for a two years fellowship in Ghana through the postdoctoral fellowship program at Noguchi Memorial Institute for Medical Research. I would like to thank Miss Deladem Mabel Tettey (Research Assistant, Department of Parasitology, NMIMR) for critical reading of this manuscript.

Funding

This work was supported by the Bill and Melinda Gates Foundation under the Postdoctoral and Postgraduate Training in Infectious Diseases Research awarded to the Noguchi Memorial Institute for Medical Research (Global Health Grant number OPP52155). The funders had no role in study design, data collection and analysis, decision to publish or preparation of the manuscript.

Authors' contributions

EMT conceptualized the topic, developed the review and wrote this manuscript. KMB, AKN, VPB, WA, DB, SK, KBAO reviewed and contributed intellectually for the improvement of the manuscript. All authors read and approved the final version of the manuscript.

Competing interests

The authors declare that they have no competing interests

Author details

[1]Noguchi Memorial Institute for Medical Research (NMIMR), College of Health Sciences, University of Ghana, PO Box LG581 Legon, Accra, Ghana. [2]Laboratory for Tuberculosis Research and Pharmacology, Biotechnology Centre, Nkolbisson, University of Yaoundé 1, Yaoundé, Cameroon. [3]Centre for Plant Medicine Research (CPMR), Akwapim, Mampong, Ghana. [4]Yaounde Emergency Centre (CURY), Yaoundé, Cameroon. [5]School of Pharmacy, College of Health sciences, University of Ghana, Accra, Ghana.

References

1. Steinmann P, Keiser J, Bos R, Tanner M, Utzinger J. Schistosomiasis and water resources development: systematic review, meta-analysis, and estimates of people at risk. Lancet Infect Dis. 2006;6(7):411–25.
2. Gryseels B. Schistosomiasis. Infect Dis Clin North Am. 2012;26(2):383–97.
3. Ezeamama AE, Friedman JF, Acosta LP, Bellinger DC, Langdon GC, Manalo DL, Olveda RM, Kurtis JD, McGarvey ST. Helminth infection and cognitive impairment among Filipino children. Am J Trop Med Hyg. 2005;72(5):540–8.
4. Fenwick A, Webster JP, Bosque-Oliva E, Blair L, Fleming FM, Zhang Y, Garba A, Stothard JR, Gabrielli AF, Clements AC, et al. The Schistosomiasis Control Initiative (SCI): rationale, development and implementation from 2002-2008. Parasitology. 2009;136(13):1719–30.
5. Fenwick A. Praziquantel: do we need another antischistosoma treatment? Future Med Chem. 2015;7(6):677–80.
6. Knopp S, Stothard JR, Rollinson D, Mohammed KA, Khamis IS, Marti H, Utzinger J. From morbidity control to transmission control: time to change tactics against helminths on Unguja Island, Zanzibar. Acta Trop. 2013;128(2):412–22.
7. Cupit PM, Cunningham C. What is the mechanism of action of praziquantel and how might resistance strike? Future Med Chem. 2015;7(6):701–5.
8. Secor WE, Montgomery SP. Something old, something new: is praziquantel enough for schistosomiasis control? Future Med Chem. 2015;7(6):681–4.
9. Pica-Mattoccia L, Cioli D. Sex- and stage-related sensitivity of Schistosoma mansoni to in vivo and in vitro praziquantel treatment. Int J Parasitol. 2004; 34(4):527–33.
10. Doenhoff MJ, Hagan P, Cioli D, Southgate V, Pica-Mattoccia L, Botros S, Coles G, Tchuem Tchuente LA, Mbaye A, Engels D. Praziquantel: its use in control of schistosomiasis in sub-Saharan Africa and current research needs. Parasitology. 2009;136(13):1825–35.
11. Pedrique B, Strub-Wourgaft N, Some C, Olliaro P, Trouiller P, Ford N, Pecoul B, Bradol JH. The drug and vaccine landscape for neglected diseases (2000-11): a systematic assessment. Lancet Glob Health. 2013;1(6):e371–379.
12. Ingram-Sieber K, Cowan N, Panic G, Vargas M, Mansour NR, Bickle QD, Wells TN, Spangenberg T, Keiser J. Orally active antischistosomal early leads identified from the open access malaria box. PLoS Negl Trop Dis. 2014;8(1):e2610.
13. Keiser J, N'Guessan NA, Adoubryn KD, Silue KD, Vounatsou P, Hatz C, Utzinger J, N'Goran EK. Efficacy and safety of mefloquine, artesunate, mefloquine-artesunate, and praziquantel against Schistosoma haematobium: randomized, exploratory open-label trial. Clin Infect Dis. 2010;50(9):1205–13.
14. Utzinger J, Xiao SH, Tanner M, Keiser J. Artemisinins for schistosomiasis and beyond. Curr Opin Investig Drugs (London, England: 2000). 2007;8(2):105–16.
15. Ramirez B, Bickle Q, Yousif F, Fakorede F, Mouries MA, Nwaka S. Schistosomes: challenges in compound screening. Expert Opin Drug Discovery. 2007;2(s1):S53–61.
16. Loker ES. A comparative study of the life-histories of mammalian schistosomes. Parasitology. 1983;87(Pt 2):343–69.
17. Peak E, Chalmers IW, Hoffmann KF. Development and validation of a quantitative, high-throughput, fluorescent-based bioassay to detect Schistosoma viability. PLoS Negl Trop Dis. 2010;4(7):e759.
18. Abdulla MH, Ruelas DS, Wolff B, Snedecor J, Lim KC, Xu F, Renslo AR, Williams J, McKerrow JH, Caffrey CR. Drug discovery for schistosomiasis: hit and lead compounds identified in a library of known drugs by medium-throughput phenotypic screening. PLoS Negl Trop Dis. 2009;3(7):e478.
19. Keiser J. In vitro and in vivo trematode models for chemotherapeutic studies. Parasitology. 2010;137(3):589–603.
20. Mansour NR, Bickle QD. Comparison of microscopy and Alamar blue reduction in a larval based assay for schistosome drug screening. PLoS Negl Trop Dis. 2010;4(8):e795.
21. Colley DG, Bustinduy AL, Secor WE, King CH. Human schistosomiasis. Lancet (London, England). 2014;383(9936):2253–64.
22. Ross AG, Bartley PB, Sleigh AC, Olds GR, Li Y, Williams GM, McManus DP. Schistosomiasis. N Engl J Med. 2002;346(16):1212–20.
23. Panic G, Flores D, Ingram-Sieber K, Keiser J. Fluorescence/luminescence-based markers for the assessment of Schistosoma mansoni schistosomula drug assays. Parasit Vectors. 2015;8:624.
24. Howe S, Zophel D, Subbaraman H, Unger C, Held J, Engleitner T, Hoffmann WH, Kreidenweiss A. Lactate as a novel quantitative measure of viability in Schistosoma mansoni drug sensitivity assays. Antimicrob Agents Chemother. 2015;59(2):1193–9.
25. Panic G, Vargas M, Scandale I, Keiser J. Activity Profile of an FDA-Approved Compound Library against Schistosoma mansoni. PLoS Negl Trop Dis. 2015;9(7):e0003962.
26. Marxer M, Ingram K, Keiser J. Development of an in vitro drug screening assay using Schistosoma haematobium schistosomula. Parasit Vectors. 2012; 5:165.
27. Manneck T, Haggenmuller Y, Keiser J. Morphological effects and tegumental alterations induced by mefloquine on schistosomula and adult flukes of Schistosoma mansoni. Parasitology. 2010;137(1):85–98.
28. Stirewalt MA. Schistosoma mansoni: cercaria to schistosomule. Adv Parasitol. 1974;12:115–82.
29. Hockley DJ, McLaren DJ. Schistosoma mansoni: changes in the outer membrane of the tegument during development from cercaria to adult worm. Int J Parasitol. 1973;3(1):13–25.
30. McLaren DJ, Hockley DJ. Schistosoma mansoni: the occurrence of microvilli on the surface of the tegument during transformation from cercaria to schistosomulum. Parasitology. 1976;73(2):169–87.
31. Tucker MS, Karunaratne LB, Lewis FA, Freitas TC, Liang Y-s. Schistosomiasis. Curr Protoc Immunol/edited by John E Coligan [et al]. 2001;0 19:Unit-19.11.
32. Samuelson JC, Caulfield JP. The cercarial glycocalyx of Schistosoma mansoni. J Cell Biol. 1985;100(5):1423–34.
33. Brink LH, McLaren DJ, Smithers SR. Schistosoma mansoni: a comparative study of artificially transformed schistosomula and schistosomula recovered after cercarial penetration of isolated skin. Parasitology. 1977;74(1):73–86.
34. Ingram K, Ellis W, Keiser J. Antischistosomal activities of mefloquine-related arylmethanols. Antimicrob Agents Chemother. 2012;56(6):3207–15.
35. Basch PF. Cultivation of Schistosoma mansoni in vitro. I. Establishment of cultures from cercariae and development until pairing. J Parasitol. 1981; 67(2):179–85.
36. de Moraes J, Nascimento C, Yamaguchi LF, Kato MJ, Nakano E. Schistosoma mansoni: in vitro schistosomicidal activity and tegumental alterations induced by piplartine on schistosomula. Exp Parasitol. 2012;132(2):222–7.
37. Protasio AV, Dunne DW, Berriman M. Comparative study of transcriptome profiles of mechanical- and skin-transformed Schistosoma mansoni schistosomula. PLoS Negl Trop Dis. 2013;7(3):e2091.
38. Milligan JN, Jolly ER. Cercarial transformation and in vitro cultivation of Schistosoma mansoni schistosomules. J Vis Exp. 2011(54):3191.
39. Molla E, Giday M, Erko B. Laboratory assessment of the molluscicidal and cercariacidal activities of Balanites aegyptiaca. Asian Pac J Trop Biomed. 2013;3(8):657–62.

40. Kiros G, Erko B, Giday M, Mekonnen Y. Laboratory assessment of molluscicidal and cercariacidal effects of *Glinus lotoides* fruits. BMC Res Notes. 2014;7:220.

41. Albagouri AH, Elegami AA, Koko WS, Osman EE, Dahab MM. *In Vitro* Anticercarial Activities of some Sudanese Medicinal Plants of the Family Combretaceae. J Forest Products Industries. 2014;3(2):93–9.

42. dos Santos AF, de Azevedo DPL, dos Santos Mata RC, de Mendonça DIMD, Sant'Ana AEG. The lethality of *Euphorbia conspicua* to adults of *Biomphalaria glabrata*, cercaria of *Schistosoma mansoni* and larvae of *Artemia salina*. Bioresour Technol. 2007;98(1):135–9.

43. Mann VH, Morales ME, Rinaldi G, Brindley PJ. Culture for genetic manipulation of developmental stages of *Schistosoma mansoni*. Parasitology. 2010;137(3):451–62.

44. Colley DG, Wikel SK. *Schistosoma mansoni*: simplified method for the production of schistosomules. Exp Parasitol. 1974;35(1):44–51.

45. Ramalho-Pinto FJ, Gazzinelli G, Howells RE, Mota-Santos TA, Figueiredo EA, Pellegrino J. *Schistosoma mansoni*: defined system for stepwise transformation of cercaria to schistosomule in vitro. Exp Parasitol. 1974;36(3): 360–72.

46. Howells RE, Ramalho-Pinto FJ, Gazzinelli G, de Oliveira CC, Figueiredo EA, Pellegrino J. *Schistosoma mansoni*: mechanism of cercarial tail loss and its significance to host penetration. Exp Parasitol. 1974;36(3):373–85.

47. Stirewalt MA, Minnick DR, Fregeau WA. Definition and collection in quantity of schistosomules of *Schistosoma mansoni*. Trans R Soc Trop Med Hyg. 1966;60(3):352–60.

48. Salafsky B, Fusco AC, Whitley K, Nowicki D, Ellenberger B. *Schistosoma mansoni*: analysis of cercarial transformation methods. Exp Parasitol. 1988;67(1):116–27.

49. Coultas KA, Zhang SM. *In vitro* cercariae transformation: comparison of mechanical and nonmechanical methods and observation of morphological changes of detached cercariae tails. J Parasitol. 2012;98(6):1257–61.

50. Skelly PJ, Shoemaker CB. Induction cues for tegument formation during the transformation of *Schistosoma mansoni* cercariae. Int J Parasitol. 2000;30(5):625–31.

51. Stirewalt MA, Uy A. *Schistosoma mansoni*: cercarial penetration and schistosomule collection in an in vitro system. Exp Parasitol. 1969;26(1):17–28.

52. Clegg JA, Smithers SR. The effects of immune rhesus monkey serum on schistosomula of *Schistosoma mansoni* during cultivation in vitro. Int J Parasitol. 1972;2(1):79–98.

53. Lazdins JK, Stein MJ, David JR, Sher A. *Schistosoma mansoni*: rapid isolation and purification of schistosomula of different developmental stages by centrifugation on discontinuous density gradients of Percoll. Exp Parasitol. 1982;53(1):39–44.

54. Mansour NR, Paveley R, Gardner JM, Bell AS, Parkinson T, Bickle Q. High Throughput Screening Identifies Novel Lead Compounds with Activity against Larval, Juvenile and Adult *Schistosoma mansoni*. PLoS Negl Trop Dis. 2016;10(4):e0004659.

55. Gold D. Assessment of the viability of *Schistosoma mansoni* schistosomula by comparative uptake of various vital dyes. Parasitol Res. 1997;83(2):163–9.

56. Wilson RA. Virulence factors of schistosomes. Microbes Infect. 2012;14(15):1442–50.

57. Skelly PJ, Alan Wilson R. Making sense of the schistosome surface. Adv Parasitol. 2006;63:185–284.

58. Peak E, Hoffmann KF. Cross-disciplinary approaches for measuring parasitic helminth viability and phenotype. An Acad Bras Cienc. 2011;83(2):649–62.

59. Gold D, Flescher E. Influence of mechanical tail-detachment techniques of schistosome cercariae on the production, viability, and infectivity of resultant schistosomula: a comparative study. Parasitol Res. 2000;86(7):570–2.

60. Nyame AK, Lewis FA, Doughty BL, Correa-Oliveira R, Cummings RD. Immunity to schistosomiasis: glycans are potential antigenic targets for immune intervention. Exp Parasitol. 2003;104(1-2):1–13.

61. Van der Linden PW, Deelder AM. *Schistosoma mansoni*: a diamidinophenylindole probe for in vitro death of schistosomula. Exp Parasitol. 1984;57(2):125–31.

62. Smout MJ, Kotze AC, McCarthy JS, Loukas A. A novel high throughput assay for anthelmintic drug screening and resistance diagnosis by real-time monitoring of parasite motility. PLoS Negl Trop Dis. 2010;4(11):e885.

63. Lalli C, Guidi A, Gennari N, Altamura S, Bresciani A, Ruberti G. Development and validation of a luminescence-based, medium-throughput assay for drug screening in *Schistosoma mansoni*. PLoS Negl Trop Dis. 2015;9(1):e0003484.

14

RECQ helicases are deregulated in hematological malignancies in association with a prognostic value

Elena Viziteu[2], Alboukadel Kassambara[1,2], Philippe Pasero[2], Bernard Klein[1,2,3] and Jerome Moreaux[1,2,3*] (iD)

Abstract

Background: RECQ helicase family members act as guardians of the genome to assure proper DNA metabolism in response to genotoxic stress. Hematological malignancies are characterized by genomic instability that is possibly related to underlying defects in DNA repair of genomic stability maintenance.

Methods: We have investigated the expression of *RECQ* helicases in different hematological malignancies and in their normal counterparts using publicly available gene expression data. Furthermore, we explored whether *RECQ* helicases expression could be associated with tumor progression and prognosis.

Results: Expression of at least one *RECQ* helicase family member was found significantly deregulated in all hematological malignancies investigated when compared to their normal counterparts. In addition, *RECQ* helicase expression was associated with a prognostic value in acute myeloid leukemia, chronic lymphocytic leukemia, lymphoma and multiple myeloma.

Conclusion: *RECQ* helicase expression is deregulated in hematological malignancies compared to their normal counterparts in association with a prognostic value. Deregulation of RECQ helicases appears to play a role in tumorigenesis and represent potent therapeutic targets for synthetic lethal approaches in hematological malignancies.

Keywords: RECQ helicases, Gene expression, Hematological malignancies, Prognostic markers, Therapeutic targets

Background

The RECQ family of DNA helicases is a family of conserved enzymes that display highly-specialized and vital roles in the maintenance of genome stability [1].

In humans, RECQ helicase family has five members with similar catalytic core: RECQ1, BLM, WRN, RECQ4 and RECQ5 [1]. Mutations in three of the five human RECQ helicases, BLM, WRN and RECQ4, lead to genetic disorders as Bloom, Rothmund-Thompson and Werner's syndromes that are associated with cancer predisposition, premature ageing and developmental abnormalities [1, 2].

The Bloom's syndrome helicase, BLM has DNA annealing and unwinding activities. Through its interaction with TOPOIIIα, BLM unwinds the short stretches of naked duplex DNA and processes homologous recombination (HR) intermediates containing a double holiday junction [1, 2]. This helicase appears to prefer specific structures including D-loops and Holliday junctions and promotes Holliday junction branch migration [3]. It may suppress hyper-sister chromatid exchange (SCE) by disruption of D-loop recombination intermediates and also might be involved in the suppression of crossing over during homology-mediated recombination [4]. BLM-mediated crossover suppression may involve synthesis-dependent strand annealing (SDSA) [3]. This helicase facilitates telomere replication by resolving G4 structures [5]. Defects in BLM are also associated with the cancer phenotype [4].

Unlike the other members of the RECQ helicase family, the Werner's syndrome helicase, WRN contains both the classical helicase activity and 3'-to 5' exonuclease activity that target multiple DNA or RNA-DNA hybrid structures [1, 2]. As BLM, WRN appears to have robust in vitro G4

* Correspondence: jerome.moreaux@igh.cnrs.fr
[1]Laboratory for Monitoring Innovative Therapies, Department of Biological Hematology, Hôpital Saint-Eloi - CHRU de Montpellier, 80, av. Augustin Fliche, 34295 Montpellier, Cedex 5, France
[2]Institute of Human Genetics, CNRS-UPR1142, Montpellier F-34396, France
Full list of author information is available at the end of the article

unwinding activity [6] and plays a specialized role in telomere replication by disruption of G-quadruplex stretches
[7]. Another specific substrate of WRN is D-loop. WRN
repress the inappropriate telomeric recombination intermediates through its ability to resolve the D-loops [8].
This helicase was found to be involved in the repair of
double strand DNA breaks and studies on Werner's syndrome fibroblasts have shown defects in recombination
intermediate resolution which suggests that WRN is involved in HR [9]. WRN can bind to NBS1 [10], a member
of the MRN complex, and to the Ku70/Ku80 heterodimer
[11], a core non-homologous end joining DNA repair
(NHEJ) complex.

RECQ1 is the shortest of the human RECQ family helicases. RECQ1 displays specific functions in branch migration and restart of reversed DNA replication forks upon
DNA topoisomerase I inhibition that is not shared by
other human RECQ helicases [12, 13]. Studies have also
shown that RECQ1 plays a role in DNA strand breaks repair, mismatch repair and resistance to replication stress
[1, 2, 13, 14]. RECQ1 can also contribute to tumor development and progression by regulating the expression of
key genes that promote cancer cell migration, invasion
and metastasis [15].

The gene encoding for RECQ5 helicase was found to
be localized on human chromosome 17q23–25, a region
associated with both breast and ovarian cancer [16].
RECQ5 was found to cause a significant increase in the
frequency of spontaneous SCE [1, 2]. As BLM, RECQ5
was shown to play an essential role in suppression of
crossovers [17]. RECQ5 was identified as a potential
proto-oncogene in mouse leukemia [18]. RECQ5 is the
only member of RECQ family associated with RNA polymerase II, maintaining genomic stability during transcription [19].

RECQ helicase are at the crossroad between replication, recombination, DNA repair and transcription and

could represent potent therapeutic targets for cancer
therapy [20]. Hematological malignancies are characterized by genomic instability that is possibly related to
underlying defects in DNA repair of genomic stability
maintenance. Since these helicases play important roles
in the maintenance of chromosomal stability [21], we focused on RECQ helicases expression in hematological
cancers compared to their normal counterparts and the
association with prognostic impact.

Results and discussion

RECQ helicase gene expression levels were analyzed in
different types of hematological malignancies and in
their normal counterparts using Oncomine Cancer
Microarray database [22] as indicated in Table 1. Abnormal expression of at least one RECQ helicase was identified in all analyzed hematological malignancies (Table 1).
RECQ1 was found to be significantly overexpressed in
mantle cell lymphoma ($P = 0.0025$) [23], in unspecified
peripheral T-cell lymphoma ($P = 0.0038$) [24], anaplastic
large lymphoma ($P = 0.0024$) [24] and angioimmunoblas-
tic large cell lymphoma ($P = 0.001$) [24] (Fig. 1a).

WRN is significantly overexpressed in primary effusion
lymphoma compared to normal B cells ($p = 0.003$) [23]
(Fig. 1a).

RECQ4 expression was increased in Burkitt Lymphoma ($P = 0.001$) [23, 25], in diffuse large B cell lymphoma ($P = 0.004$) [23] and also in primary effusion
lymphoma ($P = 0.005$) [23] compared to normal counterpart (Fig. 1a).

RECQ5 is significantly overexpressed in acute myeloid
leukemia ($P = 0,001$) [26] (Fig. 1a).

Comparing RECQ helicases expression between normal
plasma cells (BMPC), premalignant cells from MGUS patients and multiple myeloma cells (MMC) [27], BLM and
WRN were found to be significantly downregulated in
MMC compared to normal BMPC ($P = 0.002$ and $P =$

Table 1 RECQ family member expression in hematological malignancies compared to that of their normal tissue counterparts using publicly available gene expression data, including the Oncomine Cancer Microarray and Genomicscape databases

	Hematological Malignancies	Datasets	Gene overexpression compared to normal tissue counterpart				
			RECQ1	BLM	WRN	RECQ4	RECQ5
Myeloid Neoplasms	Acute Myeloid Leukemia	12	No	No	No	No	YES
B-cell neoplasms	Primary Effusion Lymphoma	8	No	No	YES	YES	No
	Chronic Lymphocyte Leukemia	11	No	No	YES	No	No
	Diffuse Large B-cell Lymphoma	8	No	No	No	YES	No
	Burkitt's Lymphoma	8	No	No	No	YES	No
	Mantle Cell Lymphoma	11	YES	No	No	No	No
	Multiple Myeloma	1	YES	YES	YES	YES	No
T-cell neoplasms	Unspecified Peripheral T-cell Lymphoma	11	YES	No	No	No	No
	Anaplastic Large Cell Lymphoma	11	YES	No	No	No	No
	Angioimmunoblastic T-Cell Lymphoma	11	YES	No	No	No	No

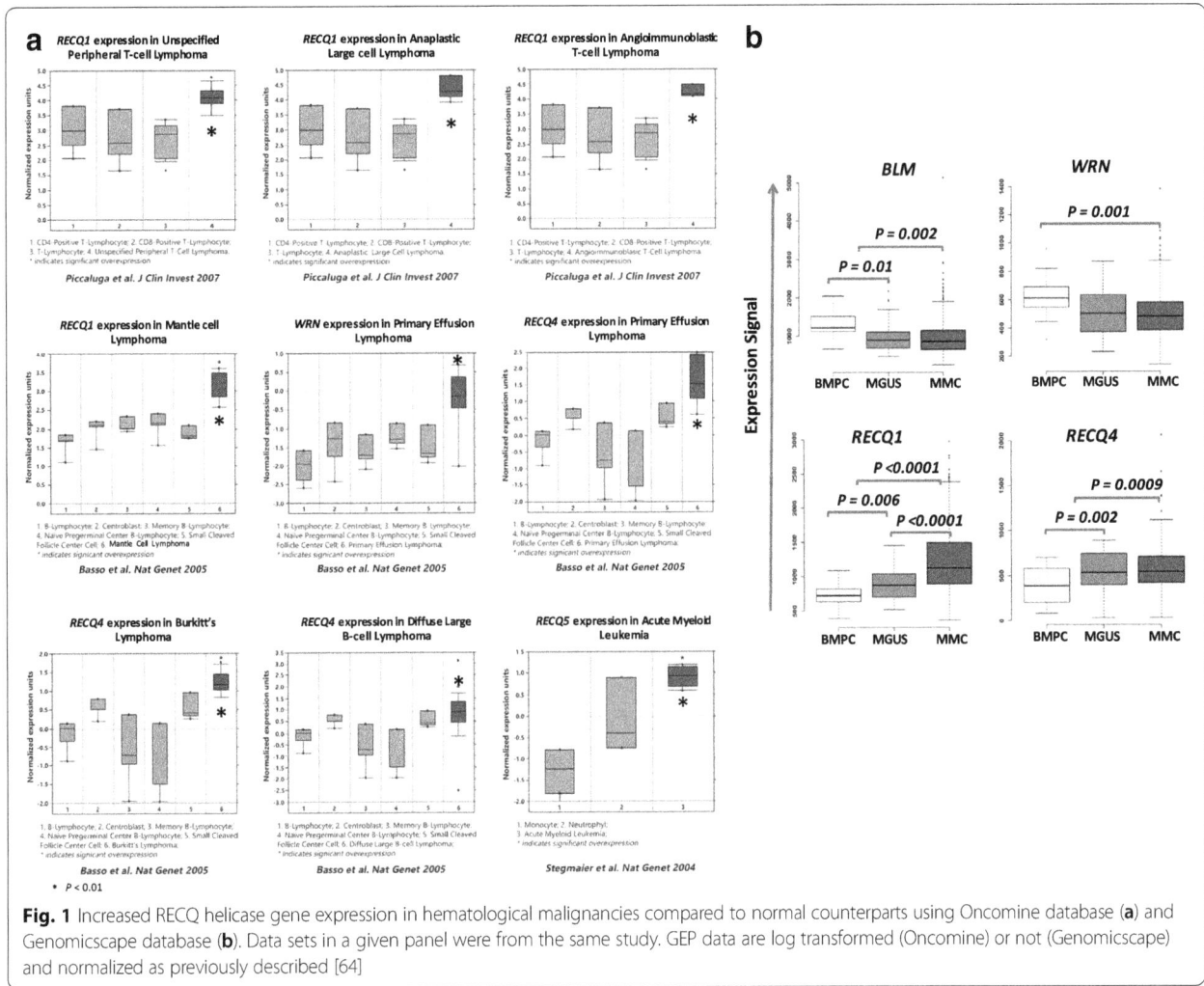

Fig. 1 Increased RECQ helicase gene expression in hematological malignancies compared to normal counterparts using Oncomine database (**a**) and Genomicscape database (**b**). Data sets in a given panel were from the same study. GEP data are log transformed (Oncomine) or not (Genomicscape) and normalized as previously described [64]

0.001 respectively) (Fig. 1b). A decreased expression of *BLM* was also observed in MGUS compared to BMPC ($P = 0.01$). *RECQ1* and *RECQ4* are overexpressed in MGUS ($P = 0.006$ and $P = 0.002$) and MMC ($P < 0.0001$ and $P = 0.0009$) compared to BMPC. Furthermore, a significant increased expression of *RECQ1* in MMC compared to MGUS was identified (Fig. 1b).

Furthermore, using the human protein atlas database [28–30], the expression of RECQ1, RECQ4 and RECQ5 could be confirmed at protein level in myeloid and lymphoid cancer cell lines (Additional file 1: Figure S1).

We investigated whether *RECQ* helicases expression could be associated with tumor progression and prognosis in hematological malignancies (Table 2).

In AML patients with abnormal karyotype (Verhaak cohort, $N = 521$ patients) [31], a high expression of *BLM* and *RECQ4* is associated with a better overall survival (OS) ($P = 0.01$ and $P = 0.003$). At the opposite, high *RECQ5* expression was linked with a poor prognosis in the same cohort of patient ($P = 0.008$) (Fig. 2a). In cox multivariate analysis, only *RECQ5*

expression kept prognostic value ($P = 0.01$, hazard ratio (HR) = 1.43).

In AML with normal karyotype, (Metzeler cohort, $N = 78$) [32], gene expression of four *RECQ* helicases out of five were identified to predict for OS. High expression of *RECQ1* ($P = 0.02$), *BLM* ($P = 0.01$) and *RECQ5* ($P = 0.03$) were found to be associated with poor prognosis. In contrast, high *RECQ4* expression was linked with a better outcome ($P = 0.03$) (Fig. 2b). When tested together in a cox multivariate analysis, only *RECQ4* expression remained significant ($P = 0.009$; HR = 0.4).

Interestingly, *RECQ5* overexpression was only identified in myeloid malignancies in association with an adverse prognosis. *RECQ5* increased expression was recently reported in JAK2V617F myeloproliferative neoplasms [33]. RECQ5 depletion in JAK2V617F-mutant cells impairs replication after hydroxyurea treatment leading to a significant increased double-stranded breaks and apoptosis [33]. RECQ5 represents a potent regulator of genome stability in myeloproliferative neoplasms in association with drug resistance

Table 2 Link between *RECQ* helicase gene expression and prognostic value in hematological malignancies

RECQ helicase	Prognostic value					
	AML		LLC	FL	DBLCL	MM
	normal karyotype	abnormal karyotype				
WRN	-	-	GOOD	GOOD	-	BAD
BLM	BAD	GOOD	-	-	-	-
RECQ1	BAD	-	-	BAD	-	BAD
RECQ4	GOOD	GOOD	-	GOOD	-	BAD
RECQ5	BAD	-	BAD	BAD	GOOD	-

GOOD : A high *RECQ* helicase expression is associated with a better outcome
BAD : A high *RECQ* helicase expression is associated with a poor prognosis

[33]. *RECQ5* overexpression could also be involved in AML pathophysiology and chemoresistance.

Even if RECQ1 mutations have been recently shown to been associated with predisposition to breast cancer [34, 35], no link between *RECQ1*, *BLM*, *WRN*, and *RECQ4* deregulation and lymphoid malignancies were previously reported.

In chronic lymphocytic leukemia (CLL), a poor prognosis was linked with high *RECQ5* expression ($P = 8E-8$) and a better outcome was associated with high *WRN* expression ($P = 0.0006$) (Fig. 3a).

In a cohort of patients with follicular lymphoma (FL) (Staudt cohort, $N = 180$) [36], high *RECQ1* and *RECQ5* expression represented adverse prognostic factors ($P = 0.003$ and $P = 0.0006$ respectively) whereas *RECQ4* expression was found to be associated with a good prognosis ($P = 0.009$) (Fig. 3b). Interestingly, *RECQ1*, *RECQ4* and *RECQ5* expresison remained independent when tested in cox multivariate analysis ($P < 0.0001$; HR = 2.8; $P = 0.002$; HR = 0.49 and $P < 0.01$; HR = 1.78 respectively).

In diffuse large B cell lymphoma (DLBCL), only *RECQ5* expression was associated with a prognostic value. Low *RECQ5* expression was a poor prognostic marker in two independent cohorts of patients ($P = 0.02$ in a cohort of patients treated by combination of cyclophosphamide, doxorubicin, vincristine and prednisone (CHOP) therapy ($N = 181$) and $P = 0.01$ in a cohort of patients treated by Rituximab combined with CHOP (R-CHOP) regimen ($N = 233$)) (Fig. 3c) [37].

In MM, high *RECQ1*, *WRN* and *RECQ4* expression are associated with an adverse prognosis in the UAMS cohort treated with total therapy 2 (Fig. 4) [27].

These data demonstrate a link between *RECQ* helicase expression and a prognostic value in different hematological malignancies.

Hematological malignancies are characterized by genomic instability that could be related to defects in DNA repair [21]. The RECQ family of DNA helicases is a family of conserved enzymes that display highly specialized and vital roles in the maintenance of genome stability. Mutations in three of the five human RECQ helicases,

BLM, WRN and RECQL4, are associated with genetic disorders characterized by chromosomal instability and increased susceptibility to cancer including leukemia [38, 39]. Mutations in *BLM* result in a dramatic lowering of *BLM* mRNA levels and premature termination of protein translation owing to nonsense-mediated mRNA decay [1, 40]. Patients with Bloom syndrome exhibit cancer predisposition including most types of cancers and particularly non-Hodgkin's lymphoma, leukemias and carcinomas of skin, breast and colon [1]. Interestingly, a low *BLM* expression is associated with a poor prognosis in AML with complex karyotypes (Fig. 2a). The cancer spectrum observed in patients with Werner's syndrome is characterized mainly by cancers of mesenchymal origin and some epithelial cancers [1, 41]. RECQ4 mutations are found in Rothmund-Thomson syndrome, RAPADILINO syndrome and Baller-Gerold syndrome [1, 41]. Rothmund-Thomson syndrome are characterized by predisposition to mainly osteosarcoma whereas RAPADILINO syndrome are linked with lymphoma and osteosarcoma predisposition [1].

Specific recurrent chromosomal translocations have been associated with DNA repair deficiencies linked with repression of DDR (DNA damage response) genes in AML [42]. In PML-RARA, PML and BLM are delocalized from the nuclear bodies into microspeckled nuclear regions [43]. All trans retinoic acid (ATRA) treatment of APL patients leads to degradation of PML-RARA and relocalization of BLM to nuclear bodies [43] suggesting that PML-RARA are involved in genomic instability in APL through disruption of BLM and PML localization and activity. Interestingly, we reported that low *BLM* and *RECQ4* expression are associated with a poor prognosis in AML with abnormal karyotype (Fig. 2a), suggesting that downregulation of RECQ helicases could be involved in leukemogenesis and genomic instability. At the opposite, in AML with normal karyotype, *RECQ1*, *BLM* and *RECQ5* high expression are associated with a poor prognosis (Fig. 2b). As reported in solid cancer, *RECQ* helicase overexpression could be a marker of chemoresistance and higher

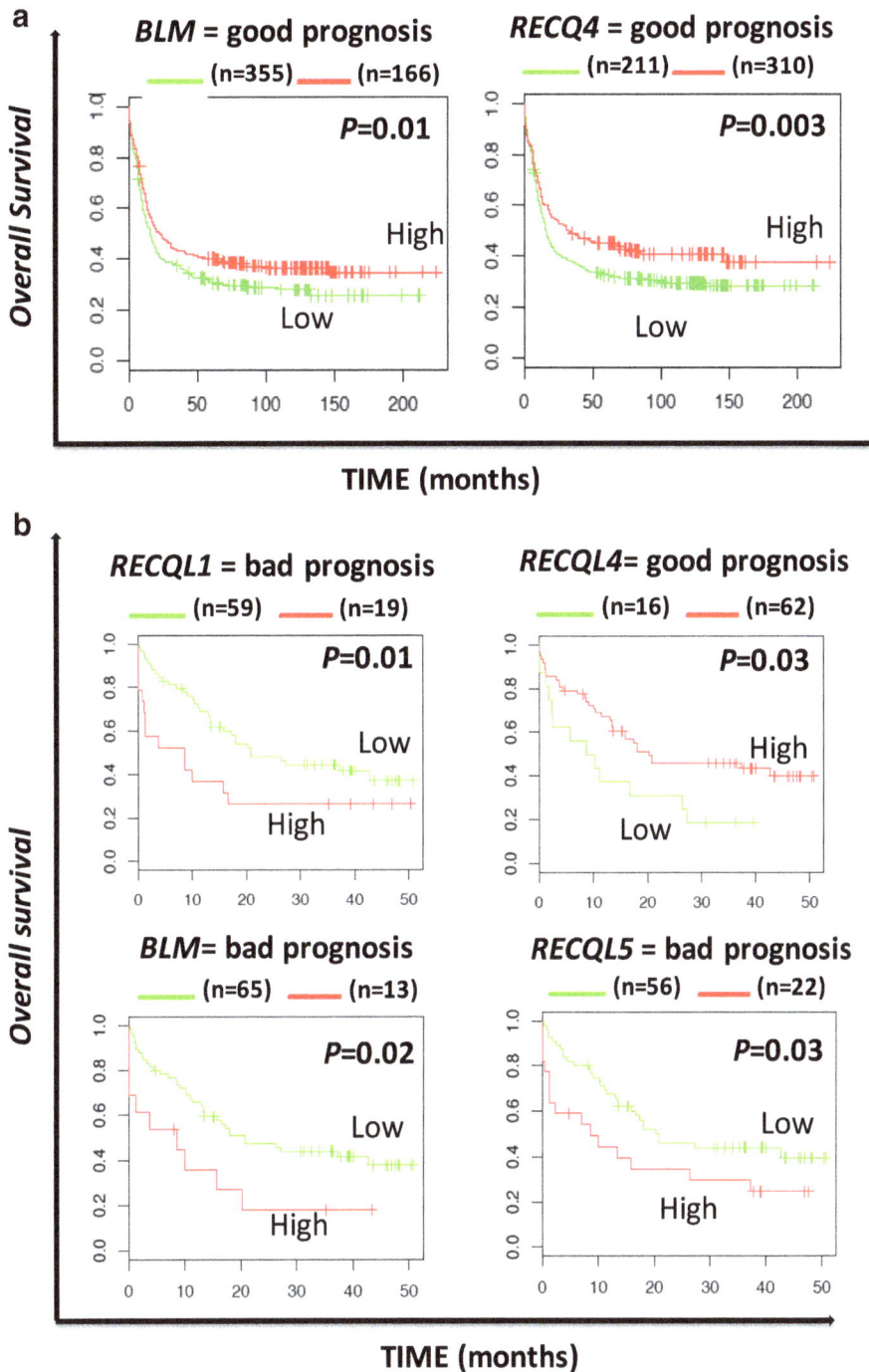

Fig. 2 Overall survival related to RECQ helicase gene expression in acute myeloid leukemia with abnormal karyotype (a) and normal karyotype (b). The prognostic value of gene expression was determined using the MaxStat R function in R software. The overall survival of subgroups of patients was compared with the log-rank test and survival curves computed with the Kaplan–Meier method (R software) [66]

proliferation helping AML cells to deal with replication stress [44, 45]. B lymphocytes are continuously produced during adult life and they undergo different genetic alterations associated with DNA breaks, including VDJ recombination, Ig class switch recombination and somatic hypermutation. These mechanisms must be tightly regulated to prevent tumorigenesis and ensure efficient immune response [46]. Collapsed DNA replication forks occurring in rapidly dividing lymphocytes leads to a restart failure and results in an interruption of the normal developmental program [47]. HR is required for lymphoid development [47]. Aberrations

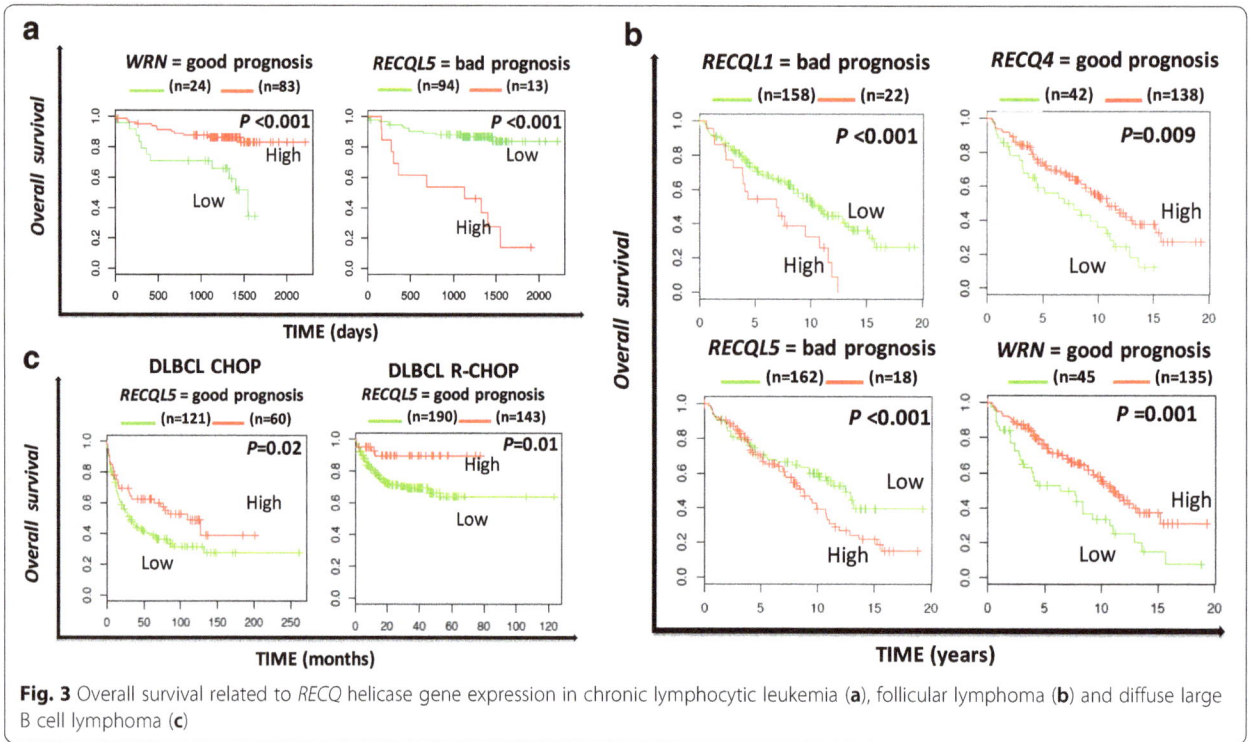

Fig. 3 Overall survival related to *RECQ* helicase gene expression in chronic lymphocytic leukemia (**a**), follicular lymphoma (**b**) and diffuse large B cell lymphoma (**c**)

affecting HR actors are correlated with genomic instability in B cell cancers [48]. By their involvement in HR and also by their ability to resolve and to continue the normal fork replication after DNA damage or replication fork arrest, WRN [49], BLM [4], RECQ1 [12] and RECQ5 [50] helicases might be crucial in lymphoid development and aberration in their expression or function can lead to cancer genesis. Interestingly, low expression of WRN in CLL and FL, low *RECQ4* expression in FL and low *RECQ5* in DLBCL are associated with a poor prognosis (Fig. 3). Furthermore, high *RECQ5* expression in CLL and FL and high *RECQ1* expression in FL are associated with a poor prognosis and could be involved in chemoresistance. In lymphoma, deregulation of DDR is associated with tumorigenesis [51, 52], poor prognosis [53, 54] and could represent a potent therapeutic target [53, 55, 56].

In MM, patients with extensive chromosomal instability and replicative stress are associated with an adverse outcome [27, 57–59]. Accordingly, high *RECQ1*, *WRN* and *RECQ4* expression is associated with a significant poor survival in MM patients (Fig. 4). Although *WRN* was found to be significantly downregulated in MMC compared to normal BMPC (Fig. 1b), patients with high expression display a poor prognosis. *WRN* is located on chromosome 8p deleted in 25 % of MM patients without prognostic value [60]. These data could explain the significant downregulation of *WRN* expression in MM compared to normal BMPC.

Recently, a set of molecule inhibitors of WRN and BLM was characterized [61, 62]. These new molecules could open up new therapeutic strategies for targeting hematological malignancies characterized by RECQ helicase deregulation and a poor prognosis.

Conclusion

The analysis reported here demonstrates that *RECQ* helicase expression is deregulated in hematological malignancies compared to their normal counterparts in association with a prognostic value in AML, CLL, lymphoma and MM. Deregulation of RECQ helicases appears to play a role in tumorigenesis and could be involved in genomic instability and chemoresistance in hematological malignances. RECQ helicases represent potent therapeutic targets for synthetic lethal approaches.

Methods

Databases: We used Oncomine Cancer Microarray database (http://www.oncomine.org) [22] and Genomicscape (http://genomicscape.com/) [63] to study gene expression of RECQ family members in nine different human hematological malignancies and their normal tissue counterpart as indicated in Table 1. To compare the gene expression of a tumor type to its normal counterpart, we used gene expression data from a same study with the same methodology. All data were log transformed, median centered per array,

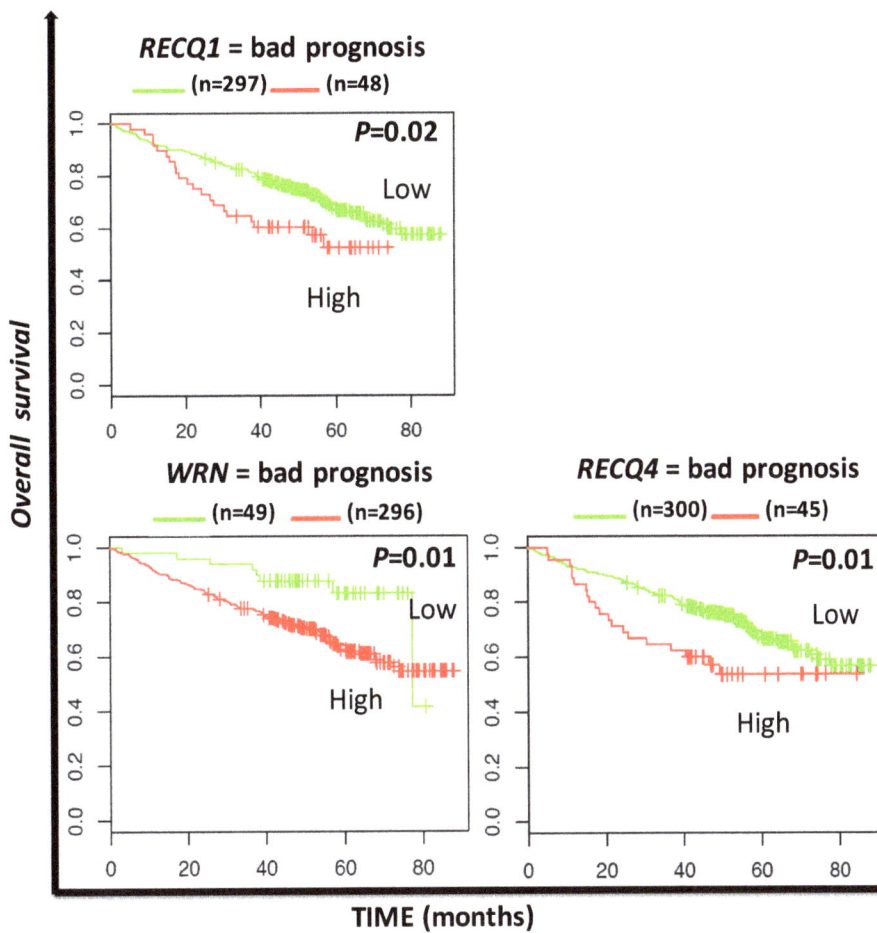

Fig. 4 Overall survival related to *RECQ* helicase gene expression in multiple myeloma

and the standard deviation was normalized to one per array [22].

Statistical comparisons were done with Mann–Whitney or Student *t*-test as previously published [64].

Prognosis values of each member of RECQ family in hematological malignancies were determined by using Maxstat R package based on publicly available data (Gene Expression Omnibus (http://www.ncbi.nlm.nih.gov/geo/); accession numbers GSE6891, GSE12417, GSE22762, GSE16131, GSE10846 and GSE4581) analyzed with Genomicscape [63] as previously reported [65].

Competing interests
The authors declare that they have no competing interests.

Authors' contributions
EV performed research, bioinformatics, and participated in the writing of the paper. AK participated in the bioinformatics. PP participated in the writing of the paper. BK participated in the research and in the writing of the paper. JM supervised the research, bioinformatics, and the writing of the paper. All authors read and approved the final manuscript.

Acknowledgements
This work was supported by grants from French INCA (Institut National du Cancer) Institute (2012-109/087437), Languedoc Roussillon CRLR (R14026FF), Fondation de France (201400047510), ITMO Cancer (MM&TT) and AXLR SATT (30041633). EV is supported by a grant from Guillaume Espoir association (Saint- Genis-Laval, France).

Author details
[1]Laboratory for Monitoring Innovative Therapies, Department of Biological Hematology, Hôpital Saint-Eloi - CHRU de Montpellier, 80, av. Augustin Fliche, 34295 Montpellier, Cedex 5, France. [2]Institute of Human Genetics, CNRS-UPR1142, Montpellier F-34396, France. [3]University of Montpellier 1, UFR de Médecine, Montpellier, France.

References
1. Chu WK, Hickson ID. RecQ helicases: multifunctional genome caretakers. Nat Rev Cancer. 2009;9(9):644–54. doi:10.1038/nrc2682.
2. Larsen NB, Hickson ID. RecQ Helicases: Conserved Guardians of Genomic Integrity. Adv Exp Med Biol. 2013;767:161–84. doi:10.1007/978-1-4614-5037-5_8.

3. Weinert BT, Rio DC. DNA strand displacement, strand annealing and strand swapping by the Drosophila Bloom's syndrome helicase. Nucleic Acids Res. 2007;35(4):1367–76. doi:10.1093/nar/gkl831.

4. Sung P, Klein H. Mechanism of homologous recombination: mediators and helicases take on regulatory functions. Nat Rev Mol Cell Biol. 2006;7(10): 739–50. 10. 1038/nrm2008.

5. Drosopoulos WC, Kosiyatrakul ST, Schildkraut CL. BLM helicase facilitates telomere replication during leading strand synthesis of telomeres. J Cell Biol. 2015;210(2):191–208. doi:10.1083/jcb.201410061.

6. Kamath-Loeb A, Loeb LA, Fry M. The Werner syndrome protein is distinguished from the Bloom syndrome protein by its capacity to tightly bind diverse DNA structures. PLoS One. 2012;7(1):e30189. doi:10.1371/journal.pone.0030189.

7. Damerla RR, Knickelbein KE, Strutt S, Liu FJ, Wang H, Opresko PL. Werner syndrome protein suppresses the formation of large deletions during the replication of human telomeric sequences. Cell Cycle. 2012;11(16):3036–44. doi:10.4161/cc.21399.

8. Opresko PL, Mason PA, Podell ER, Lei M, Hickson ID, Cech TR, et al. POT1 stimulates RecQ helicases WRN and BLM to unwind telomeric DNA substrates. J Biol Chem. 2005;280(37):32069–80. doi:10.1074/jbc.M505211200.

9. Chen L, Huang S, Lee L, Davalos A, Schiestl RH, Campisi J, et al. WRN, the protein deficient in Werner syndrome, plays a critical structural role in optimizing DNA repair. Aging Cell. 2003;2(4):191–9.

10. Kobayashi J, Okui M, Asaithamby A, Burma S, Chen BP, Tanimoto K, et al. WRN participates in translesion synthesis pathway through interaction with NBS1. Mech Ageing Dev. 2010;131(6):436–44. doi:10.1016/j.mad.2010.06.005.

11. Karmakar P, Snowden CM, Ramsden DA, Bohr VA. Ku heterodimer binds to both ends of the Werner protein and functional interaction occurs at the Werner N-terminus. Nucleic Acids Res. 2002;30(16):3583–91.

12. Berti M, Ray Chaudhuri A, Thangavel S, Gomathinayagam S, Kenig S, Vujanovic M, et al. Human RECQ1 promotes restart of replication forks reversed by DNA topoisomerase I inhibition. Nat Struct Mol Biol. 2013;20(3): 347–54. doi:10.1038/nsmb.2501.

13. Lu X, Parvathaneni S, Hara T, Lal A, Sharma S. Replication stress induces specific enrichment of RECQ1 at common fragile sites FRA3B and FRA16D. Mol Cancer. 2013;12(1):29. doi:10.1186/1476-4598-12-29.

14. Popuri V, Croteau DL, Brosh Jr RM, Bohr VA. RECQ1 is required for cellular resistance to replication stress and catalyzes strand exchange on stalled replication fork structures. Cell Cycle. 2012;11(22):4252–65. doi:10.4161/cc.22581.

15. Li XL, Lu X, Parvathaneni S, Bilke S, Zhang H, Thangavel S, et al. Identification of RECQ1-regulated transcriptome uncovers a role of RECQ1 in regulation of cancer cell migration and invasion. Cell Cycle. 2014;13(15):2431–45.

16. Sekelsky JJ, Brodsky MH, Rubin GM, Hawley RS. Drosophila and human RecQ5 exist in different isoforms generated by alternative splicing. Nucleic Acids Res. 1999;27(18):3762–9.

17. Hu Y, Lu X, Barnes E, Yan M, Lou H, Luo G. Recql5 and Blm RecQ DNA helicases have nonredundant roles in suppressing crossovers. Mol Cell Biol. 2005;25(9):3431–42. doi:10.1128/MCB.25.9.3431-3442.2005.

18. Hansen GM, Skapura D, Justice MJ. Genetic profile of insertion mutations in mouse leukemias and lymphomas. Genome Res. 2000;10(2):237–43.

19. Saponaro M, Kantidakis T, Mitter R, Kelly GP, Heron M, Williams H, et al. RECQL5 controls transcript elongation and suppresses genome instability associated with transcription stress. Cell. 2014;157(5):1037–49. doi:10.1016/j.cell.2014.03.048.

20. Rezazadeh S. RecQ helicases; at the crossroad of genome replication, repair, and recombination. Mol Biol Rep. 2011. doi:10.1007/s11033-011-1243-y

21. Economopoulou P, Pappa V, Papageorgiou S, Dervenoulas J, Economopoulos T. Abnormalities of DNA repair mechanisms in common hematological malignancies. Leuk Lymphoma. 2011;52(4):567–82. doi:10.3109/10428194.2010.551155.

22. Rhodes DR, Yu J, Shanker K, Deshpande N, Varambally R, Ghosh D, et al. ONCOMINE: a cancer microarray database and integrated data-mining platform. Neoplasia. 2004;6(1):1–6.

23. Basso K, Margolin AA, Stolovitzky G, Klein U, Dalla-Favera R, Califano A. Reverse engineering of regulatory networks in human B cells. Nat Genet. 2005;37(4):382–90. doi:10.1038/ng1532.

24. Piccaluga PP, Agostinelli C, Califano A, Rossi M, Basso K, Zupo S, et al. Gene expression analysis of peripheral T cell lymphoma, unspecified, reveals distinct profiles and new potential therapeutic targets. J Clin Invest. 2007; 117(3):823–34. doi:10.1172/JCI26833.

25. Brune V, Tiacci E, Pfeil I, Doring C, Eckerle S, van Noesel CJ, et al. Origin and pathogenesis of nodular lymphocyte-predominant Hodgkin lymphoma as revealed by global gene expression analysis. J Exp Med. 2008;205(10):2251–68. doi:10.1084/jem.20080809.

26. Stegmaier K, Ross KN, Colavito SA, O'Malley S, Stockwell BR, Golub TR. Gene expression-based high-throughput screening(GE-HTS) and application to leukemia differentiation. Nat Genet. 2004;36(3):257–63. doi:10.1038/ng1305.

27. Zhan F, Huang Y, Colla S, Stewart JP, Hanamura I, Gupta S, et al. The molecular classification of multiple myeloma. Blood. 2006;108(6):2020–8.

28. Uhlen M, Fagerberg L, Hallstrom BM, Lindskog C, Oksvold P, Mardinoglu A, et al. Proteomics. Tissue-based map of the human proteome. Science. 2015; 347(6220):1260419. doi:10.1126/science.1260419.

29. Ponten F, Jirstrom K, Uhlen M. The Human Protein Atlas–a tool for pathology. J Pathol. 2008;216(4):387–93. doi:10.1002/path.2440.

30. Uhlen M, Bjorling E, Agaton C, Szigyarto CA, Amini B, Andersen E, et al. A human protein atlas for normal and cancer tissues based on antibody proteomics. Mol Cell Proteomics. 2005;4(12):1920–32. doi:10.1074/mcp.M500279-MCP200.

31. Verhaak RG, Wouters BJ, Erpelinck CA, Abbas S, Beverloo HB, Lugthart S, et al. Prediction of molecular subtypes in acute myeloid leukemia based on gene expression profiling. Haematologica. 2009;94(1):131–4. doi:10.3324/haematol.13299.

32. Metzeler KH, Maharry K, Radmacher MD, Mrozek K, Margeson D, Becker H, et al. TET2 mutations improve the new European LeukemiaNet risk classification of acute myeloid leukemia: a Cancer and Leukemia Group B study. J Clin Oncol. 2011;29(10):1373–81. doi:10.1200/JCO.2010.32.7742.

33. Chen E, Ahn JS, Sykes DB, Breyfogle LJ, Godfrey AL, Nangalia J, et al. RECQL5 Suppresses Oncogenic JAK2-Induced Replication Stress and Genomic Instability. Cell reports. 2015;13(11):2345–52. doi:10.1016/j.celrep.2015.11.037.

34. Sun J, Wang Y, Xia Y, Xu Y, Ouyang T, Li J, et al. Mutations in RECQL Gene Are Associated with Predisposition to Breast Cancer. PLoS Genet. 2015;11(5): e1005228. doi:10.1371/journal.pgen.1005228.

35. Cybulski C, Carrot-Zhang J, Kluzniak W, Rivera B, Kashyap A, Wokolorczyk D, et al. Germline RECQL mutations are associated with breast cancer susceptibility. Nat Genet. 2015;47(6):643–6. doi:10.1038/ng.3284.

36. Leich E, Salaverria I, Bea S, Zettl A, Wright G, Moreno V, et al. Follicular lymphomas with and without translocation t(14;18) differ in gene expression profiles and genetic alterations. Blood. 2009;114(4):826–34. doi:10.1182/blood-2009-01-198580.

37. Lenz G, Wright G, Dave SS, Xiao W, Powell J, Zhao H, et al. Stromal gene signatures in large-B-cell lymphomas. N Engl J Med. 2008;359(22):2313–23. doi:10.1056/NEJMoa0802885.

38. Suhasini AN, Brosh Jr RM. Fanconi anemia and Bloom's syndrome crosstalk through FANCJ-BLM helicase interaction. Trends Genet. 2012;28(1):7–13. doi:10.1016/j.tig.2011.09.003.

39. Poppe B, Van Limbergen H, Van Roy N, Vandecruys E, De Paepe A, Benoit Y, et al. Chromosomal aberrations in Bloom syndrome patients with myeloid malignancies. Cancer Genet Cytogenet. 2001;128(1):39–42.

40. German J, Sanz MM, Ciocci S, Ye TZ, Ellis NA. Syndrome-causing mutations of the BLM gene in persons in the Bloom's Syndrome Registry. Hum Mutat. 2007;28(8):743–53. doi:10.1002/humu.20501.

41. Goto M, Miller RW, Ishikawa Y, Sugano H. Excess of rare cancers in Werner syndrome (adult progeria). Cancer Epidemiol Biomarkers Prev. 1996;5(4):239–46.

42. Esposito MT, So CW. DNA damage accumulation and repair defects in acute myeloid leukemia: implications for pathogenesis, disease progression, and chemotherapy resistance. Chromosoma. 2014;123(6):545–61. doi:10.1007/s00412-014-0482-9.

43. Zhong S, Hu P, Ye TZ, Stan R, Ellis NA, Pandolfi PP. A role for PML and the nuclear body in genomic stability. Oncogene. 1999;18(56):7941–7. doi:10.1038/sj.onc.1203367.

44. Sanada S, Futami K, Terada A, Yonemoto K, Ogasawara S, Akiba J, et al. RECQL1 DNA repair helicase: a potential therapeutic target and a proliferative marker against ovarian cancer. PLoS One. 2013;8(8):e72820. doi:10.1371/journal.pone.0072820.

45. Matsushita Y, Yokoyama Y, Yoshida H, Osawa Y, Mizunuma M, Shigeto T, et al. The level of RECQL1 expression is a prognostic factor for epithelial ovarian cancer. J Ovarian Res. 2014;7:107. doi:10.1186/s13048-014-0107-1.

46. Gennery AR, Cant AJ, Jeggo PA. Immunodeficiency associated with DNA repair defects. Clin Exp Immunol. 2000;121(1):1–7.

47. Caddle LB, Hasham MG, Schott WH, Shirley BJ, Mills KD. Homologous recombination is necessary for normal lymphocyte development. Mol Cell Biol. 2008;28(7):2295–303. doi:10.1128/MCB.02139-07.

48. Hasham MG, Donghia NM, Coffey E, Maynard J, Snow KJ, Ames J, et al. Widespread genomic breaks generated by activation-induced cytidine deaminase are prevented by homologous recombination. Nat Immunol. 2010;11(9):820–6. doi:10.1038/ni.1909.

49. Sidorova JM, Li N, Folch A, Monnat Jr RJ. The RecQ helicase WRN is required for normal replication fork progression after DNA damage or replication fork arrest. Cell Cycle. 2008;7(6):796–807.

50. Yin L. Chondroitin synthase 1 is a key molecule in myeloma cell-osteoclast interactions. J Biol Chem. 2005;280(16):15666–72.

51. Gu X, Booth CJ, Liu Z, Strout MP. AID-associated DNA repair pathways regulate malignant transformation in a murine model of BCL6-driven diffuse large B cell lymphoma. Blood. 2015. doi:10.1182/blood-2015-02-628164

52. Hathcock KS, Padilla-Nash HM, Camps J, Shin DM, Triner D, Shaffer AL, 3rd et al. ATM deficiency in absence of T cells promotes development of NF-kB-dependent murine B cell lymphomas that resemble human ABC DLBCL. Blood. 2015. doi:10.1182/blood-2015-06-654749

53. Bret C, Klein B, Cartron G, Schved JF, Constantinou A, Pasero P et al. DNA repair in diffuse large B-cell lymphoma: a molecular portrait. Br J Haematol. 2014. doi:10.1111/bjh.13206

54. Bret C, Klein B, Moreaux J. Gene expression-based risk score in diffuse large B-cell lymphoma. Oncotarget. 2012;3(12):1700–10.

55. Kwok M, Davies N, Agathanggelou A, Smith E, Petermann E, Yates E, et al. Synthetic lethality in chronic lymphocytic leukaemia with DNA damage response defects by targeting the ATR pathway. Lancet. 2015;385 Suppl 1: S58. doi:10.1016/S0140-6736(15)60373-7.

56. Bret C, Klein B, Moreaux J. Nucleotide excision DNA repair pathway as a therapeutic target in patients with high-risk diffuse large B cell lymphoma. Cell Cycle. 2013;12(12):1811–2. doi:10.4161/cc.25115.

57. Cottini F, Hideshima T, Suzuki R, Tai YT, Bianchini G, Richardson PG, et al. Synthetic Lethal Approaches Exploiting DNA Damage in Aggressive Myeloma. Cancer Discov. 2015;5(9):972–87. doi:10.1158/2159-8290.CD-14-0943.

58. Hose D, Reme T, Hielscher T, Moreaux J, Messner T, Seckinger A, et al. Proliferation is a central independent prognostic factor and target for personalized and risk-adapted treatment in multiple myeloma. Haematologica. 2011;96(1):87–95. doi:10.3324/haematol.2010.030296.

59. Kassambara A, Gourzones-Dmitriev C, Sahota S, Reme T, Moreaux J, Goldschmidt H, et al. A DNA repair pathway score predicts survival in human multiple myeloma: the potential for therapeutic strategy. Oncotarget. 2014;5(9):2487–98.

60. Walker BA, Leone PE, Chiecchio L, Dickens NJ, Jenner MW, Boyd KD, et al. A compendium of myeloma-associated chromosomal copy number abnormalities and their prognostic value. Blood. 2010;116(15):e56–65. doi:10.1182/blood-2010-04-279596.

61. Aggarwal M, Banerjee T, Sommers JA, Brosh Jr RM. Targeting an Achilles' heel of cancer with a WRN helicase inhibitor. Cell Cycle. 2013;12(20):3329–35. doi:10.4161/cc.26320.

62. Nguyen GH, Dexheimer TS, Rosenthal AS, Chu WK, Singh DK, Mosedale G, et al. A small molecule inhibitor of the BLM helicase modulates chromosome stability in human cells. Chem Biol. 2013;20(1):55–62. doi:10.1016/j.chembiol.2012.10.016.

63. Kassambara A, Reme T, Jourdan M, Fest T, Hose D, Tarte K, et al. GenomicScape: an easy-to-use web tool for gene expression data analysis. Application to investigate the molecular events in the differentiation of B cells into plasma cells. PLoS Comput Biol. 2015;11(1):e1004077. doi:10.1371/journal.pcbi.1004077.

64. Kassambara A, Klein B, Moreaux J. MMSET is overexpressed in cancers: link with tumor aggressiveness. Biochem Biophys Res Commun. 2009;379(4): 840–5. doi:10.1016/j.bbrc.2008.12.093.

65. Kassambara A, Hose D, Moreaux J, Walker BA, Protopopov A, Reme T, et al. Genes with a spike expression are clustered in chromosome (sub)bands and spike (sub)bands have a powerful prognostic value in patients with multiple myeloma. Haematologica. 2012;97(4):622–30. doi:10.3324/haematol.2011.046821.

66. Moreaux J, Kassambara A, Hose D, Klein B. STEAP1 is overexpressed in cancers: A promising therapeutic target. Biochem Biophys Res Commun. 2012;429(3-4):148–55. doi:10.1016/j.bbrc.2012.10.123.

15

NOS1-, NOS3-, PIK3CA-, and MAPK-pathways in skin following radiation therapy

Steffen Koerdt[1][*][†], Nadine Tanner[1][†], Niklas Rommel[1], Nils H. Rohleder[1], Gesche Frohwitter[1], Oliver Ristow[2], Klaus-Dietrich Wolff[1] and Marco R. Kesting[1]

Abstract

Background: Essential molecular pathways such as the MAPK pathway, NO system, or the influence of PIK3CA as an oncogene are known to regulate fundamental signalling networks. However, few knowledge about their role in the occurrence of wound healing disorders (WHD) following radiation therapy (RT) exists. This study aims to evaluate the expression profiles of specific molecular pathway marker genes.

Methods: Expression profiles of the genes encoding MAPK, NOS1, NOS3, and PIK3CA were analyzed, by RT-PCR, in specimens from patients with and without a history of RT to the head and neck. Clinical data on the occurrence of cervical WHDs were analyzed.

Results: Expression analysis of patients with postoperative WHDs revealed a significant increase in MAPK expression compared to the control group without occurrence of postoperative WHDs. PIK3CA showed a significantly increased expression in patients with a history of RT. Expression analysis of all other investigated genes did not reveal significant differences.

Conclusions: This current study is able to show the influence of RT on different molecular pathways. This underlines the crucial role of specific molecular networks, responsible for the occurrence of long-term radiation toxicity such as WHDs. Additional studies should be carried out to identify possible starting points for therapeutic interventions.

Keywords: Radiation therapy, MAPK, NOS, PIK3CA, PCR

Background

In an interdisciplinary and individual oncological treatment concept for cancers of the oral cavity, Radiation Therapy (RT) is next to the surgical resection, and chemotherapy one of the most important columns for local and regional disease control. However, RT is also accompanied with multiple side effects, which can be subdivided in short- and long-term radiation associated toxicity. In cases, when patients received RT preoperatively in a neoadjuvant setting or in cases of disease recurrence, surgeons have to deal with wound healing disorders (WHD) in previously irradiated tissue [1]. Factors, which might influence the onset of WHDs after RT appear to be immanent in terms of a reduced angiogenesis and the development of radiation-induced skin fibrosis [2–4]. Reactive oxygen and nitrogen species (RONS) in the context of oxidative stress also seem to play an important role in the pathogenesis of post-radiogenic WHDs, yet more research has to be conducted to fully understand the underlying molecular pathways and to find starting points for therapeutic interventions [5]. This current PCR-based study aims to evaluate the role of certain crucial pathways in the development of post-radiogenic WHDs following RT to the head and neck.

Nitric oxide (NO) is considered to be a short-living radical, which is involved in many important biological functions, such as vasodilation, anti-microbial activities,

---

* Correspondence: steffen.koerdt@tum.de
Steffen Koerdt and Nadine Tanner share the first-authorship.
[†]Equal contributors
[1]Department of Oral and Maxillofacial Surgery, Technical University of Munich (TUM), Ismaninger Str. 22, D-81675 Munich, Germany
Full list of author information is available at the end of the article

immunoregulation, and activities in which it functions as a neurotransmitter [6–10]. Its relevance in wound healing has been described elsewhere [11, 12]. NO is produced by nitric oxide synthase (NOS) in different isoforms. Neuronal NOS (NOS1) and endothelial NOS (NOS3), collectively referred to as cNOS are constitutively expressed depending on intracellular calcium levels [11]. The influence of comorbidities such as protein calorie malnutrition, diabetes, and steroid use, which might be accompanied with impaired wound healing have all been shown to be associated with an reduced NOS expression [13, 14]. Wang and co-workers were able to show, that NO production by dermal fibroblasts could be important during inflammatory stages of wound healing after skin injury [15].

The catalytic p110 subunit of class one phosphatidylinositol 3-kinase (PIK3CA) regulates pathways important for cell proliferation, survival, and motility [16, 17]. Samuels et al. were able to identify PIK3CA as an oncogene, with capacities as a useful marker for detection of cancers and for monitoring tumor progression [18]. The effects of UV exposure on PIK3CA mutations in skin have been described in the context of the pathogenesis of solar lentigo and benign lichenoid keratosis [19, 20].

Moreover, reports from the current literature suggest, that UVA radiation can activate mitogen-activated protein kinase (MAPK) pathway [21]. Its activation leads to activator protein-1(AP-1) induction and consequently the regulation of matrix metalloproteinase (MMP) genes. The breakdown of dermal collagen in photo-related aging has been shown to be associated with UV-induced MMPs expression, also being regulated by underlying MAPK-pathways [22, 23].

However, no distinct reports about of the influence therapeutic ionizing radiation on the MAPK pathway, NO signalling system, or PIK3CA as an essential oncogene exist in the current literature. All pathways and underlying regulatory functions build a complex network responsible for fundamental cell characteristics such as proliferation and apoptosis. This study aims to evaluate the expression of NOS isoforms, PIK3CA, and MAPK in a PCR-based study. Further understanding of essential pathways and corresponding turning points might add up to the knowledge about radiation-induced toxicity.

Methods

This study followed the Declaration of Helsinki on medical protocol and ethics, and the Institutional Review Board of the Technical University of Munich (TUM), Germany approved the study (No. 307/11). All participants were informed extensively and signed an informed consent agreement.

All patients, who met the following inclusion criteria were recruited for the study. Potential patients had to be in-patients at the Department of Oral and Maxillofacial Surgery, Technical University of Munich (TUM), Germany between January 1st, 2012 and December 31st, 2012. All study patients had to be older than 18 years, anamnestic data had to be available, and tissue specimens from the surgical access to the neck had to be available for further experiments. Clinical data (age, sex, history of RT, history of tobacco/alcohol abuse, etc.) were obtained and documented before surgery. During hospitalization, clinical data on the occurrence of cervical WHD was obtained at an interval of 30 days postoperatively.

Tissue samples from the neck were obtained from incision margins during the surgical access with approximate dimensions of 1×5 mm. Specimens were stored in Allproctect™-Solution (Qiagen, Hilden, Germany) at –80 °C for PCR analysis.

RT-PCR

Ribonucleic acid (RNA) isolation was performed by using the RNeasy® Protect Mini Kit (Qiagen). Beforehand, tissue samples were comminuted by using a rotor-stator system (Miccra, ART Labortechnik, Müllheim, Germany) and ultrasonification. After measurement of the amount of extracted RNA by means of a Biophotometer (Eppendorf, Hamburg, Germany), 1 µg isolated RNA was used for reverse transcription. Reverse transcription was performed according to the protocol of the SuperScript™ First Strand Synthesis System (Invitrogen, Carlsbad, USA). Random primers were used for RT.

For RT-PCR, 2 µl cDNA sample, 2 µl LightCycler® FastStart DNA Mater SYBR Green I reaction mix (Roche, Mannheim, Germany), 1 µl forward and reverse primers (0.5 µmol L^{-1}), 1.6 µl MgCl$_2$ (3 mmol L^{-1}), and 12.4 µl RNase-free water, resulting in a volume of 20 µl/sample were analyzed by using the LightCycler® 1.0 system (Roche). Primer specificity was tested by using electrophoretic separation of the PCR product. Primer specifications are shown in Table 1. Amplification algorithms

Table 1 Primer sequences of examined genes

Gene	Sequence 5'to 3	
MAPK	Forward	CAGTGGGATGGAATTGAAAG
	Reverse	AGCAGAAGGAATGAGTGTGC
NOS1	Forward	GACTGTTGAGATGGAAGAAC
	Reverse	ATCTTCCTGTCTCCGAGGCG
NOS3	Forward	GTGATGGCGAAGCGAGTGAAG
	Reverse	CCGAGCCCGAACACACAGAAC
PIK3CA	Forward	CTCCACGACCATCATCAGG
	Reverse	GATTACGAAGGTATTGGTT

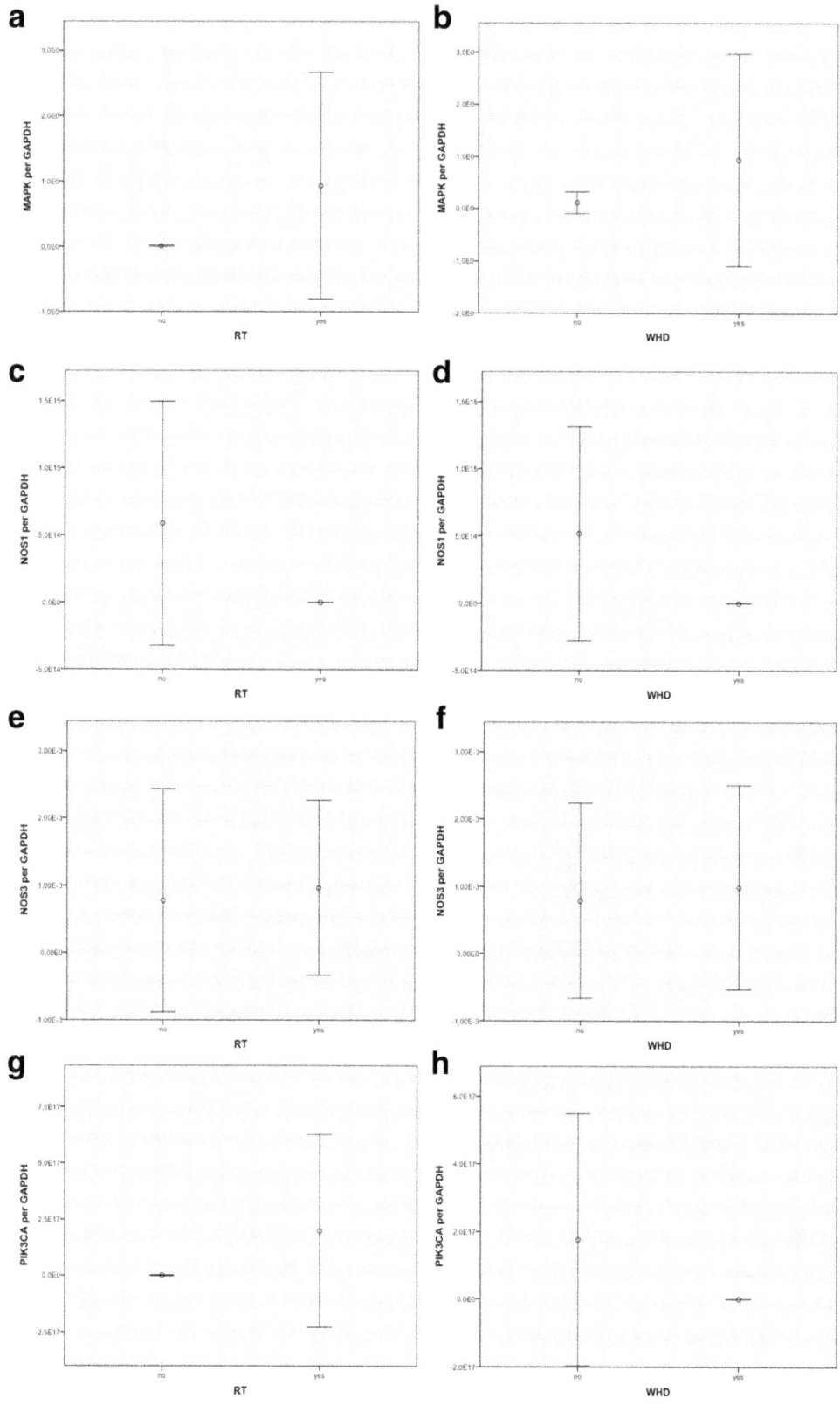

Fig. 1 (See legend on next page.)

(See figure on previous page.)
Fig. 1 Bar graph visualizing visualising the expression of the investigated genes MAPK in patients with and without a history of Radiation Therapy (RT) **a**, as well as in patients with and without the occurrence of postoperative Wound Healing Disorders (WHD) **b**. Expression levels of NOS1 **c**, **d**, NOS3 **e**, **f**, and PIK3CA **g**, **h** are displayed accordingly. Measured by real-time RT-PCR in cervical tissue samples. Given is the median value, with error bars indicating the 95% confidence interval (CI)

were as follows: 10 min at 95 °C, 40 cycles of 15 s at 94 °C, 10 s at 60 °C, and 10 s at 72 °C. A melting curve analysis was recorded in order to test for cDNA fragment consistency. The amount of RNA was automatically calculated by comparison of measured threshold cycles with standard curves and normalized with glyceraldehyde 3-phosphate dehydrogenase (GAPDH) as a housekeeping gene. A no template control was included in each run. All amplifications were carried out in triplicates.

Statistical analysis

All data were analyzed by using IBM®SPSS® for Mac (version 22.0; IBM Corp., USA). Means and standard deviation (SD) were calculated, and tests of significance were performed. For normally distributed values, t-test was performed. For values not normally distributed, the Mann–Whitney test was used. Statistical significance was defined as $\alpha = 0.05$. All p-values are local and given as two-tailed.

Results

A total of 30 patients were enrolled in the current study. Nineteen (63.3%) were male, 11 (36.7%) of were females. The mean age was 57.1 ± 10 years (minimum 43, maximum 76 years). Fifteen patients (50%) received a radiation to the head and neck at least six months before the surgical intervention took place and the tissue specimens were obtained. Patients with a history of RT were exposed to dosages of a mean of 60.0 ± 6.32 Gy (Gy) (Maximum 69.9 Gy; Minimum 50.0 Gy). Alcohol abuse could be observed in 13 patients (43.3%), nicotine abuse was observed in 19 patients (63.3%).

The results of RT-PCR analysis of the expression of MAPK are displayed in Fig. 1a and b and Table 2. No statistical significant difference could be observed in context of a preoperatively irradiated tissue ($p = .263$). Expression analysis of patients with postoperative WHDs revealed a significant increase in MAPK expression compared to the control group without occurrence of postoperative WHDs ($p = .043$). Expression of NOS1 was decreased in irradiated tissue without statistical significance ($p = .178$; Fig. 1c, Table 2). In analysis of tissue samples from patients with postoperative WHDs, a decrease of NOS1 expression could be observed ($p = .241$; Fig. 1d, Table 2). Analysis of expression profiles of NOS3 revealed increase in previously irradiated tissue ($p = .089$; Fig. 1e, Table 2) and in tissue samples from patients with postoperative WHDs ($p = .680$; Fig. 1f, Table 2). PIK3CA showed a significantly increased expression in tissue samples from patients with a history of RT ($p = .049$; Fig. 1g, Table 2). In analysis of tissue with occurrence of postoperative WHDs, an increase in samples without WHDs became obvious, even though no statistical significance could be detected ($p = .391$; Fig. 1h, Table 2).

Discussion

In an interdisciplinary and individual treatment concept in head and neck malignancies, next to the operative resection, RT with or without a concomitant chemotherapy is one of the major columns. In a clinical setting, patients with a history of RT, who are in need of a surgical intervention, regularly present with WHDs in the application field of RT. These effects have been studied before and the influence of RT on wound healing has been described

Table 2 Real-time RT-PCR results in groups with/without preoperative RT and with/without postoperative cervical WHDs

Gen	Median Expression per GAPDH			Median Expression per GAPDH		
	RT	No RT		WHD	No WHD	
	N (%)	N (%)	p Value	N (%)	N (%)	p Value
MAPK	9.32 E-01	9.65 E-03	.263	9.36 E-01	1.15 E-01	.043*
	15 (50)	15 (50)		13 (43.3)	17 (56.7)	
NOS1	6.65 E-05	5.86 E + 14	.178	7.67 E-05	5.173 E + 14	.241
	15 (50)	15 (50)		13 (43.3)	17 (56.7)	
NOS3	9.66 E-04	7.77 E-04	.089	9.86 E-04	7.84 E-04	.680
	15 (50)	15 (50)		13 (43.3)	17 (56.7)	
PIK3CA	1.99 E + 17	2.16 E + 06	.049*	6.48 E + 03	1.76 E + 17	.391
	15 (50)	15 (50)		13 (43.3)	17 (56.7)	

Abbreviations: *WHD* wound healing disorder; *RT* radiation therapy; *RT-PCR* reverse-transcription polymerase chain reaction
Data in parentheses are percentages, unless noted otherwise; *statistically significant difference at $\alpha = 0.05$

elsewhere [1–5]. Impaired wound healing is regarded to be one of the long-term side effects of RT, amongst others. However, this poses to be an increasing surgical challenge, as an increasing amount of patients with previous conservative treatments present with the need for a surgical intervention, because of tumor recurrence, local metastases, or the growth of a second primary tumor. Fundamental signalling pathways seem to play an important role in the clinical occurrence of long-term side effects related to RT. These pathways and their regulatory influence on the occurrence of post-radiogenic WHDs in particular still remain subject to further research. The identification of sign posts in this complicated network of signalling pathways could not only help to further understand the underlying mechanisms of radiation induced side effects, but might also offer starting points for therapeutic interventions in the future in order to reduce RT related side effects or to facilitate the treatment of specific side effects such as WHDs. This current study aims to evaluate different signalling pathways in previously irradiated human tissue specimens and those without any influence of ionizing radiation in a PCR-based setting.

MAPK was increased in irradiated tissues and in tissue specimens, which developed WHDs postoperatively. Kim et al. as well as Shin and colleagues described the influence of MAPK-pathways in photo-related skin aging by UV-induced MMPs expression [22, 23]. Moreover, the influence of ionizing radiation on the MAPK pathway seems to be definite, even though this study could not show any significant differences. The role of MAPK in the occurrence of radiogenic long-term toxicity should definitely be subject to further research. However, its impact could be described in this current investigation.

Evaluation of NOS systems in irradiated skin revealed an increase of NOS1 in not previously irradiated tissue and tissue specimens without occurrence of postoperative WHDs, whereas NOS3 was expressed contrariwise, however no significant differences could be observed in statistical analysis for both isoforms. NOS1 and NOS3 are together being referred to as cNOS. Influence of cNOS expression through various comorbidities has been described in the literature [13, 14]. Nevertheless, this current study describes the influence of therapeutic dosages of ionizing radiation on expression levels of cNOS. Furthermore, we were able to show that NOS1 and NOS3 seem to act contradictory.

Analysis of expression levels of PIK3CA as an essential oncogene showed a significant increase in irradiated tissues, whereas no significance could be detected in subanalysis of specimens with or without the occurrence of postoperative WHDs. The ability of PIK3CA of detecting neoplasms, its usefulness in monitoring tumor progression, as well as the influence of UV exposure on PIK3CA mutations have been subject to extensive research [18–20]. This investigation describes the influence of RT on expression levels of PIK3CA. However, gene amplifications of PIK3CA have been studied in head and neck squamous cell carcinomas by Qiu and colleagues [24]. The oncogenic properties of PIK3CA in the carcinogenesis of head and neck cancers could be described. This might be of special interest as all specimens in this current study were derived from patients with head and neck cancers. Nevertheless, as no significantly increased expression levels were found this fact seems to be crucial for carcinogenesis but not for RT associated side effects.

Taking the results of the current study into consideration, we were able to show the influence of RT on different molecular pathways. However, the influence of specific pathways in therapeutic RT and especially in long-term radiation-related side effects still remains subject to further research, this data underlines the crucial role of molecular pathways. Nevertheless, additional studies need to be carried out to identify possible starting points for novel therapies.

Conclusions

This current study is able to show the influence of RT on different molecular pathways. This underlines the crucial role of specific molecular networks, responsible for the occurrence of long-term radiation toxicity such as WHDs. Additional studies should be carried out to identify possible starting points for therapeutic interventions.

Acknowledgements

Parts of this study are published as the doctoral thesis of NT. This work was supported by the German Research Foundation (DFG) and the Technische Universität München within the funding programme.

Funding

This study was supported by internal funding.

Authors' contributions

SK, NT, NHR, and MK conceived of the study and participated in its design and coordination. NR, GF, and OR made substantial contributions to conception and design of the manuscript as well as statistical analysis. SK and NT have been involved in drafting the manuscript. KDW, and MK were involved in revising the manuscript. All authors read and approved the final manuscript.

Competing interests

The authors declare that they have no competing interests.

Author details

[1]Department of Oral and Maxillofacial Surgery, Technical University of Munich (TUM), Ismaninger Str. 22, D-81675 Munich, Germany. [2]Department of Oral and Maxillofacial Surgery, Heidelberg University Hospital, Im Neuenheimer Feld 400, D-69120 Heidelberg, Germany.

References

1. Wang J, Boerma M, Fu Q, Hauer-Jensen M. Radiation responses in skin and connective tissues: effect on wound healing and surgical outcome. Hernia. 2006;10:502–6.
2. Rohleder NH, Flensberg S, Bauer F, Wagenpfeil S, Wales CJ, Koerdt S, Wolff KD, Holzle F, Steiner T, Kesting MR. Can tissue spectrophotometry and laser doppler flowmetry help to identify patients at risk for wound healing disorders after neck dissection? Oral Surg Oral Med Oral Pathol Oral Radiol. 2014;117:302–11.
3. Koerdt S, Steinstraesser L, Stoeckelhuber M, Wales CJ, Rohleder NH, Babaryka G, Steiner T, Wolff KD, Loeffelbein DJ, Muecke T, et al. Radiotherapy for oral cancer decreases the cutaneous expression of host defence peptides. J Craniomaxillofac Surg. 2016;44(7):882–9. doi:10.1016/j.jcms.2016.04.014.
4. Koerdt S, Rohleder NH, Rommel N, Nobis C, Stoeckelhuber M, Pigorsch S, Duma MN, Wolff KD, Kesting MR. An expression analysis of markers of radiation-induced skin fibrosis and angiogenesis in wound healing disorders of the head and neck. Radiat Oncol. 2015;10:202.
5. Koerdt S, Tanner N, Rommel N, Rohleder NH, Stoeckelhuber M, Wolff KD, Kesting MR. An immunohistochemical study on the role of oxidative and nitrosative stress in irradiated skin. Cells Tissues Organs. 2016, E-pub ahead of print.
6. Benyo Z, Kiss G, Szabo C, Csaki C, Kovach AG. Importance of basal nitric oxide synthesis in regulation of myocardial blood flow. Cardiovasc Res. 1991;25:700–3.
7. Hibbs Jr JB, Taintor RR, Vavrin Z, Rachlin EM. Nitric oxide: a cytotoxic activated macrophage effector molecule. Biochem Biophys Res Commun. 1988;157:87–94.
8. Kovach AG, Szabo C, Benyo Z, Csaki C, Greenberg JH, Reivich M. Effects of NG-nitro-L-arginine and L-arginine on regional cerebral blood flow in the cat. J Physiol. 1992;449:183–96.
9. Schneemann M, Schoedon G, Frei K, Schaffner A. Immunovascular communication: activation and deactivation of murine endothelial cell nitric oxide synthase by cytokines. Immunol Lett. 1993;35:159–62.
10. Snyder SH, Bredt DS. Biological roles of nitric oxide. Sci Am. 1992;266:68–71, 74–67.
11. Lee RH, Efron D, Tantry U, Barbul A. Nitric oxide in the healing wound: a time-course study. J Surg Res. 2001;101:104–8.
12. Albina JE, Mills CD, Henry Jr WL, Caldwell MD. Temporal expression of different pathways of 1-arginine metabolism in healing wounds. J Immunol. 1990;144:3877–80.
13. Schaffer MR, Tantry U, Ahrendt GM, Wasserkrug HL, Barbul A. Acute protein-calorie malnutrition impairs wound healing: a possible role of decreased wound nitric oxide synthesis. J Am Coll Surg. 1997;184:37–43.
14. Schaffer MR, Tantry U, Efron PA, Ahrendt GM, Thornton FJ, Barbul A. Diabetes-impaired healing and reduced wound nitric oxide synthesis: a possible pathophysiologic correlation. Surgery. 1997;121:513–9.
15. Wang R, Ghahary A, Shen YJ, Scott PG, Tredget EE. Human dermal fibroblasts produce nitric oxide and express both constitutive and inducible nitric oxide synthase isoforms. J Invest Dermatol. 1996;106:419–27.
16. Phillips WA, St Clair F, Munday AD, Thomas RJ, Mitchell CA. Increased levels of phosphatidylinositol 3-kinase activity in colorectal tumors. Cancer. 1998;83:41–7.
17. Vivanco I, Sawyers CL. The phosphatidylinositol 3-Kinase AKT pathway in human cancer. Nat Rev Cancer. 2002;2:489–501.
18. Samuels Y, Wang Z, Bardelli A, Silliman N, Ptak J, Szabo S, Yan H, Gazdar A, Powell SM, Riggins GJ, et al. High frequency of mutations of the PIK3CA gene in human cancers. Science. 2004;304:554.
19. Groesser L, Herschberger E, Landthaler M, Hafner C. FGFR3, PIK3CA and RAS mutations in benign lichenoid keratosis. Br J Dermatol. 2012;166:784–8.
20. Hafner C, Stoehr R, van Oers JM, Zwarthoff EC, Hofstaedter F, Landthaler M, Hartmann A, Vogt T. FGFR3 and PIK3CA mutations are involved in the molecular pathogenesis of solar lentigo. Br J Dermatol. 2009;160:546–51.
21. Xu Q, Hou W, Zheng Y, Liu C, Gong Z, Lu C, Lai W, Maibach HI. Ultraviolet A-induced cathepsin K expression is mediated via MAPK/AP-1 pathway in human dermal fibroblasts. PLoS One. 2014;9:e102732.
22. Kim SR, Jung YR, An HJ, Kim DH, Jang EJ, Choi YJ, Moon KM, Park MH, Park CH, Chung KW, et al. Anti-wrinkle and anti-inflammatory effects of active garlic components and the inhibition of MMPs via NF-kappaB signaling. PLoS One. 2013;8:e73877.
23. Shin SW, Jung E, Kim S, Kim JH, Kim EG, Lee J, Park D. Antagonizing effects and mechanisms of afzelin against UVB-induced cell damage. PLoS One. 2013;8:e61971.
24. Qiu W, Schonleben F, Li X, Ho DJ, Close LG, Manolidis S, Bennett BP, Su GH. PIK3CA mutations in head and neck squamous cell carcinoma. Clin Cancer Res. 2006;12:1441–6.

16

The combinatorial approach of laser-captured microdissection and reverse transcription quantitative polymerase chain reaction accurately determines HER2 status in breast cancer

Elisabeth Hofmann[1†], Rita Seeboeck[1,2†], Nico Jacobi[1], Peter Obrist[2], Samuel Huter[2], Christian Klein[1], Kamil Oender[3], Christoph Wiesner[1], Harald Hundsberger[1] and Andreas Eger[1*]

Abstract

Background: HER2 expression in breast cancer correlates with increased metastatic potential, higher tumor recurrence rates and improved response to targeted therapies. Fluorescence *in situ* hybridization (FISH) and immunohistochemistry (IHC) are two methods commonly used for the analysis of HER2 in the clinic. However, lack of standardization, technical variability in laboratory protocols and subjective interpretation are major problems associated with these testing procedures.

Methods: Here we evaluated the applicability of reverse-transcription quantitative polymerase chain reaction (RT-qPCR) for HER2 testing in breast cancer. We tested thirty formaldehyde-fixed and paraffin-embedded tumor samples by RT-qPCR, FISH and IHC and analysed and compared the data from the three methods.

Results: We found that laser-captured microdissection is essential for the accurate determination of HER2 expression by RT-qPCR. When isolating RNA from total tumor tissue we obtained a significant number of false negative results. However, when using RNA from purified cancer cells the RT-qPCR data were fully consistent with FISH and IHC. In addition we provide evidence that ductal carcinomas might be further classified by the differential expression of HER3 and HER4.

Conclusions: Laser-captured microdissection in combination with RT-qPCR is a precise and cost-effective diagnostic approach for HER2 testing in cancer. The PCR assay is simple, accurate and robust and can easily be implemented and standardized in clinical laboratories.

Keywords: Breast cancer, Personalized medicine, HER2, Microdissection, Polymerase chain reaction

Background

The epidermal growth factor receptor (EGFR) family is involved in the regulation of cell proliferation, differentiation and survival [1, 2]. The family consists of four genes that have evolved from a single ancestor (HER1 or EGFR; HER2/Neu or ERBB2; HER3 or ERBB3, and HER4 or ERBB4). Functional aberrations of HER family members have been causally linked to the pathogenesis of a variety of human cancers including lung, colon, breast and ovarian carcinomas [3–5].

Approximately twenty percent of all breast cancers exhibit an amplification and overexpression of the HER2 gene [6]. Overexpression of HER2 can confer a selective growth and survival advantage on cancer cells and cause a more aggressive breast cancer phenotype [7]. Elevated expression of HER2 has been

* Correspondence: andreas.eger@fh-krems.ac.at
†Equal contributors
[1]Department Life Sciences, IMC University of Applied Sciences Krems, Piaristengasse 1, A-3500 Krems, Austria
Full list of author information is available at the end of the article

associated with poor prognosis including increased metastatic burden and higher recurrence and mortality rates, diminished response to anti-hormone and doxorubicin-based chemotherapy and increased sensitivity to anthracycline- and taxane-based chemotherapy [8–13]. Targeted inhibition of HER2 with trastuzumab (Herceptin™; Genentech), pertuzumab (Perjeta®, Genentech/Roche) or lapatinib (Tykerb™, GlaxoSmithKline) has significantly improved clinical outcome, both in the metastatic and in the adjuvant settings [14–21]. Only patients whose tumors overexpress HER2 benefit from the treatments whereas low HER2 levels indicate non-responsiveness. As a consequence the accurate quantification of HER2 expression in breast cancer is critical for selecting the right therapy and optimizing clinical treatment modalities [22–24].

Elevated HER2 protein levels are tightly associated with gene amplification. As a result HER2 status is commonly analyzed by fluorescence in situ hybridization (FISH) [25–30]. Alternatively HER2 protein levels can be semi-quantitatively assessed by immunohistochemistry (IHC) [25, 31, 32]. The rates of concordance between IHC and FISH range from eighty to ninety percent [23, 33, 34]. FISH has been reported to be more accurate, reproducible and robust than IHC [35]. However both assays are suboptimal and significant variability can arise from the lack of standardization in tissue sampling and handling, antibody diversity, chromosome 17 and CEP17 heterogeneity, instrument calibration and observer subjectivity [23, 36, 37]. Determination of HER2 mRNA levels by real-time polymerase chain reaction (qPCR) has been suggested as simple and cost-effective alternative to FISH and IHC [38]. The procedure can be fully automated, standardized and performed on small samples and biopsies. However to this day comparatively few studies have evaluated the clinical applicability of RT-qPCR for HER2 testing. The available data are conflicting and range from weak to high concordance rates with FISH and IHC [38–44]. One drawback of previous studies was that mRNA has mostly been isolated from whole tumor tissues. Abundance of non-tumorigenic stroma cells might significantly influence the overall sensitivity of the assay and yield false negative results [41, 45]. Here we assessed the HER2 status in thirty ductal carcinomas of the breast by FISH, IHC and RT-qPCR. We could demonstrate a high concordance between the three approaches when using microdissected, formaldehyde-fixed and paraffin-embedded (FFPE) tissue for RNA isolation. Moreover we could detect highly variable expression of HER3 and HER4 suggesting that both could be used as additional markers for refining predictions on prognosis and treatment response.

Methods

Formaline-fixed and paraffin-embedded (FFPE) tissue samples and laser-captured microdissection
Standard FFPE sectioning was performed with the Leica microtome RM 2255. For laser-captured microdissection 5 μm FFPE sections were prepared and mounted onto Leica FrameSlides (PET-Membrane 1.4 μm, Leica). The dried slides were subjected to a quick protocol of haematoxylin/eosin staining: the samples were incubated in xylene for 5 s, in 96 % ethanol for 30 s, in 70 % ethanol for 20 s, in ddH$_2$O for 20 s, in haematoxylin for 55 s, in ddH$_2$O for 30 s, in HCl-ethanol for 15 s, in ddH$_2$O for 20 s, in 80 % ethanol for 30 s, in eosin for 20 s, in 96 % ethanol for 25 s, in 100 % ethanol for 25 s and finally in xylene for 30 s. Tumour regions (~10 000 cells) were selected and laser cut (CryLaS FTSS 355-50, Leica) under a Leica DM6000B microscope. The study was performed according to international and regional ethical guidelines and was approved by the ethics commission of Lower Austria and the Danube University Krems, Austria (No. EK GZ 01/2015-2018).

Immunohistochemistry (IHC)
For the immunohistochemical HER2 staining, FFPE tissue sections were prepared and stained using the Dako Autostainer Universal Staining System (Dako). 2.5 μm thick sections of the FFPE samples were prepared and mounted onto silated microscopy slides (HistoSil slides, Stölzle-Oberglas). The dried slides were deparaffinated and rehydrated by immersion in xylene followed by immersion in ethanol of decreasing concentration (96 %, 80 %, 70 %). Epitope demasking was performed in a boiling citrate buffer pH 6 (Dako REAL™ Target Retrieval Solution, Dako). Staining for HER2 was performed using a rabbit polyclonal antibody directed against ERBB2/HER2 (Dako, A0485) diluted 1:500 in the EnVision™ FLEX Antibody Diluent (Dako). As a secondary antibody a horseradish peroxidase coupled polymer (EnVision+, Dako) was applied, which reacts with the substrate chromogen 3,3′-diaminobenzidinetetrahydrochloride (Liquid DAB+, Dako). Counterstaining for nuclei was performed using haematoxylin (Dako).

Fluorescent in situ hybridization (FISH)
FISH was performed on 4 μm thick FFPE sections immobilized on silated glass microscopy slides (HistoSil slides, Stölzle-Oberglas). Staining was perfomed using the Vysis TOP2A/HER2/CEP 17 FISH Probe Kit (Abbott) following the manufacturer's instructions. The pretreatment conditions were slightly changed, using a citrate buffer pH 6 (Gatt-Koller) for 70 min at 80 °C instead of a Na-SCN solution. Fluorescent signals were analysed under a Leica DM6000B microscope. FISH data

were evaluated according to the ASCO/CAP guidelines (http://www.asco.org/).

RNA extraction and reverse transcription (RT)

Total RNA was extracted from total tumor tissue sections or from microdissected (laser-captured) samples yielding only cancer cells. The RNeasy FFPE kit including an on-column DNase I digestion (Qiagen; version 09/2011) was used for RNA extraction according to the manufacturer's instructions. For deparaffinization the FFPE tissue sections were treated with xylene.

Reverse transcription was performed using total RNA according to the combined random hexamer and oligo(dT) priming protocol of the Transcriptor First Strand cDNA Synthesis Kit (Roche) in a final volume of 20 µl. Control reactions containing RNA but no reverse transcriptase were tested negative for genomic DNA contamination by qPCR.

Real-time quantitative PCR (qPCR)

Gene expression was assessed by RT-qPCR with eukaryotic translation elongation factor 1 alpha 1 (EEF1A1) as endogenous control gene. For target gene quantification pre-designed TaqMan® Gene Expression Assays (EGFR: Hs01076093_g1, HER2: Hs01001580_m1, HER3: Hs00176538_m1 and HER4: Hs00955525_m1; Life Technologies) were used. Whereas the target gene probes were labeled with 6-carboxyfluorescein (FAM), the EEF1A1 probe was labeled with Cy5 at the 5′-end and with a black-hole quencher (BHQ2) at the 3′-end (MWG Eurofins) in order to allow simultaneous quantification of EEF1A1 and HER2 in one reaction (duplex reaction). The duplex qPCR reaction mix contained a final volume of 15 µl Taqman® Gene Expression Mastermix (Life Technologies), HER2 Taqman® Gene Expression Assay, 600 nM EEF1A1 primers (MWG Eurofins), 200 nM EEF1A1 probe and 1 µl of cDNA. For HER1, HER3 and HER4 singleplex reactions were performed containing Taqman® Gene Expression Mastermix (Life Technologies), Taqman® Gene Expression Assay, and 1 µl of cDNA. Samples were measured in triplicates. All reactions were pipetted in rotor discs-100 using the Qiagility automated pipetting system (Qiagen). All qPCRs were run on a Rotor-Gene Q (Qiagen) using the following cycling conditions: 10 min at 95 °C for initial denaturation followed by 45 cycles of 95 °C for 20 s and 60 °C for 1 min. Data were analysed using the Rotor-Gene Q Series Software (Qiagen) and relative target gene expression levels were calculated according to the comparative Cq method [46]. Gene expression levels of the target genes were calculated relative to the endogenous control gene and depicted as relative expression levels in arbitrary units (AU).

Statistical analysis of RT-qPCR data

For the classification of tumors with respect to HER2-, HER3- and HER4 mRNA levels we determined cut-off values using the algorithm developed by Budczies et al., at the Charité Universitätsmedizin Berlin [47]. The statistical relevance of the difference between HER2 positive and HER2 negative samples and correlations among HER2, HER3 and HER4 expression was analysed with the Mann-Whitney test (two-tailed) using GraphPad Prism (version 6.03 for Windows, Graphpad Software, www.graphpad.com).

Results

The HER2 status in breast cancer is commonly tested by IHC and FISH. Both methods have been approved by the US Food and Drug Administration for HER2 testing in clinical laboratories [23]. The applicability of RT-qPCR for HER2 assessment has not been fully established yet. In the present study we directly compared the performance of IHC, FISH and RT-qPCR using thirty formaldehyde-fixed and paraffin-embedded (FFPE) ductal carcinoma samples selected from the archive. According to FISH and IHC twenty samples tested negative and ten positive for HER2 (Table 1). Grading of IHC assays was based on a 0, 1+, 2+ and 3+ scoring system [20]. FISH was scored positive when the HER2/CEP17 ratio exceeded 2.2 [17, 21]. Representative images of each group are shown in Fig. 1.

For RT-qPCR the RNA was isolated from two different sources. First RNA was harvested from whole FFPE tumor tissue. Second RNA was isolated exclusively from cancer cells after separating cancer cells from the tumor stroma by laser-captured microdissection. Both RNA fractions were subsequently processed for HER2 specific RT-qPCR. HER2 mRNA levels were normalized to the expression of the endogenous control gene EEF1A1 using the comparative Cq method [46]. Independent classification into HER2 positive and negative tumors was performed using the publicly available cut-off finder algorithm [47] (http://molpath.charite.de/cutoff). When RNA was isolated from total tumor tissue we could detect seven tumors with elevated HER2 mRNA levels (Fig. 2a). On the other hand when using laser-captured microdissection we could identify ten tumors with significantly increased HER2 mRNA expression (Fig. 2b).

In order to investigate the relationship among DNA amplification, mRNA and protein levels we compared the HER2 data obtained by FISH, IHC and RT-qPCR. In total tumor tissue we detected a significant discordance between RT-qPCR and the standard methods. Of the ten HER2 positive tumors identified by FISH and IHC only seven scored positive in the RT-qPCR approach when using RNA from total tumor tissue (Fig. 3a). On the

Table 1 Archive samples of ductal, invasive mammary carcinoma

Sample	Age	Grade	Stage	LN	HER2 IHC	HER2 FISH	HER2 qPCR*	HER3 qPCR*	HER4 qPCR*	EGFR qPCR*
01	58	2	pT1b	N0	0	1,0	121	46	-	5,9
02	60	3	ypT1c	yN1a	0	1,1	580	-	-	-
03	75	2	pT1b	N0	0	1,1	518	1133	215	-
04	59	2	pT1b	N0	1	0,9	474	540	439	-
05	59	2	pTa	-	2	1,2	632	-	-	-
06	70	3	pT1c	N0	1	0,9	1198	-	-	-
07	53	2	pT1b	SN0i-	1	0,9	474	680	66	-
08	68	2	pT1c	N2a	1	0,9	603	1812	281	-
09	41	2	pT1c	N1	1	1,0	305	341	133	-
10	74	2	pT1b	NX	1	1,0	473	1020	-	-
11	68	2	pT1b	N0	1	1,0	358	196	107	-
12	52	2	pT2	N0	1	1,0	598	1149	-	-
13	79	2	pT2	N1	1	1,0	186	204	145	-
14	50	2	pT1c	N0	1	1,0	796	-	-	-
15	53	2	pT2	-	1	1,0	194	687	379	-
16	76	2	pT2	N2a	1	1,0	530	440	1167	-
17	67	2	pT1b	N1a	1	1,0	172	186	93	-
18	81	2	pT2	N0	1	1,0	141	84	-	-
19	73	2	pT1c	N0	1	1,0	935	-	-	-
20	48	2	ypT2	yN0	1	1,0	294	-	-	6,4
21	74	CIN	pT1mic	-	3	2,9	15109	4350	-	-
22	26	3	pT2	N0	3	3,1	6241	149	59	0,6
23	34	3	pT2	N3a	3	4,1	7865	125	78	-
24	67	2	pT1c	N1b	3	4,3	44849	406	120	-
25	65	2	ypT2	N2a	3	5,3	12160	1053	-	-
26	59	2	pT1c	N0	3	5,4	10934	159	-	-
27	66	3	pT2	N1a	3	6,0	11866	175	-	-
28	49	DCI III	pT1mic	-	3	2,3	12609	-	-	-
29	82	2	pT3	NX	3	2,4	4541	6157	-	-
30	68	2	pT4d	N2a	3+	2,8	4019	5554	720	-

LN lymph node pathology

*relative expression of HER-family members in arbitrary units (RT-qPCR using RNA from laser-captured microdissection)

-: below the detection limit

other hand when RNA was isolated exclusively from cancer cells the RT-qPCR data were fully consistent with FISH and IHC (Fig. 3b). Even though the sample size is rather small one can conclude that RT-qPCR results in high false-negative rates when RNA is extracted from total tumor tissue (three out of ten). Hence laser-captured microdissection prior to RT-qPCR strongly improved the accuracy of HER2 mRNA quantification in the tumor.

HER1, HER2 and HER3 were all implicated in the development and progression of cancer [4, 48]. To quantitatively assess the expression of HER1, HER3 and HER4 in the breast cancer samples we performed RT-qPCR using RNA derived from microdissected FFPE tissues. Significant but very low expression of HER1 (EGFR) was detected only in ten percent of the tumors (Table 1). HER4 expression could be found in around fifty percent of the breast cancer samples (Table 1 and Fig. 4a). The tumors could be separated into two groups expressing either low or high HER4 mRNA levels (Fig. 4a). However, the amount of HER4 mRNA varied stochastically in the HER2-negative and HER2-positive tumors (Table 1 and Fig. 4a). HER3 was expressed in the majority of the breast cancer samples. Ninety percent of the HER2-positive and around seventy percent of the HER2-negative cells expressed HER3 mRNA (Table 1). Analogous to HER4

a IHC

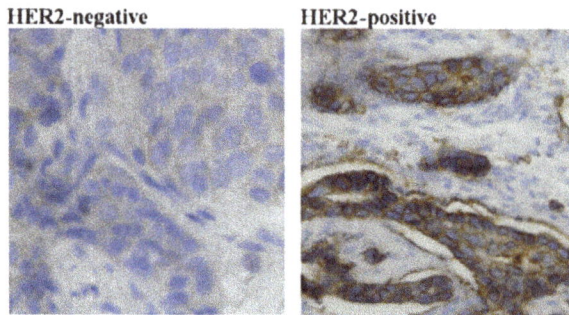

b FISH

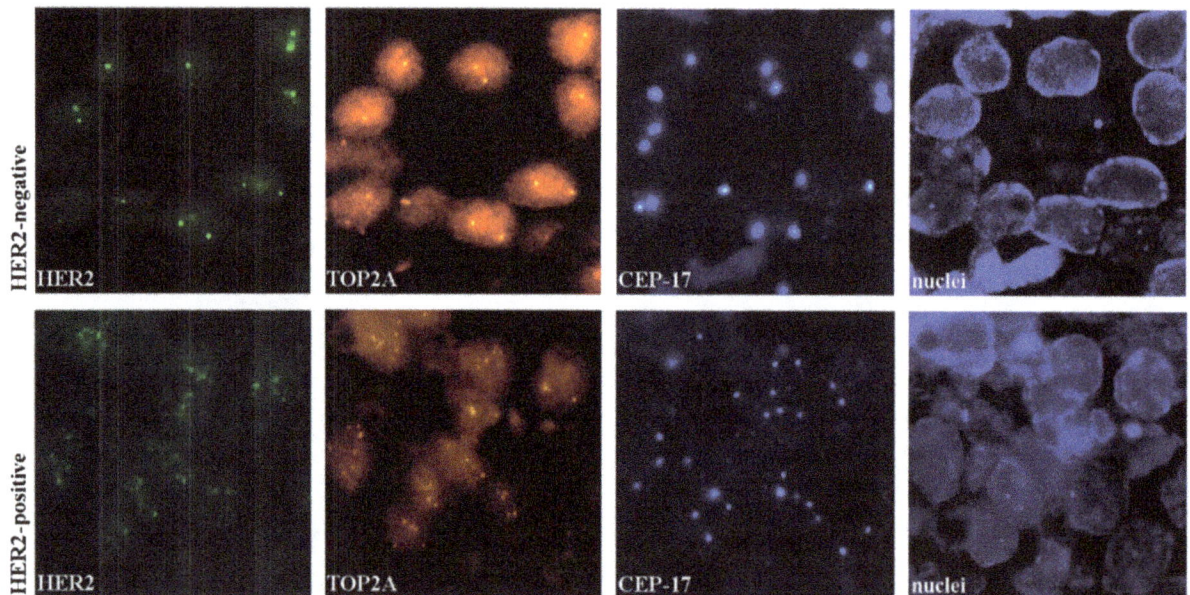

Fig. 1 Representative images of HER2-negative and HER2-positive breast cancer specimen. **a** Tumor sections were subjected to IHC using HER2 specific antibodies and were counterstained for nuclei using haematoxylin (*blue*). Brown colour indicates subcellular localization of HER2. **b** Determination of HER2 amplification by FISH. Specific probes for HER2 (*green*) TOP2A (*orange*) and CEP-17 (*blue*) were used. The nuclei were selectively stained with DAPI

we could separate the tumors into either low or high HER3 expressing subpopulations (Fig. 4b). Interestingly all HER2 negative cancer cells showed also low HER3 expression. On the other hand in the HER2- positive samples we could detect a significant fraction of tumors that additionally expressed very high levels of HER3 mRNA (Fig. 4b and Table 1).

Discussion

Personalized oncology is expected to significantly improve patient care and disease outcome in the near future [49]. Precision therapy requires biomarkers to select the right patients for the right treatment [50, 51]. Technological advances in genomics, proteomics and systems biology have identified a large number of biomarkers with potential clinical value [52–54]. This

wealth of information needs to be translated to the clinic. Translation and clinical validation requires experimental tools that allow the accurate and simultaneous analysis of a large number of biomarkers. Genetic testing is superior to immunological and protein- or cell-based technologies [53, 55–57]. Nucleic acids are easily accessible and can be isolated in sufficient quantity and quality from small amounts of archived FFPE samples or biopsies. qPCR is presently the gold standard method for assessing genetic biomarkers. Precise mutational analysis or quantification of gene expression can be performed in a standardized and automated manner. As a consequence the clinical validation of RT-qPCR methods for biomarker assessment is of prime importance in personalized oncology.

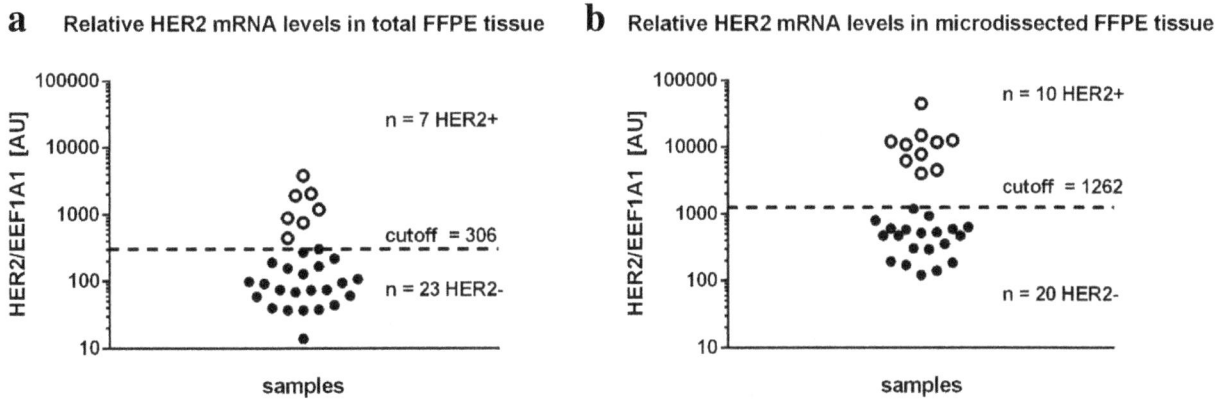

Fig. 2 HER2 mRNA levels in breast cancer specimen. Expression levels of HER2 relative to the endogenous control gene EEF1A1 in arbitrary units (AU) (**a**) Total FFPE tissue (**b**) microdissected FFPE tissue. HER2- negative and positive samples were identified using the publicly available cutoff finder algorithm [47]

The HER2 biomarker is instrumental for selecting breast cancer patients that respond to the targeted HER2 inhibitors trastuzumab, pertuzumab and lapatinib [22, 51]. Despite the clinical importance of HER2 the present diagnostic methods for its detection in the tumor are only semi-quantitative, difficult to standardize and prone to subjective interpretation [23]. Here we analysed the applicability of RT-qPCR for the accurate quantification of HER2 expression in breast cancer. When isolating the RNA from total tumor tissue we found that RT-qPCR gives rather high false-negative results. In line with these findings concerns have also been raised by other groups regarding the sensitivity and accuracy of the qPCR approach [41, 45]. However, when combining RT-qPCR with laser-captured microdissection we could demonstrate that RT-qPCR is fully

consistent with FISH and IHC. The focused isolation of RNA from cancer cells significantly improved the sensitivity and accuracy of the qPCR approach.

Signaling by HER family members is a complex and highly integrated network with crosstalk, redundancy and feedback controls and interactions with different effector molecules [4]. Overexpression of different members and complex homo- and heterodimerization is likely to influence the clinical efficacy of targeted HER inhibitors. Here we additionally examined the expression of HER1 (EGFR), HER3 and HER4 in the breast cancer samples by RT-qPCR.

HER1 mRNA levels were extremely low and expression was found in a small fraction of the samples. This is consistent with previous IHC studies that demonstrated HER1 overexpression in only a subset of ductal breast

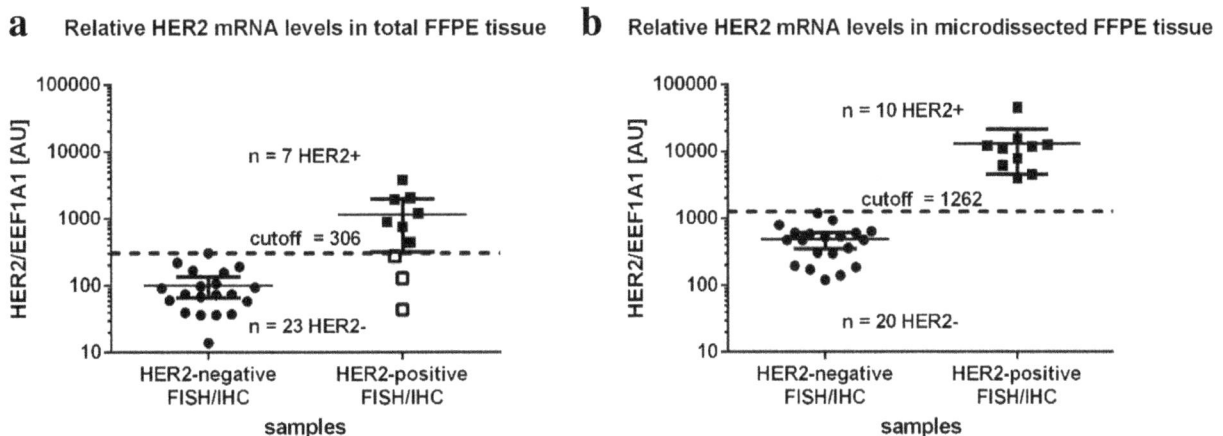

Fig. 3 Assessment of HER2 status using RT-qPCR, FISH and IHC. Relative expression levels of HER2/EEF1A1 in arbitrary units (AU) were calculated for (**a**) total tumor tissue and (**b**) microdissected tumor tissue and compared to the HER2 status as determined by IHC and FISH. Mean values and the 95 % confidence interval for the mean is separately indicated for HER2- positive and negative samples. Significantly higher HER2 mRNA levels were detected in IHC/FISH HER2-positive samples with $p < 0.001$ and $p < 0.0001$ for total FFPE tissue and microdissected FFPE tissue, respectively

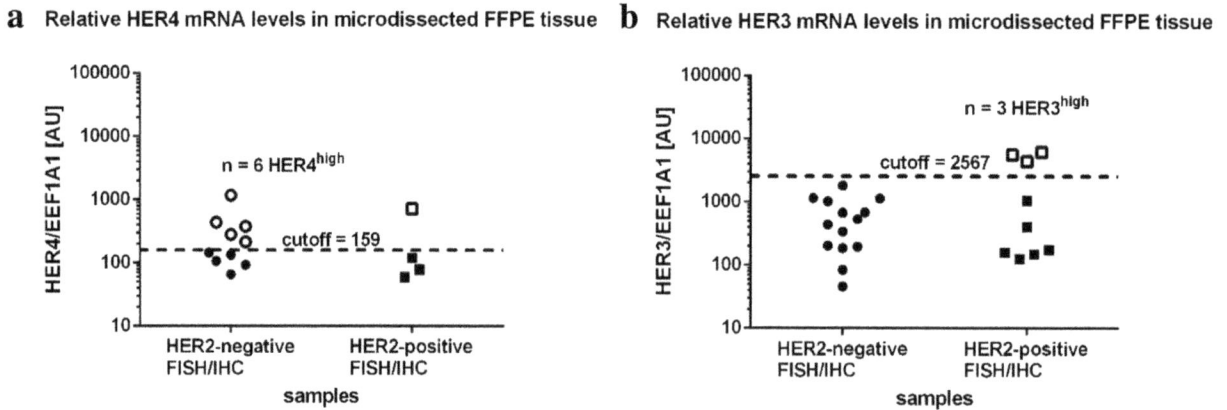

a Relative HER4 mRNA levels in microdissected FFPE tissue   **b** Relative HER3 mRNA levels in microdissected FFPE tissue

Fig. 4 Relative HER4 and HER3 mRNA levels in breast cancer specimen. **a** HER3- and (**b**) HER4-high (*open circles*) and -low (*filled circles*) expressing tumors were identified using the cutoff algorithm [47]. The differences between high and low HER3 and HER4 expression are significant with $p < 0.01$ for HER3 and $p < 0.001$ for HER4

carcinomas [58]. HER4 was expressed in approximately fifty percent of the tumors, and expression levels varied irrespective of whether HER2 was present or not. Previous data on HER4 in breast carcinoma are conflicting. There is evidence that the receptor is a negative regulator of cell proliferation [4]. In some studies HER4 expression has been directly correlated to improved overall survival and diminished tumor grade, metastasis and disease recurrence [4]. Here we could not detect any significant correlation between HER4 expression and tumor differentiation, size or metastatic potential.

HER3 is the preferred hetero-dimerization partner of HER2 in different cancer types [48]. The HER2-HER3 heterodimer was found to be critically involved in tumor initiation and progression and is considered the most active signalling dimer of the HER family in cancer [48, 59, 60]. In our study we could identify two distinct tumor populations that expressed either high or low levels of HER3. Interestingly the highest expression of HER3 was detected in the HER2 positive samples. Overexpression of both HER2 and HER3 might critically influence oncogenic signalling, oncogene addiction and responsiveness to drugs targeting HER and HER-related RTKs. Presently we are planning a large-scale retrospective study for assessing the clinical usability of HER biomarker profiles for predicting therapy response and patient outcome in ductal carcinomas of the breast and in non-small cell lung cancer.

In the future advances in high-throughput PCR and massive parallel sequencing will allow the cost-effective analyses of genetic alterations in cancer cells on a larger scale [61, 62]. Massive parallel sequencing can provide both, information on mutations and genetic rearrangements as well as gene expression (mRNA) levels [63, 64]. These technologies will facilitate the analysis of the genetic make-up of a large panel of genes at a time and

thus will have a strong impact on clinical decision making, including the determination of familial predispositions, cancer subclasses, cancer progression, prognosis, therapy selection and tumor recurrence [61]. For the genetic analyses only few cancer cells are necessary making it also an ideal tool for the molecular characterization of circulating cancer cells in the peripheral blood. Massive parallel sequencing will be possible without amplification of the DNA or RNA in the near future [65, 66]. Thus the cost-effective and routine analyses of large gene panels or whole genomes and transcriptomes will be feasible in the clinic on a daily basis. However, when using mRNA levels as indicators for protein expression pilot studies are necessary for each signaling molecule in order to demonstrate a clear correlation between RNA and protein amounts in different cancer types. Here we could demonstrate that the expression of HER2 mRNA and protein levels were only matching when mRNA was isolated specifically from cancer cells after laser-captured microdissection of ductal carcinomas of the breast. Laser-captured microdissection can easily be standardized and implemented into daily clinical practice and yields mRNA of sufficient quality for qPCR or quantitative sequencing [67]. In addition it offers the advantage for analyzing subpopulations of cancer cells in the tumor to determine tumor heterogeneity and cancer stem cell properties. Both might be critical determinants for therapy selection, treatment success and tumor recurrence.

Conclusion

Considering the present data we suggest that laser-captured microdissection in combination with RT-qPCR is an accurate diagnostic approach for HER2 testing in cancer. In contrast to FISH and IHC the qPCR-based assays are simple, accurate and robust, easily standardized and automatized and display high sensitivity, specificity and reproducibility. However, additional and larger clinical studies are needed to fully validate the value of RT-qPCR for the assessment of HER family members in cancer.

The clinical validation of genetic biomarkers is of prime importance in oncology. Large numbers of validated genetic markers could be simultaneously tested in large-scale studies using high-throughput qPCR or massive parallel sequencing technologies. Comprehensive and multi-parametric genetic profiling of tumors will further advance personalized medicine, improve the efficacy of targeted therapeutics and decrease morbidity and mortality rates in cancer.

Competing interests

None of the authors have any competing interests in the manuscript.

Authors' contributions

EH: first author, laser-captured microdissection, RT-qPCR, FISH and IHC, data analysis and interpretation, preparation of manuscript, design of figures. RS: first author, laser-captured microdissection, RT-qPCR, FISH and IHC, data analysis and interpretation, preparation of manuscript, design of figures. NJ: co-author, establishment of protocols for laser-captured microdissection, optimization of RT-qPCR. PO: co-author, selection of samples, pathological assessment, study design. SH: laser-captured microdissection. CK: co-author, statistical analysis. KO: co-author, FISH. CW: co-author, IHC. HH: co-author, IHC. AE: corresponding author, acquisition of funding, conception, design and supervision of the work, establishment of experimental methods, analysis and interpretation of data, literature and data mining, design and lay-out of figures, preparation and writing of manuscript. All authors read and approved the final manuscript.

Acknowledgements

This work was supported with funds received from the Lower Austria Research and Education Fund (NÖ Forschungs- und Bildungsges.m.b.H., NFB), project number LS09-023 and LS11-013.

Author details

[1]Department Life Sciences, IMC University of Applied Sciences Krems, Piaristengasse 1, A-3500 Krems, Austria. [2]Pathology Laboratory Obrist and Brunhuber, Klostergasse 1, A-6511 Zams, Austria. [3]Research Program for Rational Drug Design in Dermatology and Rheumatology, Department of Dermatology, Paracelsus Medical University of Salzburg, Müllner Hauptstraße 48, A-5020 Salzburg, Austria.

References

1. Avraham R, Yarden Y. Feedback regulation of EGFR signalling: decision making by early and delayed loops. Nat Rev Mol Cell Biol. 2011;12(2):104–17.
2. Yarden Y, Pines G. The ERBB network: at last, cancer therapy meets systems biology. Nat Rev Cancer. 2012;12(8):553–63.
3. Hynes NE, Lane HA. ERBB receptors and cancer: the complexity of targeted inhibitors. Nat Rev Cancer. 2005;5(5):341–54.
4. Roskoski Jr R. The ErbB/HER family of protein-tyrosine kinases and cancer. Pharm Res. 2014;79:34–74.
5. Tebbutt N, Pedersen MW, Johns TG. Targeting the ERBB family in cancer: couples therapy. Nat Rev Cancer. 2013;13(9):663–73.
6. Ross JS, Slodkowska EA, Symmans WF, Pusztai L, Ravdin PM, Hortobagyi GN. The HER-2 receptor and breast cancer: ten years of targeted anti-HER-2 therapy and personalized medicine. Oncologist. 2009;14(4):320–68.
7. Neve RM, Lane HA, Hynes NE. The role of overexpressed HER2 in transformation. Ann Oncol. 2001;12 Suppl 1:S9–13.
8. Gabos Z, Sinha R, Hanson J, Chauhan N, Hugh J, Mackey JR, Abdulkarim B. Prognostic significance of human epidermal growth factor receptor positivity for the development of brain metastasis after newly diagnosed breast cancer. J Clin Oncol Off J Am Soc Clin Oncol. 2006;24(36):5658–63.
9. Paik S, Bryant J, Park C, Fisher B, Tan-Chiu E, Hyams D, Fisher ER, Lippman ME, Wickerham DL, Wolmark N. erbB-2 and response to doxorubicin in patients with axillary lymph node-positive, hormone receptor-negative breast cancer. J Natl Cancer Inst. 1998;90(18):1361–70.
10. Paik S, Bryant J, Tan-Chiu E, Yothers G, Park C, Wickerham DL, Wolmark N. HER2 and choice of adjuvant chemotherapy for invasive breast cancer: National Surgical Adjuvant Breast and Bowel Project Protocol B-15. J Natl Cancer Inst. 2000;92(24):1991–8.
11. Pritchard KI, Messersmith H, Elavathil L, Trudeau M, O'Malley F, Dhesy-Thind B. HER-2 and topoisomerase II as predictors of response to chemotherapy. J Clin Oncol. 2008;26(5):736–44.
12. Seshadri R, Firgaira FA, Horsfall DJ, McCaul K, Setlur V, Kitchen P. Clinical significance of HER-2/neu oncogene amplification in primary breast cancer. The South Australian Breast Cancer Study Group. J Clin Oncol. 1993;11(10):1936–42.
13. Slamon DJ, Clark GM, Wong SG, Levin WJ, Ullrich A, McGuire WL. Human breast cancer: correlation of relapse and survival with amplification of the HER-2/neu oncogene. Science. 1987;235(4785):177–82.
14. Baselga J, Cortes J, Kim SB, Im SA, Hegg R, Im YH, Roman L, Pedrini JL, Pienkowski T, Knott A. Pertuzumab plus trastuzumab plus docetaxel for metastatic breast cancer. N Engl J Med. 2012;366(2):109–19.
15. Cobleigh MA, Vogel CL, Tripathy D, Robert NJ, Scholl S, Fehrenbacher L, Wolter JM, Paton V, Shak S, Lieberman G. Multinational study of the efficacy and safety of humanized anti-HER2 monoclonal antibody in women who have HER2-overexpressing metastatic breast cancer that has progressed after chemotherapy for metastatic disease. J Clin Oncol. 1999;17(9):2639–48.
16. Geyer CE, Forster J, Lindquist D, Chan S, Romieu CG, Pienkowski T, Jagiello-Gruszfeld A, Crown J, Chan A, Kaufman B. Lapatinib plus capecitabine for HER2-positive advanced breast cancer. N Engl J Med. 2006;355(26):2733–43.
17. Piccart-Gebhart MJ, Procter M, Leyland-Jones B, Goldhirsch A, Untch M, Smith I, Gianni L, Baselga J, Bell R, Jackisch C. Trastuzumab after adjuvant chemotherapy in HER2-positive breast cancer. N Engl J Med. 2005;353(16):1659–72.
18. Romond EH, Perez EA, Bryant J, Suman VJ, Geyer Jr CE, Davidson NE, Tan-Chiu E, Martino S, Paik S, Kaufman PA. Trastuzumab plus adjuvant chemotherapy for operable HER2-positive breast cancer. N Engl J Med. 2005;353(16):1673–84.
19. Sjogren S, Inganas M, Lindgren A, Holmberg L, Bergh J. Prognostic and predictive value of c-erbB-2 overexpression in primary breast cancer, alone and in combination with other prognostic markers. J Clin Oncol. 1998;16(2):462–9.
20. Slamon D, Eiermann W, Robert N, Pienkowski T, Martin M, Press M, Mackey J, Glaspy J, Chan A, Pawlicki M. Adjuvant trastuzumab in HER2-positive breast cancer. N Engl J Med. 2011;365(14):1273–83.
21. Slamon DJ, Leyland-Jones B, Shak S, Fuchs H, Paton V, Bajamonde A, Fleming T, Eiermann W, Wolter J, Pegram M. Use of chemotherapy plus a monoclonal antibody against HER2 for metastatic breast cancer that overexpresses HER2. N Engl J Med. 2001;344(11):783–92.
22. Montemurro F, Scaltriti M. Biomarkers of drugs targeting HER-family signalling in cancer. J Pathol. 2014;232(2):219–29.
23. Perez EA, Cortes J, Gonzalez-Angulo AM, Bartlett JM. HER2 testing: current status and future directions. Cancer Treat Rev. 2014;40(2):276–84.
24. van de Vijver MJ. Molecular tests as prognostic factors in breast cancer. Virchows Archiv. 2014;464(3):283–91.
25. Bofin AM, Ytterhus B, Martin C, O'Leary JJ, Hagmar BM. Detection and quantitation of HER-2 gene amplification and protein expression in breast carcinoma. Am J Clin Pathol. 2004;122(1):110–9.
26. Kallioniemi OP, Kallioniemi A, Kurisu W, Thor A, Chen LC, Smith HS, Waldman FM, Pinkel D, Gray JW. ERBB2 amplification in breast cancer analyzed by fluorescence in situ hybridization. Proc Natl Acad Sci U S A. 1992;89(12):5321–5.
27. Mass RD, Press MF, Anderson S, Cobleigh MA, Vogel CL, Dybdal N, Leiberman G, Slamon DJ. Evaluation of clinical outcomes according to HER2 detection by fluorescence in situ hybridization in women with metastatic breast cancer treated with trastuzumab. Clin Breast Cancer. 2005;6(3):240–6.
28. Pauletti G, Godolphin W, Press MF, Slamon DJ. Detection and quantitation of HER-2/neu gene amplification in human breast cancer archival material using fluorescence in situ hybridization. Oncogene. 1996;13(1):63–72.
29. Persons DL, Borelli KA, Hsu PH. Quantitation of HER-2/neu and c-myc gene amplification in breast carcinoma using fluorescence in situ hybridization. Mod Pathol. 1997;10(7):720–7.

30. Press MF, Bernstein L, Thomas PA, Meisner LF, Zhou JY, Ma Y, Hung G, Robinson RA, Harris C, El-Naggar A. HER-2/neu gene amplification characterized by fluorescence in situ hybridization: poor prognosis in node-negative breast carcinomas. J Clin Oncol. 1997;15(8):2894–904.

31. Portier BP, Wang Z, Downs-Kelly E, Rowe JJ, Patil D, Lanigan C, Budd GT, Hicks DG, Rimm DL, Tubbs RR. Delay to formalin fixation 'cold ischemia time': effect on ERBB2 detection by in-situ hybridization and immunohistochemistry. Mod Pathol. 2013;26(1):1–9.

32. Ross JS, Fletcher JA, Bloom KJ, Linette GP, Stec J, Clark E, Ayers M, Symmans WF, Pusztai L, Hortobagyi GN. HER-2/neu testing in breast cancer. Am J Clin Pathol. 2003;120(Suppl):S53–71.

33. Dybdal N, Leiberman G, Anderson S, McCune B, Bajamonde A, Cohen RL, Mass RD, Sanders C, Press MF. Determination of HER2 gene amplification by fluorescence in situ hybridization and concordance with the clinical trials immunohistochemical assay in women with metastatic breast cancer evaluated for treatment with trastuzumab. Breast Cancer Res Treat. 2005; 93(1):3–11.

34. Perez EA, Press MF, Dueck AC, Jenkins RB, Kim C, Chen B, Villalobos I, Paik S, Buyse M, Wiktor AE. Immunohistochemistry and fluorescence in situ hybridization assessment of HER2 in clinical trials of adjuvant therapy for breast cancer (NCCTG N9831, BCIRG 006, and BCIRG 005). Breast Cancer Res Treat. 2013;138(1):99–108.

35. Press MF, Slamon DJ, Flom KJ, Park J, Zhou JY, Bernstein L. Evaluation of HER-2/neu gene amplification and overexpression: comparison of frequently used assay methods in a molecularly characterized cohort of breast cancer specimens. J Clin Oncol. 2002;20(14):3095–105.

36. Sorscher SM. HER-2 overexpression in breast tumors lacking gene amplification. J Clin Oncol. 2004;22(20):4232. author reply 4232-4233.

37. Vanden Bempt I, Van Loo P, Drijkoningen M, Neven P, Smeets A, Christiaens MR, Paridaens R, Wolf-Peeters C. Polysomy 17 in breast cancer: clinicopathologic significance and impact on HER-2 testing. J Clin Oncol. 2008;26(30):4869–74.

38. Lehmann-Che J, Amira-Bouhidel F, Turpin E, Antoine M, Soliman H, Legres L, Bocquet C, Bernoud R, Flandre E, Varna M. Immunohistochemical and molecular analyses of HER2 status in breast cancers are highly concordant and complementary approaches. Br J Cancer. 2011;104(11):1739–46.

39. Baehner FL, Achacoso N, Maddala T, Shak S, Quesenberry Jr CP, Goldstein LC, Gown AM, Habel LA. Human epidermal growth factor receptor 2 assessment in a case-control study: comparison of fluorescence in situ hybridization and quantitative reverse transcription polymerase chain reaction performed by central laboratories. J Clin Oncol. 2010;28(28):4300–6.

40. Cuadros M, Talavera P, Lopez FJ, Garcia-Perez I, Blanco A, Concha A. Real-time RT-PCR analysis for evaluating the Her2/neu status in breast cancer. Pathobiology. 2010;77(1):38–45.

41. Dabbs DJ, Klein ME, Mohsin SK, Tubbs RR, Shuai Y, Bhargava R. High false-negative rate of HER2 quantitative reverse transcription polymerase chain reaction of the Oncotype DX test: an independent quality assurance study. J Clin Oncol. 2011;29(32):4279–85.

42. Nistor A, Watson PH, Pettigrew N, Tabiti K, Dawson A, Myal Y. Real-time PCR complements immunohistochemistry in the determination of HER-2/neu status in breast cancer. BMC Clin Pathol. 2006;6:2.

43. Noske A, Loibl S, Darb-Esfahani S, Roller M, Kronenwett R, Muller BM, Steffen J, Toerne C, Wirtz R, Baumann I. Comparison of different approaches for assessment of HER2 expression on protein and mRNA level: prediction of chemotherapy response in the neoadjuvant GeparTrio trial (NCT00544765). Breast Cancer Res Treat. 2011;126(1):109–17.

44. Park S, Wang HY, Kim S, Ahn S, Lee D, Cho Y, Park KH, Jung D, Kim SI, Lee H. Quantitative RT-PCR assay of HER2 mRNA expression in formalin-fixed and paraffin-embedded breast cancer tissues. Int J Clin Exp Pathol. 2014; 7(10):6752–9.

45. Bartlett JM, Starczynski J. Quantitative reverse transcriptase polymerase chain reaction and the Oncotype DX test for assessment of human epidermal growth factor receptor 2 status: time to reflect again? J Clin Oncol. 2011;29(32):4219–21.

46. Schmittgen TD, Livak KJ. Analyzing real-time PCR data by the comparative C(T) method. Nat Protoc. 2008;3(6):1101–8.

47. Budczies J, Klauschen F, Sinn BV, Gyorffy B, Schmitt WD, Darb-Esfahani S, Denkert C. Cutoff Finder: a comprehensive and straightforward Web application enabling rapid biomarker cutoff optimization. PLoS One. 2012; 7(12):e51862.

48. Baselga J, Swain SM. Novel anticancer targets: revisiting ERBB2 and discovering ERBB3. Nat Rev Cancer. 2009;9(7):463–75.

49. Gonzalez de Castro D, Clarke PA, Al-Lazikani B, Workman P. Personalized cancer medicine: molecular diagnostics, predictive biomarkers, and drug resistance. Clin Pharmacol Ther. 2013;93(3):252–9.

50. Dienstmann R, Rodon J, Tabernero J. Biomarker-driven patient selection for early clinical trials. Curr Opin Oncol. 2013;25(3):305–12.

51. Patani N, Martin LA, Dowsett M. Biomarkers for the clinical management of breast cancer: international perspective. Int J Cancer. 2013;133(1):1–13.

52. Kulasingam V, Diamandis EP. Strategies for discovering novel cancer biomarkers through utilization of emerging technologies. Nat Clin Pract Oncol. 2008;5(10):588–99.

53. Pasic MD, Samaan S, Yousef GM. Genomic medicine: new frontiers and new challenges. Clin Chem. 2013;59(1):158–67.

54. Pasic MD, Yousef GM, Diamandis EP. The proteomic revolution in laboratory medicine. Clin Biochem. 2013;46(6):397–8.

55. Altman RB. Personal genomic measurements: the opportunity for information integration. Clin Pharmacol Ther. 2013;93(1):21–3.

56. Bartlett G, Zgheib N, Manamperi A, Wang W, Hizel C, Kahveci R, Yazan Y. Pharmacogenomics in primary care: a crucial entry point for global personalized medicine? Curr Pharmacogenomics Person Med. 2012;10(2):101–5.

57. Dienstmann R, Rodon J, Barretina J, Tabernero J. Genomic medicine frontier in human solid tumors: prospects and challenges. J Clin Oncol. 2013;31(15): 1874–84.

58. Lewis S, Locker A, Todd JH, Bell JA, Nicholson R, Elston CW, Blamey RW, Ellis IO. Expression of epidermal growth factor receptor in breast carcinoma. J Clin Pathol. 1990;43(5):385–9.

59. Siegel PM, Ryan ED, Cardiff RD, Muller WJ. Elevated expression of activated forms of Neu/ErbB-2 and ErbB-3 are involved in the induction of mammary tumors in transgenic mice: implications for human breast cancer. EMBO J. 1999;18(8):2149–64.

60. Travis A, Pinder SE, Robertson JF, Bell JA, Wencyk P, Gullick WJ, Nicholson RI, Poller DN, Blamey RW, Elston CW. C-erbB-3 in human breast carcinoma: expression and relation to prognosis and established prognostic indicators. Br J Cancer. 1996;74(2):229–33.

61. Tucker T, Marra M, Friedman JM. Massively parallel sequencing: the next big thing in genetic medicine. Am J Hum Genet. 2009;85:142–54.

62. Gingras I, Sonnenblick A, De Azambuja E, Paesmans M, Delaloge S, Aftimos P, Piccart MJ, Sotiriou C, Ignatiadis M, Azim HA. The current use and attitudes towards tumor genome sequencing in breast cancer. Sci Rep. 2016;6:22517.

63. Roychowdhury S, Chinnaiyan AM. Translating cancer genomes and transcriptomes for precision oncology. CA Cancer J Clin. 2016;66:75–88.

64. Costa V, Angelini C, De Feis I, Ciccodicola A. Uncovering the complexity of transcriptomes with RNA-Seq. J Biomed Biotechnol. 2010;2010:853916.

65. Wang Y, Yang Q, Wang Z. The evolution of nanopore sequencing. Front Genet. 2015;5:449.

66. Metzker ML. Sequencing technologies-the next generation. Nat Rev Genet. 2010;11(1):31–46.

67. Fend F, Raffeld M. Laser capture microdissection in pathology. J Clin Pathol. 2000;53:666–72.

17

Circulating tumor cell clusters-associated gene plakoglobin is a significant prognostic predictor in patients with breast cancer

Wataru Goto[1], Shinichiro Kashiwagi[1*], Yuka Asano[1], Koji Takada[1], Katsuyuki Takahashi[2], Takaharu Hatano[3], Tsutomu Takashima[1], Shuhei Tomita[2], Hisashi Motomura[3], Masahiko Ohsawa[4], Kosei Hirakawa[1] and Masaichi Ohira[1]

Abstract

Background: Circulating tumor cells (CTCs) are linked to metastatic relapse and are regarded as a prognostic marker for human cancer. High expression of plakoglobin, a cell adhesion protein, within the primary tumor is positively associated with CTC clusters in breast cancer. In this study, we investigated the correlation between plakoglobin expression and survival of breast cancer.

Methods: We evaluated 121 breast cancer patients treated with neoadjuvant chemotherapy. Expression of plakoglobin was identified by immunohistochemical staining in the cell membrane. We also examined the relation between the expression of plakoglobin and E-cadherin, an epithelial–mesenchymal transition (EMT) marker.

Results: Patients with high plakoglobin expression had significantly worse distant-metastasis-free survival (DMFS) ($P = 0.016$, log rank). Plakoglobin expression had no correlation with pathological complete response rate ($P = 0.627$). On univariate analysis with respect to distant metastasis, high plakoglobin expression showed worse prognosis than low plakoglobin expression [$P = 0.036$, hazard ratio (HR) = 3.719]. Multivariate analysis found the same result ($P = 0.013$, HR = 5.052). In addition, there was a significant relationship between the expression of plakoglobin and E-cadherin ($P = 0.023$).

Conclusions: Plakoglobin expression is an independent prognostic factor in patients with breast cancer, particularly for DMFS, and this is related to EMT.

Keywords: Plakoglobin, Circulating tumor cells, Neoadjuvant chemotherapy, Breast cancer, Predictive marker

Background

Breast cancer is the most common and deadly form of cancer worldwide in women. Although treatment with neoadjuvant chemotherapy (NAC) increases the rate of breast-conserving surgery and reduces the risk of postoperative recurrence in patients with resectable breast cancer [1–4], recurrence and metastasis remain major problems for cure [5]. NAC requires tailoring; particularly by exploring biomarkers using genetic approaches or establishing therapeutic strategies based on the response to early treatment.

Haematogenous metastasis occurs by circulating tumor cells (CTCs) that detach from primary tumor tissues and circulate in the bloodstream and reach distant sites after extravasation [6]. CTCs are regarded as a useful prognostic marker in patients with breast cancer [7]. Some studies reported that clusters of CTCs were detected within the circulation of patients with metastatic epithelial cancers, and that those clusters had greater metastatic potential than single CTCs [8]. Cell–cell adhesion is a determinant of CTCs in single or clustered cells, and plakoglobin, a cell adhesion protein, is a key mediator of tumor-cell clustering, which is expressed in a heterogeneous pattern within the primary tumor [8]. High plakoglobin expression enables tumor cells to stick together and move in clusters in the bloodstream,

* Correspondence: spqv9ke9@view.ocn.ne.jp
[1]Department of Surgical Oncology, Osaka City University Graduate School of Medicine, 1-4-3 Asahi-machi, Abeno-ku, Osaka 545-8585, Japan
Full list of author information is available at the end of the article

allowing more chance of metastasis and resulting in worse survival of breast cancer [9]. Also, tumor cells with high plakoglobin levels show low motility and result in the inhibition of invasion [10].

The association between plakoglobin and malignancy remains controversial. Epithelial–mesenchymal transition (EMT) is observed when cancer spreads, and promotes cancer infiltration and metastasis by facilitating cancer cell motility and breakdown of the extracellular matrix [11]. Plakoglobin is related to EMT, because it can be a linker between E-cadherin and α-catenin in cell–cell adhesion [12]. Insufficient expression of plakoglobin could therefore promote EMT [9]. In this study, we aimed to evaluate plakoglobin as a possible marker for predicting outcome and treatment response in breast cancer, and to investigate the relationship between plakoglobin and E-cadherin expression.

Methods

Patient background

A total of 121 patients with resectable, early-stage breast cancer diagnosed as stage IIA (T1, N1, M0 or T2, N0, M0), IIB (T2, N1, M0 or T3, N0, M0), or IIIA (T1–2, N2, M0 or T3, N1–2, M0) were treated with NAC between 2007 and 2013. Tumor stage and T and N factors were stratified based on the TNM Classification of Malignant Tumors, UICC 7th Edition [13]. Breast cancer was confirmed histologically by core needle biopsy and staged by systemic imaging studies using computed tomography (CT), ultrasonography (US), and bone scintigraphy. Breast cancer was classified into subtypes according to the immunohistochemical expression of estrogen receptor (ER), progesterone receptor (PgR), human epidermal growth factor receptor (HER) 2, and Ki67.

All patients received a standardised protocol of NAC consisting of four courses of FEC100 (500 mg m^{-2} fluorouracil, 100 mg m^{-2} epirubicin, and 500 mg m^{-2} cyclophosphamide) every 3 weeks, followed by 12 courses of 80 mg m^{-2} paclitaxel administered weekly [14, 15]. Thirty-five patients had HER2-positive breast cancer and were additionally administered weekly (2 mg kg^{-1}) or tri-weekly (6 mg kg^{-1}) trastuzumab during paclitaxel treatment [16]. All patients underwent chemotherapy as outpatients. Therapeutic anti-tumor effects were assessed according to the Response Evaluation Criteria in Solid Tumors (RECIST) criteria [17]. Pathological complete response (pCR) was defined as the complete disappearance of the invasive component of the lesion, with or without intraductal components, including in the lymph nodes. Patients underwent mastectomy or breast-conserving surgery after NAC. All patients who underwent breast-conserving surgery were administered postoperative radiotherapy to the remnant breast. Overall survival (OS) time was the period from the initiation of NAC to the time of

death from any cause. Disease-free survival (DFS) was defined as freedom from all local, locoregional, and distant recurrences. Distant metastasis-free survival (DMFS) time was defined as time to distant metastasis or death if the latter event occurred before a distant metastasis was diagnosed. All patients were followed up by physical examination every 3 months, US every 6 months, and CT and bone scintigraphy annually. The median follow-up period for the assessment of OS was 3.5 years (range, 0.6–7.6 years), 3.3 years (range, 0.1–7.6 years) for DFS, and 3.4 years (range, 0.1–7.6 years) for DMFS.

This study was conducted at Osaka City University Graduate School of Medicine, Osaka, Japan, according to the Reporting Recommendations for Tumor Marker prognostic Studies (REMARK) guidelines and a retrospectively written research, pathological evaluation, and statistical plan. The design of this study is a retrospective chart review study. Written informed consent was obtained from all patients. This research conformed to the provisions of the Declaration of Helsinki of 2013. The study protocol was approved by the Ethics Committee of Osaka City University (#926).

Immunohistochemistry

All patients underwent a core needle biopsy prior to NAC, and they underwent curative surgery involving mastectomy or conservative surgery with axillary lymph node dissection after NAC. Immunohistochemical studies were performed as previously described on core needle biopsy specimens [18, 19]. Tumor specimens were fixed in 10% formaldehyde solution and embedded in paraffin, and 4-µm-thick sections were mounted on glass slides. Slides were deparaffinised in xylene and heated for 20 min (105 °C, 0.4 kg m^{-2}) in an autoclave in Target Retrieval Solution (Dako, Carpinteria, CA, USA). Specimens were incubated with 3% hydrogen peroxide in methanol for 15 min to block endogenous peroxidase activity, and then incubated in 10% normal goat or rabbit serum to block non-specific reactions.

Primary monoclonal antibodies directed against ER (clone 1D5, dilution 1:80; Dako), PgR (clone PgR636, dilution 1:100; Dako), HER2 (HercepTest™; Dako), Ki67 (clone MIB-1, dilution 1:00; Dako), plakoglobin (clone 4C12, dilution 1:200; Abcam, Cambridge, UK), E-cadherin (clone #3195, dilution 1:400; Cell Signaling Technology, Danvers, MA, USA) and β-catenin (clone #9562, dilution 1:400; CST, Danvers, USA) and were used. Tissue sections were incubated with each antibody for 70 min at room temperature or overnight at 4 °C, and then with horseradish-peroxidase-conjugated anti-rabbit or anti-mouse immunoglobulin secondary antibodies (HISTOFINE (PO)™ Kit; Nichirei, Tokyo, Japan). Slides were subsequently treated with streptavidin–peroxidase reagent and incubated in phosphate-buffered

Circulating tumor cell clusters-associated gene plakoglobin is a significant prognostic...

151

saline–diaminobenzidine and 1% hydrogen peroxide (v/v), followed by counterstaining with Mayer's haematoxylin. Positive and negative controls for each marker were used according to the supplier's data sheet.

Immunohistochemical scoring

Immunohistochemical scoring was performed by two pathologists specialised in mammary gland pathology, using the blind method to confirm the objectivity and reproducibility of diagnosis. The cutoffs for ER and PgR positivity were both ≥1% positive tumor cells with nuclear staining [20]. Tumors with 3+ HER2 on immunohistochemical staining were considered to show HER2 overexpression; tumors with 2+ HER2 were further analysed by fluorescence in situ hybridisation; and those with HER2/ centromeric probe for chromosome (CEP) 17 ≥ 2.0 were also considered to exhibit HER2 overexpression [21]. A Ki67-labeling index ≥14% tumor cells with nuclear staining was determined to be positive [22]. To evaluate plakoglobin, E-cadherin and β-catenin expression, three fields of view (FOVs) in darkly stained areas were selected, and the percentage of cancer cells showing membrane positivity in each FOV was measured microscopically at 400× magnification. The value of plakoglobin expression was categorised as follows: 0 = no cells; 1+ = 1–25% cells (Fig. 1a); 2+ = 26–75% of cells; and 3+ = >75% of cells (Fig. 1b) [23]. Plakoglobin expression was considered high if the score was 3, and low when score was ≤2. The value of E-cadherin expression was categorised as follows: 0 = no cells; 1+ = 1–30% of cells (Fig. 1c); 2+ = 31–70% of cells; and 3+ = >70% of cells (Fig. 1d) [24, 25]. E-cadherin expression was considered high if the score was ≥2, and low when the score was ≤1. β-catenin expression was considered high if cells were ≥30% (Additional file 1: Figure S1A), and low when cells were <30% (Additional file 1: Figure S1B).

Statistical analysis

Statistical analysis was performed using JMP11 software (SAS Institute, Cary, NC, USA). The associations between plakoglobin, E-cadherin and clinicopathological variables were evaluated using the χ^2 test (or Fisher's exact test when necessary). The Kaplan–Meier method was used to estimate OS, DFS and DMFS. The association with survival was analysed by Kaplan–Meier plot and log-rank test. The Cox proportional hazards model was used to compute univariate and multivariate hazards ratios (HRs) for the study parameters with 95% confidence interval (CI). A P value <0.05 was considered significant.

Results

Clinicopathological response of primary breast cancer to NAC

The subtype in 121 patients who received NAC was triple negative breast cancer (TNBC) in 39 (32.2%) patients and non-TNBC in 82 (67.8%) patients. Regarding treatment response, 48 (39.7%) patients had a pCR, and 73 (60.3%) had a non-pCR. According to subtype, 19 (48.7%) TNBC patients and 29 (35.4%) non-TNBC patients had a pCR (Additional file 2: Table S1).

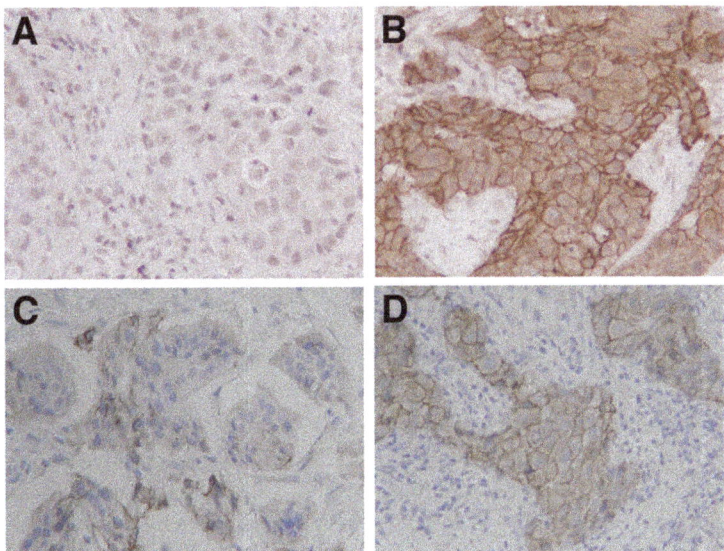

Fig. 1 Immunohistochemical determination of plakoglobin and E-cadherin. Plakoglobin and E-cadherin were observed at cell–cell boundaries of breast cancer cells. Plakoglobin expression was categorised as follows: 0 = no cells; 1+ = 1–25% of cells (**a**); 2+ = 26–75% of cells; 3+ = >75% of cells (**b**). E-cadherin expression was categorised as follows: 0 = no cells; 1+ = 1–30% of cells (**c**); 2+ = 31–70% of cells; 3+ = >70% of cells (**d**) (400×)

Table 1 Correlation between clinicopathological features and plakoglobin and E-cadherin expression in 121 patients with breast cancer

Parameters	plakoglobin		p value	E-cadherin		p value
	High (n = 21)	Low (n = 100)		High (n = 71)	Low (n = 50)	
HR and HER2 status						
TNBC	4 (19.0%)	35 (35.0%)	0.203	15 (21.1%)	24 (48.0%)	0.003
non-TNBC	17 (81.0%)	65 (65.0%)		56 (78.9%)	26 (52.0%)	
HER2 status						
negative	16 (76.2%)	70 (70.0%)		47 (66.2%)	39 (78.0%)	0.222
positive	5 (23.8%)	30 (30.0%)	0.792	24 (33.8%)	11 (22.0%)	
Age at operation						
≤ 56	12 (57.1%)	45 (45.0%)	0.344	34 (47.9%)	23 (46.0%)	0.855
> 56	9 (42.9%)	55 (55.0%)		37 (52.1%)	27 (54.0%)	
Menopause						
Negative	10 (47.6%)	38 (38.0%)	0.466	28 (39.4%)	20 (40.0%)	0.950
Positive	11 (52.4%)	62 (62.0%)		43 (60.6%)	30 (60.0%)	
Tumor size						
≤ 2 cm	2 (9.5%)	15 (15.0%)	0.734	9 (12.7%)	8 (16.0%)	0.607
> 2 cm	19 (90.5%)	85 (85.0%)		62 (87.3%)	42 (84.0%)	
Lymph node status						
Negative	8 (38.1%)	27 (27.0%)	0.304	23 (32.4%)	12 (24.0%)	0.416
Positive	13 (61.9%)	73 (73.0%)		48 (67.6%)	38 (76.0%)	
Nuclear grade						
1, 2	16 (76.2%)	78 (78.0%)	0.857	54 (76.1%)	40 (80.0%)	0.663
3	5 (23.8%)	22 (22.0%)		17 (23.9%)	10 (20.0%)	
Ki67						
≤ 14%	6 (28.6%)	45 (45.0%)	0.225	30 (42.3%)	21 (42.0%)	0.978
> 14%	15 (71.4%)	55 (55.0%)		41 (57.7%)	29 (58.0%)	
Pathological response						
pCR	7 (33.3%)	41 (41.0%)	0.627	39 (54.9%)	34 (68.0%)	0.187
non-pCR	14 (66.7%)	59 (59.0%)		32 (45.1%)	16 (32.0%)	
Plakoglobin						
Low	Not	Not		54 (76.1%)	46 (92.0%)	0.023
High	determined	determined		17 (23.9%)	4 (8.0%)	
E-cadherin						
Negative	4 (19.0%)	46 (46.0%)	0.023	Not	Not	
Positive	17 (81.0%)	54 (54.0%)		determined	determined	

HER2 human epidermal growth factor receptor 2; *HR* hormone receptor; *pCR* pathological complete response; *TNBC* triple-negative breast cancer

Plakoglobin and E-cadherin expression in all breast cancer

There were 21 (17.4%) patients with high plakoglobin expression (score: 3) and 100 (82.6%) with low plakoglobin expression (score: ≤2). There were 71 (58.7%) patients with high E-cadherin expression (score: ≥2) and 50 (41.3%) with low E-cadherin expression (score: ≤1).

Evaluation based on clinicopathological features showed that plakoglobin was significantly correlated with E-cadherin (*P* = 0.023) (Table 1). There was no significant correlation between plakoglobin and any other tested clinicopathological parameter, including pCR (*P* = 0.627). Patients with low E-cadherin expression had a significantly higher rate of TNBC (*P* = 0.003), and patients with high E-cadherin expression in TNBC tended to have a high pCR rate (*P* = 0.105) (Table 2).

DMFS was significantly worse in patients with high compared with low plakoglobin expression (*P* = 0.016,

Table 2 Correlation between pCR and plakoglobin and E-cadherin expression in 39 TNBC and 82 non-TNBC.

	Parameters	plakoglobin		p value	E-cadherin		p value
		High (n = 4)	Low (n = 35)		High (n = 15)	Low (n = 24)	
TNBC (n = 39)	Pathological response						
	pCR	3 (75.0%)	16 (45.7%)	0.342	10 (66.7%)	9 (37.5%)	0.105
	non-pCR	1 (25.0%)	19 (54.3%)		5 (33.3%)	15 (62.5%)	
non-TNBC (n = 82)		High (n = 17)	Low (n = 65)		High (n = 56)	Low (n = 26)	
	Pathological response						
	pCR	4 (23.5%)	25 (38.5%)	0.393	22 (39.3%)	7 (26.9%)	0.328
	non-pCR	13 (76.5%)	40 (61.5%)		34 (60.7%)	19 (73.1%)	

pCR pathological complete response; TNBC triple-negative breast cancer

log-rank) (Fig. 2a). DFS and OS did not differ significantly between patients with low or high plakoglobin expression (P = 0.052, log rank) (P = 0.063, log rank) (Figs. 2b, c). OS was significantly longer in patients with high compared with low E-cadherin expression (P = 0.002, log rank), while DFS and DMFS tended to be longer in the high-E-cadherin group (P = 0.171, log rank) (P = 0.162, log rank) (Fig. 3a–c).

The correlations between DMFS, OS and the various clinicopathological factors are shown in Table 3. According to the results of univariate analysis, DMFS exhibited significant relationships with age (P = 0.006), tumor size (P = 0.049) and plakoglobin (P = 0.036), and OS exhibited significant relationships with age (p = 0.020) and E-cadherin (P = 0.002). Multivariate analysis indicated that age (HR = 6.543, 95% CI: 1.563–47.40, P = 0.008), lymph node (HR = 7.035, 95% CI: 1.195–137.4, P = 0.028), nuclear grade (HR = 12.79, 95% CI: 1.591–163.3, P = 0.016), Ki67 (HR = 13.99, 95% CI: 2.063–203.4, P = 0.005), and plakoglobin (HR = 7.371, 95% CI: 1.596–44.23, P = 0.011) were independent prognostic factors for DMFS, and that age (HR = 6.525, 95% CI: 1.437–52.39, P = 0.013), nuclear grade (HR = 7.513, 95% CI: 1.047–84.10, P = 0.045), plakoglobin (HR = 8.232, 95% CI: 1.428–63.37, P = 0.019), and E-cadherin (HR = 15.62, 95% CI: 2.425–172.9, P = 0.003) were independent prognostic factor for OS (Additional file 3: Table S2).

According to the results of univariate analysis, DMFS exhibited significant relationships with tumor size (P = 0.049) and plakoglobin (P = 0.036), and OS exhibited significant relationships with E-cadherin (P = 0.002). Multivariate analysis indicated that tumor size (>2) (HR = 5.511, 95% CI: 1.223–46.08, P = 0.032) and plakoglobin (HR = 5.052, 95% CI: 1.449–16.41, P = 0.013) were independent prognostic factors for DMFS, and that E-cadherin (HR = 8.045, 95% CI: 2.014–53.84, P = 0.002) was an independent prognostic factor for OS (Additional file 3: Table S2).

Combination of plakoglobin and E-cadherin

Only four patients had a combination of high plakoglobin and low E-cadherin expression. Compared with patients with other combinations, those with high plakoglobin and low E-cadherin expression had significantly worse OS (P < 0.001, log rank), DFS (P < 0.001, log rank), and DMFS (P < 0.001, log rank) (Fig. 4a–c).

In addition, we evaluated β-catenin expression of patients with high plakoglobin and low E-cadherin expression. They all exhibited high β-catenin expression.

Discussion

Stephen Paget proposed in 1889 that cancer metastasis depends on the concept of "seed and soil". With regard to the ability of the seed, the physical characteristics of

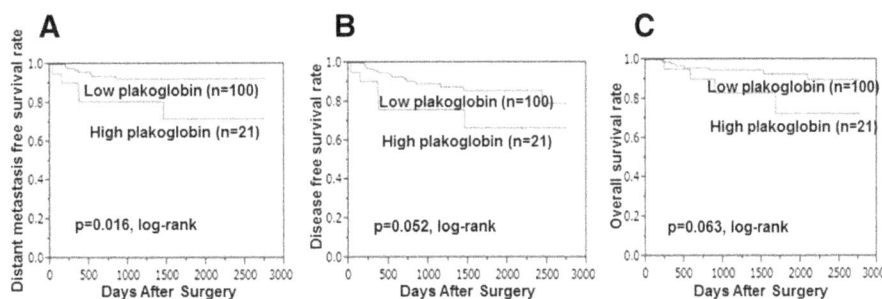

Fig. 2 Kaplan–Meier stratified by plakoglobin expression in breast cancer. DMFS was significantly worse in the high- compared with low-plakoglobin group (P = 0.016, log rank) (**a**). DFS and OS did not differ significantly between patients with low or high plakoglobin expression (P = 0.052, log rank) (**b**) (P = 0.063, log rank) (**c**). Abbreviations: DFS = disease-free survival; DMFS = distant-metastasis-free survival; OS = overall survival

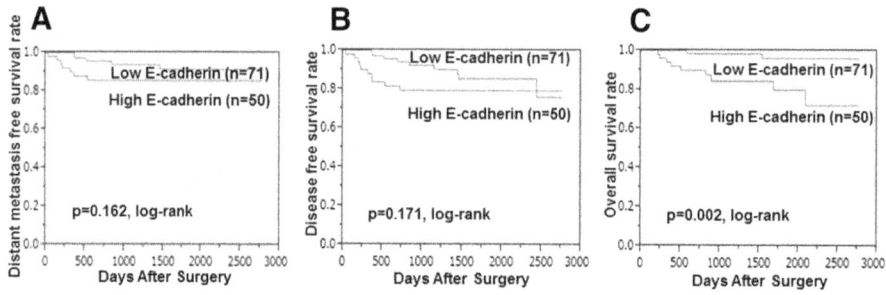

Fig. 3 Kaplan–Meier stratified by E-cadherin expression in breast cancer. Compared with those with low E-cadherin, patients with high expression had superior overall survival (*P* = 0.002) (**c**), disease-free survival (*P* = 0.171) (**b**), and distant-metastasis-free survival (*P* = 0.162) (**a**)

single and clustered CTCs may also contribute to metastatic propensity [26]. CTC clusters are more rapidly cleared from the circulation than single CTCs, therefore, clusters account for only 2–5% of all observed CTCs. However, CTC clusters have 23–50 times greater metastatic potential than single CTCs; have more resistance to apoptosis than single CTCs; and contribute to shorter survival in patients with breast cancer [8]. Aceto et al. [8] found that CTC clusters had higher plakoglobin expression than single CTCs and that patients with high plakoglobin expression in primary tumors had significantly worse DMFS.

Plakoglobin (also known as γ-catenin) is a member of the Armadillo family of proteins and a homologue of β-catenin, and an important component of both the adherens junctions and desmosomes [27]. High plakoglobin expression makes tumor cells move in clusters in the circulation, which have a greater tendency to form distant metastasis than single CTCs have [9]. Plakoglobin interacts directly with E-cadherin and plays a fundamental role as a link between desmosomal cadherin and the intermediate filament cytoskeletons [12]. Insufficient desmosomal assembly leads to cytoskeletal reorganisation and loss of polarity of epithelial cells, thereby promoting EMT

[28, 29]. This study also showed that patients with low plakoglobin expression had a significantly longer DMFS, and patients with high plakoglobin expression had significantly higher E-cadherin expression.

However, unlike plakoglobin, high E-cadherin expression was an independent prognostic factor. Therefore, the combination of low E-cadherin and high plakoglobin expression meant that EMT was promoted and there were more CTC clusters. Although only a few patients had that combination, they had remarkably high metastatic potential and poor outcome. Also, patients with low E-cadherin expression had a significantly higher rate of TNBC. Some studies demonstrated that Wnt/β-catenin signaling activation was preferentially found in TNBC [30, 31]. Though there was no significant correlation between plakoglobin and TNBC, patients with high plakoglobin and low E-cadherin expression all exhibited high β-catenin expression. It suggests that the reason why the combination of high plakoglobin and low E-cadherin expression induced significantly poor outcome may relate to Wnt/β-catenin signaling activation.

Emerging evidence suggests that EMT contributes to chemoresistance [32, 33]. The present study also showed that patients with high E-cadherin expression in TNBC

Table 3 Univariate and multivariate analysis with respect to distant metastasis-free survival in 121 patients with breast cancer

Parameter		Univariable analysis			Multivariable analysis		
		Hazard ratio	95% CI	p value	Hazard ratio	95% CI	p value
Intrinsic subtype	TNBC vs non-TNBC	1.053	0.281–3.344	0.933	0.632	0.137–2.710	0.535
Intrinsic subtype	HER2 vs non-HER2	2.060	0.543–13.41	0.314	1.721	0.353–12.53	0.517
Age at operation	≤56 vs >56	6.096	1.606–39.67	0.006	6.543	1.563–47.40	0.008
Tumor size (cm)	≤2 vs >2	3.234	0.445–40.56	0.049	2.811	0.874–46.08	0.062
Lymph node status	Negative vs Positive	4.493	0.873–82.10	0.077	7.035	1.195–137.4	0.028
Nuclear grade	1–2 vs 3	1.805	0.482–5.730	0.353	12.79	1.591–163.3	0.016
Ki67 (%)	≤14 vs >14	2.048	0.652–6.942	0.218	13.99	2.063–203.4	0.005
Pathological response	pCR vs non-pCR	2.075	0.619–9.357	0.248	1.561	0.301–10.34	0.609
plakoglobin	High vs Low	3.719	1.100–11.66	0.036	7.371	1.596–44.23	0.011
E-cadherin	Low vs High	2.223	0.709–7.517	0.169	5.003	0.966–35.14	0.055

HER2 human epidermal growth factor receptor 2; *CI* confidence interval; *pCR* pathological complete response; *TNBC* triple-negative breast cancer

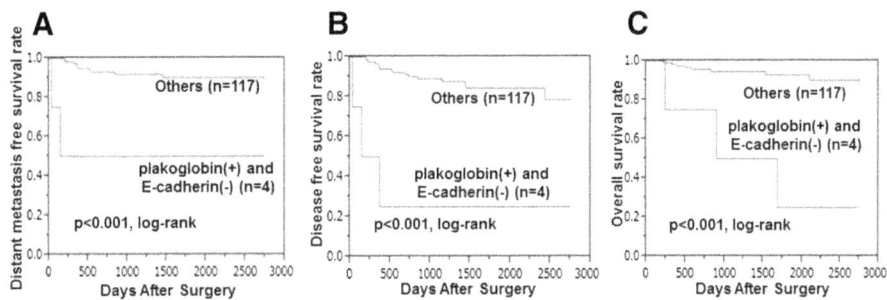

Fig. 4 Kaplan–Meier stratified by combination of plakoglobin and E-cadherin expression in breast cancer. Compared with those with high plakoglobin and low E-cadherin expression, patients with others had superior overall survival (*P* < 0.001) (**c**), disease-free survival (*P* < 0.001) (**b**), and distant-metastasis-free survival (*P* < 0.001) (**a**)

tended to have a high pCR rate. However, plakoglobin expression did not significantly affect response to NAC in breast cancer. This may be because plakoglobin is not only involved in cell adhesion. It has been reported that plakoglobin plays both positive and negative roles in diverse malignancies [34–36]. It suggests that the microenvironment and the activated signalling pathways decide whether plakoglobin acts as an oncogene or tumor suppressor. In other words, the correlation between high plakoglobin expression and more distant metastatic potential of breast cancer may have nothing to do with either oncogene or tumor suppressor. While E-cadherin is one of EMT-markers, it is thought that plakoglobin is more useful prognostic factor for distant metastasis. As a potential limitation, the sample size of our study was small, and the numbers of combination of high plakoglobin and low E-cadherin expression were thus even smaller.

Conclusions

In conclusion, plakoglobin expression in primary tumor is useful as a biomarker to predict DMFS in breast cancer. It may offer an opportunity for therapeutic intervention. Further studies are therefore warranted to investigate which transcription factors regulate the expression of plakoglobin.

Abbreviations

CEP: Centromeric probe for chromosome; CI: Confidence interval; CT: Computed tomography; CTC: Circulating tumor cells; DFS: Disease-free survival; DMFS: Distant-metastasis-free survival; EMT: Epithelial–mesenchymal transition; ER: Estrogen receptor; FOV: Fields of view; HER: Human epidermal growth factor receptor; HR: Hazards ratios; NAC: Neoadjuvant chemotherapy; OS: Overall survival; pCR: Pathological complete response; PgR: Progesterone receptor; RECIST: Response Evaluation Criteria in Solid Tumors; REMARK: Reporting Recommendations for Tumor Marker prognostic Studies; TNBC: Triple negative breast cancer; US: Ultrasonography

Acknowledgements
We thank Yayoi Matsukiyo and Tomomi Ohkawa (Department of Surgical Oncology, Osaka City University Graduate School of Medicine) for helpful advice regarding data management.

Funding
This study was supported in part by Grants-in Aid for Scientific Research (KAKENHI, Nos. 25,461,992 and 26,461,957) from the Ministry of Education, Science, Sports, Culture and Technology of Japan.

Authors' contributions
All authors were involved in the preparation of this manuscript. WG collected the data, and wrote the manuscript. SK, YA, KTakada, KTakahashi, TH and TT performed the operation and designed the study. WG, SK and ST summarized the data and revised the manuscript. MOhsawa performed the pathological diagnosis. HM, KH and MOhira substantial contribution to the study design, performed the operation, and revised the manuscript. All authors read and approved the final manuscript.

Competing interests
The authors declare that they have no competing interests.

Author details
[1]Department of Surgical Oncology, Osaka City University Graduate School of Medicine, 1-4-3 Asahi-machi, Abeno-ku, Osaka 545-8585, Japan. [2]Department of Pharmacology, Osaka City University Graduate School of Medicine, 1-4-3 Asahi-machi, Abeno-ku, Osaka 545-8585, Japan. [3]Department of Plastic and Reconstructive Surgery, Osaka City University Graduate School of Medicine, 1-4-3 Asahi-machi, Abeno-ku, Osaka 545-8585, Japan. [4]Department of Diagnostic Pathology, Osaka City University Graduate School of Medicine, 1-4-3 Asahi-machi, Abeno-ku, Osaka 545-8585, Japan.

References

1. Mayer EL, Carey LA, Burstein HJ. Clinical trial update: implications and management of residual disease after neoadjuvant therapy for breast cancer. Breast Cancer Res. 2007;9(5):110.
2. Sachelarie I, Grossbard ML, Chadha M, Feldman S, Ghesani M, Blum RH. Primary systemic therapy of breast cancer. Oncologist. 2006;11(6):574–89.
3. van der Hage JA, van de Velde CJ, Julien JP, Tubiana-Hulin M, Vandervelden C, Duchateau L. Preoperative chemotherapy in primary operable breast cancer: results from the European Organization for Research and Treatment of cancer trial 10902. J Clin Oncol. 2001;19(22):4224–37.
4. Wolmark N, Wang J, Mamounas E, Bryant J, Fisher B. Preoperative chemotherapy in patients with operable breast cancer: nine-year results from National Surgical Adjuvant Breast and bowel project B-18. J Natl Cancer Inst Monogr. 2001;30:96–102.
5. Carlson RW, Allred DC, Anderson BO, Burstein HJ, Edge SB, Farrar WB, Forero A, Giordano SH, Goldstein LJ, Gradishar WJ, et al. Metastatic breast cancer, version 1.2012: featured updates to the NCCN guidelines. J Natl Compr Cancer Netw. 2012;10(7):821–9.
6. Hanahan D, Weinberg RA. Hallmarks of cancer: the next generation. Cell. 2011;144(5):646–74.
7. Zhang L, Riethdorf S, Wu G, Wang T, Yang K, Peng G, Liu J, Pantel K. Meta-analysis of the prognostic value of circulating tumor cells in breast cancer. Clin Cancer Res. 2012;18(20):5701–10.
8. Aceto N, Bardia A, Miyamoto DT, Donaldson MC, Wittner BS, Spencer JA, Yu M, Pely A, Engstrom A, Zhu H, et al. Circulating tumor cell clusters are oligoclonal precursors of breast cancer metastasis. Cell. 2014;158(5):1110–22.
9. Lu L, Zeng H, Gu X, Ma W. Circulating tumor cell clusters-associated gene plakoglobin and breast cancer survival. Breast Cancer Res Treat. 2015;151(3):491–500.
10. Rieger-Christ KM, Ng L, Hanley RS, Durrani O, Ma H, Yee AS, Libertino JA, Summerhayes IC. Restoration of plakoglobin expression in bladder carcinoma cell lines suppresses cell migration and tumorigenic potential. Br J Cancer. 2005;92(12):2153–9.
11. Thiery JP, Acloque H, Huang RY, Nieto MA. Epithelial-mesenchymal transitions in development and disease. Cell. 2009;139(5):871–90.
12. Fukunaga Y, Liu H, Shimizu M, Komiya S, Kawasuji M, Nagafuchi A. Defining the roles of beta-catenin and plakoglobin in cell-cell adhesion: isolation of beta-catenin/plakoglobin-deficient F9 cells. Cell Struct Funct. 2005;30(2):25–34.
13. Greene FL, Sobin LH. A worldwide approach to the TNM staging system: collaborative efforts of the AJCC and UICC. J Surg Oncol. 2009;99(5):269–72.
14. Mauri D, Pavlidis N, Ioannidis JP. Neoadjuvant versus adjuvant systemic treatment in breast cancer: a meta-analysis. J Natl Cancer Inst. 2005; 97(3):188–94.
15. Mieog JS, van der Hage JA, van de Velde CJ. Preoperative chemotherapy for women with operable breast cancer. Cochrane Database Syst Rev. 2007;2: CD005002.
16. Buzdar AU, Valero V, Ibrahim NK, Francis D, Broglio KR, Theriault RL, Pusztai L, Green MC, Singletary SE, Hunt KK, et al. Neoadjuvant therapy with paclitaxel followed by 5-fluorouracil, epirubicin, and cyclophosphamide chemotherapy and concurrent trastuzumab in human epidermal growth factor receptor 2-positive operable breast cancer: an update of the initial randomized study population and data of additional patients treated with the same regimen. Clin Cancer Res. 2007;13(1):228–33.
17. Eisenhauer EA, Therasse P, Bogaerts J, Schwartz LH, Sargent D, Ford R, Dancey J, Arbuck S, Gwyther S, Mooney M, et al. New response evaluation criteria in solid tumors: revised RECIST guideline (version 1.1). Eur J Cancer. 2009;45(2):228–47.
18. Asano Y, Kashiwagi S, Onoda N, Kurata K, Morisaki T, Noda S, Takashima T, Ohsawa M, Kitagawa S, Hirakawa K. Clinical verification of sensitivity to preoperative chemotherapy in cases of androgen receptor-expressing positive breast cancer. Br J Cancer. 2016;114(1):14–20.
19. Kashiwagi S, Yashiro M, Takashima T, Aomatsu N, Kawajiri H, Ogawa Y, Onoda N, Ishikawa T, Wakasa K, Hirakawa K. C-kit expression as a prognostic molecular marker in patients with basal-like breast cancer. Br J Surg. 2013; 100(4):490–6.
20. Umemura S, Kurosumi M, Moriya T, Oyama T, Arihiro K, Yamashita H, Umekita Y, Komoike Y, Shimizu C, Fukushima H, et al. Immunohistochemical evaluation for hormone receptors in breast cancer: a practically useful evaluation system and handling protocol. Breast Cancer. 2006;13(3):232–5.
21. Wolff AC, Hammond ME, Hicks DG, Dowsett M, McShane LM, Allison KH, Allred DC, Bartlett JM, Bilous M, Fitzgibbons P, et al. Recommendations for human epidermal growth factor receptor 2 testing in breast cancer: American Society of Clinical Oncology/College of American Pathologists clinical practice guideline update. Arch Pathol Lab Med. 2014;138(2):241–56.
22. Goldhirsch A, Wood WC, Coates AS, Gelber RD, Thurlimann B, Senn HJ, Panel m: Strategies for subtypes–dealing with the diversity of breast cancer: highlights of the St. Gallen international expert consensus on the primary therapy of early breast cancer 2011. Ann Oncol 2011, 22(8):1736-1747.
23. Sivrikoz ON, Doganay L, Sivrikoz UK, Karaarslan S, Sanal SM. Distribution of CXCR4 and gamma-catenin expression pattern in breast cancer subtypes and their relationship to axillary nodal involvement. Pol J Pathol. 2013;64(4):253–9.
24. Kashiwagi S, Yashiro M, Takashima T, Aomatsu N, Ikeda K, Ogawa Y, Ishikawa T, Hirakawa K. Advantages of adjuvant chemotherapy for patients with triple-negative breast cancer at stage II: usefulness of prognostic markers E-cadherin and Ki67. Breast Cancer Res. 2011;13(6):R122.
25. Kashiwagi S, Yashiro M, Takashima T, Nomura S, Noda S, Kawajiri H, Ishikawa T, Wakasa K, Hirakawa K. Significance of E-cadherin expression in triple-negative breast cancer. Br J Cancer. 2010;103(2):249–55.
26. Mathot L, Stenninger J. Behavior of seeds and soil in the mechanism of metastasis: a deeper understanding. Cancer Sci. 2012;103(4):626–31.
27. Aktary Z, Pasdar M. Plakoglobin: role in tumorigenesis and metastasis. Int J Cell Biol. 2012;2012:189521.
28. Gosavi P, Kundu ST, Khapare N, Sehgal L, Karkhanis MS, Dalal SN. E-cadherin and plakoglobin recruit plakophilin3 to the cell border to initiate desmosome assembly. Cell Mol Life Sci. 2011;68(8):1439–54.
29. Kundu ST, Gosavi P, Khapare N, Patel R, Hosing AS, Maru GB, Ingle A, Decaprio JA, Dalal SN. Plakophilin3 downregulation leads to a decrease in cell adhesion and promotes metastasis. Int J Cancer. 2008;123(10):2303–14.
30. Khramtsov AI, Khramtsova GF, Tretiakova M, Huo D, Olopade OI, Goss KH. Wnt/beta-catenin pathway activation is enriched in basal-like breast cancers and predicts poor outcome. Am J Pathol. 2010;176(6):2911–20.
31. Geyer FC, Lacroix-Triki M, Savage K, Arnedos M, Lambros MB, MacKay A, Natrajan R. Reis-Filho JS: beta-Catenin pathway activation in breast cancer is associated with triple-negative phenotype but not with CTNNB1 mutation. Mod Pathol. 2011;24(2):209–31.
32. Fischer KR, Durrans A, Lee S, Sheng J, Li F, Wong ST, Choi H, El Rayes T, Ryu S, Troeger J, et al. Epithelial-to-mesenchymal transition is not required for lung metastasis but contributes to chemoresistance. Nature. 2015;527(7579):472–6.
33. Singh A, Settleman J. EMT, cancer stem cells and drug resistance: an emerging axis of evil in the war on cancer. Oncogene. 2010;29(34):4741–51.
34. Hakimelahi S, Parker HR, Gilchrist AJ, Barry M, Li Z, Bleackley RC, Pasdar M. Plakoglobin regulates the expression of the anti-apoptotic protein BCL-2. J Biol Chem. 2000;275(15):10905–11.
35. Kolligs FT, Kolligs B, Hajra KM, Hu G, Tani M, Cho KR. Fearon ER: gamma-catenin is regulated by the APC tumor suppressor and its oncogenic activity is distinct from that of beta-catenin. Genes Dev. 2000;14(11):1319–31.
36. Shiina H, Breault JE, Basset WW, Enokida H, Urakami S, Li LC, Okino ST, Deguchi M, Kaneuchi M, Terashima M, et al. Functional loss of the gamma-catenin gene through epigenetic and genetic pathways in human prostate cancer. Cancer Res. 2005;65(6):2130–8.

18

Investigation of HNF-1B as a diagnostic biomarker for pancreatic ductal adenocarcinoma

Michelle X. Yang[1,7*], Ryan F. Coates[1], Abiy Ambaye[1], Juli-Anne Gardner[1], Richard Zubarick[2], Yuan Gao[3], Joan Skelly[4], James G. Liu[5] and Mari Mino-Kenudson[6]

Abstract

Background: Diagnosing pancreatic ductal adenocarcinoma (PDAC) in the setting of metastasis with an unknown primary remains very challenging due to the lack of specific biomarkers. HNF-1B has been characterized as an important transcription factor for pancreatic development and was reported as a biomarker for clear cell subtype of PDAC.

Methods: To investigate the diagnostic role of HNF-1B for PDAC, we used tissue microarray (TMA) and immunohistochemistry (IHC) to characterize HNF-1B expression in a large cohort of carcinomas, including 127 primary PDACs, 47 biliary adenocarcinomas, 17 metastatic PDACs, and 231 non-pancreaticobiliary carcinomas.

Results: HNF-1B was expressed in 107 of 127 (84.3%) of PDACs, 13 of 15 (86.7%) of cholangiocarcinomas, 13 of 18 (72%) of ampullary carcinomas, and 13 of 14 (92.9%) of gallbladder adenocarcinomas. Notably, HNF-1B was expressed in 16 of 17 (94.1%) of metastatic PDACs. Among the non-pancreaticobiliary cancers, HNF-1B was expressed in ~ 77% clear cell carcinomas of the kidney and ovarian clear cell carcinomas. Gastroesophageal, lung, and prostate adenocarcinomas occasionally expressed HNF-1B in up to 37% cases. HNF-1B was completely negative in hepatocellular, colorectal, breast, and lung squamous cell carcinomas. The sensitivity, specificity, positive predictive value, negative predictive value, and accuracy of HNF-1B for primary pancreaticobiliary carcinoma is 84, 68, 66, 85, and 75%, respectively. HNF-1B expression was not significantly associated with overall survival in patients with PDAC, but tumor size ≥2 cm and high tumor grade were significantly associated with worse overall survival in multivariate analyses.

Conclusions: HNF-1B may be used in surgical pathology to aid the diagnosis of metastatic pancreatic and biliary carcinoma with a panel of other markers to exclude lung, kidney, prostate, and Müllerian origins.

Keywords: HNF-1B, Pancreatic, Pancreaticobiliary, Adenocarcinoma, Tissue microarray, Immunohistochemistry

Background

Pancreatic ductal adenocarcinoma (PDAC) consists of approximately 85% of cancers arising in the pancreas, and is one of the most lethal malignancies in the world. Despite new generations of neoadjuvant and adjuvant therapies, the 5-year overall survival rate remains less than 5%, and patients with PDAC often present with metastatic disease of an unknown primary [1, 2]. An accurate diagnosis of PDAC on biopsy specimens remains challenging due to the lack of specific biomarkers [3, 4]. Investigating additional markers to improve the diagnosis of PDAC is of paramount important in daily practice for surgical pathologists.

Hepatocyte nuclear factor 1B (HNF-1B) has been well-characterized as one of the transcription factors involved in the early development of liver, pancreas, and kidney [5–7]. In animal models, HNF-1B gene was required for the morphogenesis of both ventral and dorsal pancreatic buds [8, 9]. In human subjects, mutations in HNF-1B caused severe pancreatic agenesis or hypoplasia, maturity-onset diabetes of the young (MODY) type 5, multi-cystic renal dysplasia, and hepatobiliary tract and Müllerian tract abnormalities [10–14]. In human adenocarcinomas,

* Correspondence: michelle.yang@umassmemorial.org
[1]Department of Pathology and Laboratory Medicine, University of Vermont Medical Center, 111 Colchester Avenue, Burlington, VT, USA
[7]Present address: Department of Pathology, University of Massachusetts Medical Center, 1 Innovation Drive, Worcester, MA 01605, USA
Full list of author information is available at the end of the article

HNF-1B was highly expressed in ovarian clear cell carcinomas and has been recognized as a useful molecular biomarker for this entity [15–17]. Interestingly, a recent study showed that PDAC with clear cell morphology strongly expressed HNF-1B, in contrast to the conventional type PDAC with only weak (61%) to moderate (24%) staining [18]. Due to the essential role of HNF-1B in pancreatic development, we hypothesized that HNF-1B was expressed in all cancers arising from the pancreatic ductal epithelium regardless of the histomorphology, and its expression may serve as a diagnostic marker of these cancers. Using immunohistochemistry (IHC) and tissue microarray (TMA), we investigated HNF-1B protein expression in 127 primary PDACs, 47 biliary tract adenocarcinomas, 17 metastatic PDACs, and 231 common non-pancreaticobiliary carcinomas, and calculated its sensitivity and specificity. The utility of HNF-1B to aid the diagnosis of pancreaticobiliary adenocarcinoma was discussed.

Methods

Study population

A total of 127 primary PDAC resections and 17 known metastatic PDACs were retrospectively retrieved from formalin fixed paraffin embedded (FFPE) blocks. Among the 127 primary PDACs, 10 cases received neoadjuvant therapy and 112 cases had negative resection margins (R0). A total of 85 cases had complete survival data with at least 2 years of follow-up after resection. Among the 17 metastatic PDACs, metastatic sites included liver ($N = 13$), celiac lymph nodes ($N = 2$), peritoneum ($N = 1$), and bone ($N = 1$). In addition, 47 adenocarcinomas from the biliary tract and 231 non-pancreaticobiliary carcinomas that morphologically mimic PDAC (mimickers) were also evaluated for comparison, including those of the ampulla, intrahepatic and extrahepatic biliary tract, gallbladder, colorectal, esophagus, stomach, hepatocellular carcinoma, lung (both adenocarcinoma and squamous cell carcinoma), bladder (urothelial carcinoma), breast (ductal and lobular), kidney (mainly clear cell carcinoma), prostate, ovarian surface epithelial, and endometrial. This study was approved by our Institutional Review Board (IRB # 17–0009).

Histological evaluation and tissue microarray (TMA) construction

All tumor slides of the 127 primary PDAC resections were reviewed, and the size of the tumor, tumor (pT) and nodal (pN) stages, tumor grade, tumor morphology (cytoplasmic clearing), lymphovascular invasion (LVI), perineural invasion (PNI), and resection margin status were extracted from the electronic pathologic record. The death status were extracted from the Tumor Registry data set. The final stage of PDAC was diagnosed in accordance with the American Joint Committee on Cancer (AJCC), 7th edition [19]. Two-millimeter core TMAs

were constructed with two cores each from the FFPE tumor tissue or adjacent non-neoplastic pancreas (as control) of primary PDAC resections or 278 non-pancreatic cancers (Beecher Instruments Inc., Sun Prairie, WI). Eleven of 17 metastatic PDACs were also included in the duplicated 2-mm core TMA, and the remaining 6 metastatic PDACs were biopsies that were mounted onto individual slides.

Immunohistochemistry (IHC)

Polyclonal anti-HNF-1B (Sigma, St. Louis, MO, HPA002083, 1:200 dilutions) was validated in non-neoplastic pancreatic tissue sections. Antigen retrieval was obtained for HNF-1B in H1 buffer (Leica Biosystems, Buffalo Grove, IL) for 10 min, All IHCs were performed in Leica BOND-III automated IHC stainer. Localization of staining – nuclear, cytoplasmic and/or membranous – was recorded in each case, and the case was recorded as positive if any amount of tumor cells had any pattern of HNF-1B expression. A two-tier scale was applied to all positive cases for HNF-1B: "strong", if the stain was clearly visualized at 20× low magnification, and "weak", if the stain was clearly visualized at 100× magnification with less intensity.

As comparison, a monoclonal antibody (Abnova, clone CL0374, 1:200 dilution) was validated under the same conditions mentioned above and showed nuclear reactivity in normal pancreatic ductal epithelium, but not in the acinar cells or islet cells, which was consistent with the result of polyclonal antibody. All cancer TMAs were investigated with the HNF-1B expression using the polyclonal antibody.

Statistical analysis

All demographic and clinicopathological measures were screened for ranges and appropriate codes. Eighty five of the 127 primary PDAC patients had complete demographic and clinicopathological measures and had survival data with at least 2 years of follow-up after the resection. For these 85 patients, descriptive statistics for these measures were calculated. The association between HNF-1B protein expression and clinicopathological features was examined using 2×2 contingency tables with Fisher's extract tests. Univariate Cox proportional hazard function models were used to examine the association of each of the clinicopathological measures with overall survival. The significant measures were included in a stepwise modeling procedure to determine a final model. The expression rate of HNF-1B in PDAC was compared to the rate in each of the other cancer types using Fisher's exact tests. The sensitivity, specificity and other measures of HNF-1B in classifying pancreaticobiliary and non-pancreaticobiliary carcinomas were calculated with 95% confidence intervals. All statistical analyses were conducted using SAS 9.3 software (SAS Institute, Cary NC). Statistical significant was determined by $P < .05$.

Results

Demographics and clinicopathologic features of PDAC

Among the 85 primary PDAC patients with complete clinicopathologic data, the mean age was 65 years (SD = 10), 55 were male (65%) (Table 1). Sixty eight (80%) had positive HNF-1B expression. Fisher's exact tests found no significant associations between HNF-1B expression and the clinicopathologic parameters. In univariate analysis, only tumor size ≥ 2 cm (P = .03) and high tumor grade (P = .02) were significantly associated with worse overall survival. HNF-1B protein expression did not demonstrate significant association with the overall survival. In multivariate analysis, tumor size ≥ 2 cm (P = .03) and high tumor grade (P = .02) remained significantly associated with worse overall survival (Table 2).

HNF-1B expression in non-neoplastic pancreatic and biliary epithelium

In non-neoplastic adult pancreas, HNF-1B was expressed in the ductal epithelium and centroacinar ductal cells with predominant nuclear and faint cytoplasmic staining (Fig. 1a). Since HNF-1B is also a transcription factor for liver development, we investigated HNF-1B immunostaining in normal liver and gallbladder. Interestingly, HNF-1B showed

Table 1 Demographics and clinicopathological parameters in patients with PDAC

Variables	PDAC (N = 85)
Age: Mean ± SD (years)	65 ± 10
Gender	
Male	55 (65%)
Female	30 (35%)
Tumor size	
≤ 2 cm	18 (21%)
> 2 cm	67 (79%)
Tumor location	
Head	63 (74%)
Tail	22 (26%)
LN metastasis	54 (64%)
LVI	40 (48%)
PNI	61 (72%)
No neoadjuvant	75 (88%)
Stage	
Stage I, II	24 (28%)
Stage III, IV	61 (72%)
Tumor grade	
Low grade (1/2)	56 (66%)
High grade (3)	29 (34%)

Abbreviations: *PDAC* pancreatic ductal adenocarcinoma;
SD standard deviation, *LVI* lymphovascular invasion;
LN lymph node, *PNI* perineural invasion

Table 2 Overall survival and clinicopathological variables in 85 patients with PDAC

Variables	Hazard ratio (95% CI)	p-value
Univariate analysis		
Age (< 65 vs ≥65)	0.98 (0.59–1.62)	.94
Gender (male vs. female)	1.13 (0.68–1.88)	.65
Tumor size (< 2 cm vs. ≥ 2 cm)	2.11 (1.07–4.16)	**.03**
Stage (I/II vs. III/IV)	0.74 (0.44–1.26)	.28
Grade (low vs. high)	1.84 (1.11–3.05)	**.02**
PNI	1.18 (0.70–2.01)	.54
LVI	1.46 (0.90–2.40)	.13
LN metastasis	1.31 (0.77–2.21)	.32
HNF-1B (negative vs. positive)	1.34 (0.70–2.57)	.38
No neoadjuvant	1.14 (0.41–1.14)	.80
Multivariate analysis		
Tumor size (< 2 cm vs. ≥ 2 cm)	2.10 (1.06–4.16)	**.03**
Grade (low vs. high)	1.83 (1.10–3.06)	**.02**

Abbreviations: PDAC, pancreatic ductal adenocarcinoma; VS, versus;
SD standard deviation, *LVI* lymphovascular invasion;
LN lymph node, *PNI* perineural invasion
Bold: Statistically significant

predominant nuclear staining in the gallbladder epithelium (Fig. 1b), in contrast to a predominant cytoplasmic staining in non-neoplastic intrahepatic ductal and extrahepatic ductal epithelium (Fig. 1c).

Morphological variation of primary and metastatic PDAC

In a previous study, Kim et al. reported that HNF-1B was strongly expressed in PDAC with cytoplasmic clearing and only weakly to moderately expressed in PDAC with conventional histomorphology.[18] We reviewed the morphology specifically the cytoplasmic clearing for all the PDAC cases in this cohort and separated them into 3 categories: 1) Conventional- if > 95% of tumors cells demonstrated no cytoplasmic clearing (Fig. 2a); 2) Prominent clearing- if > 75% tumor cells demonstrated cytoplasmic clearing (Fig. 2b); and 3) mixed features- if 5–75% tumor cells demonstrated cytoplasmic clearing (Fig. 2c). Among the 127 primary PDACs, 84 cases (66.1%) were conventional PDAC, and 43 cases (33.9%) showed variable cytoplasmic clearing in the tumor cells, including 10 cases (7.9%) with prominent clearing, and 33 cases (26%) with mixed features. In 17 metastatic PDACs, 1 case showed prominent cytoplasmic clearing, 2 cases had mixed features, and the remaining showed conventional morphology.

Variable expression pattern of HNF-1B in primary and metastatic PDAC

Although HNF-1B was characterized as a nuclear transcription factor, HNF-1B was expressed in a total of 107 (84.3%) PDACs with multiple staining patterns, including

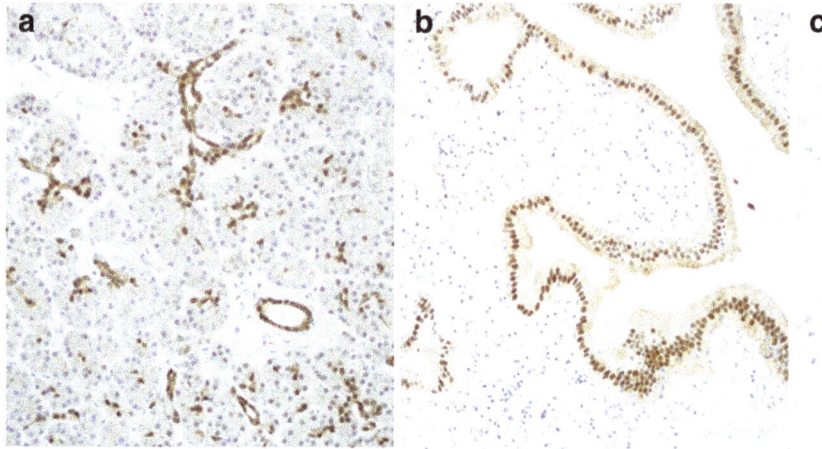

Fig. 1 HNF-1B expression pattern by IHC in non-neoplastic pancreaticobiliary epithelium, including (**a**) Pancreas, (**b**) Gallbladder, and (**c**) intrahepatic bile duct. Original magnification, 200×

cytoplasmic staining in 64 (59.8%) cases (Fig. 3a), nuclear staining in 32 (29.9%) cases (Fig. 3b), nuclear and cytoplasmic staining in 6 (5.6%) cases (Fig. 3c), and cytoplasmic and membranous staining in 5 (4.7%) cases (Fig. 3d). Among the 107 HNF-1B positive PDAC cases, 90 cases (70.9%) showed strong staining, while 17 (13.4%) showed weak staining pattern. There was no significant association of HNF-1B staining pattern or intensity with cytoplasmic clearing of the tumor cells.

Sixteen of 17 (94.1%) metastatic PDACs were positive for HNF-1B, including 13 cases (76.5%) with strong staining and 3 cases (17.6%) showed weak staining. Interestingly, 12 metastatic PDACs (70.6%) showed predominantly nuclear immunoreactivity with or without cytoplasmic staining (Fig. 3e, f).

HNF-1B expression in non-pancreatic carcinomas

In order to investigate whether HNF-1B protein expression was restricted to the adenocarcinomas of pancreatic ductal origin, HNF-1B IHC was performed on a total of 278 common carcinomas from other organ systems,

including cholangiocarcinoma (intrahepatic and extrahepatic biliary tracts), ampullary region, gallbladder, colorectum, distal esophagus, stomach, hepatocellular, lung adenocarcinoma, lung squamous cell carcinoma, breast, prostate, ovary, uterus, bladder urothelial, and kidney.

Not surprisingly, HNF-1B was strongly immunoreactive with nuclear and/or cytoplasmic patterns in 13 of 15 (86.7%) intrahepatic and extrahepatic cholangiocarcinomas, 13 of 18 (72.2%) ampullary adenocarcinomas, and 13 of 14 (92.9%) gallbladder adenocarcinomas. In addition, strong nuclear immunoreactivity of HNF-1B was observed in 16 of 21 (76.1%) clear cell carcinomas of the kidney, 10 of 14 (71.4%) ovarian clear cell carcinomas, 6 of 24 (25%) lung adenocarcinomas, and 4 of 15 (26.7%) prostate adenocarcinomas. Weak nuclear with or without cytoplasmic HNF-1B expression was seen in 3 of 11 (27.3%) esophageal adenocarcinomas, 9 of 14 (64.3%) stomach adenocarcinomas, 7 of 18 bladder urothelial (38.9%), and 10 of 21 (42.8%) non-clear cell type Müllerian carcinomas. HNF-1B was completely negative in all colorectal cancer, breast cancer, hepatocellular carcinoma, and lung squamous cell

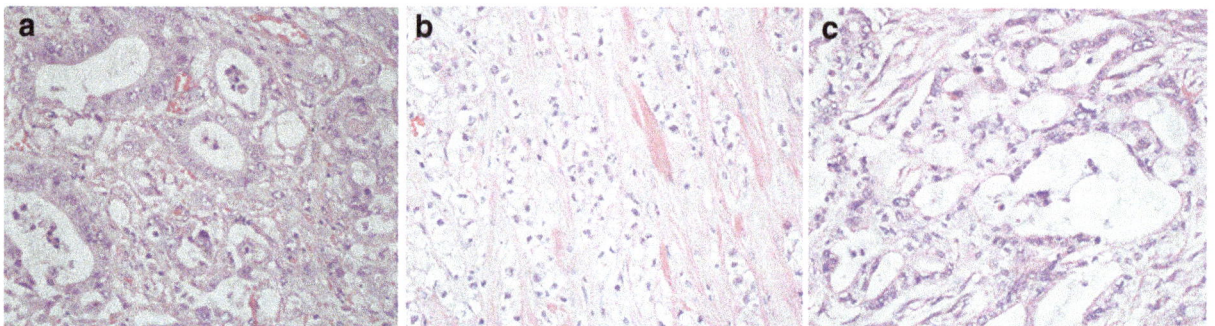

Fig. 2 Histomorphological variation of PDAC on hematoxylin and eosin (HE) staining, including (**a**) conventional, (**b**) clear cell variant, and (**c**) mixed features. Original magnification, 400×

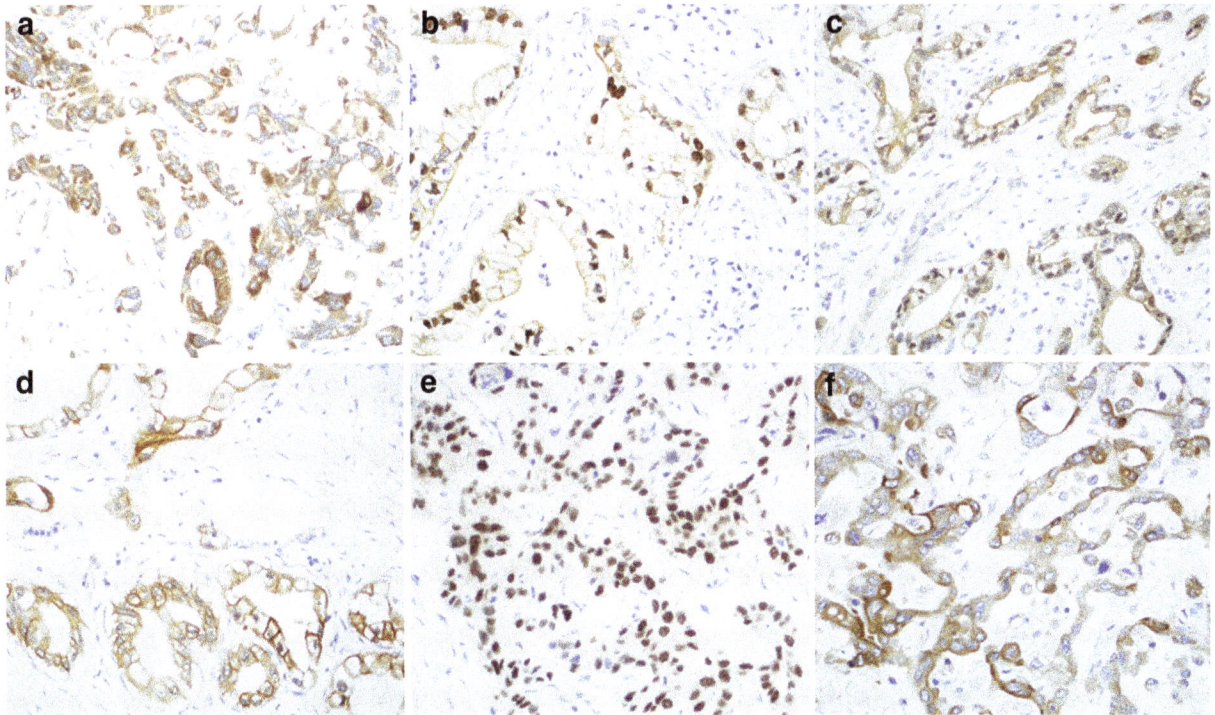

Fig. 3 Variable expression pattern of HNF-1B by IHC in primary and metastatic PDACs. (**a**) Primary PDAC with cytoplasmic staining, (**b**) Primary PDAC with nuclear staining, (**c**) Primary PDAC with nuclear and cytoplasmic staining, (**d**) Primary PDAC with cytoplasmic and membranous staining, (**e**) Metastatic PDAC with nuclear staining, and (**f**) Metastatic PDAC with cytoplasmic staining. Original magnification, 400×

Table 3 Immunoreactivity of HNF-1B in PDAC and non-pancreatic carcinomas

Cancer type	Total No.	HNF-1B +	Stain pattern	Fisher's exact p-value
Pancreatic primary	127	107 (84.3%)	C, N, M	ref
Cholangiocarcinoma	15	13 (86.7%)	C, N, M	.81
Ampullary	18	13 (72%)	C, N, M	.21
Gallbladder	14	13 (92.9%)	C, N, M	.69
Colorectal	39	0	–	<.001
Hepatocellular	20	0	–	<.001
Esophagus	11	3 (27.3%)	C, N	<.001
Stomach	14	9 (64.3%)	C, N	.13
Lung adenocarcinoma	24	6 (25%)	C, N	<.001
Lung Squamous cell	10	0	–	<.001
Breast	20	0	–	<.001
Bladder	18	7 (38.9%)	C, N	<.001
Prostate	15	4 (26.7%)	C, N	<.001
Kidney	21	16 (76.2%)	N	.35
Ovary	18	14 (77.8%)	N, C	.50
Uterus	21	10 (47.6%)	N, C	<.001
Metastatic PDAC	17	16 (94.1%)	N, C	
Total No.	422			

Abbreviations: PDAC, pancreatic ductal adenocarcinoma;
SCC squamous cell carcinoma, *C* cytoplasmic, *N* nuclear, *M* membranous

carcinoma (Table 3). Fisher's exact tests showed significantly lower HNF-1B expression rate in the colorectal, hepatocellular, esophageal, lung, breast, bladder, prostate, and uterine carcinomas ($P < .001$, Table 3).

Sensitivity and specificity of HNF-1B in pancreaticobiliary carcinomas

Since we observed that HNF-1B was expressed in the majority of carcinomas arising from the pancreatic and biliary epithelium, we calculated the sensitivity, specificity, positive predictive value, negative predictive value, and accuracy with 95% confidence interval (95% CI) of HNF-1B for all primary pancreaticobiliary carcinomas in comparison to non-pancreaticobiliary carcinomas. The results were summarized in Table 4. Overall, HNF-1B showed high sensitivity (84%) and high negative predictive value (85%) for primary pancreaticobiliary carcinomas with moderate specificity and accuracy (68 and 75%, respectively).

Discussion

We investigated the protein expression pattern of HNF-1B in 127 primary PDACs, 47 biliary adenocarcinomas, 17 metastatic PDACs, and 231 other common carcinomas that may mimic PDAC. HNF-1B was highly expressed in adenocarcinomas along the pancreaticobiliary tract, including PDAC, intrahepatic and extrahepatic cholangiocarcinomas, ampullary adenocarcinomas, and gallbladder adenocarcinomas with nuclear and/or cytoplasmic staining pattern. Importantly, HNF-1B expression was expressed in 94.1% of metastatic PDAC with predominantly nuclear staining.

KRAS mutation is a frequent molecular abnormality that is identified in up to 90% of PDACs [20]. Interestingly, a recent study showed that mutated KRAS can induce abnormal regulations of pancreatic transcription factors including HNF-1B, which in turn causes abnormal cell growth and proliferation that leads to pancreatic cancer [21]. These findings were consistent with the fundamental pathophysiological role of HNF-1B in the pancreaticobiliary system. The other group has also reported cytoplasmic and/or nuclear expression of HNF-1B in PDAC [18]. Although transcription factors are translated in the cytoplasm, they are generally translocated into the nucleus to regulate downstream target genes in active physiological state. During inactive regulation or with aberrantly excessive expression, transcription factors may form complex with other proteins and remain in the cytoplasm and/or cell membrane. This might explain why HNF-1B showed variable nuclear, cytoplasmic and/or membranous staining patterns in PDAC and other carcinomas.

Among non-pancreaticobiliary carcinomas, clear cell carcinomas of the kidney showed predominantly nuclear HNF-1B expression, while Müllerian origin, including ovarian and endometrial clear cell carcinoma showed nuclear and/or cytoplasmic HNF-1B expression. The expression of HNF-1B in carcinomas of kidney and Müllerian origin also indicates its pathophysiological role in these organs. Interestingly, silencing of HNF-1B expression secondary to promoter methylation appears to promote disease progression via epithelial-to-mesenchymal transition in both prostate and ovarian cancers [22]. In contrast to the association of HNF-1B with poor prognosis in PDAC observed by Kim et al. [18], HNF-1B seemed to have tumor-suppressor role in both prostate and kidney cancers [22, 23]. Thus, a biological role(s) of HNF-1B as well as the significance of its aberrant cytoplasmic and membranous expressions in different types of cancer needs to be investigated in the future.

Conclusions

Our data suggested that HNF-1B may serve as a useful diagnostic biomarker for tumors of the pancreaticobiliary origin with high sensitivity and negative predictive value, but moderate specificity and accuracy for these tumors. Since HNF-1B can also be expressed less frequently in variable tumors of the non-pancreaticobiliary origin, especially of the kidney, Müllerian tract, lung, gastroesophageal, bladder, and prostate carcinomas, the concurrent use of other markers such as TTF-1, PAX-8, WT-1, CAIX, NKX3.1, p40, and PSA as a panel to rule out other organ primaries, and correlation with imaging studies and/or endoscopic findings are important to refine the diagnosis.

Table 4 Sensitivity and specificity of HNF-1B in pancreaticobiliary carcinomas

Measure	Proportion	95% CI
Sensitivity	0.84	(0.79, 0.90)
Specificity	0.68	(0.62, 0.74)
Positive Predictive Value	0.66	(0.60, 0.73)
Negative Predictive Value	0.85	(0.80, 0.90)
Accuracy	0.75	(0.71, 0.79)

Abbreviation: *CI* confidence interval

Abbreviations
CAIX: Carbonic anhydrase 9; FFPE: Formalin fixed paraffin embedded; HE: Hematoxylin and eosin; HNF-1B: Hepatocyte nuclear factor 1B; IHC: Immunohistochemistry; MODY: Maturity-onset diabetes of the young; NKX3.1: NK3 Homeobox 1; PAX-8: Paired box gene 8; PDAC: Pancreatic ductal adenocarcinoma; PSA: Prostate specific antigen; SD: Standard deviation; TMA: Tissue microarray; TTF-1: Thyroid transcription factor 1; WT-1: Wilms' tumor 1

Acknowledgements
We are very grateful for the technical support from Valerie M Cortright, Jeannette M Mitchell, and Alexa Buskey of the Department of Pathology and Laboratory Medicine, University of Vermont Medical Center, Burlington, VT 05401.

Funding

This work was supported by funding from the University of Vermont Medical Group Research Award to M.X.Y for the proposal entitled "delineating tumors of pancreatic origin" (MG171).

Authors' contributions

MXY initiated the design of this project. AA, AG, YG, RZ, JGL, and MMK all participated in the design of this study. RFC collected clinical data. JS performed the statistics. MXY and RFC interpreted the protein expression and wrote the manuscript. All authors read, revised and approved the final manuscript.

Competing interests

The authors declare that they have no competing interests.

Author details

[1]Department of Pathology and Laboratory Medicine, University of Vermont Medical Center, 111 Colchester Avenue, Burlington, VT, USA. [2]Gastroenterology, University of Vermont Medical Center, 111 Colchester Avenue, Burlington, VT, USA. [3]Department of Gastrointestinal Surgery, Nanjing Medical University affiliated Changzhou 2nd People's Hospital, Changzhou, Jiangsu, China. [4]University of Vermont Medical Biostatistics Department, Burlington, VT, USA. [5]Applied Pathology Systems, Worcester, MA, USA. [6]Department of Pathology, Massachusetts General Hospital, Boston, MA, USA. [7]Present address: Department of Pathology, University of Massachusetts Medical Center, 1 Innovation Drive, Worcester, MA 01605, USA.

References

1. Siegel RD, Naishadham D, Jemal A. Cancer statistics, 2012. CA Cancer J Clin. 2012;62(1):10–29.
2. Yu J, Blackford AL, Molin MD, Wolfgang CL, Goggins M. Time to progression of pancreatic ductal adenocarcinoma from low-to-high tumour stages. Gut. 2015;64(11):1783–9.
3. Malaguarnera G, Giordano M, Paladina I, et al. Markers of bile duct tumors. World J Gastrointest Oncol. 2011;3(4):49–59.
4. Lin F, Chen ZE, Wang HL. Utility of immunohistochemistry in the pancreatobiliary tract. Arch Pathol Lab Med. 2015;139(1):24–38.
5. Bach I, Mattei MG, Cereghini S, Yaniv M. Two members of an HNF1 homeoprotein family are expressed in human liver. Nucleic Acids Res. 1991; 19(13):3553–9.
6. Cereghini S, Ott MO, Power S, Maury M. Expression patterns of vHNF1 and HNF1 homeoproteins in early postimplantation embryos suggest distinct and sequential developmental roles. Development. 1992;116(3):783–97.
7. Reichert M, Rustgi AK. Pancreatic ductal cells in development, regeneration, and neoplasia. J Clin Invest. 2011;121(12):4572–8.
8. Haumaitre C, Barbacci E, Jenny M, Ott MO, Gradwohl G, Cereghini S. Lack of TCF2/vHNF1 in mice leads to pancreas agenesis. Proc Natl Acad Sci U S A. 2005;102(5):1490–5.
9. De Vas MG, Kopp JL, Heloit C, Sander M, Cereghini S, Haumaitre C. Hnf1b controls pancreas morphogenesis and the generation of Ngn3+ endocrine progenitors. Development. 2015;142(5):871–82.
10. Body-Bechou D, Loget P, D'Herve D, et al. TCF2/HNF-1beta mutations: 3 cases of fetal severe pancreatic agenesis or hypoplasia and multicystic renal dysplasia. Prenat Diagn. 2014;34(1):90–3.
11. Haumaitre C, Fabre M, Cormier S, Baumann C, Delezoide AL, Cereghini S. Severe pancreas hypoplasia and multicystic renal dysplasia in two human fetuses carrying novel HNF1beta/MODY5 mutations. Hum Mol Genet. 2006; 15(15):2363–75.
12. Kitanaka S, Miki Y, Hayachi Y, Igarashi T. Promoter-specific repression of hepatocyte nuclear factor (HNF)-1 beta and HNF-1 alpha transcriptional activity by an HNF-1 beta missense mutant associated with type 5 maturity-onset diabetes of the young with hepatic and biliary manifestations. J Clin Endocrinol Metab. 2004;89(3):1369–78.
13. Haldorsen IS, Vesterhus M, Raeder H, et al. Lack of pancreatic body and tail in HNF1B mutation carriers. Diabet Med. 2008;25(7):782–7.
14. Teo AK, Lau HH, Valdez IA, et al. Early developmental perturbations in a human stem cell model of MODY5/HNF1B pancreatic hypoplasia. Stem Cell Reports. 2016;6(3):357–67.
15. Tsuchiya A, Sakamoto M, Yasuda J, et al. Expression profiling in ovarian clear cell carcinoma: identification of hepatocyte nuclear factor-1 beta as a molecular marker and a possible molecular target for therapy of ovarian clear cell carcinoma. Am J Pathol. 2003;163(6):2503–12.
16. Huang W, Cheng XM, Ji J, Zhang J, Li Q. The application value of HNF-1beta transcription factor in the diagnosis of ovarian clear cell carcinoma. Int J Gynecol Pathol. 2016;35(1):66–71.
17. Kato N, Sasou S, Motoyama T. Expression of hepatocyte nuclear factor-1beta (HNF- 1beta) in clear cell tumors and endometriosis of the ovary. Mod Pathol. 2006;19(1):83–9.
18. Kim L, Liao J, Zhang M, et al. Clear cell carcinoma of the pancreas: histopathologic features and a unique biomarker: hepatocyte nuclear factor-1beta. Mod Pathol. 2008;21(9):1075–83.
19. Edge SB, Compton CC. The American joint committee on Cancer: the 7th edition of the AJCC cancer staging manual and the future of TNM. Ann Surg Oncol. 2010;17(6):1471–4.
20. Miglio U, Oldani A, Mezzapelle R, et al. KRAS mutational analysis in ductal adenocarcinoma of the pancreas and its clinical significance. Pathol Res Pract. 2014;210(5):307–11.
21. Naqvi AAT, Hasan GM, Hassan MI. Investigating the role of transcription factors of pancreas development in pancreatic cancer. Pancreatology. 2018; 18(2):184–90.
22. Ross-Adams H, Ball S, Lawrenson K, et al. HNF1B variants associate with promoter methylation and regulate gene networks activated in prostate and ovarian cancer. Oncotarget. 2016;7(46):74734–46.
23. Buchner A, Castro M, Hennig A, et al. Downregulation of HNF-1B in renal cell carcinoma is associated with tumor progression and poor prognosis. Urology. 2010;76(2):507 e6–11.

19

Comparative analysis of cerebrospinal fluid metabolites in Alzheimer's disease and idiopathic normal pressure hydrocephalus in a Japanese cohort

Yuki Nagata[1]* , Akiyoshi Hirayama[2], Satsuki Ikeda[2], Aoi Shirahata[2], Futaba Shoji[2], Midori Maruyama[2], Mitsunori Kayano[3], Masahiko Bundo[4], Kotaro Hattori[5], Sumiko Yoshida[5], Yu-ichi Goto[5], Katsuya Urakami[6], Tomoyoshi Soga[2], Kouichi Ozaki[1] and Shumpei Niida[1]

Abstract

Background: Alzheimer's disease (AD) is a most common dementia in elderly people. Since AD symptoms resemble those of other neurodegenerative diseases, including idiopathic normal pressure hydrocephalus (iNPH), it is difficult to distinguish AD from iNPH for a precise and early diagnosis. iNPH is caused by the accumulation of cerebrospinal fluid (CSF) and involves gait disturbance, urinary incontinence, and dementia. iNPH is treatable with shunt operation which removes accumulated CSF from the brain ventricles.

Methods: We performed metabolomic analysis in the CSF of patients with AD and iNPH with capillary electrophoresis-mass spectrometry. We assessed metabolites to discriminate between AD and iNPH with Welch's t-test, receiver operating characteristic (ROC) curve analysis, and multiple logistic regression analysis.

Results: We found significant increased levels of glycerate and N-acetylneuraminate and significant decreased levels of serine and 2-hydroxybutyrate in the CSF of patients with AD compared to the CSF of patients with iNPH. The ROC curve analysis with these four metabolites showed that the area under the ROC curve was 0.90, indicating good discrimination between AD and iNPH.

Conclusions: This study identified four metabolites that could possibly discriminate between AD and iNPH, which previous research has shown are closely related to the risk factors, pathogenesis, and symptoms of AD. Analyzing pathway-specific metabolites in the CSF of patients with AD may further elucidate the mechanism and pathogenesis of AD.

Keywords: Alzheimer's disease, Idiopathic normal pressure hydrocephalus, Diagnostic marker, Cerebrospinal fluid, Serine, Glycerate, N-acetylneuraminate, 2-hydroxybutyrate

Background

Alzheimer's disease (AD) is the most common type of dementia in the world, which concerns approximately 60–70% cases of dementia, and it is becoming a significant social issue because of the growing aging population.

In general, AD is diagnosed based on the presence of cognitive impairment and by neuropsychological testing according to the National Institute of Neurological and Communicative Disorders and Stroke and the Alzheimer's Disease and Related Disorders Association criteria [1]. Currently, there is no curative or radical treatment for AD, although some medicines have been developed to reduce the symptoms [2]. However, some symptoms of AD are similar to those of other neurodegenerative diseases, such as idiopathic normal pressure hydrocephalus (iNPH). iNPH is caused by the accumulation of cerebrospinal fluid (CSF) in the brain and causes gait disturbance, urinary incontinence, and dementia. In

* Correspondence: nagata@ncgg.go.jp
[1]Medical Genome Center, National Center for Geriatrics and Gerontology, 7-430 Morioka-cho, Obu, Aichi 474-8511, Japan
Full list of author information is available at the end of the article

contrast to other dementias, iNPH is treatable by shunt operation that removes the accumulated CSF [3]. Therefore, a precise diagnosis that discriminates patients with AD from patients with iNPH is essential for proper treatment at the early stages of these diseases. Presently, increased phosphate tau (p-tau) and decreased amyloid-beta 1-42 (Aβ42) in the CSF are used as established AD diagnostic markers [4]. However, p-tau accumulates after synaptic degeneration and Aβ42 is difficult to accurately quantify. Therefore, we tried to find additional biomarkers, capable of precisely detecting AD before neurodegeneration progresses.

Recently, accumulated evidence has indicated that AD is a type of metabolic disease in the brain [5, 6]. The brain is the most energy-consuming organ and glucose is an essential and dominant energy source for the brain [7]. Progressive regional cerebral glucose metabolism reduction, correlated with the symptom severity, has been found in the brain of patients with AD [8, 9]. Mills et al. (2013) performed RNA-Seq analysis in the parietal cortex of patients with AD and reported that two enzymes, ACOT1 and ACOT2, which are involved in lipid metabolism, were upregulated. They also found a downregulation of TERC, which is involved in the synthesis of very long chain fatty acids [10]. In addition, impairment of the insulin response, as is seen in diabetes mellitus and metabolic syndrome, was revealed as a risk factor for AD [11–13]. These reports suggested that the pathomechanism of AD is strongly related to a disturbance in brain energy metabolism and homeostasis. The disturbance could induce metabolite alterations in the body fluids of patients with AD, such as in the plasma, serum, and CSF. Therefore, metabolome analysis of body fluids in AD has been actively performed to identify new diagnostic markers. Especially, the CSF is thought to be a superior analyte than other body fluids because it is in direct contact with the extracellular space of the brain and thus directly reflects the biological changes in the pathological brain processes in AD.

So far, several pertinent reports have been published and several diagnostic markers for AD have been suggested. For example, D' Aniello et al. (2005) conducted high performance liquid chromatography (HPLC) analysis and found L-glutamine was increased and L-asparate was decreased in the CSF of patients with AD than in the CSF of controls [14]. Czech et al. (2012) reported that increased cysteine with decreased uridine was the optimal combination to identify mild AD, and increased cortisol levels were associated with the progression of AD in a European cohort [15]. Ibanez et al. (2012) performed capillary electrophoresis-mass spectrometry (CE-MS) to investigate metabolome changes in the CSF of patients

at different AD stages and found that choline, dimethylarginine, arginine, valine, proline, serine, histidine, creatine, carnitine, and suberylglycine could be possible disease progression markers [16]. Furthermore, they conducted ultra-high-performance liquid chromatography-time-of-flight mass spectrometry (TOFMS) and found uracil and uridine were good candidate biomarkers for AD, as has been previously described [15, 17].

However, different metabolomic platforms and methods detect different metabolites, thus utilizing multiple types of metabolomic platforms would provide a wider perspective of metabolomics information under study. In addition, differences in ethnicity, culture, and education may influence decision making regarding the diagnosis, symptoms, and severity of AD [18]. Accordingly, accumulating information related to AD pathology from differential ethnoracial cohorts and with differential methods is essential.

From these points of view, we performed metabolomic analysis of the CSF of patients with AD or iNPH in Japanese cohorts with capillary electrophoresis-TOFMS (CE-TOFMS). Our present findings would support the utility of metabolomics analysis for discriminate between AD and iNPH.

Methods

Subjects

The characteristics of the study patients with AD and iNPH are summarized in Table 1. AD and iNPH were diagnosed according to previously published criteria [1, 19]. Bioresources were largely obtained from the biobank of the National Center for Geriatrics and Gerontology (NCGG, Aichi, Japan) and partly donated by the National Center of Neurology and Psychiatry (NCNP, Tokyo, Japan) and the Department of Biological Regulation, School of Medicine, Tottori University (Tottori, Japan). All samples were obtained with the written informed consent of the patients before sampling between 2011 and 2015. This study was reviewed and approved by the ethics committees of all participating institutes and biobanks.

Table 1 Subject characteristics.

	Metabolomics		Validation	
	AD	iNPH	AD	iNPH
Subject No.	39	19	42	38
Mean age (SD)	73.5 (9.8)	77.8 (4.5)	74.1 (9.6)	77.9 (5.6)
Age range	47-86	70-86	47-86	57-87
P-value	0.03		0.03	
Male/female	14/25	9/10	15/27	22/16
P-value	0.24		0.09	
Mean MMSE (SD)	21.4 (5.1)	23.5 (2.9)	21.2 (5.0)	22.1 (3.1)
P-value	0.08		0.46	
Missing values	6	0	6	0

Collection of CSF

CSF was collected by lumbar puncture and centrifuged to remove debris. The supernatant was aliquoted into low protein-binding tubes and immediately frozen in liquid nitrogen and stored at −80 °C until use.

Measurement of p-tau and Aβ42

To detect the concentration of *p*-tau and Aβ42 in the CSF, the enzyme-linked immunosorbent assay systems of INNOTEST β-AMYLOID$_{(1-42)}$ and INNOTEST PHOSPHO-TAU$_{(181P)}$ were used according to the manufacturer's instructions (Fujibireo Inc., Tokyo, Japan).

Metabolites extraction from CSF

Frozen CSF samples were thawed and 40 μL aliquots were placed into 360 μL of methanol containing internal standards (20 μmol/L each of methionine sulfone and D-camphor-10-sulfonic acid). The solutions were thoroughly mixed, and then both 400 μL of chloroform and 160 μL of Milli-Q water were added, followed by centrifugation at 10,000 × *g* for 3 min at 4 °C. The aqueous layer was transferred to a 5-kDa-cutoff filter (Human Metabolome Technologies, Tsuruoka, Japan) to remove proteins. The filtrate was dried using a centrifuge concentrator and reconstituted with 50 μL of Milli-Q water containing reference compounds (200 μmol/L each of 3-aminopyrrolidine and trimesic acid) prior to CE-TOFMS analysis.

Metabolome analysis by CE-TOFMS

All CE-TOFMS experiments were performed using an Agilent 1600 Capillary Electrophoresis system (Agilent technologies, Santa Clara, CA), an Agilent 6220 TOF LC/MS system, an Agilent 1200 series isocratic HPLC pump, a G1603A Agilent CE-MS adapter kit, and a G1607A Agilent CE-electrospray ionization (ESI)-MS sprayer kit. In the anionic metabolites analysis, ESI sprayer was replaced with a platinum needle instead of the initial stainless steel needle [20]. The other conditions relating to the CE-ESI-MS sprayer were identical as received. For CE-MS system control and data acquisition, we used the Agilent MassHunter software.

Cationic metabolome analysis

For cationic metabolome analysis, a fused-silica capillary (50 μm i.d. × 100 cm) filled with 1 mol/L formic acid as the electrolyte was used [21]. A new capillary was flushed with the electrolyte for 20 min, and the capillary was equilibrated for 4 min by flushing with the electrolyte before each run. Sample solution was injected at 5 kPa for 3 s and a positive voltage of 30 kV was applied. The temperatures of the capillary and sample trays were maintained at 20 °C and 4 °C, respectively. Methanol/water (50% *v/v*) containing 0.1 μmol/L hexakis(2,2-difluoroethoxy)phosphazene was

delivered as sheath liquid at 10 L/min. ESI-TOFMS was operated in the positive ion mode, and the capillary voltage was set at 4 kV. The flow rate of heated nitrogen gas (heater temperature, 300 °C) was maintained at 10 psig. In TOFMS, the fragmentor, skimmer, and Oct RF voltages were set at 75, 50, and 125 V, respectively. Automatic recalibration of each acquired spectrum was performed using the masses of reference standards ([^{13}C isotopic ion of protonated methanol dimer (2CH$_3$OH + H)]$^+$, *m/z* 66.06306) and ([hexakis(2,2-difluoroethoxy)phosphazene + H]$^+$, *m/z* 622.02896). Exact mass data were acquired at the rate of 1.5 cycles/s over a 50 to 1000 *m/z* range.

Anionic metabolome analysis

For the anionic metabolome analysis, a COSMO(+) capillary (50 μm i.d. × 105 cm, Nacalai Tesque, Kyoto, Japan) filled with 50 mmol/L ammonium acetate (pH 8.5) as the electrolyte was used [20]. Before the first use, a new capillary was successively flushed with the electrolyte, 50 mmol/L acetic acid (pH 3.4), and then the electrolyte again for 10 min each. Before each run, the capillary was equilibrated by flushing with 50 mmol/L acetic acid (pH 3.4) for 2 min and then with the electrolyte for 5 min. Sample was injected at 5 kPa for 30 s and a negative voltage of 30 kV was applied. The temperatures of the capillary and sample trays were maintained at 20 °C and 4 °C, respectively. Ammonium acetate (5 mmol/L) in 50% (*v/v*) methanol/water solution that contained 0.1 μmol/L hexakis(2,2-difluoroethoxy)phosphazene was delivered as sheath liquid at 10 μL/min. ESI-TOFMS was operated in the negative ion mode, and the capillary voltage was set at 3.5 kV. The flow rate of heated nitrogen gas (heater temperature, 300 °C) was maintained at 10 psig. In TOFMS, the fragmentor, skimmer, and Oct RF voltages were set at 100, 50, and 200 V, respectively. Automatic recalibration of each acquired spectrum was performed using the masses of reference standards ([^{13}C isotopic ion of deprotonated acetate dimer (2CH$_3$COOH − H)]$^-$, *m/z* 120.03841) and ([hexakis(2,2-difluoroethoxy)phosphazene + deprotonated acetate(CH$_3$COOH − H)]$^-$, *m/z* 680.03554). Exact mass data were acquired at the rate of 1.5 cycles/s over a 50 to 1000 *m/z* range.

Statistical analyses

Comprehensive metabolic data were processed using our proprietary software (MasterHands) [22–24]. The peaks were identified by matching *m/z* values and normalized migration times of corresponding authentic standard compounds. Statistical analysis was performed using Welch's *t*-test, receiver operating characteristic (ROC) curve analysis, and Pearson's correlation analysis in R version 3.3.2 (2016-10-31) [25]. Multiple logistic regression analysis was performed with Statflex ver. 6 (Artech

Co., Ltd., Osaka, Japan). A *P*-value <0.05 was considered to be significant.

Results

First, we performed comprehensive metabolic analysis of the CSF to identify characteristic metabolites in the patients with AD and iNPH with the screening subjects indicated in Table 1 (column: Metabolomics). Eighty-three anionic and 60 cationic metabolites were detected in this analysis (Additional file 1). Among these, 18 metabolites showed a *P*-value <0.05 and an area under the ROC curve (AUC) > 0.7 between AD and iNPH with several missing values (Table 2). Therefore, to validate the concentration of these metabolites in the CSF of patients with AD and iNPH, we repeated CE-TOFMS with additional samples (Table 1, column: Validation). Undecanoate (PubChem ID: 8180) and N-acetylhistidine (PubChem ID: 273,260) were excluded from further analysis as false positives because they are not metabolized in the human brain [26]. Nine metabolites indicated *P*-value <0.05 and an AUC > 0.7 between AD and iNPH without missing values (Table 3). Of these metabolites, glycerate (PubChem ID: 752) and N-acetylneuraminate (Neu5Ac, PubChem ID: 3568) were

increased in the CSF of patients with AD than of patients with iNPH, while the other seven metabolites were decreased.

Next, we performed multiple logistic regression analysis with these nine metabolites, setting age as a covariate. Using stepwise regression, we found statistical significance for four metabolites, serine (PubChem ID: 617), glycerate, Neu5Ac, and 2-hydroxybutylate (2-HB, PubChem ID: 11,266) (Fig. 1 and Table 4). Formulation of the regression coefficient of these four metabolites was as follows; $(-0.1198) \times$ age $+ (-0.2508) \times$ serine $+ (0.05715) \times$ glycerate $+ (0.37226) \times$ Neu5Ac $+ (-0.1705) \times$ 2-HB $+ 12.3001$. When the cutoff value was set to 9.73, sensitivity and specificity were highest (Fig. 2, AUC = 0.90, sensitivity = 0.86, specificity = 0.84, and the odds ratio was 32.0).

Further, we examined the correlation between *p*-tau, Aβ42, and these four metabolites. Correlation coefficient values were −0.33, 0.35, 0.55, and −0.27 between *p*-tau and serine, glycerate, Neu5Ac, and 2-HB, respectively, showing a weak to moderate correlation between *p*-tau and the four metabolites (Fig. 3). On the other hand, the correlation coefficients between Aβ42 and the four metabolites were 0.10, −0.35, 0.18, and 0.01 for serine, glycerate, Neu5Ac, and 2-HB, respectively, showing weak or absent correlations for the first three metabolites and a negative correlation for glycerate (Fig. 4).

Table 2 Statistically significant metabolites between AD and iNPH in the metabolomics

PubChem ID	Metabolite	Mean concentration, μmol/L (SD)				Welch's t-test	ROC	AD/iNPH	Valid value		Missing value	
		AD		iNPH		*P*-value	AUC	Fold change	AD	iNPH	AD	iNPH
752	Glycerate	60.61	(30.94)	26.23	(6.22)	6.E-07	0.88	2.31	32	16	7	3
1060	Pyruvate	45.22	(13.45)	68.34	(12.95)	1.E-04	0.89	0.66	12	16	27	3
3441	2-Oxoisopentanoate	4.29	(1.19)	5.64	(1.29)	0.001	0.78	0.76	30	19	9	0
3568	N-Acetylneuraminate	16.75	(3.89)	13.35	(3.2)	0.001	0.76	1.25	39	19	0	0
617	Serine	24.63	(3.9)	30.12	(6.15)	0.002	0.77	0.82	39	19	0	0
273,260	N-Acetylhistidine[a]	1.19	(0.88)	0.88	(0.92)	0.002	0.72	1.36	39	19	0	0
8180	Undecanoate[a]	0.54	(0.17)	0.71	(0.09)	0.003	0.81	0.76	17	7	22	12
3,527,278	4-Methyl-2-oxopentanoate	2.64	(0.85)	3.51	(0.98)	0.003	0.74	0.75	39	19	0	0
11,266	2-Hydroxybutyrate	18.08	(5.98)	23.14	(6.06)	0.005	0.74	0.78	39	19	0	0
525	Malate	1.17	(0.33)	1.54	(0.46)	0.005	0.73	0.76	39	19	0	0
602	Alanine	32.03	(8.53)	42.82	(14.42)	0.006	0.77	0.75	39	19	0	0
876	Methionine	2.79	(1.08)	3.67	(1.07)	0.006	0.76	0.76	39	19	0	0
205	Threonine	27.56	(6.43)	34.81	(9.53)	0.006	0.73	0.79	39	19	0	0
232	Arginine	23.08	(4.5)	26.79	(4.6)	0.006	0.71	0.86	39	19	0	0
64,969	3-Methylhistidine	1.12	(0.88)	1.81	(0.92)	0.010	0.79	0.62	39	19	0	0
1081	Citramalate	1.20	(0.96)	0.57	(0.12)	0.010	0.74	2.12	19	8	20	11
1175	Urate	20.84	(11.36)	30.61	(15.74)	0.023	0.73	0.68	39	19	0	0
866	Lysine	30.00	(5.84)	36.35	(10.66)	0.023	0.72	0.82	39	19	0	0

[a]Undecanoate and N-Acetylhistidine were excluded from further analysis
AD Alzheimer's disease, *iNPH* idiopathic normal pressure hydrocephalus, *AUC* area under the curve, *ROC* receiver operator characteristic

Table 3 Statistically significant metabolites between AD and iNPH in the validation

Metabolite	Mean concentration, μmol/L (SD)				Welch's t-test P-value[a]	ROC AUC	AD/iNPH Fold change
	AD		iNPH				
Serine	29.1	(5.3)	34.5	(4.9)	1.6E-04	0.78	0.84
Glycerate	54.6	(22.2)	37.3	(12.9)	2.0E-04	0.71	1.46
3-Methylhistidine	1.1	(0.9)	2.1	(1.2)	6.4E-04	0.82	0.52
Threonine	29.0	(7.0)	39.4	(12.9)	7.4E-04	0.77	0.74
Methionine	2.6	(1.0)	3.6	(1.2)	9.4E-04	0.77	0.71
Urate	19.9	(8.6)	28.7	(9.9)	1.3E-03	0.78	0.70
N-Acetylneuraminate	16.1	(3.9)	12.9	(3.2)	1.9E-03	0.75	1.25
Alanine	33.0	(8.4)	42.4	(12.6)	3.9E-03	0.73	0.78
2-Hydroxybutyrate	17.5	(4.6)	22.2	(6.7)	0.009	0.72	0.79

[a]Bonferroni correction was applied

AD Alzheimer's disease, *iNPH* idiopathic normal pressure hydrocephalus, *AUC* area under the curve, *ROC* receiver operator characteristic

When ROC curve analysis was performed between AD and iNPH with p-tau and Aβ42, the AUC values were 0.94 and 0.71 for p-tau and Aβ42, respectively (Fig. 5). These results indicate that these metabolites combined may have a discriminatory power equal to that of *p*-tau.

Discussion

We found the combination of four metabolites, serine, glycerate, Neu5Ac, and 2-HB could contribute to distinguishing AD from iNPH (Table 4, Fig. 2). We searched the KEGG Pathway Database [27] (http://www.genome.jp/

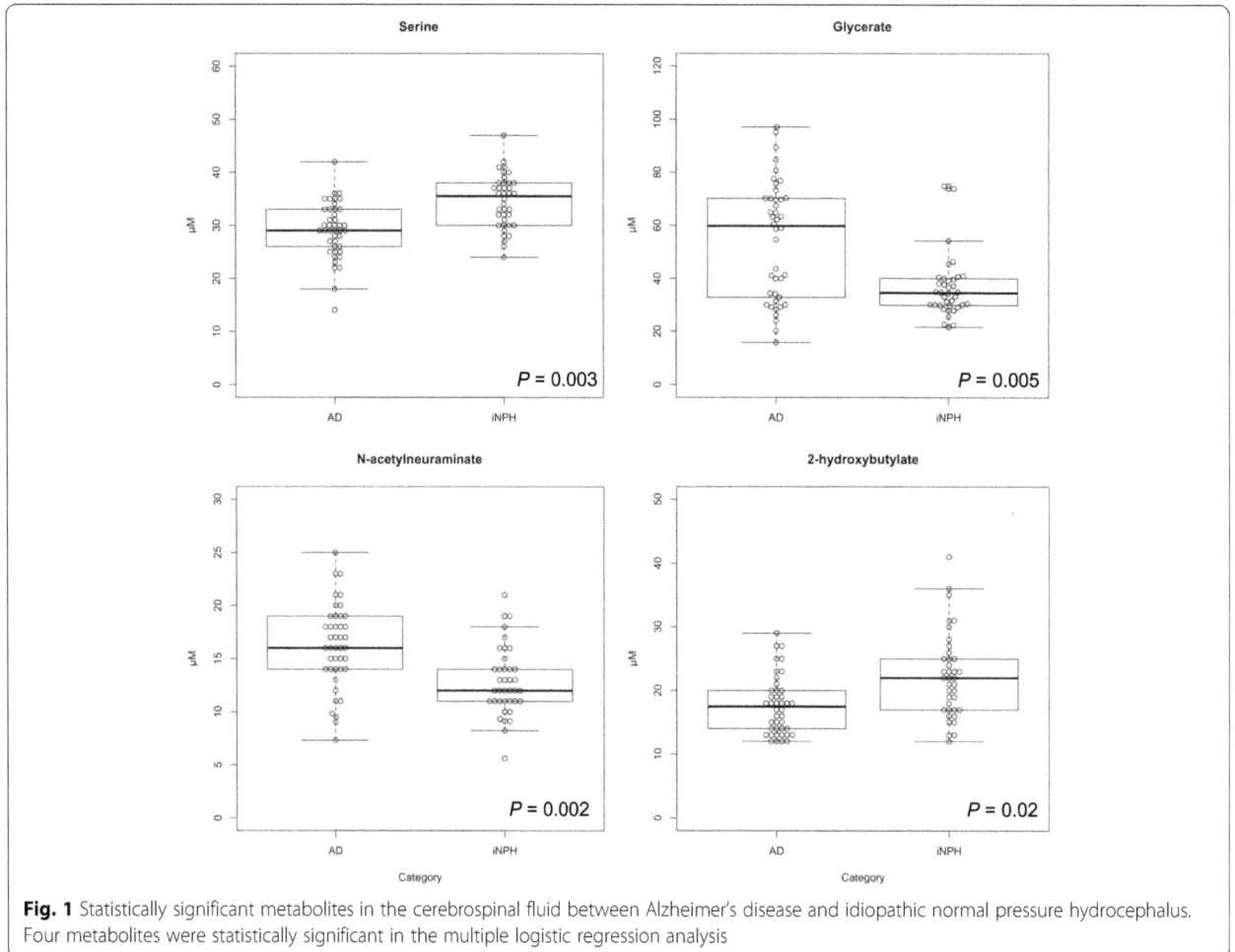

Fig. 1 Statistically significant metabolites in the cerebrospinal fluid between Alzheimer's disease and idiopathic normal pressure hydrocephalus. Four metabolites were statistically significant in the multiple logistic regression analysis

Table 4 Statistically significant metabolites in multiple logistic regression analysis

Metabolite	P-value	Odds ratio	CI 95%
Serine	0.002	0.78	0.66-0.91
Glycerate	0.009	1.06	1.01-1.10
N-Acetylneuraminate	0.003	1.45	1.14-1.85
2-Hydroxybutyrate	0.034	0.84	0.72-0.99

Age was used as a covariate

kegg/pathway.html) and found that glycerate is the intermediate metabolite in the pentose phosphate pathway (PPP, KEGG ID: map00030), amino acid metabolism (KEGG ID: map00260), and glycerolipid metabolism (KEGG ID: map00561) in humans.

PPP is one of the glucose metabolic pathways generating pentose and nicotinamide adenine dinucleotide phosphate (NADPH). NADPH has an antioxidant reducing activity and an important role in opposing oxidative stress [28]. In the brain of patients with AD, oxidative stress signatures are observed at the very early stage of the disease [29–31] and PPP is activated to provide NAPDH to counteract oxidative stress [32, 33]. In addition, in the state of hypoxia, which is reportedly a risk factor for AD [34], the PPP preferentially metabolizes glucose instead of the common glycolysis pathway [35], also suggesting the activation of PPP in the brain of patients with AD. Together, increased glycerate in the

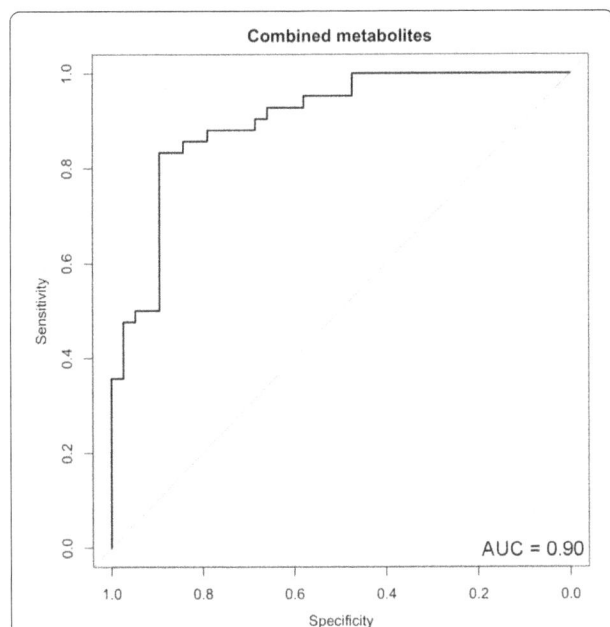

Fig. 2 Receiver operator characteristic (ROC) curve analysis of statistically significant metabolites in the cerebrospinal fluid between Alzheimer's disease (AD) and idiopathic normal pressure hydrocephalus (iNPH). ROC curve analysis was performed to compare the predictive power of AD and iNPH with the combined metabolites

CSF of patients with AD may reflect the activation of PPP to compensate for the failure in brain functions that accompany AD progression.

Glycerate is also generated in amino acid metabolism, glycine, serine, and threonine. Some reports have indicated alterations in amino acid metabolism in AD [36–38]. Especially, Madeira et al. reported increased levels of D-serine and total serine concentrations in the CSF of patients with AD [39]. They indicated that the amyloid beta oligomer activated serine racemase, an enzyme which converts L-serine to D-serine. In our study, although we did not detect D-serine sole concentration, total serine concentration was decreased in the patients with AD (Fig. 1). However, as we included patients with iNPH as controls, it is difficult to directly compare our results to those of the other studies, which included healthy individuals as controls. However, there is a report indicating phosphatidylserine synthase (PSS) was activated in the aging rat brain [40]. PSS incorporates serine into phosphatidylethanolamine or phosphatidylcholine and generates phosphatidylserine. As aging is a risk factor for AD [40] and phosphatidylserine administration improved several cognitive measures in AD [41], serine reduction in the CSF of patients with AD may reflect the neuroprotective role of PSS. Moreover, serine is converted to hydroxypyruvate by transamination, followed by conversion to glycerate by glycerate dehydrogenase [42]. Additionally, glycerate is generated in the serine degradation pathway [43, 44]. Therefore, increased glycerate and decreased serine in the CSF of patients with AD seem to be justifiable.

Another group indicated that there was no statistically significant difference in serine concentration between the CSF of patients with AD and that of controls [14, 45]. However, these studies were performed with relatively small sample sizes and amino acids concentration in the CSF seemingly influenced by the content of daily diet [46], further studies with larger sample sizes are needed to elucidate the relations between serine concentration in the CSF and AD.

Glycerate is also produced during glycerolipid metabolism. Malaisse et al. indicated that triglyceride species were increased in the brain tissue of Type II diabetic rats [47]. Type II diabetes is known as a risk factor for AD [48, 49] and AD is known as the Type III diabetes [50], suggesting glycerolipid metabolism accelerated in the AD brain and may result in the accumulation of glycerate in the CSF.

Other than glycerate, Neu5Ac was increased in the CSF of AD. Neu5Ac is the most abundant sialic acid in nature and a component of gangliosides [51]. Gangliosides are abundant in neural cell membranes and have important roles in the organization of lipid rafts [52]. Lipid rafts are

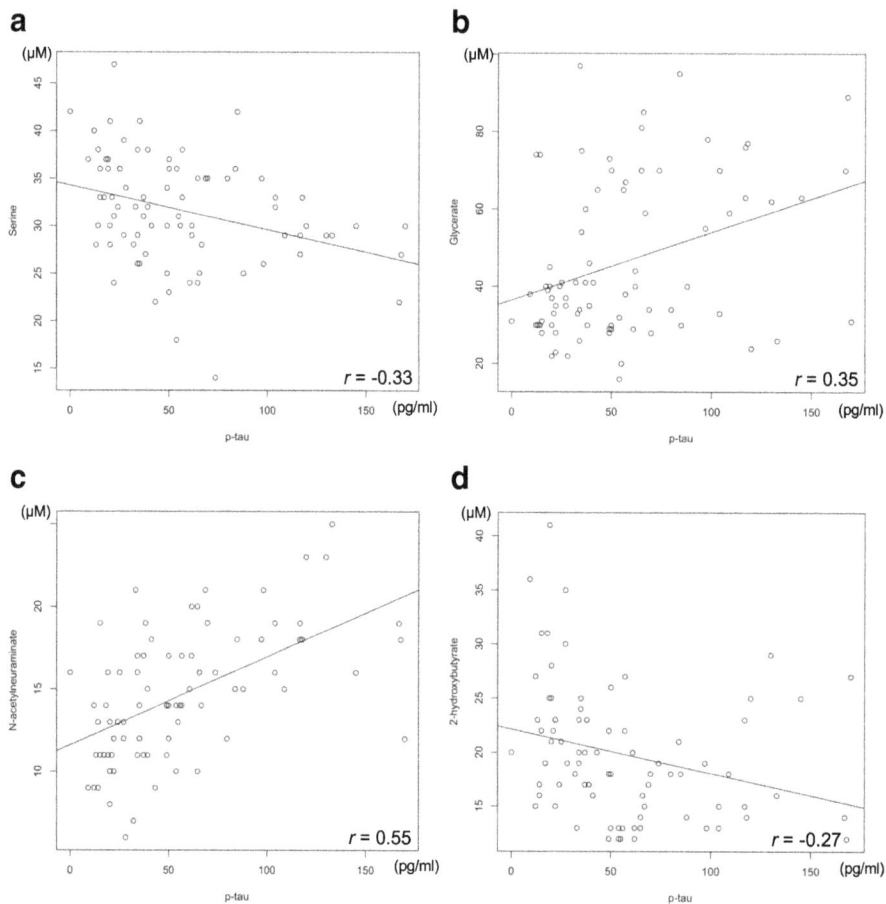

Fig. 3 Correlation diagram of p-tau versus the four metabolites. (**a**) serine, (**b**) glycerate, (**c**) Neu5Ac, and (**d**) 2-HB with regression lines are indicated

the subdomains of the plasma membrane that integrate numerous types of lipid proteins having important roles in cell signaling, cell-cell adhesion, and intracellular vesicular trafficking. There are some reports indicating that lipid rafts contain many types of AD associated proteins [53–56] and aberrations in the structure of the lipid rafts are considered to lead to AD [57]. Kracun et al. indicated that there was significant decrease of gangliosides in the brain of patients with AD and in the aging population, suggesting accelerated degradation of gangliosides accompanied by neuronal cell death [58]. Hence, the increased level of Neu5Ac in the CSF of patients with AD may reflect that neuronal and lipid raft destruction may accompany AD progression.

In this study, 2-HB was decreased in the CSF of patients with AD. 2-HB is derived from 2-ketobutyrate (2-KB) dehydration by lactate dehydrogenase (LDH) [59]. 2-KB is an important intermediate metabolite of amino acid metabolism, which is reportedly altered in AD [36–38]. In addition, in the brain of AD model mice, LDH expression was decreased [60], which may

result in decreased 2-HB production. Hence, the four metabolites detected in this study are likely related to AD risk factors, pathogenesis, and/or symptoms (Fig. 6). Also, all these metabolites are found at the first time as the AD related ones in the CSF.

The metabolites described here likely participate in several pathways; however, we could not find other statistically significant metabolites included in these pathways. Easily detectable metabolites differ from metabolomic platforms and methods; therefore, other metabolites participating in the pathways indicated here could not be detected in this study. Further analyses with several metabolomic platforms are needed to complement metabolomic information for AD.

Recently, fluorodeoxyglucose (FDG)-positron emission tomography (PET), which detects the cerebral metabolic rates of glucose, has been used to diagnose AD [61], indicating the usefulness of measuring metabolic pathways for diagnosing AD. Other than glucose metabolic rates, several studies have indicated numerous types of metabolic pathways to be influenced relatively early in AD progression [6, 12, 62]. However, it is still difficult to make a precise and early diagnosis for AD at present. To

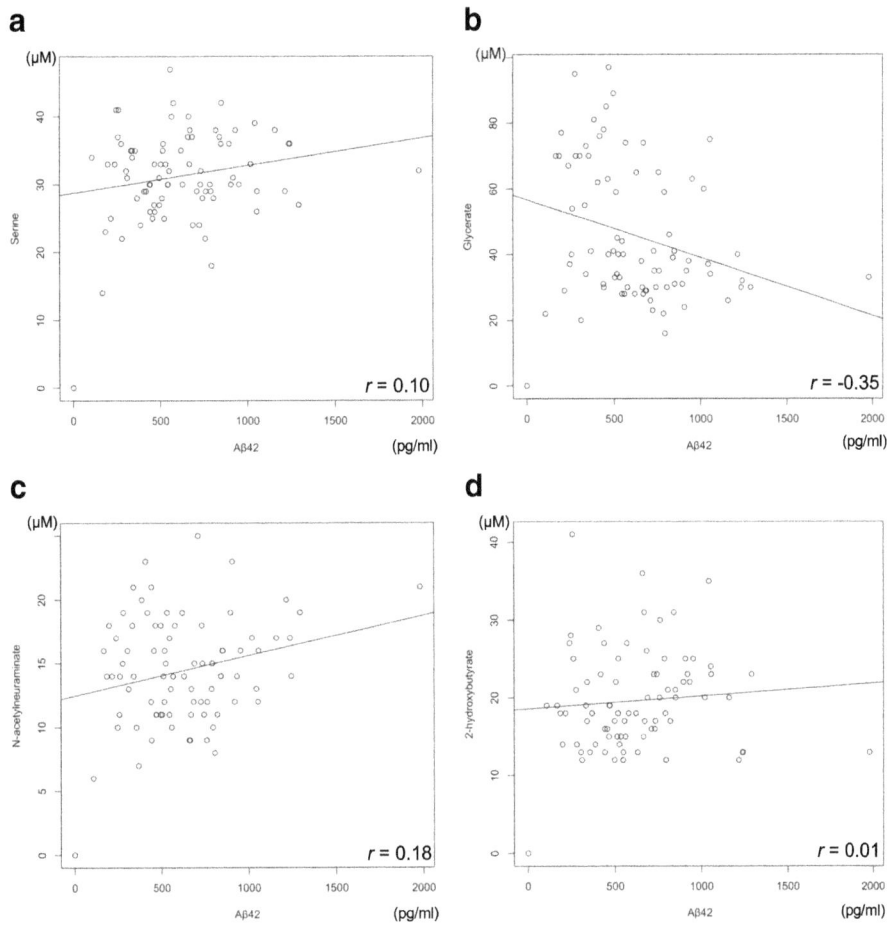

Fig. 4 Correlation diagram of Aβ42 versus the four metabolites. (**a**) serine, (**b**) glycerate, (**c**) Neu5Ac, and (**d**) 2-HB with regression lines are indicated

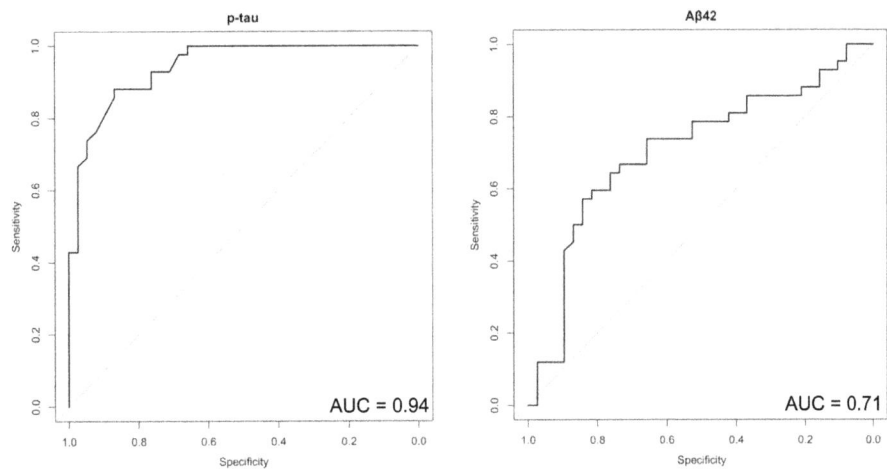

Fig. 5 Receiver operator characteristic (ROC) curve analysis of *p*-tau and Aβ42 in the cerebrospinal fluid between Alzheimer's disease and idiopathic normal pressure hydrocephalus. ROC curve analysis was performed to compare the predictive power of p-tau (left) and Aβ42 (right)

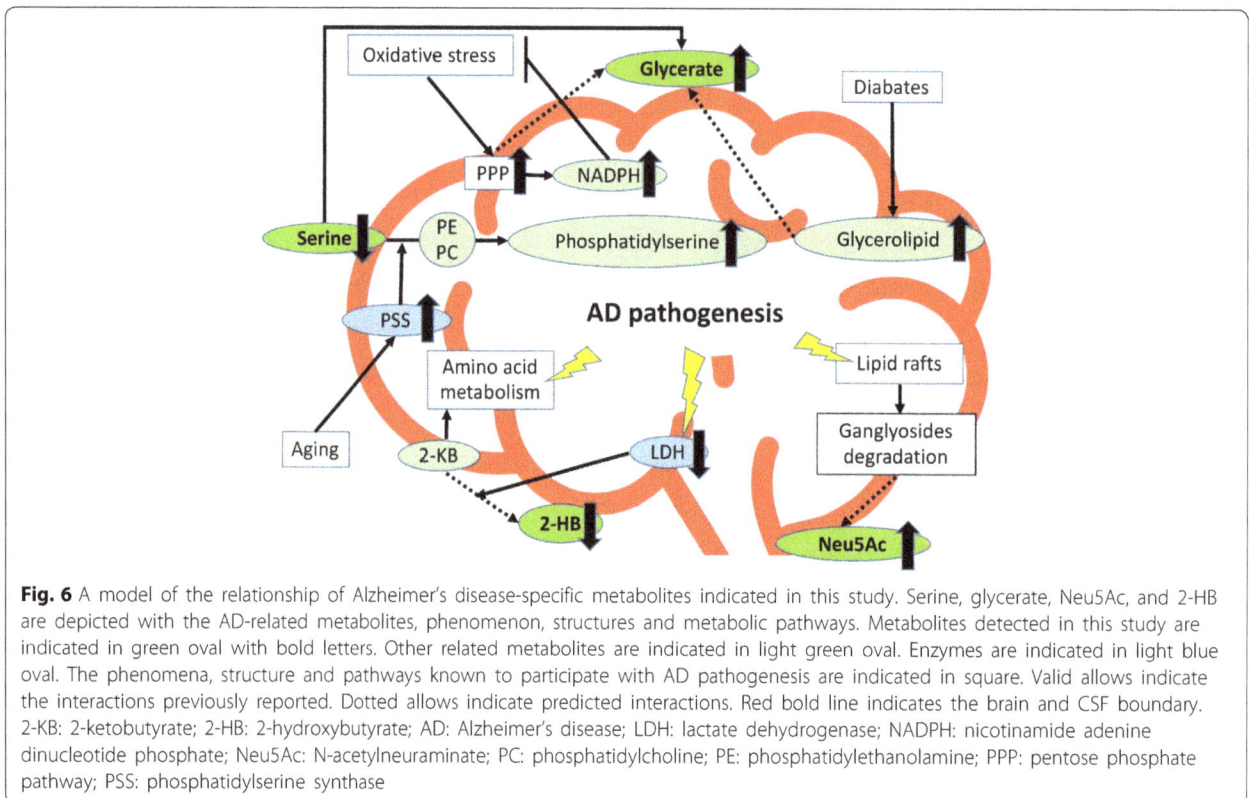

Fig. 6 A model of the relationship of Alzheimer's disease-specific metabolites indicated in this study. Serine, glycerate, Neu5Ac, and 2-HB are depicted with the AD-related metabolites, phenomenon, structures and metabolic pathways. Metabolites detected in this study are indicated in green oval with bold letters. Other related metabolites are indicated in light green oval. Enzymes are indicated in light blue oval. The phenomena, structure and pathways known to participate with AD pathogenesis are indicated in square. Valid allows indicate the interactions previously reported. Dotted allows indicate predicted interactions. Red bold line indicates the brain and CSF boundary. 2-KB: 2-ketobutyrate; 2-HB: 2-hydroxybutyrate; AD: Alzheimer's disease; LDH: lactate dehydrogenase; NADPH: nicotinamide adenine dinucleotide phosphate; Neu5Ac: N-acetylneuraminate; PC: phosphatidylcholine; PE: phosphatidylethanolamine; PPP: pentose phosphate pathway; PSS: phosphatidylserine synthase

establish the methods of precise and early diagnosis, comprehensive analyses for the pathway specific metabolites altered in AD would be effective.

In this study, the concentration of the four metabolites and established AD biomarker, p-tau, in the CSF were weakly correlated, although another established AD biomarker, Aβ42, did not show similarly significant results (Figs. 3, 4). In addition, according to the AUC value, the four metabolites and p-tau showed the same power in discriminating AD from iNPH (Figs. 2, 5). Since p-tau is expected to be a good surrogate marker for AD progression [63], the four metabolites indicated here could also be additional surrogate markers. Moreover, metabolic alterations are reportedly seen at a relatively early stage of AD [6, 12, 62], and the four metabolites could be capable of detecting AD earlier than p-tau may detect it.

To validate these results and speculations, utilizing differential metabolite detection methods with additional larger sample size including healthy persons, patients with AD at an early stage, and/or mild cognitive impairment will reveal further information for AD pathogenesis and early diagnosis. We believe that the integration and combination of such information could contribute to developing new diagnostic markers for AD and to expanding the understanding of AD.

Conclusions

In this study, we found four metabolites that closely participate in the PPP, glycerolipid metabolism, amino acid metabolism, and lipid raft integration were significantly altered in the CSF of patients with AD compared to the CSF of patients with iNPH. All these biological pathways have been demonstrated to be associated with AD in previous reports. Additionally, the combination of these metabolites could discriminate between AD and iNPH with a power equal to that of p-tau and indicated moderate correlation with p-tau. In future studies, the combination of these and additional metabolites included in the metabolic pathways altered in AD would be useful to classify potential patients with AD earlier and with greater precision.

Abbreviations
2-HB: 2-hydroxybutyrate; AD: Alzheimer's disease; AUC: Area under the ROC curve; CE-ESI-MS: Capillary electrophoresis-electrospray ionization-mass spectrometry; CE-MS: Capillary electrophoresis-mass spectrometry; CE-TOFMS: Capillary electrophoresis-time-of-flight-mass spectrometry; CSF: Cerebrospinal fluid; HPLC: High performance liquid chromatography; iNPH: Idiopathic normal pressure hydrocephalus; Neu5Ac: N-acetylneuraminate; PSS: Phosphatidylserine synthase

Acknowledgements
We thank Nobuyoshi Shimoda, Ph.D. for helpful discussions. We thank Editage (www.editage.jp) for English language editing.

Funding
This research was supported by the Program for Promotion of Fundamental Studies in Health Sciences of the National Institute of Biomedical Innovation of Japan (10-45), The Research Funding for Longevity Sciences (26-20), "Development of Diagnostic Technology for Detection of miRNA in Body Fluids" grant from the Japan Agency for Medical Research and Development and New Energy and Industrial Technology Development Organization.

Authors' contributions
YN and SN designed the experiments. AH, SI, AS, FS, MM, and TS performed the metabolome analysis. YN and AH wrote the initial draft, KO reviewed the results and performed critical reading and editing of the manuscript. MK performed the statistical analyses. MB, KH, SY, YG, and KU collected the CSF samples and provided the medical records. All authors read and approved the final manuscript.

Competing interests
The authors declare that they have no competing interests.

Author details
[1]Medical Genome Center, National Center for Geriatrics and Gerontology, 7-430 Morioka-cho, Obu, Aichi 474-8511, Japan. [2]Institute for Advanced Biosciences, Keio University, 246-2 Mizukami, Kakuganji, Tsuruoka, Yamagata 997-0052, Japan. [3]Research Center for Global Agromedicine, Obihiro University of Agriculture and Veterinary Medicine, 2-11 Inada-cho, Obihiro, Hokkaido 080-8555, Japan. [4]Department of Experimental Neuroimaging, National Center for Geriatrics and Gerontology, Obu, Aichi 474-8511, Japan. [5]Medical Genome Center, National Center of Neurology and Psychiatry, Kodaira, Tokyo 187-8551, Japan. [6]Department of Biological Regulation, School of Health Science, Faculty of Medicine, Tottori University, Yonago, Tottori 683-8503, Japan.

References
1. Dubois B, Feldman HH, Jacova C, Dekosky ST, Barberger-Gateau P, Cummings J, Delacourte A, Galasko D, Gauthier S, Jicha G, et al. Research criteria for the diagnosis of Alzheimer's disease: revising the NINCDS-ADRDA criteria. Lancet Neurol. 2007;6:734–46.
2. Yiannopoulou KG, Papageorgiou SG. Current and future treatments for Alzheimer's disease. Ther Adv Neurol Disord. 2013;6:19–33.
3. Adams RD, Fisher CM, Hakim S, Ojemann RG, Sweet WH. Symptomatic occult hydrocephalus with normal cerebrospinal-fluid pressure. New Engl J Med. 1965;273:117–26.
4. Kanai M, Matsubara E, Isoe K, Urakami K, Nakashima K, Arai H, Sasaki H, Abe K, Iwatsubo T, Kosaka T, et al. Longitudinal study of cerebrospinal fluid levels of tau, a beta1-40, and a beta1-42(43) in Alzheimer's disease: a study in Japan. Ann Neurol. 1998;44:17–26.
5. Chen Z, Zhong C. Decoding Alzheimer's disease from perturbed cerebral glucose metabolism: implications for diagnostic and therapeutic strategies. Prog Neurobiol. 2013;108:21–43.
6. Cunnane S, Nugent S, Roy M, Courchesne-Loyer A, Croteau E, Tremblay S, Castellano A, Pifferi F, Bocti C, Paquet N, et al. Brain fuel metabolism, aging, and Alzheimer's disease. Nutrition. 2011;27:3–20.
7. Bouzier-Sore AK, Voisin P, Bouchaud V, Bezancon E, Franconi JM, Pellerin L. Competition between glucose and lactate as oxidative energy substrates in both neurons and astrocytes: a comparative NMR study. Eur J Neurosci. 2006;24:1687–94.
8. Mosconi L. Brain glucose metabolism in the early and specific diagnosis of Alzheimer's disease. FDG-PET studies in MCI and AD. Eur J Nucl Med Mol Imaging. 2005;32:486–510.
9. Mosconi L, Tsui WH, De Santi S, Li J, Rusinek H, Convit A, Li Y, Boppana M, de Leon MJ. Reduced hippocampal metabolism in MCI and AD: automated FDG-PET image analysis. Neurology. 2005;64:1860–7.
10. Mills JD, Nalpathamkalam T, Jacobs HI, Janitz C, Merico D, Hu P, Janitz M. RNA-Seq analysis of the parietal cortex in Alzheimer's disease reveals alternatively spliced isoforms related to lipid metabolism. Neurosci Lett. 2013;536:90–5.
11. Arvanitakis Z, Wilson RS, Bienias JL, Evans DA, Bennett DA. Diabetes mellitus and risk of Alzheimer disease and decline in cognitive function. Arch Neurol. 2004;61:661–6.
12. Pasinetti GM, Eberstein JA. Metabolic syndrome and the role of dietary lifestyles in Alzheimer's disease. J Neurochem. 2008;106:1503–14.
13. Leibson CL, Rocca WA, Hanson VA, Cha R, Kokmen E, O'Brien PC, Palumbo PJ. Risk of dementia among persons with diabetes mellitus: a population-based cohort study. Am J Epidemiol. 1997;145:301–8.
14. D'Aniello A, Fisher G, Migliaccio N, Cammisa G, D'Aniello E, Spinelli P. Amino acids and transaminases activity in ventricular CSF and in brain of normal and Alzheimer patients. Neurosci Lett. 2005;388:49–53.
15. Czech C, Berndt P, Busch K, Schmitz O, Wiemer J, Most V, Hampel H, Kastler J, Senn H. Metabolite profiling of Alzheimer's disease cerebrospinal fluid. PLoS One. 2012;7:e31501.
16. Ibanez C, Simo C, Martin-Alvarez PJ, Kivipelto M, Winblad B, Cedazo-Minguez A, Cifuentes A. Toward a predictive model of Alzheimer's disease progression using capillary electrophoresis-mass spectrometry metabolomics. Anal Chem. 2012;84:8532–40.
17. Ibanez C, Simo C, Barupal DK, Fiehn O, Kivipelto M, Cedazo-Minguez A, Cifuentes A. A new metabolomic workflow for early detection of Alzheimer's disease. J Chromatogr A. 2013;1302:65–71.
18. Chin AL, Negash S, Hamilton R. Diversity and disparity in dementia: the impact of Ethnoracial differences in Alzheimer's disease. Alzheimer Dis Assoc Disord. 2011;25:187–95.
19. Mori E, Ishikawa M, Kato T, Kazui H, Miyake H, Miyajima M, Nakajima M, Hashimoto M, Kuriyama N, Tokuda T, et al. Guidelines for management of idiopathic normal pressure hydrocephalus: second edition. Neurol Med Chir (Tokyo). 2012;52:775–809.
20. Soga T, Igarashi K, Ito C, Mizobuchi K, Zimmermann HP, Tomita M. Metabolomic profiling of anionic metabolites by capillary electrophoresis mass spectrometry. Anal Chem. 2009;81:6165–74.
21. Soga T, Heiger DN. Amino acid analysis by capillary electrophoresis electrospray ionization mass spectrometry. Anal Chem. 2000;72:1236–41.
22. Hirayama A, Kami K, Sugimoto M, Sugawara M, Toki N, Onozuka H, Kinoshita T, Saito N, Ochiai A, Tomita M, et al. Quantitative metabolome profiling of colon and stomach cancer microenvironment by capillary electrophoresis time-of-flight mass spectrometry. Cancer Res. 2009;69:4918–25.
23. Sugimoto M, Kawakami M, Robert M, Soga T, Tomita M. Bioinformatics tools for mass spectroscopy-based Metabolomic data processing and analysis. Curr Bioinforma. 2012;7:96–108.
24. Sugimoto M, Wong DT, Hirayama A, Soga T, Tomita M. Capillary electrophoresis mass spectrometry-based saliva metabolomics identified oral, breast and pancreatic cancer-specific profiles. Metabolomics. 2010;6:78–95.
25. Ihaka R and Gentleman R. R: a language for data analysis and graphics. J Comp Graph Stat. 1996;5:299-314.
26. Wishart DS, Tzur D, Knox C, Eisner R, Guo AC, Young N, Cheng D, Jewell K, Arndt D, Sawhney S, et al. HMDB: the human Metabolome database. Nucleic Acids Res. 2007;35:D521–6.

27. Kanehisa M, Furumichi M, Tanabe M, Sato Y, Morishima K. KEGG: new perspectives on genomes, pathways, diseases and drugs. Nucleic Acids Res. 2017;45:D353–d361.

28. Grant CM. Metabolic reconfiguration is a regulated response to oxidative stress. J Biol. 2008;7:1.

29. Ansari MA, Scheff SW. Oxidative stress in the progression of Alzheimer disease in the frontal cortex. J Neuropathol Exp Neurol. 2010;69:155–67.

30. Nunomura A, Perry G, Aliev G, Hirai K, Takeda A, Balraj EK, Jones PK, Ghanbari H, Wataya T, Shimohama S, et al. Oxidative damage is the earliest event in Alzheimer disease. J Neuropathol Exp Neurol. 2001;60:759–67.

31. Zhu X, Lee HG, Casadesus G, Avila J, Drew K, Perry G, Smith MA. Oxidative imbalance in Alzheimer's disease. Mol Neurobiol. 2005;31:205–17.

32. Palmer AM. The activity of the pentose phosphate pathway is increased in response to oxidative stress in Alzheimer's disease. J Neural Transm (Vienna). 1999;106:317–28.

33. Russell RL, Siedlak SL, Raina AK, Bautista JM, Smith MA, Perry G. Increased neuronal glucose-6-phosphate dehydrogenase and sulfhydryl levels indicate reductive compensation to oxidative stress in Alzheimer disease. Arch Biochem Biophys. 1999;370:236–9.

34. Sun X, He G, Qing H, Zhou W, Dobie F, Cai F, Staufenbiel M, Huang LE, Song W. Hypoxia facilitates Alzheimer's disease pathogenesis by up-regulating BACE1 gene expression. Proc Natl Acad Sci U S A. 2006;103:18727–32.

35. Hakim AM, Moss G, Gollomp SM. The effect of hypoxia on the pentose phosphate pathway in brain. J Neurochem. 1976;26:683–8.

36. Ghauri FY, Nicholson JK, Sweatman BC, Wood J, Beddell CR, Lindon JC, Cairns NJ. NMR spectroscopy of human post mortem cerebrospinal fluid: distinction of Alzheimer's disease from control using pattern recognition and statistics. NMR Biomed. 1993;6:163–7.

37. Kaddurah-Daouk R, Rozen S, Matson W, Han X, Hulette CM, Burke JR, Doraiswamy PM, Welsh-Bohmer KA. Metabolomic changes in autopsy-confirmed Alzheimer's disease. Alzheimers Dement. 2011;7:309–17.

38. Nicoli F, Vion-Dury J, Confort-Gouny S, Maillet S, Gastaut JL, Cozzone PJ. Cerebrospinal fluid metabolic profiles in multiple sclerosis and degenerative dementias obtained by high resolution proton magnetic resonance spectroscopy. C R Acad Sci III. 1996;319:623–31.

39. Madeira C, Lourenco MV, Vargas-Lopes C, Suemoto CK, Brandao CO, Reis T, Leite RE, Laks J, Jacob-Filho W, Pasqualucci CA, et al. D-serine levels in Alzheimer's disease: implications for novel biomarker development. Transl. Psychiatry. 2015;5:e561.

40. Giusto NM, Salvador GA, Castagnet PI, Pasquare SJ, Ilincheta de Boschero MG. Age-associated changes in central nervous system glycerolipid composition and metabolism. Neurochem Res. 2002;27:1513–23.

41. Crook T, Petrie W, Wells C, Massari DC. Effects of phosphatidylserine in Alzheimer's disease. Psychopharmacol Bull. 1992;28:61–6.

42. Van Schaftingen E. D-glycerate kinase deficiency as a cause of D-glyceric aciduria. FEBS Lett. 1989;243:127–31.

43. Snell K. The duality of pathways for serine biosynthesis is a fallacy. Trends Biochem Sci. 1986;11:241–3.

44. Hart CE, Race V, Achouri Y, Wiame E, Sharrard M, Olpin SE, Watkinson J, Bonham JR, Jaeken J, Matthijs G, Van Schaftingen E. Phosphoserine aminotransferase deficiency: a novel disorder of the serine biosynthesis pathway. Am J Hum Genet. 2007;80:931–7.

45. Biemans EA, Verhoeven-Duif NM, Gerrits J, Claassen JA, Kuiperij HB, Verbeek MM. CSF d-serine concentrations are similar in Alzheimer's disease, other dementias, and elderly controls. Neurobiol Aging. 2016;42:213–6.

46. Grimes MA, Cameron JL, Fernstrom JD. Cerebrospinal fluid concentrations of large neutral and basic amino acids in Macaca Mulatta: diurnal variations and responses to chronic changes in dietary protein intake. Metabolism. 2009;58:129–40.

47. Malaisse WJ, Zhang Y, Louchami K, Sener A, Portois L, Carpentier YA. Brain phospholipid and triglyceride fatty acid content and pattern in type 1 and type 2 diabetic rats. Neurosci Lett. 2006;409:75–9.

48. Janson J, Laedtke T, Parisi JE, O'Brien P, Petersen RC, Butler PC. Increased risk of type 2 diabetes in Alzheimer disease. Diabetes. 2004;53:474–81.

49. Biessels GJ, Kappelle LJ. Increased risk of Alzheimer's disease in type II diabetes: insulin resistance of the brain or insulin-induced amyloid pathology? Biochem Soc Trans. 2005;33:1041–4.

50. de la Monte SM, Wands JR. Alzheimer's disease is type 3 diabetes–evidence reviewed. J Diabetes Sci Technol (Online). 2008;2:1101–13.

51. Sonnino S, Mauri L, Chigorno V, Prinetti A. Gangliosides as components of lipid membrane domains. Glycobiology. 2007;17:1r–13r.

52. Cantu L, Del Favero E, Sonnino S, Prinetti A. Gangliosides and the multiscale modulation of membrane structure. Chem Phys Lipids. 2011;164:796–810.

53. Ehehalt R, Keller P, Haass C, Thiele C, Simons K. Amyloidogenic processing of the Alzheimer beta-amyloid precursor protein depends on lipid rafts. J Cell Biol. 2003;160:113–23.

54. Harris B, Pereira I, Parkin E. Targeting ADAM10 to lipid rafts in neuroblastoma SH-SY5Y cells impairs amyloidogenic processing of the amyloid precursor protein. Brain Res. 2009;1296:203–15.

55. Hur JY, Welander H, Behbahani H, Aoki M, Franberg J, Winblad B, Frykman S, Tjernberg LO. Active gamma-secretase is localized to detergent-resistant membranes in human brain. FEBS J. 2008;275:1174–87.

56. Parkin ET, Turner AJ, Hooper NM. Amyloid precursor protein, although partially detergent-insoluble in mouse cerebral cortex, behaves as an atypical lipid raft protein. Biochem J. 1999;344(Pt 1):23–30.

57. Furukawa K, Ohmi Y, Ohkawa Y, Tokuda N, Kondo Y, Tajima O, Furukawa K. Regulatory mechanisms of nervous systems with glycosphingolipids. Neurochem Res. 2011;36:1578–86.

58. Kracun I, Rosner H, Drnovsek V, Heffer-Lauc M, Cosovic C, Lauc G. Human brain gangliosides in development, aging and disease. Int J Dev Biol. 1991; 35:289–95.

59. Rosalki SB, Wilkinson JH. Reduction of alpha-ketobutyrate by human serum. Nature. 1960;188:1110–1.

60. Newington JT, Rappon T, Albers S, Wong DY, Rylett RJ, Cumming RC. Overexpression of Pyruvate Dehydrogenase Kinase 1 and lactate Dehydrogenase a in nerve cells confers resistance to Amyloid β and other toxins by decreasing mitochondrial respiration and reactive oxygen species production. J Biol Chem. 2012;287:37245–58.

61. Mosconi L, Berti V, Glodzik L, Pupi A, De Santi S, de Leon MJ. Pre-clinical detection of Alzheimer's disease using FDG-PET, with or without Amyloid imaging. J Alzheimers Dis. 2010;20:843–54.

62. Cruz T, Gleizes M, Balayssac S, Mornet E, Marsal G, Millan JL, Malet-Martino M, Nowak LG, Gilard V, Fonta C. Identification of altered brain metabolites associated with TNAP activity in a mouse model of hypophosphatasia using untargeted NMR-based metabolomics analysis. J Neurochem. 2017;140:919–40.

63. Blennow K, Zetterberg H, Minthon L, Lannfelt L, Strid S, Annas P, Basun H, Andreasen N. Longitudinal stability of CSF biomarkers in Alzheimer's disease. Neurosci Lett. 2007;419:18–22.

20

Protein kinase inhibitors for acute leukemia

Yuan Ling, Qing Xie, Zikang Zhang and Hua Zhang*

Abstract

Conventional treatments for acute leukemia include chemotherapy, radiation therapy, and intensive combined treatments (including bone marrow transplant or stem cell transplants). Novel treatment approaches are in active development. Recently, protein kinase inhibitors are on clinical trials and offer hope as new drugs for acute leukemia treatment. This review will provide a brief summary of the protein kinase inhibitors in clinical applications for acute leukemia treatment.

Keywords: Protein kinase inhibitor, Acute lymphocyte leukemia, Acute myeloid leukemia

Background

Acute leukemia is subdivided into acute myelocytic leukemia (AML) and acute lymphoblastic leukemia (ALL) [1, 2]. AML accounts for about 90% of all acute leukemias in adults, and the cure rates are 35–40% in patients under 60 years old and 5–15% in those over 60 years old respectively [3]. The elderly always have poor prognosis with a median survival of 5–10 months. ALL is the most common subtype found in childhood with a peak incidence in 2–5 years. Although more than 80% of children with ALL receive positive effect after treatments, there are only 20%–40% of adults ALL [4]. Philadelphia-positive acute lymphoblastic leukemia (Ph + ALL) has poor prognosis which is the most frequent genetic subtype of adult ALL and, in the elderly, Ph + ALL accounts for approximately 30% of cases [5, 6]. To date, chemotherapy is still the main treatment strategy for leukemia. Although hematopoietic stem cell transplantation (HSCT) is also sometimes used as front-line therapy for patients with high-risk leukemia, usually, it is considered when induction chemotherapy fails or leukemia relapses [7, 8]. Cancer cells typically evade the immune surveilence and have genetic heterogeneity with mutant targets [9]. Currently, emerging molecular targeted therapy is being used in clinic, such as inhibitors of FMS-like tyrosine kinase 3 (FLT3) and mammalian target of rapamycin (mTOR) in acute leukemia [10].

Besides, new inhibitors specific to novel targets like IDH1/2, PP2A, DOCK2, PAK1 have been developed [11].

Thus, targeted inhibitors have been developed as replacements for conventional chemotherapy and provide a less toxic and more effective way than the conventional chemotherapy. Here, we will provide a comprehensive overview of the main protein kinase inhibitors (PKIs) used or being developed in acute leukemia.

Protein kinase inhibitors in acute leukemia

Protein kinases are conventionally divided into five classes: protein tyrosine kinase, protein serine/threonine kinase, tryptophan protein kinase, histidine protein kinase and protein aspartyl/glutamoyl kinase. It has been proved that the abnormal activity of protein kinases is associated with many diseases like, inflammation immune system disease, and cancer including leukemia [12]. The main protein kinases particularly involve the phosphatidyl-inositol 3-kinase/v-akt murine thymoma viral oncogene homolog 1 (PI3K/AKT), mitogenactivated protein kinase/extracellular signal regulated kinase (MAPK/ERK), janus kinase signal transducer and activator of transcription (JAK-STAT) and signal transducer and activator of transcription 5 (STAT5) in AML observed to be aberrantly activated in a variety of malignancies, including pre-B-ALL, T cell ALL, and AML [13, 14]. Other targets have been reported, such as FLT3, Bruton's tyrosine kinase (BTK), mTOR, AKT, poly (ADP-ribose) polymerase (PARP), histone deacetylase (HDAC), etc. [15]. Thus, protein kinases have become new focus and PKIs have been developed as new anti-

* Correspondence: huazhang@gdmu.edu.cn
Guangdong Provincial Key Laboratory of Medical Molecular Diagnostics, Institute of Laboratory Medicine, Guangdong Medical University, Dongguan 523808, China

tumor drugs to disrupt the abnormal signal transduction in the therapy of acute leukemia.

As we all know the ABL-inhibitor imatinib became the first Food and Drug Administration (FDA)-approved small molecule protein kinase blocker. However, due to the emergence of many new mutation sites of protein kinase, the drug resistance to imatinib is more and more serious. Other pharmacological inhibitors including dasatinib and nilotinib, which are significantly more potent than imatinib and may overcome resistance have been developed. Imatinib and dasatinib, are registered for the treatment of Ph + ALL in adults [16]. On the other hand, imatinib and sunitinib reduce AML cell by blocking the activity of c-KIT pharmacologically [17, 18]. Many molecular changes are being studied the prognitic impact in acute leukemia. However, only FMS-like tyrosine kinase 3 internal tandem duplications (FLT3-ITDs), Nucleophosmin (NPM1), CCAAT/enhancer-binding protein-α (C/EBP-α) and c-KIT have been currently incorporated in validated international risk stratification schema [19]. FLT3-ITDs is associated with worse prognosis in AML and several FLT3 inhibitors have undergone clinical trials [20]. Here, we summarized some PKIs are being used or under clinical evaluation at phase I, II and III clinical trials in acute leukemia (Table 1).

Tyrosine protein kinase inhibitors
FLT3 inhibitors
Quizartinib (AC220)

Quizartinib is a second-generation FLT3 inhibitor and selectively inhibits class III receptor tyrosine kinases including FLT3, stem cell factor receptor (SCFR), colony-stimulating factor 1 receptor (CSF1R) and platelet derived growth factor receptors (PDGFRs), thus usually results in a better complete remissions in relapsed/refractory (r/r) AML [21]. Other studies also showed that quizartinib can lead to favorable prognosis for the treatment of AML [22, 23].

Midostaurin

Midostaurin, a multi-target protein kinase inhibitor with anti-FLT3 activity which also combined with conventional induction and consolidation therapies, has been found to significantly prolong survival of FLT3-mutated AML patients in the phase III clinical trial [15]. After successful Phase II clinical trials, midostaurin was approved by the FDA for the treatment of adult AML patients of FLT3 positive usually combining with chemotherapy or for companion diagnose to detect the FLT3 mutation in patients with AML [24]. Notably, the combination of midostaurin and chemotherapy for AML patients had 23% improvement in overall survival (OS) [25].

Sunitinib

Sunitinib (SU11248), the first FLT3 inhibitor studied in the clinic, plays a role in inhibiting both tumor angiogenesis and tumor cell proliferation, and usually is used with cytarabine against AML cell lines with FL3-ITD mutation. However, sunitinib is a multi-targeted receptor tyrosine kinase (RTK) inhibitor and was proved to target platelet-derived growth factor (PDGF-Rs), vascular endothelial growth factor receptors (VEGFRs), and CD117 (c-KIT) receptor tyrosine kinases except for FLT3 [26]. Sunitinib has been recommended as a second-line drug for patients resistant to imatinib due to c-KIT mutations or those who can not tolerate sunitinib [27].

Lestaurtinib

Lestaurtinib (rINN, codenamed CEP-701) is an inhibitor of the kinases FLT3, tropomyosin receptor kinase A/B/C (TrkA/B/C), Janus kinase 2 (JAK2) [28]. It is quite non-selective like inhibiting other tyrosine kinases like Janus kinase 2 (JAK2), and tropomycin receptor kinase (TRK) [29]. Previous studies have shown that lestaurtinib has the potential to promote apoptosis in FLT3-ITD leukemic cells [30]. Currently, lestaurtinib is being investigated to be combined with chemotherapy in infants and young children [31].

Tandutinib (MLN518)

Tandutinib, can supress the autophosphorylation of FLT3, c-KIT and PDGF (platelet-derived growth factor) receptor tyrosine kinases, thereby inhibiting cellular proliferation and inducing apoptosis in AML [32]. Tandutinib can improve the CR rate to 90% in primarily diagonosed AML patients when used with daunorubicin and cytarabine [33].

Gilteritinib (ASP2215)

Gilteritinib, a pyrazinecarboxamide derivative, is on trial at phase I-II-III and a promising novel inhibitor of FLT3 inhibitors for its potential activity against all classes of FLT3-activating mutations [34]. In addition, a trial of gilteritinib as maintenance therapy for the first remission patients receiving HSCT are to be investigated [35].

Crenolanib (PLX-3397)

Crenolanib, the third generation agent, is an orally available drug that selectively and potently inhibits signaling of class III receptor tyrosine kinases (RTK) FLT3 and platelet-derived growth factor receptor α/β (PDGFR α/β). Unlike most RTK inhibitors, crenolanib can be applied to the induction chemotherapy in AML [36].

Bortezomib (PS-341)

Bortezomib, a reversible 26S proteasome inhibitor, can interfere with the transcription and induce the early

Table 1 The therapeutic protein kinase inhibiors in acute leukemia

Targets	Inhibitors	Comments	Main side effects	Phase
FLT3	Quizartinib	An anti-FLT3 TKI, was investigated in ALL or AML	Nausea, anemia, vomiting, etc	I-II-III [70]
	Midostaurin	It is an oral multi-targeted kinase inhibitor to inihibit leukemia cells including ALL and FLT3-positive AML	Diarrhhoea, nausea, headache, etc.	I-II-III [71]
	Sunitinib	Sunitinib inhibits leukemia cells survival and angiogenesis	Cardiotoxic, dyspnea, etc.	II [72]
	Lestaurtinib	Lestaurtinib might inhibit the activity of FLT3 kinase and it is more appropriate during intensive chemotherapy	Gastrointestinal reaction, etc.	I-II-III [73]
	Tandutinib	It inhibits the FLT3 ITD-positive rather than the ITD-negative patients with AML.	Bone pain, nausea, etc.	I-II-III
	Gilteritinib	Gilteritinib is a kind of favourable safety agent and is being on trial at 120 mg/day	Diarrhea, etc.	I-II -III
	Crenolanib	Crenolanib is a potential selective inhibitor of FLT3-ITDs and PDGFRα/β	Vomiting, headache, etc	II
	Bortezomib	It is associated with apoptotic and autophagic cell death of AML	Gastro-intestinal, asthenia, etc	I-II-III [74]
BTK	Ibrutinib	Although ibrutinib has its own unique toxicity, it usually causes fewer infections	Pneumonia, sinusitis, headache upper respiratory tract infection, etc.	II
	Acalabrutinib	It has received accelerated approval for the treatment of cell lymphoma	Headache, diarrhea, weight gain skin rash, severe diarrhea, etc.	I-II
JAK-STAT	Ruxolitinib	The JAK1/JAK2 inhibitor, is more effective against JAK-STAT pathway	Nausea, anemia, vomiting, ect.	III
	Pacritinib (SB1518)	It is potent inhibitor FLT3-ITDs, JAK2, JAK2V617F in phase III development	Anemia, ect.	I-II-III [75]
	Everolimus	Everolimus is combined with MK-2206, particularly important in the setting of resistance to therapeutic drugs	Cardiac failure, respiratory failure septic shock, etc.	I-II [76]
	Temsirolimus	Temsirolimus combines with etoposide, cyclophosphamide and dexamethasone for relapsed pediatric ALL in adults	Nausea, etc.	I-II [77]
mTOR	Sirolimus	Sirolimus is an mTOR inhibitor, but it has a similar suppressive effect on the immune system	Abdominal pain, nausea, etc.	II [78]
	AZD8055	AZD8055 inhibits the phosphorylation of mTORC1 with p70S6K and 4E–BP1 and downstream proteins	Anorexia, etc.	I
	Ciclopirox	Ciclopirox enhances the effect of the preclinical antileukemia while irritation	Itching, blistering, swelling, etc.	I
MEK	Pimasertib	It is a novel, selective, orally bioavailable MEK1/2	Bleeding risk, etc.	II
	GSK690693	It inhibits apoptosis in sensitive ALL cell lines	Not clearly	I
AKT	MK-2206	An orally inhibitor of the PI3K/Akt pathway which can inhibit tumor cell proliferation	Fatigue, vomiting, anorexia, etc	I-II
	T315I	The mutation of T315I occurs to patients even when second- and third-genneration on trails	Nausea, swelling, rash, etc.	II-III
	Gefitinib	A third-line agent and also is an EGFR inhibitor	Diarrhoea, vomiting, anorexia, etc.	II [79]
	Ponatinib	It is a multi-targeted tyrosine-kinase inhibitor often with hypertension	Hypertension, rash, abdominal pain, fatigue, etc.	I-II
Bcr-Abl	Dasatinib	It also inhibits the Src kinase family	Anemia, diarrhea, swelling, rash, etc	II
	ABL001	ABL001 is taken orally and the high does of it can be given safely to patients	Not clearly	I
	BEZ235	BEZ-235 is a PI3K inhibitor. It also inhibits mTOR. It is being investigated as a possible leukemia treatment.	Anemia, vomiting, etc	I-II
PI3K	Idelalisib	Idelalisib is effective in leukemia patients who have p53 mutation	Fever, fatigue, nausea, cough abdominal, pain, rash, chills, etc.	on trial
	PKI-587	Gedatolisib is an agent targeting the PI3K/mTOR pathway	Nausea, etc.	I
PLK1	Volasertib	It has been reported the volasertib inhibits PLK1 in both cancer and normal cells	Anaema, throm bocytopenia, nausea febrile neutropenia, etc.	I-II

degradation of FLT3 internal tandem duplications (FLT3-ITD) through autophagy against ALL [37]. In addition, bortezomib can trigger the inhibition of MAPK/ERK, PI3K/AKT and STAT5 pathways in the AML [38, 39]. Evidence showed that bortezomib could potentiate the cytotoxic effects of combination chemotherapy in patients with leukemia.

BTK inhibitors
Ibrutinib (Imbruvica)
Ibrutinib inhibits pre-BCR+ B-cell by targeting Bruton's tyrosine kinase (BTK) and B lymphocyte kinase (BLK), while selectively targets FLT3-ITD in mutant FLT3-positive in AML [40]. Clinical trials studies have demonstrated its tolerability in malignant B cells and has progressed into phase III trials. The combination treatment of ibrutinib with vincristine or dexamethasone demonstrated valid activity during the therapy of ALL [41].

Acalabrutinib (ACP-196)
Acalabrutinib, a second generation BTK inhibitor, has been shown to be better than ibrutinib for improved targeting specificity for BTK [42]. Large clinical samples and longer follow-up are still needed to ascertain these potential advantages.

JAK-STAT inhibitors
Ruxolitinib
The JAK-STAT cell signaling pathway mainly regulates gene transcription. And the combination of ruxolitinib with nilotinib usually inhibits the proliferation of leukemia cells especially in Ph + ALL [43].

Pacritinib (SB1518)
Pacritinib (SB1518) was found to inhibit JAK2/FLT3 with a great potential for its less side effects in advanced myeloid malignancies, myelofibrosis and myeloproliferative neoplasms during phase I/II study [44].

Other inhibitors
Gefitinib (ZD1839)
Gefitinib is the third generation agent, and the first selective inhibitor of epidermal growth factor receptor (EGFR) tyrosine kinase domain. Although gefitinib can induce differentiation in AML cells, a phase II trial has shown that conventional use of gefitinib as a single agent for AML is not yet clear. Therefore, additional clinical trails are currently recruiting [45].

Ponatinib
Ponatinib (previously AP24534), the third-generation TKI, is an oral TKI drug developed for the treatment of T315I-positive Ph + ALL, however, it's appilcation may be limited for some ALL patients particularly with imatinib-resistance and multiple mutations [46].

Protein serine/threonine kinase inhibitors
mTOR inhibitors
Everolimus
Everolimus can inhibit the mTORC1, and contributes to a high activation of the kinase AKT. Everolimus has important effect on the function of cell proliferation and the combination with azacitidine has shown promising clinical activity in AML [47].

Temsirolimus
Temsirolimus, a specific inhibitor of mTOR, interferes with cell growth. Currently, it is also found to be converted to sirolimus (rapamycin) in vivo [48]. Furthermore, the combination of temsirolimus with ibrutinib resulted in the cell growth reduction during the B-cell receptor pathway [49].

Sirolimus
Sirolimus, also known as rapamycin, inhibits activation of T cells and B cells. In vitro, it has also been found that sirolimus inhibits cell growth and even promotes cell death in B-precursor ALL [50, 51].

AZD8055
AZD8055 can inhibit mTORC1, mTORC2 and its downstream proteins through phosphorylation and markedly increase the survival of AML transplanted mice due to supress tumor growth [52]. Synergistic combinations of chemotherapy with low-dose AZD8055 could be more effective.

Ciclopirox
Ciclopirox, also an anti-fungal agent, is proved to be a novel specific mTOR kinase inhibitor and the combination with parthenolide which has been applied into preclinical anti-leukemia in AML and ciclopirox demonstrates greater availability against AML than treatment with either compound alone [53]. Besides ciclopirox could enhance the efficiency of compound parthenolide.

MEK inhibitors
Pimasertib, a MEK1/2 inhibitor, is efficient to target many hematologic malignancies including ALL and AML, however, the probability of clinical benefit and more effective clinical trials still remains to be warranted [54, 55].

AKT inhibitors
GSK690693
GSK690693 is a novel ATP-competitive Akt kinase inhibitor and selective for the Akt isoforms, while it also

can inhibit additional members of the AGC kinase family [56].

Mk-2206

MK-2206 is another kind of oral inhibitor of Akt1/2/3 that promotes apoptosis and cell cycle arrest in AML [57]. During the trials of diffuse large B-cell lymphoma (DLBCL), MK-2206 significantly decreased p-AKT and downstream targets of AKT signaling [58].

T315I

T315I is an integrin-linked kinase (ILK) inhibitor, which downregulates protein kinase B (Akt) and p-Akt and decreases cell activity of AML [59]. The T315I is a unique mutation because of its resistance to the approved BCR-ABL inhibitors. The BCR-ABL fusion gene is a driver oncogene in chronic myeloid leukemia and 30–50% of cases of adult ALL [60, 61]. Introduction of ABL1 kinase inhibitors like imatinib has markedly improved patient survival, but drug resistance still remains a challenge.

Other inhibitor

Alvocidib, also known as flavopiridol or HMR-1275, is a multi-serine threonine cyclin-dependent kinase inhibitor and mainly downregulates CDK7 and CDK9 to inhibit c-MYC, cyclin D1, and MCL-1. Alvocidib has currently been examined in a phase II study for the treatment of intermediate- and high-risk AML combined with othet effective agents [62].

Potential inhibitors in acute leukemia
Volasertib

Volasertib, also known as BI 6727, is a small molecule inhibitor of the polo-like kinase 1 (PLK1) protein, and being developed as an anti-cancer agent with the potential combination therapy for those untreated patients who are ineligible for intensive induction therapy [63]. Volasertib is currently undergoing investigation in phase I and II trials and has not yet been licensed by the FDA.

Dasatinib

Dasatinib, former BMS 354825, is an orally available small-molecule multi-kinase inhibitor. It potently inhibits BCR-ABL and SRC-family kinases as well as PDGFR α/β, c-KIT, and ephrin receptor kinase [64]. Dasatinib is approved for the treatment of Ph + ALL resistant or intolerant to imatinib.

BEZ235

BEZ235 is a dual PI3K/mTOR inhibitor and used in combination with dexamethasone in ALL. Inhibition of the PI3K/AKT/mTOR pathway with the dual PI3K/mTOR inhibitor BEZ235 enhanced dexamethasone-

induced anti-leukemic activity both in vitro and in vivo models of T-ALL [65, 66].

Idelalisib

Idelalisib is a promising treatment option for B-cell precursor acute lymphoblastic leukemia (BCP-ALL) patients with TCF3-PBX1 (E2A-PBX1), whereas other drugs could be useful depending on the genetic context of individual patients [67].

PKI-587

PKI-587 is a selective inhibitor to suppress T-ALL cells proliferation and colony formation through PI3K/mTOR pathway. It has been reported that PKI-587 could delay tumor progression and enhance the survival rate during the mouse xenograft models [68].

ABL001

ABL001, also named asciminib, could bind to the myristoyl pocket of ABL1 and induces the formation of kinase conformation. ABL001 is a potent and selective ABL1 inhibitor that is undergoing clinical development testing in patients with CML and Ph + acute lymphoblastic leukemia [69].

Conclusions

In summary, molecular targeted therapy has demonstrated impressive efficacy and the development of PKIs has promising impact on acute leukemia patients. With the rapid development of biological information technology, multiple new types of PKIs have been selected to treat acute leukemia patients separately or jointly with traditional treatments. However, there are still some challenges to overcome, such as the off-target effects and stability of the PKIs, the mutations of protein kinases, the best dose for individual patient, the drug-resistance for PKIs, and the evolved immune escape, etc. Thus, screening new targets and seeking novel effective PKIs are necessary and will provide more options for acute leukemia treatment.

Abbreviations

ALL: Acute lymphoblastic leukemia; AML: Acute myelocytic leukemia; BCP-ALL: B-cell precursor acute lymphoblastic leukemia; BLK: B lymphocyte kinase; BTK: Bruton's tyrosine kinase; C/EBP-α: CCAAT/enhancer-binding protein-α; CSF1R: Colony-stimulating factor 1 receptor; DLBCL: Iffuse large B-cell lymphoma; EGFR: Epidermal Growth Factor Receptor; FDA: Food and Drug Administration; FLT3: FMS-like tyrosine kinase 3; FLT3-ITD: FLT3 internal tandem duplications; FLT3-ITDs: FMS-like tyrosine kinase 3 internal tandem duplications; HDAC: Histone deacetylase; HSCT: Hematopoietic stem cell transplantation; ITD: Internal tandem duplication; JAK2: Janus kinase 2; JAK-STAT: Janus kinase signal transducer and activator of transcription; MAPK/

ERK: Mitogenactivated protein kinase/extracellular signal regulated kinase; mTOR: Mammalian target of rapamycin; NPM1: Nucleophosmin; OS: Overall survival; PARP: Poly (ADP-ribose) polymerase; PDGFR α/β: Platelet-derived growth factor receptor α/β; PDGFRs: Platelet derived growth factor receptors; PDGF-Rs: Platelet-derived growth factor; Ph + ALL: Philadelphia-positive acute lymphoblastic leukemia; PI3K/AKT: Phosphatidyl-inositol 3-kinase/v-akt murine thymoma viral oncogene homolog 1; PKIs: Protein kinase inhibitors; PLK1: Polo-like kinase 1; RTK: Receptor tyrosine kinases; SCFR: Stem cell factor receptor; STAT5: Signal transducer and activator of transcription 5; TRK: Tropomycin receptor kinase; TrkA/B/C: Tropomyosin receptor kinase A/B/C; VEGFRs: Vascular endothelial growth factor receptors

Acknowledgements
Not applicable.

Funding
This work was supported by National Natural Science Foundation of China (81300398), Natural Science Foundation of Guangdong Province, China (2015A030313528), and 2013 Sail Plan "the Introduction of the Shortage of Top-Notch Talent" Project (YueRenCaiBan [2014] 1).

Authors' contributions
All authors have contributed to write and revise the manuscripts. All authors have read and approved the final version.

Competing interests
The authors declare that they have no competing interests.

References
1. Ma M, Wang X, Tang J, Xue H, Chen J, Pan C, et al. Early T-cell precursor leukemia: a subtype of high risk childhood acute lymphoblastic leukemia. Front Med. 2012;6(4):416–20.
2. Yang X, Wang J. Precision therapy for acute myeloid leukemia. J Hematol Oncol. 2018;11(1):3.
3. Dohner H, Weisdorf DJ, Bloomfield CD. Acute Myeloid Leukemia. N Engl J Med. 2015;373(12):1136–52.
4. Zhang E, Xu H. A new insight in chimeric antigen receptor-engineered T cells for cancer immunotherapy. J Hematol Oncol. 2017;10(1):1.
5. Granacher NCP, Berneman ZN, Schroyens W, Van de Velde ALR, Verlinden A, Gadisseur APA. Adult acute precursor B-cell lymphoblastic leukemia presenting as hypercalcemia and osteolytic bone lesions. Exp Hematol Oncol. 2017;6:9.
6. Chiaretti S, Foa R. How has the management of Ph+ acute lymphoblastic leukemia (ALL) changed over the years. Rinsho Ketsueki. 2016;57(10):2038–48.
7. Yang J. SALL4 as a transcriptional and epigenetic regulator in normal and leukemic hematopoiesis. Biomark Res. 2018;6(1)
8. Testa U, Lo-Coco F. Targeting of leukemia-initiating cells in acute promyelocytic leukemia. Stem Cell Investig. 2015;2:8.
9. Vezzalini M, Mafficini A, Tomasello L, Lorenzetto E, Moratti E, Fiorini Z, et al. A new monoclonal antibody detects downregulation of protein tyrosine phosphatase receptor type gamma in chronic myeloid leukemia patients. J Hematol Oncol. 2017;10(1):129.
10. Wang AY, Weiner H, Green M, Chang H, Fulton N, Larson RA, et al. A phase I study of selinexor in combination with high-dose cytarabine and mitoxantrone for remission induction in patients with acute myeloid leukemia. J Hematol Oncol. 2018;11(1):4.
11. Dominguez-Berrocal L, Zhang X, Zini JM, Fominaya J, Rebollo A, Bravo J. Evaluation of caspase-9b and PP2Acalpha2 as potential biomarkers for chronic lymphocytic leukemia. Biomark Res. 2016;4:9.
12. Grant SK. Therapeutic protein kinase inhibitors. Cell Mol Life Sci. 2009;66(7):1163–77.
13. Wang J, Liu X, Qiu Y, Shi Y, Cai J, Wang B, et al. Cell adhesion-mediated mitochondria transfer contributes to mesenchymal stem cell-induced chemoresistance on T cell acute lymphoblastic leukemia cells. J Hematol Oncol. 2018;11(1):11.
14. Lim SY, Lee JH, Welsh SJ, Ahn SB, Breen E, Khan A, et al. Evaluation of two high-throughput proteomic technologies for plasma biomarker discovery in immunotherapy-treated melanoma patients. Biomark Res. 2017;5:32.
15. Man LM, Morris AL, Keng M. New therapeutic strategies in acute lymphocytic leukemia. Curr Hematol Malig Rep. 2017;12(3):197–206.
16. Malagola M, Papayannidis C, Baccarani M. Tyrosine kinase inhibitors in Ph+ acute lymphoblastic leukaemia: facts and perspectives. Ann Hematol. 2016; 95(5):681–93.
17. An N, Cen B, Cai H, Song JH, Kraft A, Kang Y. Pim1 kinase regulates c-kit gene translation. Exp Hematol Oncol. 2016;5:31.
18. Saygin C, Carraway HE. Emerging therapies for acute myeloid leukemia. J Hematol Oncol. 2017;10(1):93.
19. Heidrich K, Thiede C, Schäfer-Eckart K, Schmitz N, Aulitzky WE, Krämer A, et al. Allogeneic hematopoietic cell transplantation in intermediate risk acute myeloid leukemia negative for FLT3-ITD, NPM1- or biallelic CEBPA mutations. Ann Oncol. 2017;28(11):2793–8.
20. Chen Y, Pan Y, Guo Y, Zhao W, Ho WT, Wang J, et al. Tyrosine kinase inhibitors targeting FLT3 in the treatment of acute myeloid leukemia. Stem Cell Investig. 2017;4:48.
21. An X, Liu J, Wang N, Wang D, Huang L, Zhang L, et al. AC220 and AraC cause differential inhibitory dynamics in patient-derived M5-AML with FLT3-ITD and, thus, ultimately distinct therapeutic outcomes. Exp Hematol. 2017; 45:36–44.
22. Cortes JE, Kantarjian H, Foran JM, Ghirdaladze D, Zodelava M, Borthakur G, et al. Phase I study of quizartinib administered daily to patients with relapsed or refractory acute myeloid leukemia irrespective of FMS-like tyrosine kinase 3-internal tandem duplication status. J Clin Oncol. 2013; 31(29):3681–7.
23. Zhang Y, Xue D, Wang X, Lu M, Gao B, Qiao X. Screening of kinase inhibitors targeting BRAF for regulating autophagy based on kinase pathways. Mol Med Rep. 2014;9(1):83–90.
24. DeAngelo DJ, George TI, Linder A, Langford C, Perkins C, Ma J, et al. Efficacy and safety of midostaurin in patients with advanced systemic mastocytosis: 10-year median follow-up of a phase II trial. Leukemia. 2017; https://doi.org/10.1038/leu.2017.234.
25. Hassanein M, Almahayni MH, Ahmed SO, Gaballa S, Fakih El. R. FLT3 inhibitors for treating acute myeloid leukemia. Clin Lymphoma Myeloma Leuk. 2016;16(10):543–9.
26. Gan HK, Seruga B, Knox JJ. Sunitinib in solid tumors. Expert Opin Investig Drugs. 2009;18(6):821–34.
27. Fiedler W, Kayser S, Kebenko M, Janning M, Krauter J, Schittenhelm M, et al. A phase I/II study of sunitinib and intensive chemotherapy in patients over 60 years of age with acute myeloid leukaemia and activating FLT3 mutations. Br J Haematol. 2015;169(5):694–700.
28. Knapper S, Burnett AK, Littlewood T, Kell WJ, Agrawal S, Chopra R, et al. A phase 2 trial of the FLT3 inhibitor lestaurtinib (CEP701) as first-line treatment for older patients with acute myeloid leukemia not considered fit for intensive chemotherapy. Blood. 2006;108(10):3262–70.
29. Shabbir M, Stuart R. Lestaurtinib, a multitargeted tyrosine kinase inhibitor: from bench to bedside. Expert Opin Investig Drugs. 2010;19(3):427–36.
30. Wei G, Wang J, Huang H, Novel ZY. Immunotherapies for adult patients with B-lineage acute lymphoblastic leukemia. J Hematol Oncol. 2017;10(1):150.
31. Al-Jamal HA, Mat JS, Hassan R, Johan MF. Enhancing SHP-1 expression with 5-azacytidine may inhibit STAT3 activation and confer sensitivity in lestaurtinib (CEP-701)-resistant FLT3-ITD positive acute myeloid leukemia. BMC Cancer. 2015;15:869.
32. Cheng Y, Paz K. Tandutinib, an oral, small-molecule inhibitor of FLT3 for the treatment of AML and other cancer indications. IDrugs. 2008;11(1):46–56.
33. Friedman R. The molecular mechanism behind resistance of the kinase FLT3 to the inhibitor quizartinib. Proteins. 2017;85(11):2143–52.
34. Perl AE, Altman JK, Cortes J, Smith C, Litzow M, Baer MR, et al. Selective inhibition of FLT3 by gilteritinib in relapsed or refractory acute myeloid leukaemia: a multicentre, first-in-human, open-label, phase 1-2 study. Lancet Oncol. 2017;18(8):1061–75.
35. Hackl H, Astanina K, Molecular WR. Genetic alterations associated with therapy resistance and relapse of acute myeloid leukemia. J Hematol Oncol. 2017;10(1):51.

36. Momparler RL. Optimization of cytarabine (ARA-C) therapy for acute myeloid leukemia. Exp Hematol Oncol. 2013;2:20.

37. Horton TM, Pati D, Plon SE, Thompson PA, Bomgaars LR, Adamson PC, et al. A phase 1 study of the proteasome inhibitor bortezomib in pediatric patients with refractory leukemia: a Children's oncology group study. Clin Cancer Res. 2007;13(5):1516–22.

38. Fan M, Li M, Gao L, Geng S, Wang J, Wang Y, et al. Chimeric antigen receptors for adoptive T cell therapy in acute myeloid leukemia. J Hematol Oncol. 2017;10(1):151.

39. Horton TM, Gannavarapu A, Blaney SM, D'Argenio DZ, Plon SE, Berg SL. Bortezomib interactions with chemotherapy agents in acute leukemia in vitro. Cancer Chemother Pharmacol. 2006;58(1):13–23.

40. Collett L, Howard DR, Munir T, McParland L, Oughton JB, Rawstron AC, et al. Assessment of ibrutinib plus rituximab in front-line CLL (FLAIR trial): study protocol for a phase III randomised controlled trial. Trials. 2017;18(1):387.

41. Lichtenegger FS, Krupka C, Haubner S, Köhnke T, Recent SM. Developments in immunotherapy of acute myeloid leukemia. J Hematol Oncol. 2017;10(1):142.

42. Wu J, Zhang M, Liu D. Acalabrutinib (ACP-196): a selective second-generation BTK inhibitor. J Hematol Oncol. 2016;9:21.

43. Kong Y, Wu YL, Song Y, Shi MM, Cao XN, Zhao HY, et al. Ruxolitinib/nilotinib cotreatment inhibits leukemia-propagating cells in Philadelphia chromosome-positive ALL. J Transl Med. 2017;15(1):184.

44. Verstovsek S, Odenike O, Singer JW, Granston T, Al-Fayoumi S, Phase DHJ. 1/2 study of pacritinib, a next generation JAK2/FLT3 inhibitor, in myelofibrosis or other myeloid malignancies. J Hematol Oncol. 2016;9(1):137.

45. Yadav M, Singh AK, Kumar H, Rao G, Chakravarti B, Gurjar A, et al. Epidermal growth factor receptor inhibitor cancer drug gefitinib modulates cell growth and differentiation of acute myeloid leukemia cells via histamine receptors. Biochim Biophys Acta. 2016;1860(10):2178–90.

46. Tojo A, Kyo T, Yamamoto K, Nakamae H, Takahashi N, Kobayashi Y, et al. Ponatinib in Japanese patients with Philadelphia chromosome-positive leukemia, a phase 1/2 study. Int J Hematol. 2017;106(3):385–97.

47. Tan P, Tiong IS, Fleming S, Pomilio G, Cummings N, Droogleever M, et al. The mTOR inhibitor everolimus in combination with azacitidine in patients with relapsed/refractory acute myeloid leukemia: a phase Ib/II study. Oncotarget. 2017;8(32):52269–80.

48. Qin L, Zhao R, Li P. Incorporation of functional elements enhances the antitumor capacity of CAR T cells. Exp Hematol Oncol. 2017;6:28.

49. Zoellner AK, Bayerl S, Hutter G, Zimmermann Y, Hiddemann W, Temsirolimus DM. Inhibits cell growth in combination with inhibitors of the B-cell receptor pathway. Leuk Lymphoma. 2015;56(12):3393–400.

50. Mathias MD, Ortiz MV, Magnan H, Ambati SR, Slotkin EK, Chou AJ, et al. A case report of concurrent embryonal rhabdomyosarcoma and diffuse large B-cell lymphoma in an adult without identifiable cancer predisposition. Biomark Res. 2017;5:7.

51. Brown VI, Fang J, Alcorn K, Barr R, Kim JM, Wasserman R, et al. Rapamycin is active against B-precursor leukemia in vitro and in vivo, an effect that is modulated by IL-7-mediated signaling. Proc Natl Acad Sci U S A. 2003;100(25):15113–8.

52. Yates JWT, Holt SV, Logie A, Payne K, Woods K, Wilkinson RW, et al. A pharmacokinetic-pharmacodynamic model predicting tumour growth inhibition after intermittent administration with the mTOR kinase inhibitor AZD8055. Br J Pharmacol. 2017;174(16):2652–61.

53. Sen S, Hassane DC, Corbett C, Becker MW, Jordan CT, Guzman ML. Novel mTOR inhibitory activity of ciclopirox enhances parthenolide antileukemia activity. Exp Hematol. 2013;41(9):799–807.

54. Ravandi F, Pigneux A, DeAngelo DJ, Raffoux E, Delaunay J, Thomas X, et al. Clinical, pharmacokinetic and pharmacodynamic data for the MEK1/2 inhibitor pimasertib in patients with advanced hematologic malignancies. Blood Cancer J. 2015;5:e375.

55. Leonard JT, Raess PW, Dunlap J, Hayes-Lattin B, Tyner JW, Traer E. Functional and genetic screening of acute myeloid leukemia associated with mediastinal germ cell tumor identifies MEK inhibitor as an active clinical agent. J Hematol Oncol. 2016;9:31.

56. Brown JR. How I treat CLL patients with ibrutinib. Blood. 2018;131(4):379-86.

57. Wang J, Xu-Monette ZY, Jabbar KJ, Shen Q, Manyam GC, Tzankov A, et al. AKT Hyperactivation and the potential of AKT-targeted therapy in diffuse large B-cell lymphoma. Am J Pathol. 2017;187(8):1700–16.

58. Larsen JT, Shanafelt TD, Leis JF, LaPlant B, Call T, Pettinger A, et al. Akt inhibitor MK-2206 in combination with bendamustine and rituximab in relapsed or refractory chronic lymphocytic leukemia: results from the N1087 alliance study. Am J Hematol. 2017;92(8):759–63.

59. Xu P, Guo D, Shao X, Peng M, Chen B. Characteristics and mutation analysis of Ph-positive leukemia patients with T315I mutation receiving tyrosine kinase inhibitors. Onco Targets Ther. 2017;10:4731–8.

60. Diggs LP, Hsueh EC. Utility of PD-L1 immunohistochemistry assays for predicting PD-1/PD-L1 inhibitor response. Biomark Res. 2017;5:12.

61. Ghelli LDRA, Iacobucci I, Martinelli G. The cell cycle checkpoint inhibitors in the treatment of leukemias. J Hematol Oncol. 2017;10(1):77.

62. LaCerte C, Ivaturi V, Gobburu J, Greer JM, Doyle LA, et al. Exposure-response analysis of Alvocidib (Flavopiridol) treatment by bolus or hybrid Administration in Newly Diagnosed or relapsed/refractory acute leukemia patients. Clin Cancer Res. 2017;23(14):3592–600.

63. Schnerch D, Schüler J, Follo M, Felthaus J, Wider D, Klingner K, et al. Proteasome inhibition enhances the efficacy of volasertib-induced mitotic arrest in AML in vitro and prolongs survival in vivo. Oncotarget. 2017;8(13):21153–66.

64. Talpaz M, Shah NP, Kantarjian H, Donato N, Nicoll J, Paquette R, et al. Dasatinib in imatinib-resistant Philadelphia chromosome-positive leukemias. N Engl J Med. 2006;354(24):2531–41.

65. Deng L, Jiang L, Lin XH, Tseng KF, Liu Y, Zhang X, et al. The PI3K/mTOR dual inhibitor BEZ235 suppresses proliferation and migration and reverses multidrug resistance in acute myeloid leukemia. Acta Pharmacol Sin. 2017;38(3):382–91.

66. Wei G, Ding L, Wang J, Hu Y, Huang H. Advances of CD19-directed chimeric antigen receptor-modified T cells in refractory/relapsed acute lymphoblastic leukemia. Exp Hematol Oncol. 2017;6:10.

67. Coelho H, Badior M, Melo T. Sequential kinase inhibition (Idelalisib/Ibrutinib) induces clinical remission in B-cell prolymphocytic leukemia harboring a 17p deletion. Case Rep Hematol. 2017;2017:8563218.

68. Neri LM, Cani A, Martelli AM, Simioni C, Junghanss C, Tabellini G, et al. Targeting the PI3K/Akt/mTOR signaling pathway in B-precursor acute lymphoblastic leukemia and its therapeutic potential. Leukemia. 2014;28(4):739–48.

69. Wylie AA, Schoepfer J, Jahnke W, Cowan-Jacob SW, Loo A, Furet P, et al. The allosteric inhibitor ABL001 enables dual targeting of BCR-ABL1. Nature. 2017;543(7647):733–7.

70. Yamaura T, Nakatani T, Uda K, Ogura H, Shin W, Kurokawa N, et al. A novel irreversible FLT3 inhibitor, FF-10101, shows excellent efficacy against AML cells with FLT3 mutations. Blood. 2018;131(4):426-38.

71. Garcia JS, Percival ME. Midostaurin for the treatment of adult patients with newly diagnosed acute myeloid leukemia that is FLT3 mutation-positive. Drugs Today (Barc). 2017;53(10):531–43.

72. Cooper SL, Sandhu H, Hussain A, Mee C, Maddock H. Involvement of mitogen activated kinase kinase 7 intracellular signalling pathway in Sunitinib-induced cardiotoxicity. Toxicology. 2018;394:72–83.

73. Knapper S, Russell N, Gilkes A, Hills RK, Gale RE, Cavenagh JD, et al. A randomized assessment of adding the kinase inhibitor lestaurtinib to first-line chemotherapy for FLT3-mutated AML. Blood. 2017;129(9):1143–54.

74. YH M, Gaynon PS, Sposto R, van der Giessen J, Eckroth E, Malvar J, et al. Bortezomib with chemotherapy is highly active in advanced B-precursor acute lymphoblastic leukemia: Therapeutic Advances in Childhood Leukemia & Lymphoma (TACL) Study. Blood. 2012;120(2):285–90.

75. Verstovsek S, Komrokji RS. A comprehensive review of pacritinib in myelofibrosis. Future Oncol. 2015;11(20):2819–30.

76. Kolb EA, Gorlick R, Houghton PJ, Morton CL, Neale G, Keir ST, et al. Initial testing (stage 1) of AZD6244 (ARRY-142886) by the pediatric preclinical testing program. Pediatr Blood Cancer. 2010;55(4):668–77.

77. Rheingold SR, Tasian SK, Whitlock JA, Teachey DT, Borowitz MJ, Liu X, et al. A phase 1 trial of temsirolimus and intensive re-induction chemotherapy for 2nd or greater relapse of acute lymphoblastic leukaemia: a Children's oncology group study (ADVL1114). Br J Haematol. 2017;177(3):467–74.

78. Wasko JA, Westholder JS, Jacobson PA. Rifampin-sirolimus-voriconazole interaction in a hematopoietic cell transplant recipient. J Oncol Pharm Pract. 2017;23(1):75–9.

79. Weber C, Schreiber TB, Daub H. Dual phosphoproteomics and chemical proteomics analysis of erlotinib and gefitinib interference in acute myeloid leukemia cells. J Proteome. 2012;75(4):1343–56.

21

Fibronectin protein expression in renal cell carcinoma in correlation with clinical stage of tumour

Sandeep Kondisetty[1]* (iD), Krishnakumar N. Menon[2] and Ginil Kumar Pooleri[1]

Abstract

Background: Carcinogenesis is a multistep process which involves interplay between the tumour cells and the matrix proteins. This occurs by adherence between the tumour cells and proteins in the extracellular matrix. VHL mutation affects through the hypoxia inducible factor (HIF) and causes changes in various tissue proteins like VEGF, PDGF, TGF, Fibronectin and others. As not much literature is available, we aim to quantify the changes of fibronectin protein in renal cell carcinoma (RCC) tissue.

Methods: This Prospective unbalanced case control study was conducted over a period of 18 months from April 2016 to September 2017. The patients undergoing nephrectomy for the diagnosis of RCC were included in the study after obtaining written informed consent. Patients were excluded from study, if normal renal tissue could not be identified in the resected kidney and if the artery clamp time to retrieval of tissue was more than 30 min. Fibronectin protein is estimated in the tumour tissue by gel electrophoresis and western blotting which is compared with that of normal kidney tissue of the same kidney. Results have been expressed as absolute values with standard deviation and relative expression (RE).

Results: Of the 21 patients analysed 15 showed an increase in fibronectin expression in the renal tumour tissue while 6 did not. The mean expression of Fibronectin protein has increased 1.5 times in the tumour tissue when compared with the normal tissue. The increase was 1.54 times in early tumours compared to 1.37 times in advanced tumours of RCC.

Conclusions: Fibronectin showed a 1.5 times increase in the tumour compared to normal. This increase is more in Stage 1&2 tumours when compared to the Stage 3&4 tumours.

Keywords: Fibronectin, Renal cell carcinoma, VHL disease

Background

Renal cell carcinoma (RCC) is the most common renal malignancy and accounts to 3% of all human cancers [1]. There is a substantial increase in the RCC in the recent few years. The incidence of RCC is more in Western countries compared to India and other Eastern countries. There were about 12,500 new cases of renal tumours in the UK in 2014 with an incidence of 25/100,000. In India, the incidence of RCC was estimated at 2/100,000 population among males and about 1/100,000 population among females [2].

With increasing incidence, to combat the disease new modalities of treatment are mainly targeting the VEGF and VHL pathways. Von Hippel-Lindau (VHL) disease is an autosomal dominant hereditary disorder characterized by many tumours including clear cell renal cell carcinoma [3]. The frequency of VHL mutation event ranges from 46 to 82% of sporadic cases of RCC. Vikkath et al. has screened 30 VHL patients and found that RCC is the presenting manifestation in 7 (22.6%) patients [4]. VHL mutation affects through the hypoxia inducible factor (HIF) and causes changes in various tissue proteins like VEGF, PDGF, TGF, Fibronectin and others.

---

* Correspondence: docsunnyhyd@yahoo.com
[1]Department of Urology, Amrita Institute of Medical Sciences, Amrita Vishwa Vidyapeetham, Ponekkara, Kochi, Kerala, India
Full list of author information is available at the end of the article

As not much is known about the changes in FN in renal cancers, we had decided to study FN protein in early and advanced stages of RCC. Already drugs targeting VEGF are available but there is no drug in clinical use targeting FN. Other drugs in clinical use are tyrosine kinase inhibitors and mTOR inhibitors.

Carcinogenesis is a multistep process which involves interplay between the tumour cells and the matrix proteins. This occurs by adherence between the tumour cells and proteins in the extracellular matrix. Among the many extracellular matrix proteins which were identified, Fibronectin (FN) a glycoprotein seems to be involved in adhesion and migration processes of the cancer cells [5]. He et al. [6] was investigating the changes which happen by VHL mutation in RCC tumour tissue. He found in a RCC patient there was HIF-1α diffuse granular staining in cytoplasm of tumour cells if there is presence of von Hippel-Lindau (VHL) gene mutation and no staining in the absence of VHL mutation. At the same time distribution of FN in tissue changes in the presence of VHL mutation. In presence of VHL mutation the matrix fibronectin has decreased with presence of FN at varying levels in the cytoplasm of tumour cells. In the absence of VHL mutation in the RCC the matrix FN is strong with absence of FN in the tumour cell cytoplasm [6]. This suggests that FN protein changes in the tumour cells and the surrounding matrix play a role in all patients of RCC especially with VHL mutations.

Methods
Patients
This Prospective unbalanced case control study was conducted in the Department of Urology at Amrita Institute of Medical Sciences, Kochi, India over a period of 18 months from April 2016 to September 2017. The patients undergoing Partial / Radical Nephrectomy for the diagnosis of RCC were included in the study after obtaining written informed consent. Patients were excluded from study, if normal renal tissue could not be identified in the resected kidney particularly in partial nephrectomy and if the artery clamp time to retrieval of tissue was more than 30 min. Tumor tissue samples were grouped based on TNM (tumour-node-metastasis) classification 7th edition as proposed by Union International Cancer Control (UICC) and American Joint Committee on Cancer (AJCC) in 2009 and nuclear grading according to the Fuhrman grading system [7]. Histological types were based on the consensus classification of renal cell neoplasia [8]. As the tumour stromal percentage (TSP) is coming up as novel independent predictor in many solid organ tumours we have attempted to classify the tumours based on stromal content into 3 groups. The first is less than 10%, second 10–50% and

lastly more than 50%. Gujam et al. has studied on the outcome of breast cancer based on different tumour stromal percentage [9]. Patient data was collected from the hospital electronic medical records system and subsequently analysed using a microsoft excel program. The study was approved by the institutional ethics committee and scientific review committee.

Tissue specimens
The renal tissue was collected immediately after surgery for RCC by taking a small fragment minimum of 5 mm from macroscopically appearing tumour tissue and another from the surrounding normal appearing tissue which is the control for protein estimation analysis for further fibronectin protein level determination using immunoblotting experiments. After confirming the tissue by frozen section with haematoxylin and eosin staining, the tissue was labelled and immediately stored at – 80 degrees Celsius within 30 min from devascularisation. The tissue was homogenised with gentle MACS Dissociator with the lysate buffer. Lysate buffer was made with 6 g of Urea, 2.5 g of SDS in 50 ml of PBS. To 200 mg of the tissue 1.7 ml of Lysate Buffer was added and homogenized with 40 µl of Protease Inhibitor 50X. Then the total protein was estimated in both the tissues by using the Bradford protein estimation method [10]. The mean protein in the tumour was 8.95 ± 1.36 mg/ml while that in the normal renal tissue was 8.29 ± 2.39 mg/ml. This shows that there is no significant difference in the total protein of RCC tumour or the renal normal tissue (p value = 0.23).

Laboratory procedure
The homogenate was used for further fibronectin analysis. Gel electrophoresis (SDS-PAGE) was done using 4–15% Mini-PROTEAN® TGX™ Precast Protein Gels, 15-well, 15 µl and Mini-PROTEAN® Tetra Vertical Electrophoresis Cell. 30µgm of protein was loaded in each well for the electrophoresis. The gels were western blotted for further probing using specific antibodies against fibronectin. The antibody used was rabbit polyclonal IgG antibody from Santa Cruz Biotechnology Fibronectin Antibody (H-300). This antibody recognises the protein FN at 220 kDa. Following chemiluminiscent reaction the membrane was exposed and image was captured using ChemiDoc XRS+ system. The expression of proteins was analysed quantitatively by densitometric analysis using ImageJ software (National Institutes of Health) which is one of free software available. Actin staining (Additional file 1) was done to normalize the immunoblots and served as loading controls. Results have been expressed as absolute values with standard deviation and relative expression (RE) considering the ratio between the optical densities of protein band under

study to corresponding actin band optical density multiplied by the average of actin bands.

Statistical analysis

All data collected was entered in Microsoft excel program and analyzed by using IBM SPSS software version 20. All the continuous variables were expressed using mean and standard deviation and categorical variables were presented using frequency and percentage. To test the statistical significance of mean protein changes from normal to tumour based on tumour size, clinical stage, furhman's grade, tumour stromal percentage and histological type, Wilcoxon signed ranks test was used. To test the statistical significant changes in tumour between Stage 1&2 and Stage 3&4 Mann-Whitney U test was used. To test the statistical significant difference in increase or decrease protein between tumour and normal Chi-square test/ Fisher's exact test was used. A p value < 0.05 was considered statistically significant.

Results

A total of 21 patients were included in the study, the Fibronectin levels were quantified from both the tumour tissue and the adjacent normal kidney tissue. The clinicopathological data of all the patients included in the study were given in Table 1.

Western blot analysis to detect Fibronectin (FN) levels (Fig. 1) showed that mean expression levels of fibronectin in tumour tissue is 141.75 ± 75.11 while in normal tissue the mean expression is 93.59 ± 38.29 which is statistically significant (p value = 0. 002) ($n = 21$) (Fig. 2). The mean expression of Fibronectin protein has increased 1.5 times in the tumour tissue when compared with the normal tissue. Of the 21 patients analysed 15 showed an increase in fibronectin expression in the renal tumour tissue while 6 did not. The increase is noted in both tumours with clear cell histology and also the non-clear cell tumours.

The mean expression of fibronectin in Clear cell tumours is 131.62 ± 80.86 while in normal tissue the mean expression is 85.14 ± 38.13 which is statistically significant (p value = 0.023). The mean expression of fibronectin in non-clear cell tumours is 167.06 ± 56.41 while in normal tissue the mean expression is 114.72 ± 32.29 which is also statistically significant (p value = 0.046) (Table 2). The increase is 1.55 times in clear cell tumours and 1.46 times in non-clear cell tumours. The mean expression of fibronectin in tumours with tumour stromal percentage (TSP) < 10% is 141.9 ± 77.06 when compared to normal tissue which has 92.62 ± 39.02. The increase in these tumours is 1.53 times which was statistically significant (p value = 0.002). The mean expression of fibronectin in tumour ($n = 1$) with tumour stromal percentage (TSP) > 50% is 138.66 when compared to

Table 1 Clinicopathological data regarding the patients from whom the sample both tumour and normal was collected

	Clinicopathological variables	
	Number of patients ($n = 21$)	Percentage of patientspercentage of patientspercentage of patients
Age ($n = 21$)		
< 50	6	28.57
50–60	8	38.1
60–70	4	19.05
> 70	3	14.28
Sex ($n = 21$)		
Male	14	66.67
Female	7	33.33
Surgery ($n = 21$)		
Partial nephrectomy	10	47.61
Radical nephrectomy	11	52.39
Histology type by H & E staining ($n = 21$)		
Clear cell carcinoma	15	71.43
Papillary carcinoma	3	14.29
Chromophobe carcinoma	2	9.52
Others / Multilocular cystic renal cell neoplasm	1	4.76
Furhmann's grade by H & E staining ($n = 19$)		
1	1	5.26
2	12	63.16
3	6	31.58
T – Primary tumour ($n = 21$)		
T1a	5	23.81
T1b	9	42.86
T2b	2	9.52
T3a	5	23.81
Lymph node metastasis ($n = 21$)		
Absent	21	100
Distant metastasis ($n = 21$)		
Absent	20	95.24
Present	1	4.76
Stage ($n = 21$)		
I	14	66.67
II	2	9.52
III	4	19.05
IV	1	4.76
Tumour stroma percentage / TSP ($n = 21$)		
< 10%	20	95.24
> 50%	1	4.76

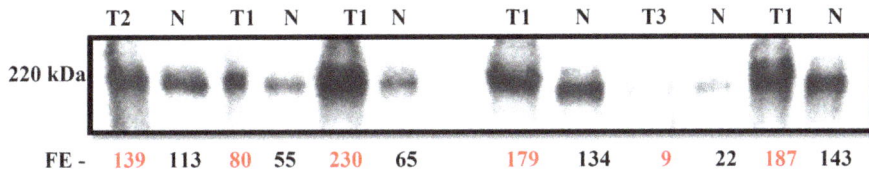

Fig. 1 Western Blot showing-Fibronectin Protein Bands resolved at 220 kDa in SDS PAGE. Fibronectin Expression(FE) of tumour showed in red and normal tissue showed in black. T1- Tumour stage I, T2- Tumour stage II, T3- Tumour stage III

normal issue which has 113. The increase in this tumour is 1.23 times only but cannot draw any conclusions as this was only one in the group.

The mean expression of fibronectin in Stage 1 &2 tumours is 159.18 ± 65.47 while in normal tissue the mean expression is 103.21 ± 32.5 which is statistically significant (p value = 0. 004). The mean expression of fibronectin in Stage 3 & 4 tumours is 85.95 ± 83.79 while in normal tissue the mean expression is 62.83 ± 42.61 which is not statistically significant (p value = 0. 686) (Table 2). The increase was 1.54 times in early tumours compared to 1.37 times in advanced tumours of RCC. In early renal tumours fibronectin is increased in 13 cases but decreased in 3 cases while in advanced renal tumours it is increased in only 2 cases but decreased in 3 cases (p = 0.115, Fisher's exact test).

Discussion

FN plays a critical role in mediating cell adhesion and migration, and also has a role in the process of apoptosis in certain tissues [11]. Waalkes et al. [12] compared 109 RCC tissue with 86 adjacent normal tissue by doing mRNA detection and concluded a notable increase in expression of fibronectin mRNA in RCC when compared to normal renal tissue. In their study both organ-confined and advanced disease showed significant higher levels of fibronectin mRNA expression compared to normal renal tissue. At the same time they concluded that the increase in FN is higher as the stage of disease advances. In our study the protein expression was found to be increased in all stages of renal tumours but the early stages showed a higher expression of fibronectin when compared to advanced tumours which is a new finding. This is in contrast to what was shown before by Waalkes et al. [12]. It has to be noted that presence of mRNA not necessarily always leads to translation into protein. Therefore identification of FN protein presence is more relevant in the functional context.

Steffens et al. [13] collected 270 clear cell RCC tissue specimens of patients who had surgery for the disease and did immunohistochemistry on the tissue. They found to have no significant association between cytoplasmic FN staining and patient characteristics such as age, gender, tumor differentiation and visceral metastasis. As they evaluated survival rates both tumor-specific as well as overall survival rate in 153 patients, they concluded mortality rate in patients with increased cytoplasmic FN expression, indicating a possible role of FN in the prognosis of RCC. This is a large volume study after the He et al. [6] who also used immunohistochemistry of the

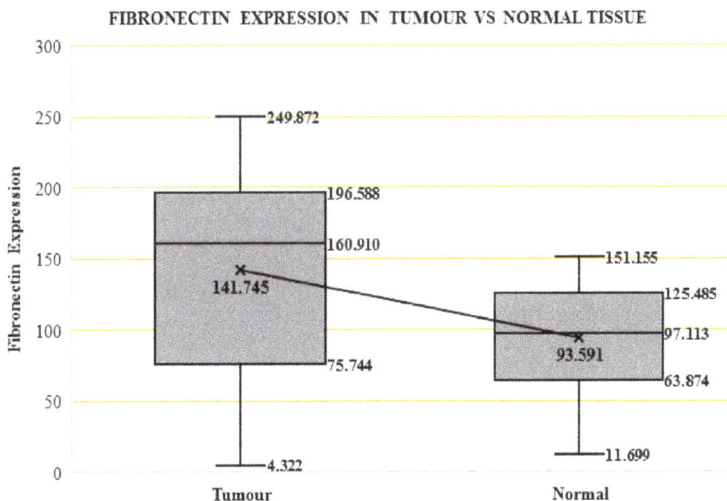

Fig. 2 Box-Whisker Plot showing changes in Fibronectin Expression in Tumour vs Normal Tissue

Table 2 Changes in Fibronectin protein in RCC tumour against normal renal tissue

	Fibronectin expression			
	RCC tissue	Normal renal tissue	Relative increase	p-value
All specimens n = 21	141.75 ± 75.11	93.59 ± 38.29	1.5	0.002
Clear cell tumours n = 15	131.62 ± 80.86	85.14 ± 38.13	1.55	0.023
Non clear cell tumours n = 6	167.06 ± 56.41	114 ± 32.29	1.46	0.046
Stage I and II n = 16	159.18 ± 65.47	103.21 ± 325	1.54	0.004
Stage III and IV n = 5	85.95 ± 83.79	62.83 ± 42.62	1.37	0.686

tumour tissue to determine the FN content. Indeed, in our study we show that early tumors tend to have higher expression of FN compared to late stage indicating that FN may play a role in the progression of tumor and that once it reaches a late stage levels do not change.

Till date there are no drugs against Fibronectin in clinical use. Pharmacological agents targeting FN will be a hope of future as animal experiments by Chaves et al. with endostatin gene therapy shows a promising result [14]. This group has studied the murine model of metastatic RCC in lungs. After endostatin gene therapy the FN levels were 80% less than the control groups who did not receive the therapy. In this model they used densitometric quantification of the immunoblot for the estimation of FN and a similar quantification technique was used by us. In this context, identification of differential expression of FN in normal vs early stage tumor in our study may have potential prognostic value in preferential endostatin therapy to patients who are overexpressing FN.

Conclusion

On western blot protein analysis of 21 RCC tissue and the normal kidney tissue of the same patient, fibronectin showed a 1.5 times increase in the tumour compared to normal. This increase is more in Stage 1&2 tumours when compared to the Stage 3&4 tumours. Although the number is the limitation the relative decrease in FN in advanced disease may be interesting finding for further refinement.

Abbreviations
FN: Fibronectin; RCC: Renal cell carcinoma; SDS-PAGE: Sodium dodecyl sulfate polyacrylamide gel electrophoresis; TSP: Tumour stromal percentage; VEGF: Vascular endothelial growth factor; VHL: Von Hippel-Lindau

Acknowledgements
The success and final outcome of this project required a lot of guidance and assistance from many people and I am extremely privileged to have got this all along the completion of my project. I would not forget to remember my wife Dr. Pallavi Vijay Borkar for her timely support.

Funding
This study was not funded by a company or Institution.

Authors' contributions
KS: designed the study, collected and analyzed the data and wrote the manuscript; GP: came with idea of study and participation in manuscript preparation and review; KM: collected and analyzed the data and reviewed the manuscript. All authors read and approved the final manuscript.

Competing interests
The authors declare that they have no competing interests.

Author details
[1]Department of Urology, Amrita Institute of Medical Sciences, Amrita Vishwa Vidyapeetham, Ponekkara, Kochi, Kerala, India. [2]Center for Nanosciences and Molecular Medicine, Amrita Institute of Medical Sciences, Amrita Vishwa Vidyapeetham, Ponekkara, Kochi, Kerala, India.

References
1. Schrader A, Sevinc S, Olbert P, et al. Urologe. 2008;47:1182.
2. Abraham G, Cherian T, Mahadevan P, Avinash T, George D, Manuel E. Detailed study of survival of patients with renal cell carcinoma in India. Indian J Cancer. 2016;53:572–4.
3. Lonser RR, Glenn GM, Walther M, et al. von Hippel-Lindau disease. Lancet. 2003;361(9374):2059–67.
4. Vikkath N, Valiyaveedan S, Nampoothiri S, et al. Familial Cancer. 2015;14:585.
5. Wilson CB, Leopard J, Cheresh DA, Nakamura RM. Extracellular matrix and integrin composition of the normal bladder wall. World J Urol. 1996;14:S30–7.
6. He Z, Liu S, Guo M, Mao J, Hughson MD. Expression of fibronectin and HIF-1alpha in renal cell carcinomas: relationship to von Hippel-Lindau gene inactivation. Cancer Genet Cytogenet. 2004;152:89–94.
7. Fuhrman SA, Lasky LC, Limas C. Prognostic significance of morphologic parameters in renal cell carcinoma. Am J Surg Pathol. 1982;6:655–63.
8. Stenzl A, De Kernion JB. Pathology, biology, and clinical staging of renal cell carcinoma. Semin Oncol. 1989;16(Suppl 1):3–11.
9. Gujam FJA, Edwards J, Mohammed ZMA, Going JJ, McMillan DC. The relationship between the tumour stroma percentage, clinicopathological characteristics and outcome in patients with operable ductal breast cancer. Br J Cancer. 2014;111(1):157–65.
10. Bradford MM. A rapid and sensitive method for the quantitation of microgram quantities of protein utilizing the principle of protein-dye binding. Anal Biochem. 1976;72:248–54.

11. De la Fuente MT, Casanova B, Garcia-Gila M, Silva A, Garcia-Pardo A. Fibronectin interaction with alpha4beta1 integrin prevents apoptosis in B cell chronic lymphocytic leukemia: correlation with Bcl-2 and Bax. Leukemia. 1999;13:266–74.

12. Waalkes S, Atschekzei F, Kramer MW, et al. Fibronectin 1 mRNA expression correlates with advanced disease in renal cancer. BMC Cancer. 2010;10:503.

13. Steffens S, Schrader AJ, Vetter G, et al. Fibronectin 1 protein expression in clear cell renal cell carcinoma. Oncol Lett. 2012;3(4):787–90.

14. Chaves KC, Turaça LT, Pesquero JB, et al. Fibronectin expression is decreased in metastatic renal cell carcinoma following endostatin gene therapy. Biomed Pharmacother. 2012;66(6):464–8.

22

Biomarkers of cytokine release syndrome and neurotoxicity related to CAR-T cell therapy

Zhenguang Wang and Weidong Han[*]

Abstract: Severe cytokine release syndrome (CRS) and neurotoxicity following chimeric antigen receptor T cell (CAR-T) therapy can be life-threatening in some cases, and management of those toxicities is still a great challenge for physicians. Researchers hope to understand the pathophysiology of CRS and neurotoxicity, and identify predictive biomarkers that can forecast those toxicities in advance. Some risk factors for severe CRS and/or neurotoxicity including patient and treatment characteristics have been identified in multiple clinical trials of CAR-T cell therapy. Moreover, several groups have identified some predictive biomarkers that are able to determine beforehand which patients may suffer severe CRS and/or neurotoxicity during CAR-T cell therapy, facilitating testing of early intervention strategies for those toxicities. However, further studies are needed to better understand the biology and related risk factors for CRS and/or neurotoxicity, and determine if those identified predictors can be extrapolated to other series. Herein, we review the pathophysiology of CRS and neurotoxicity, and summarize the progress of predictive biomarkers to improve CAR-T cell therapy in cancer.

Keywords: Chimeric antigen receptor, CAR-T, CRS, Neurotoxicity, Biomarker

Background

In past year, three CD19-directed chimeric antigen receptor T cell (CAR-T) programs, including Novartis's CTL019, Kite's KTE-C19, and Juno's JCAR015, were racing to become the first-ever approved by the US Food and Drug Administration (FDA). Novartis's CTL019 has been approved recently under the name tisagenlecleucel (KYMRIAH™) by FDA for the treatment of relapsed or refractory (r/r) patients with B-cell acute lymphoblastic leukemia (B-ALL) up to 25 years of age [1]; Kite's KTE-C19 has also been approved under the name axicabtagene ciloleucel (YESCARTA™) by FDA for the treatment of adult patients with certain types of large B-cell lymphoma who have not responded to or who have relapsed after at least two other kinds of treatment [2]. In contrast, Juno Therapeutics abandoned its CAR-T frontrunner JCAR015 after deaths of five patients due to cerebral edema, a neurologic adverse event seen in the pivotal phase II trial(ROCKET) of JCAR015 for adult patients with B-ALL [3]. The extreme consequences of JCAR015 highlights the challenge of how to control the toxicities of CAR-T cell therapy.

In contrast to traditional cancer therapies, CAR-T cells can be considered as 'living drugs' which undergo a marked proliferation (100–100,000 fold) in vivo upon antigen engagement [4]. In addition to the potent anti-tumor activity, these CAR-T cells can also give rise to significant side effects. The two most common and concerning toxicities with CAR-T cells are cytokine release syndrome (CRS) and neurotoxicity [5–8]. In the phase II trial of tisangenlecleucel for r/r B-ALL, severe CRS and neurotoxicity were reported in 47% and 15% of patients who received tisangenlecleucel [9]; while in the pivotal trial of axicabtagene ciloleucel for aggressive B-cell non-Hodgkin lymphoma (B-NHL), severe CRS and neurotoxicity occurred in 13% and 28% of patients who received axicabtagene ciloleucel [10]. Guidelines to manage those toxicities with agents that include Interleukin (IL)-6 receptor inhibitor tocilizumab alone or with steroids have been established and incorporated into some of the CAR-T clinical trials [8, 11]. In general, those two toxicities are manageable in most patients, however, it can be life-threatening in some cases, and management of those conditions can be highly challenging [12–15] .

---
* Correspondence: hanwdrsw69@yahoo.com
Molecular & Immunological Department, Bio-therapeutic Department,
Chinese PLA General Hospital, No. 28 Fuxing Road, Beijing 100853, China

It is critical to understand the pathophysiology of CRS and neurotoxicity for early detection and better management of those conditions. Moreover, it is essential to identify predictive characteristics and biomarkers in patients with severe CRS and neurotoxicity so that it may be possible to risk stratify patients for the development of these complications during CAR-T cell therapy. A few risk factors associated with CRS and neurotoxicity have been identified in the various clinical trials of CAR-T cell therapy conducted so far. Some studies have been able to verify biomarkers that can predict the development and severity of CRS and/or neurotoxicity [13, 14, 16, 17]. Screening patients for high risk of CRS and neurotoxicity can be highly beneficial as these patients can be monitored closely or even be prophylactically treated with preemptive anti-cytokine directed treatment which would effectively mitigate severe CRS and neurotoxicity. In this minireview, we discuss the pathophysiology of CRS and neurotoxicity, and summarize the progress of biomarkers as aids to CAR-T cell therapy in cancer.

Manifestations of CRS related to CAR-T cell therapy

CRS is a clinical constellation of symptoms including fever, nausea, fatigue, myalgias, malaise, hypotension, hypoxia, coagulopathy and capillary leak, and/or multiorgan toxicity, which has been reported to occur in 30–94% of patients, including grade ≥3 CRS in 1–48% [9, 10, 13, 18–25]. CRS typically occurs 1 to 22 days after CAR-T cell infusion, the median time to onset of CRS is 2–3 days [26, 27].Severe CRS usually starts earlier than the CRS that is not severe [13, 28]. The first clinical sign of CRS in most of patients is high fever, which can even rise to more than 40 °C in some patients [13, 29–31]. Notably, in a large cohort of 133 patients with B-cell malignancies who received anti-CD19 CAR-T cell (JCAR014) following lymphodepletion chemotherapy, the investigators showed that fever in patients with grade ≥ 4 CRS not only presented and peaked earlier after CAR-T cell infusion, but also reached a higher maximum temperature and was of longer duration than that of in patients with grade<4 CRS [13]. Besides the constitutional symptoms such as high fever, myalgias, malaise, some severe cases can experience significant hemodynamic instability and capillary leak with hypotension, tachycardia, hypoxia, tachypnea, hemophagocytic lymphohistiocytosis/macrophage activation syndrome, and or other organ toxicity [8, 11, 32]. Mild-to moderate CRS usually is self-limited, and can be managed with close observation and supportive care. Severe CRS must require intensive medical management with tocilizumab alone or with steroids. Nonetheless, resistant CRS, characterized by no clinical improvement or worsening at any time despite use of tocilizumab and steroids [27, 33], may occur in a small number of patients, and in

whom the mortality risk is very high [13, 34, 35]. The time to resolution of CRS is variable, can be ranged from 1 to 60 days after CAR-T cell infusion, and the median time to resolution of CRS is about a week [26, 27]. It must be emphasized is that patients with severe CRS presented delayed hematopoietic recovery [13], potentially increasing the chances of infection, especially in the setting of using tocilizumab that is able to worsen the neutropenia. Empiric antibiotic therapy should be initiated at the beginning of the lymphodepletion chemotherapy.

The cytokine profiles involved in CRS following CAR-T cell therapy encompass not only the effector cytokines such as interferon (IFN)-γ, IL-2, soluble IL-2Rα, IL-6, soluble IL-6R and granulocyte-macrophage colony-stimulating factor (GM-CSF), but also the cytokines mainly secreted by the monocytes and/or macrophages such as IL-1,IL-6, IL-8,IL-10,IL-12, tumor necrosis factor (TNF)-α, IFN-α, monocyte chemotactic protein (MCP)-1, macrophage inflammatory protein (MIP) 1α etc. [36–41]. In addition, some serum biochemical markers, including C-reactive protein (CRP) and ferritin levels are always elevated in patients who experienced CRS after CAR-T cell therapy [13, 28–30, 37, 42, 43]. Monitoring the changes of those laboratory markers after CAR-T cell infusion can give insight in to CRS, and investigational cytokine activation profiles that are associated with CRS have been documented in several CAR-T clinical trials [4, 13, 29]. Of note, the diagnoses, grading and management of CRS are mainly based on abovementioned clinical signs and symptoms rather than those laboratory markers [8, 11, 43, 44].

Pathophysiology of CRS related to CAR-T cell therapy

CRS is not restricted to CAR-T cell therapy and is associated with therapeutic monoclonal antibodies such as anti-CD3 (OKT3) [45], anti-CD20 (rituximab) [46],anti-CD28 (TGN1412) [47], anti-CD52 (alemtuzumab) [48], CD3/CD19 bispecific antibody (blinatumomab) [49] and anti-PD-1 (nivolumab) [50]. CRS is also known as another similar term: cytokine storm, which highlights the state of the immune system gone awry and inflammatory response flaring out of control [51]. The two terms are used interchangeably in some literature [47, 52, 53], but some researchers use the term cytokine storm to refer to the severe case of CRS. In general, there is a balance between the proinflammatory and anti-inflammatory mechanisms, which determines the intensity of the inflammatory response and maintains the immune homeostasis [51, 54]. The proinflammatory and anti-inflammatory cytokines are regulated by complex regulatory networks involving lymphocytes (B cells, T cells, and/or natural killer cells), myeloid cells (macrophages, dendritic cells, and monocytes) and endothelial cells

[55]. Moreover, each cytokine also can exert inductive and inhibitive effects to other cytokines, making a cytokine matrix that is responsible for balance regulation [56]. If this delicate balance ever fails and proinflammatory cytokines prevail, then the outcome may contribute to a cytokine storm.

CRS is a direct result of overproduction of inflammatory cytokines caused by supraphysiological levels of immune activation. However, the detailed mechanism remains poorly defined. Significantly, recent findings in this area may shed light on the underlying mechanism of CAR-T cell induced CRS. (1) CAR is major histocompatibility complex-independent receptor and, thus can function in CD4 and CD8 T cells [57], enabling the biology of CAR-T cells is distinct from that of classic T-lymphocytes. Several preclinical studies have shown that CD4+ CAR-T cells alone have the comparable anti-tumor activity to CD8+ CAR-T cells, and can undergo stronger expansion as well as produce higher amounts of immune-stimulatory cytokines, such as IFN-γ, TNF-α, IL-2 etc. [58, 59]. This unique feature may contribute to the prompt and high cytokine secretion by CAR-T cells upon engagement of the target antigen in either tumor cells or nonmalignant cells. IFN-γ released by the activated CD4+ CAR-T cells and CD8+ CAR-T cells can stimulate macrophages activation and inducing high level of proinflammatory cytokines including IL-12, IL-6, TNF-α,IL-1β, IL-15 and low level of anti-inflammatory cytokines including IL-4,IL-10 to further promote subsequent immune response [60, 61]. IFN-γ–assisted macrophage activation has a direct positive effect on maintaining and enhancing the intensity of the immune response, potentially increasing the likelihood of CRS. The interaction between macrophages and T cells via cytokines may explain why macrophage activation syndrome can occur in a subset of patients who received CAR-T cells [48, 49], and why the cytokine profiles and clinical manifestations of macrophage activation syndrome overlap with those of CRS [50]. (2) Recent two clinical studies have demonstrated that vascular endothelial activation or dysfunction is associated with severe CRS [13, 15]. The data from a study of 133 patients treated with JCAR014 have indicated that biomarkers of endothelial activation including von Willebrand Factor (VWF) and angiopoietin (Ang)-2 are elevated during severe CRS, which is consistent with the presentation of vascular instability, capillary leak, and consumptive coagulopathy in severe CRS [15]. Moreover, the study also has demonstrated that patients with preexisting endothelial activation before infusion of CAR-T cells are prone to develop sever CRS. It is noteworthy that investigators from University of Pennsylvania (Upenn) have confirmed that endothelial cells, in particular blood-vessel endothelial cells, are the key source of IL-6 in

CRS by using dual RNA ISH to examination of the IL-6 expression level of lymph node tissue from a patient who succumbed to the CRS after CTL019 infusion [15]. Thus, there may be a possible cascade that progressively amplifies endothelial activation, where, the high concentrations of systemic cytokines such as IFN-γ, IL-6 and TNF-α released by the hyper-activation of CAR-T cells and non-CAR-T cells induce endothelial cell activation, and then the activated endothelial cells produce more IL-6. The high levels of IL-6 may initiate a proinflammatory IL-6-mediated signaling cascade [11], exacerbating the imbalance of proinflammatory and anti-inflammatory cytokines. This observation from Upenn may be informative for elucidating the mechanism of tocilizumab in alleviating CRS.

Manifestations of neurotoxicity related to CAR-T cell therapy

Neurotoxicity is another prominent toxicity with published reports of 20–64%, including grade ≥3 in 13–52%, and the most common symptoms include encephalopathy, headache, delirium, anxiety, tremor, aphasia; other manifestations of neurotoxicity such as decreased level of consciousness, confusion, seizures and cerebral edema have also been observed in clinical trials of CAR-T cells [5, 9, 10, 14, 18, 19, 22, 30, 62, 63]. The median onset of neurologic events occurs on 4–5 days after CAR-T cell infusion, it can be concurrent with CRS, following resolution of CRS or occur alone [14, 26, 27]. In general, the mild clinical signs are self-limited and resolve within days; more severe symptoms may require supportive care alone or with dexamethasone, and can be complete resolved within 4 weeks. However, some deaths caused by this unexpected toxicity have been documented [14, 21, 64, 65], requiring immediate attention to neurotoxicity management. Similar neurotoxicity has also been reported after administration of blinatumomab [66], a CD3/CD19 bispecific antibody that can result in robust T-cell activation as does the CAR-T cells [67, 68].

Pathophysiology of neurotoxicity related to CAR-T cell therapy

Thus far, the exact mechanism of CAR-T associated neurotoxicity has not been completely elucidated, and several probable mechanisms may contribute to the development of neurotoxicity. (1) CAR-T cells directly mediate toxicity on central nervous system (CNS) tissues that may have the yet-to-be-detected expression of targeted antigen. To date, the main understanding regarding the CAR-T cell induced neurotoxicity is gained from the trials involving CD19. Multiple anti-CD19 CAR-T cell programs have observed that intravenously infused CAR-T cells can cross the blood-brain barrier (BBB) to a sufficient degree, irrespective of CNS malignancy status at the time of CAR-T cell therapy [28, 29, 34, 42, 69–71]. These CAR-T cells trafficking to cerebrospinal fluid (CSF) are able to eradicate the CNS malignancy efficiently in a subset of patients [42, 70]. However, there is so far no experimental evidence to prove the CD19 expression in CNS tissues. An alternative approach to prove that the CD19 antigen is not involved is using CARs targeting antigens other than CD19, such as CD20 or CD22, and then testing if similar neurotoxicity can be seen in these trials. Recently, Fry and colleges have reported that several patients experience reversible neurologic events including transient visual hallucinations, mild unresponsiveness, mild disorientation, and mild–moderate pain among the first 16 patients with B-ALL who received anti-CD22 CAR-T cells [63]. Davila et al. have documented that no detectable CAR-T cells are found in the CSF of patients who exhibited neurotoxicity [29]. Taken together, these findings provide moderate evidence to disprove this hypothesis; however, the contribution from the direct toxicity effect of CAR-T cells on CNS normal cells expressing targeted antigen cannot be excluded until the conclusive evidence to prove or disprove this hypothesis has been showed. More studies are needed to examine the validity of this hypothesis by using beyond CD19 CAR-T cell products. (2) CNS endothelial cell activation emerges as a driver of CAR-T cell-associated neurotoxicity [72]. Recently, Gust et al. have observed endothelial dysfunction and increased BBB permeability in patients who had neurotoxicity, and constructed a plausible pathophysiologic model to elucidate the development of neurotoxicity; Moreover, they have shown that patients with evidence of endothelial activation before lymphodepletion may be at increased risk of neurotoxicity [14]. In this large cohort of 133 adults with B-cell malignancies(62 B-NHL,47 B-ALL and 24 chronic lymphocytic leukemia) who received lymphodepletion chemotherapy followed by JCAR014, the overall incidence of neurotoxicity is 40%(53 of 133); grade ≥3 neurotoxicity occurs in 21%(28 of 133), including 5 grade 5 neurotoxicity. Gust and colleagues have found that patients who developed grade ≥ 3 neurotoxicity have more severe vascular dysfunction including vascular leak and disseminated inravascular coagulation, which is consistent with widespread endothelial activation evidenced by the elevated serum Ang-2, VWF after CAR-T cell infusion. Moreover, they have also demonstrated that neurotoxicity is associated with early onset of high concentrations of serum cytokines including those that activate endothelial cells, such as IL-6, IFN-γ, and TNF-α. Those high levels of inflammatory cytokines induce endothelial cell activation, resulting in release of Ang-2 and VWF from endothelial Weibel-Palade bodies, and the released VWF binds activated endothelium and sequesters platelets. Increased permeability of the BBB due to the endothelium activation allows transit into CSF of high concentrations of serum cytokines, including IFN-γ and TNF-α, initiating a feed-forward loop of continued endothelial cell and pericyte activation. In the most severe case, this feed-forward loop can cause breakdown of the parenchymal basement membrane and vascular disruption, with cerebral edema, hemorrhage, infarction, and necrosis, and neuronal death as observed in autopsy studies of 2 patients who had fatal neurotoxicity. It must be emphasized that IL-6 may play a crucial role in this feed-forward loop. Significantly, they have shown that an earlier peak of the IL-6 serum concentration is associated with a higher risk of grade ≥ 4 neurotoxicity. In fact, markedly elevated IL-6 levels in CSF and serum of patients experiencing mild encephalopathy with a reversible splenial lesion have been reported [73]. Our group has also observed that IL-6 levels in serum of a patient with B-ALL is highly elevated 1 day after CD19/CD20 bi-specific CAR-T cell infusion, just at the onset of grade 3 neurotoxicity (unpublished data). Furthermore, the National Cancer Institute (NCI) has observed that administration of tocilizumab results in the onset of neurotoxicity in a subset of patients receiving CAR-T cells, which should be attributable to a transient elevated IL-6 level due to the inhibition of IL-6 receptor-mediated clearance by tocilizumab [11]. In short, the work by Gust and colleagues provides the first detailed clinico-pathological insights in to the CAR-T cell-associated neurotoxicity, and the confirmation in other CAR-T cell trials is required.

Risk factors for CRS and neurotoxicity related to CAR-T cell therapy

Based on the above analysis, CRS and neurotoxicity should not be seen as two completely unrelated adverse events, but be proposed as overlapping off-target toxicities resulted from the excessive immune activation either CAR-T cells or non-CAR-T cells. Although neurotoxicity can occur alone in a small number of patients, neurotoxicity severity tracked largely with CRS severity, and both correlated with enhanced CAR-T cell expansion [72]. Any factors that can increase in vivo CAR-T cell numbers, including high disease burden, higher infused CAR-T cell dose, high intensity lymphodepletion regimen, as well as some patient characteristics including preexisting endothelial activation, severe thrombocytopenia may increase the risk of CRS and/or neurotoxicity(Fig. 1). Significantly, as observed in the ROCKET trial [74], patients who have all of these factors or almost all of these factors may be at an extremely high risk of severe CRS and/or neurotoxicity.

Disease burden

Disease burden is associated with the peak expansion of CAR-T cells in vivo [75, 76], which should be the underlying mechanism of disease burden effect on the

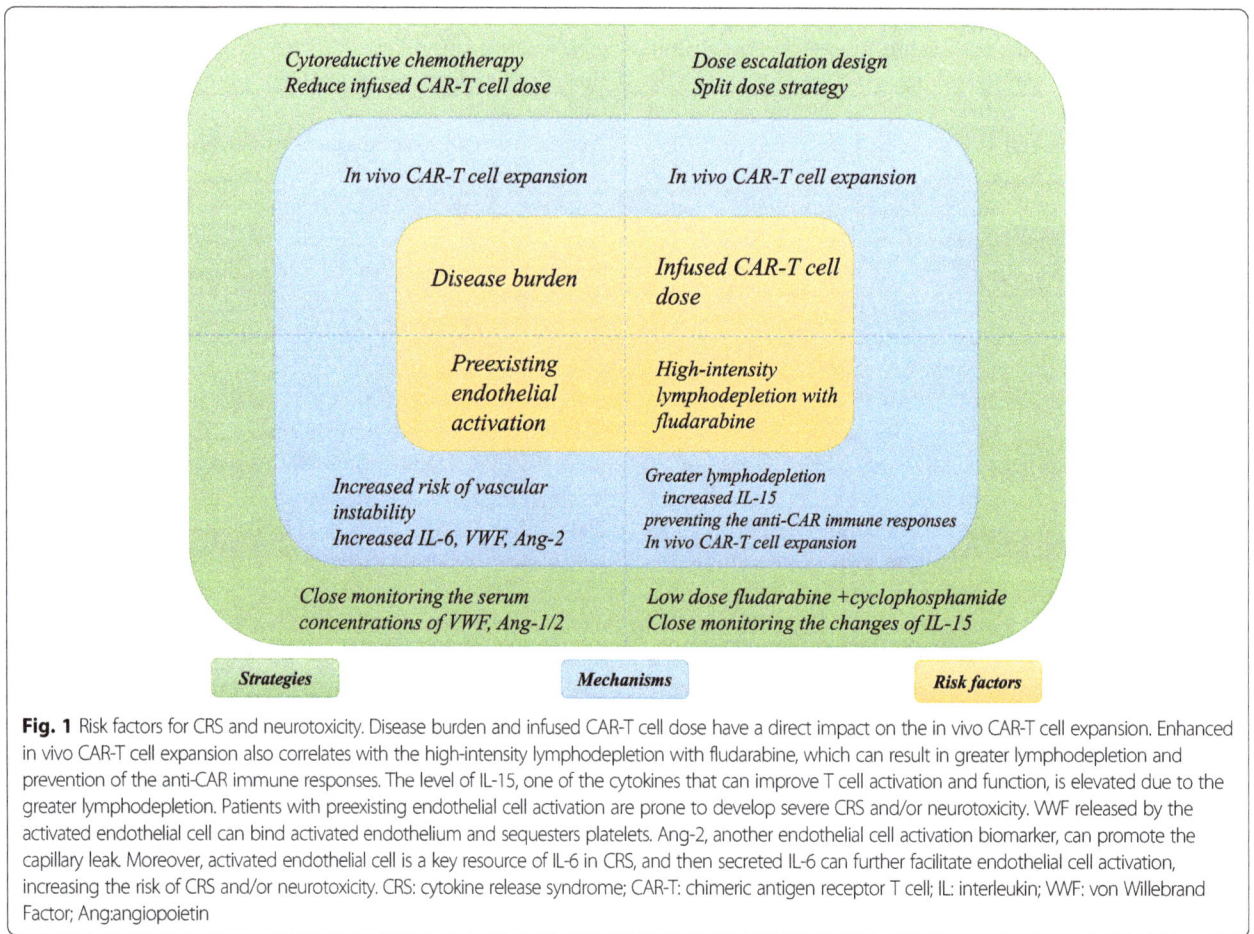

Fig. 1 Risk factors for CRS and neurotoxicity. Disease burden and infused CAR-T cell dose have a direct impact on the in vivo CAR-T cell expansion. Enhanced in vivo CAR-T cell expansion also correlates with the high-intensity lymphodepletion with fludarabine, which can result in greater lymphodepletion and prevention of the anti-CAR immune responses. The level of IL-15, one of the cytokines that can improve T cell activation and function, is elevated due to the greater lymphodepletion. Patients with preexisting endothelial cell activation are prone to develop severe CRS and/or neurotoxicity. VWF released by the activated endothelial cell can bind activated endothelium and sequesters platelets. Ang-2, another endothelial cell activation biomarker, can promote the capillary leak. Moreover, activated endothelial cell is a key resource of IL-6 in CRS, and then secreted IL-6 can further facilitate endothelial cell activation, increasing the risk of CRS and/or neurotoxicity. CRS: cytokine release syndrome; CAR-T: chimeric antigen receptor T cell; IL: interleukin; VWF: von Willebrand Factor; Ang:angiopoietin

occurrence and severity of CRS and neurotoxicity. Disease burden has been a consistent risk factor for CRS following CAR-T cell infusion [19, 28, 29, 42, 75–78], and strong correlation between the severity of CRS and disease burden at the time of CAR-T cell infusion has been noted in multiple clinical trials of CAR-T cell therapy of hematological malignancies [28, 29, 42, 75, 77]. In our phase I trial of CART-20 cells for B-NHL, we have observed that those patients with bulky disease burden defined as the lesions with a maximum diameter greater than 5 cm or more than three lesions have increased risk of CRS [77, 79]. In addition, the association between disease burden and neurotoxicity has also been reported by several programs [14, 16, 80, 81]. For example, Memorial Sloan Kettering Cancer Center (MSKCC) group has identified that the bone marrow leukemic blasts>50% is significantly associated with sever neurotoxicity in the trial of JCAR015 for B-ALL [16].Therefore, debulking therapy such as chemotherapy or radiotherapy to decrease the disease burden is essential to controlling the risk of toxicity following CAR-T cell therapy in the case of high disease burden. A cytoreductive chemotherapy regimen aiming to not only reduce disease burden but

also effect a preconditioning regimen has been adopted by our and other groups as an indispensable portion of the CAR-T cell clinical trial protocol [31, 38, 79, 82, 83]. Moreover, using a lower CAR-T cell dose for patients with high disease burden, a strategy called "risk-stratified CAR-T cell dosing" has been successfully implemented by Fred Hutchinson Cancer Research Center (FHCRC) group in a trial of JCAR014 for B-ALL, by which the incidence of neurotoxicity in patients with high disease burden (bone marrow leukemic blasts>20%) is decreased,while the disease response is not impaired [76]. Modifying the CAR-T cell dose seems feasible in B-ALL, but may reduce nodal response in other tumors, and therefore can be proposed as an alternative if necessary [13]. In conclusion, it is a challenge to treat a patient with a high disease burden, and decreasing disease burden before CAR-T cell infusion is worthy of consideration.

Infused CAR-T cell dose
Although there is no clear dose-toxicity relationship between the number of CAR T cell infused and the occurrence and severity of CRS and/or neurotoxicity, several groups have observed that infused CAR-T cell dose

indeed impacts the severity of CRS and/or neurotoxicity [13, 14, 19, 42, 63]. In the abovementioned trial of 133 patients treated with lymphodepletion chemotherapy and JCAR014 at 1 of 3 dose levels (2×10^5, 2×10^6 or 2×10^7 JCAR014 cells/kg), six of seven patients who developed grade ≥ 4 neurotoxicity were treated during the dose-escalation phase of the protocol and received JCAR014 at a dose level of 2×10^7 JCAR014 cells/kg, while only 1 of 79 patients treated after completion of the CAR-T cell dose-escalation phase and receiving JCAR014 at a dose level of 2×10^6 JCAR014 cells/kg developed grade ≥ 4 neurotoxicity [14]. This remarkable effect of infused CAR-T cell dose on the severity of toxicity highlights the necessity of the dose escalation design when testing a new CAR-T cell product.

High-intensity lymphodepletion with fludarabine
Turtle and colleagues have reproted that addition of fludarabine (Flu) to cyclophosphamide (Cy) in lymphodepletion enhances in vivo CAR-T cell expansion, which may be attribute to greater lymphodepletion and delaying or preventing the anti-CAR immune responses [76, 84]. Greater lymphodepletion can lead to increased levels of homeostatic cytokines, including IL-15, one of the cytokines that support T cell proliferation and enhance T-cell function [85–87]. Kochenderfe et al. have documented that serum IL-15 levels of all 22 patients are elevated after lymphodepletion chemotherapy and are strongly associated with the peak levels of CAR-T cells in vivo, and associated with the neurotoxicity [88]. Similar to that reported by Kochenderfe, Gilbert has also demonstrated that early and rapid CAR- T cell expansion and a rise in IL-15 levels are primary contributors to the high rates of cerebral edema seen with JCAR015 in the phase II ROCKET trial. Moreover, he has noted that the early and rapid expansion of CAR-T cells appears to correlate with higher levels of IL-15, which are increased before commencing CAR-T cell infusion due to the combined use of Flu and Cy [74]. Together, it is not surprising that addition of Flu at any given CAR-T cell dose will increase the risk of CRS and neurotoxicity, as observed by investigators from FHCRC in the larger cohort of 133 patients treated with lymphodepletion followed by JCAR014 infusion [13, 14].

Preexisting endothelial activation
As discussed above, patients with preexisting endothelial activation before infusion of CAR-T cells are at higher risk of developing sever CRS and/or neurotoxicity, suggesting that preexisting endothelial activation might be a previously unrecognized risk factor for severe CRS and/or neurotoxicity [13, 14]. Notably, severe thrombocytopenia before lymphodepletion chemotherapy is associated with higher risk of developing CRS [13]. MSKCC group have

showed that low platelet (platelet<60) is significantly correlated with severe neurotoxicity [16]. These findings imply that patients with severe thrombocytopenia might be prone to endothelial activation given the fact that platelets are one of the few sources of the endothelial stabilizing cytokine, Ang-1 [13].Thus, close examination of endothelial activation biomarkers such as VWF, Ang-2 before and after CAR-T cell infusion should be recommended, which may make sense for clinical management during CAR-T cell therapy. However, more studies are required to further explore the association between preexisting endothelial activation and higher risk of CRS and/or neurotoxicity.

Other risk factors
Preexisting neurologic comorbidities may be a risk factor for neurotoxicity [14]. Moreover, neurotoxicity is more frequent in younger patients [14, 74] and non-heavily pretreated patients [74]; a plausible reason this phenomenon may be that the expansion ability of CAR-T cells from those patients is not compromised.

Predictive biomarkers of CRS and neurotoxicity related to CAR-T cell therapy
An area of ongoing research is whether the early changes of cytokine profiles or serum biochemical markers can be applied to forecast severity of CRS and/or neurotoxicity, so as to guiding the preemptive anti-cytokine directed treatment. It is plausible that serum cytokine levels serve as biomarkers due to the natural feature of CRS characterized by significant systemic inflammation with elevated inflammatory cytokines [11].Positive significant correlation between serum cytokine levels after CAR-T cell infusion and severity of CRS has been identified across different institutions [4, 80, 89]. Recently, Teachey and colleagues have reported that they could accurately predict which patients would develop severe CRS with the forward-selected logistic regression model including three cytokines. Particularly in the pediatric patients, the modeling analyses based on evaluating the IFN-γ, IL-13, MIP1α concentrations within the 72 h of infusion are highly accurate with sensitivity of 100% and specificity of 96%, and are validated in an independent cohort of 12 pediatric patients [4]. Their work highlights that an optimal predictive biomarker for CRS must meet the following requirements: (1) significant association is not enough; it must be able to predict the onset of severe CRS with a high sensitivity and specificity. For instance, CRP and ferritin are associated with CRS, but both of these biomarkers fail to predict development of severe CRS [4]; (2) evaluating cytokines must be early. 72 h appears longer, given severe CRS can occur 24 to 72 h after CAR-T cell infusion in a subset of patients. In contrast to the model constructed by Teachey and colleagues, investigators from FHCRC have developed an more simple and timely classification tree modeling

including fever and single cytokine for earlier identification of patients at high risk of grade ≥ 4 CRS. The best sensitivity and specificity are obtained by testing serum MCP-1 in patients with fever ≥38.9 °C within 36 h of infusion [13]; Moreover, by combination of IL-6 ≥ 16 pg/mL in the first 36 h after CAR-T cell infusion, this algorithm can be used as a predictive biomarker for grade ≥ 4 neurotoxicity with sensitivity of 100% and specificity of 94% [14]. Of note, MSKCC group has demonstrated that some baseline characteristics of patients can be proposed as a predictive biomarker for severe neurotoxicity with 95% sensitivity and 70% specificity, including baseline blood platelet level<60 or mean corpuscular hemoglobin concentration>33.2% and morphologic disease (>5% blasts) [16]. It is not yet clear if these predictive models will be generalizable, confirmation is required in further studies. Moreover, it is a challenge for testing for cytokines such as MCP-1, MIP1α that cannot be readily available in most clinical hospitals currently [11]. Therefore, modeling using combination of clinical parameters may be more widely used in practice.

How to decrease the CRS and neurotoxicity related to CAR-T cell therapy

Strategies for decreasing CRS and/or neurotoxicity fall into two categories, prevention strategy aiming to lessen the occurrence of severe toxicities, and remedy strategy in an effort to minimize the toxicity once the fatal toxicities associated to CAR-T cells occur.

Based on the risk factors described above, prevention strategies mainly encompass using debulking chemotherapy to reduce the disease burden prior CAR-T cell infusion, and reducing the CAR-T cell dose in patients with high disease burden, particularly in the patients with B-ALL. More importantly, intervention early in those patients at highest risk identified by close monitoring those predictive biomarkers. Currently, in the case of management of severe or life-threatening CRS occurring after CAR-T cell therapy, tocilizumab 8 mg/kg I.V (maximum dosage per infusion does not exceed 800 mg) is recommended [8].This recommendation may be also suitable for the early intervention with CRS, as evidenced by the observation by the Seattle group that early intervention with tocilizumab ±dexamethasone appears to decrease the rates of severe CRS while not jeopardizing the efficacy [90]. Of note, at the 2017 annual meeting of the American Society of Hematology, Locke and colleges have presented that prophylactic 8 mg/kg of tocilizumab on day 2 post KTE-C19 infusion plus 750 mg of levetiracetam twice a day on day 0 reduce the incidence of severe CRS but not neurotoxicity in a safety expansion cohort of ZUMA-1, providing a preliminary supporting evidence for prophylactic tocilizumab to lessen the occurrence of severe CRS [91]. However, it seems

that prophylactic or early tocilizumab has not beneficial effect on neurotoxicity, highlighting the necessity of development of preemptive therapies rather than tocilizumab for management of neurotoxicity.

Best-in-class example of remedy strategy is the addition of "suicide" or "elimination" genes in to CAR-T cells, enabling the selective depletion of CAR-T cells in the event that severe toxicity occurs [92, 93]. Inducible caspase-9 (iCasp9) enzyme can be activated and leads to the rapid death of T cells expressing it when exposed to a synthetic dimerizing drug AP1903 [94], and several clinical trials evaluating iCasp9-modified CAR-T cells are enrolling patients (NCT02274584 and NCT02414269) [92]. However, the dimerizing drug AP1903/Rimiducid cannot be available in china, potentially limiting the widespread use of this suicide system in CAR-T cells. This selective depletion can also be mediated by the clinically approved therapeutic antibody(cetuximab or rituximab) when the transduced cells are engineered to express the antibody targeted cell surface antigen such as truncated EGFR (tEGFR) [95] or RQR8(combining target epitopes from both CD34 and CD20 antigens) [96].tEGFR has been used by Juno therapeutics in its anti-CD19 CAR-T cell products including JCAR014 and JCAR017 [19, 76], while RQR8 has been incorporated by Celletics company in to its universal anti-CD19 CAR-T cell product [97]. Nonetheless, it is a concern whether this cell ablation through antibody-dependent cellular cytotoxicity can rapidly start in case of severe toxicity.

Conclusions

CRS and neurotoxicity are two potentially life-threatening complications of CAR-T cell therapy, and a gradually growing body of research supports that both of these two toxicities are associated with the enhanced in vivo CAR-T cell expansion, implying the pathophysiology of these two distinct clinical syndromes is intertwined. Endothelial cell activation radically expands our understanding of CRS and neurotoxicity. Some simple and timely predictive biomarkers such as the combination of fever and MCP-1 make sense of early intervention for the patients at high risk of CRS and/or neurotoxicity, but confirmation is required in further clinical studies. The optimal pre-emptive therapy of high-risk patients is unknown. Prophylactic or early tocilizumab seems to benefit CRS but not neurotoxicity; endothelial stabilizing agents may be effective in neurotoxicity. Systematic investigations are necessary to determine whether those early interventions affect the antitumor activity of CAR-T cells. Efforts to further elucidate the pathologic characteristics of thes two toxicities, identification of related biomarkers, and optimize management strategies for those syndromes will make great sense to safely deliver CAR-T cell therapy.

Abbreviations

Ang: Angiopoietin; B-ALL: B cell acute lymphoblastic leukemia; BBB: Blood–brain barrier; B-NHL: B-cell non-Hodgkin lymphoma; CAR-T: Chimeric antigen receptor T cell; CNS: Central nervous system; CRP: C-reactive protein; CRS: Cytokine release syndrome; CSF: Cerebrospinal fluid; Cy: Cyclophosphamide; FDA: US Food and Drug Administration; FHCRC: Fred Hutchinson Cancer Research Center; Flu: Fludarabine; GM-CSF: Granulocyte-macrophage colony-stimulating factor; iCasp9: Inducible caspase-9; IFN: Interferon; IL: Interleukin; MCP: Monocyte chemotactic protein; MIP: Macrophage inflammatory protein; MSKCC: Memorial Sloan Kettering cancer center; NCI: National Cancer Institute; r/r: Relapsed or refractory; TNF: Tumor necrosis factor; Upenn: University of Pennsylvania; VWF: Von Willebrand factor

Acknowledgements

None.

Funding

This research was supported by the grants from the Science and Technology Planning Project of Beijing City (No. Z151100003915076 to WDH), and the National Key Research and Development Program of China (No.2016YFC1303501 and 2016YFC1303504 to WDH).

Authors' contributions

WH designed the study. ZW drafted the manuscript and figure. All authors read and approved the final manuscript.

Competing interests

The authors declare that they have no competing interests.

References

1. First-Ever CAR. T-cell therapy approved in U.S. Cancer Discov; 2017. https://doi.org/10.1158/2159-8290.CD-NB2017-126.
2. FDA Approves Second CAR T-cell Therapy. Cancer Discov; 2017. https://doi.org/10.1158/2159-8290.cd-nb2017-155.
3. DeFrancesco L. CAR-T's forge ahead, despite Juno deaths. Nat Biotechnol. 2017;35:6–7.
4. Teachey DT, Lacey SF, Shaw PA, Melenhorst JJ, Maude SL, Frey N, et al. Identification of predictive biomarkers for cytokine release syndrome after Chimeric antigen receptor T-cell therapy for acute lymphoblastic leukemia. Cancer Discov. 2016;6:664–79.
5. Wang Z, Guo Y, Han W. Current status and perspectives of chimeric antigen receptor modified T cells for cancer treatment. Protein Cell; 2017. https://doi.org/10.1007/s13238-017-0400-z.
6. Dai H, Wang Y, Lu X, Han W. Chimeric antigen receptors modified T-cells for cancer therapy. J Natl Cancer Inst. 2016;108:djv439.
7. Brudno JN, Kochenderfer JN. Chimeric antigen receptor T-cell therapies for lymphoma. Nat Rev Clin Oncol; 2017. https://doi.org/10.1038/nrclinonc.2017.128.
8. Neelapu SS, Tummala S, Kebriaei P, Wierda W, Gutierrez C, Locke FL, et al. Chimeric antigen receptor T-cell therapy - assessment and management of toxicities. Nat Rev Clin Oncol; 2017. https://doi.org/10.1038/nrclinonc.2017.148.
9. Buechner J, Grupp SA, Maude SL, Boyer M, Bittencourt H, Laetsch TW, et al. Global registration trial of efficacy and safety of CTL019 in pediatric and young adult patients with relapsed/refractory (R/R) acute lymphoblastic leukemia (ALL): update to the interim analysis. Clinical Lymphoma Myeloma Leuk. 2017;17:S263–4.
10. Neelapu SS, Locke FL, Bartlett NL, Lekakis LJ, Miklos DB, Jacobson CA, et al. Axicabtagene Ciloleucel CAR T-cell therapy in refractory large B-cell lymphoma. N Engl J Med; 2017. https://doi.org/10.1056/NEJMoa1707447.
11. Lee DW, Gardner R, Porter DL, Louis CU, Ahmed N, Jensen M, et al. Current concepts in the diagnosis and management of cytokine release syndrome. Blood. 2014;124:188–95.
12. Fitzgerald JC, Weiss SL, Maude SL, Barrett DM, Lacey SF, Melenhorst JJ, et al. Cytokine release syndrome after Chimeric antigen receptor T cell therapy for acute lymphoblastic leukemia. Crit Care Med. 2017;45:e124–31.
13. Hay KA, Hanafi LA, Li D, Gust J, Liles WC, Wurfel MM, et al. Kinetics and biomarkers of severe cytokine release syndrome after CD19 Chimeric antigen receptor-modified T cell therapy. Blood; 2017. https://doi.org/10.1182/blood-2017-06-793141.
14. Gust J, Hay KA, Hanafi LA, Li D, Myerson D, Gonzalez-Cuyar LF, et al. Endothelial activation and blood-brain barrier disruption in neurotoxicity after adoptive immunotherapy with CD19 CAR-T cells. Cancer Discov. 2017; 7:1404–19.
15. Obstfeld AE, Frey NV, Mansfield K, Lacey SF, June CH, Porter DL, et al. Cytokine release syndrome associated with chimeric-antigen receptor T-cell therapy; clinicopathological insights. Blood. 2017; https://doi.org/10.1182/blood-2017-08-802413.
16. Park JH, Santomasso B, Riviere I, Senechal B, Wang X, Purdon T, et al. Baseline and early post-treatment clinical and laboratory factors associated with severe neurotoxicity following 19-28z CAR T cells in adult patients with relapsed B-ALL. J Clin Oncol. 2017;35:7024.
17. Frey N. Cytokine release syndrome: who is at risk and how to treat. Best Pract Res Clin Haematol. 2017;30:336–40.
18. Schuster SJ, Bishop MR, Tam C, Waller EK, Borchmann P, McGuirk J, et al. Global pivotal phase 2 trial of the Cd19-targeted therapy Ctl019 in adult patients with relapsed or refractory (R/R) diffuse large B-cell lymphoma (Dlbcl)-an interim analysis. Hematol Oncol. 2017;35:27.
19. Gardner RA, Finney O, Annesley C, Brakke H, Summers C, Leger K, et al. Intent-to-treat leukemia remission by CD19 CAR T cells of defined formulation and dose in children and young adults. Blood. 2017;129:3322–31.
20. Schuster SJ, Svoboda J, Chong EA, Nasta SD, Mato AR, Anak Ö, et al. Chimeric antigen receptor T cells in refractory B-cell lymphomas. N Engl J Med; 2017. https://doi.org/10.1056/NEJMoa1708566.
21. DeAngelo DJ, Ghobadi A, Park JH, Dinner SN, Mannis GN, Lunning MA, et al. 32nd Annual Meeting and Pre-Conference Programs of the Society for Immunotherapy of Cancer (SITC 2017): Part One National Harbor, MD, USA. 8-12 November 2017 Abstracts. J Immunother Cancer. 2017;5(Suppl 2):P217.
22. Abramson JS, Palomba ML, Gordon LI, Arnason JE, Wang M, et al. High durable CR rates in relapsed/refractory (R/R) aggressive B-NHL treated with the CD19-directed CAR T cell product JCAR017 (TRANSCEND NHL 001): defined composition allows for dose-finding and definition of pivotal cohort. Blood. 2017;130:581.
23. Hu Y, Wu Z, Yu J, Wang J, Wei G, Wu W, et al. Efficacy of CD19-targeted chimeric antigen receptor T cells in the treatment of relapsed extramedullary B-cell acute lymphoblastic leukemia (B-ALL) and diffuse large B-cell lymphoma (DLBCL). J Clin Oncol. 2017;35:-e14549.
24. Xiao L, Huang H, Huang X, Ke X, Hu Y, Li J, et al. Efficacy of anti-CD19 chimeric antigen receptor modified T(CAR-T) cell therapy in Chinese patients with relapsed/refractory acute lymphocytic leukemia in a multicenter trial. J Clin Oncol. 2017;35:7028.
25. Wang Y, Chen M, Wu Z, Tong C, Huang J, Lv H, et al. CD133-redirected chimeric antigen receptor engineered autologous T-cell treatment in patients with advanced and metastatic malignancies. J Clin Oncol. 2017;35:3042.
26. Yescarta (axicabtagene ciloleucel) suspension for intravenous infusion prescribing information, Kite Pharma, Inc, October 2017. Available at https://www.fda.gov/BiologicsBloodVaccines/CellularGeneTherapyProducts/ApprovedProducts/ucm581222.htm. Accessed 7 Nov 2017.
27. Kymriah (tisagenlecleucel) suspension for intravenous infusion prescribing information, Novartis Pharmaceuticals Corp; 2017. Available at www.fda.gov/downloads/BiologicsBloodVaccines/CellularGeneTherapyProducts/ApprovedProducts/UCM573941.pdf. Accessed 6 Sept 2017.
28. Maude SL, Frey N, Shaw PA, Aplenc R, Barrett DM, Bunin NJ, et al. Chimeric antigen receptor T cells for sustained remissions in leukemia. N Engl J Med. 2014;371:1507–17.

29. Davila ML, Riviere I, Wang X, Bartido S, Park J, Curran K, et al. Efficacy and toxicity management of 19-28z CAR T cell therapy in B cell acute lymphoblastic leukemia. Sci Transl Med. 2014;6:224ra225.

30. Mei H, Jiang H, Wu Y, Guo T, Xia L, Jin R, et al. Neurological toxicities and coagulation disorders in the cytokine release syndrome during CAR-T therapy. Br J Haematol; 2017. https://doi.org/10.1111/bjh.14680.

31. Dai H, Zhang W, Li X, Han Q, Guo Y, Zhang Y, et al. Tolerance and efficacy of autologous or donor-derived T cells expressing CD19 chimeric antigen receptors in adult B-ALL with extramedullary leukemia. Oncoimmunology. 2015;4:e1027469.

32. Brudno JN, Kochenderfer JN. Toxicities of chimeric antigen receptor T cells: recognition and management. Blood. 2016;127:3321–30.

33. Ishii K, Shalabi H, Yates B, Delbrook C, Mackall CL, Fry TJ, et al. Tocilizumab-refractory cytokine release syndrome (CRS) triggered by Chimeric antigen receptor (CAR)-Transduced T cells may have distinct cytokine profiles compared to typical CRS. Blood. 2016;128:3358.

34. Mueller KT, Maude SL, Porter DL, Frey N, Wood P, Han X, et al. Cellular kinetics of CTL019 in relapsed/refractory B-cell acute lymphoblastic leukemia and chronic lymphocytic leukemia. Blood; 2017. https://doi.org/10.1182/blood-2017-06-786129.

35. Frey NV, Levine BL, Lacey SF, Grupp SA, Maude SL, Schuster SJ, et al. Refractory cytokine release syndrome in recipients of Chimeric antigen receptor (CAR) T cells. Blood. 2014;124:2296.

36. Xu XJ, Tang YM. Cytokine release syndrome in cancer immunotherapy with chimeric antigen receptor engineered T cells. Cancer Lett. 2014;343:172–8.

37. Zhang Y, Zhang W, Dai H, Wang Y, Shi F, Wang C, et al. An analytical biomarker for treatment of patients with recurrent B-ALL after remission induced by infusion of anti-CD19 chimeric antigen receptor T (CAR-T) cells. Sci China Life Sci. 2016;59:379–85.

38. Wang CM, Wu ZQ, Wang Y, Guo YL, Dai HR, Wang XH, et al. Autologous T cells expressing CD30 Chimeric antigen receptors for relapsed or refractory Hodgkin lymphoma: an open-label phase I trial. Clin Cancer Res. 2017;23:1156–66.

39. O'Hara MH, Stashwick C, Plesa G, Tanyi JL. Overcoming barriers of car T-cell therapy in patients with mesothelin-expressing cancers. Immunotherapy. 2017;9:767–80.

40. Brentjens R, Yeh R, Bernal Y, Riviere I, Sadelain M. Treatment of chronic lymphocytic leukemia with genetically targeted autologous T cells: case report of an unforeseen adverse event in a phase I clinical trial. Mol Ther. 2010;18:666–8.

41. Cai B, Guo M, Wang Y, Zhang Y, Yang J, Guo Y, et al. Co-infusion of haplo-identical CD19-chimeric antigen receptor T cells and stem cells achieved full donor engraftment in refractory acute lymphoblastic leukemia. J Hematol Oncol. 2016;9:131.

42. Lee DW, Kochenderfer JN, Stetler-Stevenson M, Cui YK, Delbrook C, Feldman SA et al. T Cells expressing CD19 chimeric antigen receptors for acute lymphoblastic leukaemia in children and young adults: a phase 1 dose-escalation trial. Lancet (London Engl). 2015; 385:517-528.

43. Porter DL, Hwang WT, Frey NV, Lacey SF, Shaw PA, Loren AW, et al. Chimeric antigen receptor T cells persist and induce sustained remissions in relapsed refractory chronic lymphocytic leukemia. Sci Transl Med. 2015;7:303ra139.

44. Frey NV, Porter DL. Cytokine release syndrome with novel therapeutics for acute lymphoblastic leukemia. Hematol Am Soc Hematol Educ Program. 2016;2016:567–72.

45. Norman DJ, Chatenoud L, Cohen D, Goldman M. Consensus statement regarding OKT3-induced cytokine-release syndrome and human antimouse antibodies. Transplant Proc. 1993;25:89–92.

46. Winkler U, Jensen M, Manzke O, Schulz H, Diehl V, Engert A. Cytokine-release syndrome in patients with B-cell chronic lymphocytic leukemia and high lymphocyte counts after treatment with an anti-CD20 monoclonal antibody (rituximab, IDEC-C2B8). Blood. 1999;94:2217–24.

47. Suntharalingam G, Perry MR, Ward S, Brett SJ, Castello-Cortes A, Brunner MD, et al. Cytokine storm in a phase 1 trial of the anti-CD28 monoclonal antibody TGN1412. N Engl J Med. 2006;355:1018–28.

48. Wing MG, Moreau T, Greenwood J, Smith RM, Hale G, Isaacs J, et al. Mechanism of first-dose cytokine-release syndrome by CAMPATH 1-H: involvement of CD16 (FcgammaRIII) and CD11a/CD18 (LFA-1) on NK cells. J Clin Invest. 1996;98:2819–26.

49. Teachey DT, Rheingold SR, Maude SL, Zugmaier G, Barrett DM, Seif AE, et al. Cytokine release syndrome after blinatumomab treatment related to abnormal macrophage activation and ameliorated with cytokine-directed therapy. Blood. 2013;121:5154–7.

50. Rotz SJ, Leino D, Szabo S, Mangino JL, Turpin BK, Pressey JG. Severe cytokine release syndrome in a patient receiving PD-1-directed therapy. Pediatr Blood Cancer; 2017. https://doi.org/10.1002/pbc.26642.

51. Tisoncik JR, Korth MJ, Simmons CP, Farrar J, Martin TR, Katze MG. Into the eye of the cytokine storm. Microbiol Mol Biol Rev. 2012;76:16–32.

52. Bugelski PJ, Achuthanandam R, Capocasale RJ, Treacy G, Bouman-Thio E. Monoclonal antibody-induced cytokine-release syndrome. Expert Rev Clin Immunol. 2009;5:499–521.

53. Walker M, Makropoulos D, Achuthanandam R, Bugelski PJ. Recent advances in the understanding of drug-mediated infusion reactions and cytokine release syndrome. Curr Opin Drug Discov Devel. 2010;13:124–35.

54. Opal SM, DePalo VA. Anti-inflammatory cytokines. Chest. 2000;117:1162–72.

55. Balkwill FR, Burke F. The cytokine network. Immunol Today. 1989;10:299–304.

56. Yiu HH, Graham AL, Stengel RF. Dynamics of a cytokine storm. PLoS One. 2012;7:e45027.

57. Harris DT, Kranz DM. Adoptive T cell therapies: a comparison of T cell receptors and Chimeric antigen receptors. Trends Pharmacol Sci. 2016;37:220–30.

58. Yang Y, Kohler ME, Chien CD, Sauter CT, Jacoby E, Yan C, et al. TCR engagement negatively affects CD8 but not CD4 CAR T cell expansion and leukemic clearance. Sci Transl Med; 2017. https://doi.org/10.1126/scitranslmed.aag1209.

59. Adusumilli PS, Cherkassky L, Villena-Vargas J, Colovos C, Servais E, Plotkin J, et al. Regional delivery of mesothelin-targeted CAR T cell therapy generates potent and long-lasting CD4-dependent tumor immunity. Sci Transl Med. 2014;6:261ra151.

60. Wu C, Xue Y, Wang P, Lin L, Liu Q, Li N, et al. IFN-γ primes macrophage activation by increasing Phosphatase and Tensin homolog via Downregulation of miR-3473b. J Immunol. 2014;193:3036–44.

61. Martinez FO, Helming L, Gordon S. Alternative activation of macrophages: an immunologic functional perspective. Annu Rev Immunol. 2009;27:451–83.

62. Prudent V, Breitbart WS. Chimeric antigen receptor T-cell neuropsychiatric toxicity in acute lymphoblastic leukemia. Palliat Support Care. 2017;15:499–503.

63. Fry TJ, Shah NN, Orentas RJ, Stetler-Stevenson M, Yuan CM, Ramakrishna S, et al. CD22-targeted CAR T cells induce remission in B-ALL that is naive or resistant to CD19-targeted CAR immunotherapy. Nat Med; 2017. https://doi.org/10.1038/nm.4441.

64. Hawkes N. Trial of novel leukaemia drug is stopped for second time after two more deaths. BMJ. 2016;355:i6376.

65. Abbasi J, Amid FDA. Approval filings, another CAR-T therapy patient death. JAMA. 2017;317:2271.

66. Topp MS, Gökbuget N, Stein AS, Zugmaier G, O'Brien S, Bargou RC, et al. Safety and activity of blinatumomab for adult patients with relapsed or refractory B-precursor acute lymphoblastic leukaemia: a multicentre, single-arm, phase 2 study. Lancet Oncol. 2015;16:57.

67. Wu J, Fu J, Zhang M, Liu D. Blinatumomab: a bispecific T cell engager (BiTE) antibody against CD19/CD3 for refractory acute lymphoid leukemia. J Hematol Oncol. 2015;8:104.

68. Fan G, Wang Z, Hao M, Li J. Bispecific antibodies and their applications. J Hematol Oncol. 2015;8:130.

69. O'Rourke DM, Nasrallah MP, Desai A, Melenhorst JJ, Mansfield K, Morrissette JJD, et al. A single dose of peripherally infused EGFRvIII-directed CAR T cells mediates antigen loss and induces adaptive resistance in patients with recurrent glioblastoma. Sci Transl Med; 2017. https://doi.org/10.1126/scitranslmed.aaa0984.

70. Abramson JS, McGree B, Noyes S, Plummer S, Wong C, Chen YB, et al. Anti-CD19 CAR T cells in CNS diffuse large-B-cell lymphoma. N Engl J Med. 2017;377:783–4.

71. Hu Y, Sun J, Wu Z, Yu J, Cui Q, Pu C, et al. Predominant cerebral cytokine release syndrome in CD19-directed chimeric antigen receptor-modified T cell therapy. J Hematol Oncol. 2016;9:70.

72. Mackall CL, Miklos DB. CNS endothelial cell activation emerges as a driver of CAR T cell-associated neurotoxicity. Cancer Discov. 2017;7:1371–3.

73. Kometani K, Kawatani M, Ohta G, Okazaki S, Ogura K, Yasutomi M, et al. Marked elevation of interleukin-6 in mild encephalopathy with a reversible splenial lesion (MERS) associated with acute focal bacterial nephritis caused by Enterococcus faecalis. Brain and Development. 2014;36:551–3.

74. Inman S. JCAR015 Experience Informs Future CAR-T Studies. OncLive; 2017. http://www.onclive.com/web-exclusives/jcar015-experience-informs-future-cart-studies . Accessed 10 Nov 2017.

75. Turtle CJ, Hay KA, Hanafi LA, Li D, Cherian S, Chen X, et al. Durable molecular remissions in chronic lymphocytic leukemia treated with CD19-

specific Chimeric antigen receptor-modified T cells after failure of Ibrutinib. J Clin Oncol. 2017;35:3010–20.

76. Turtle CJ, Hanafi LA, Berger C, Gooley TA, Cherian S, Hudecek M, et al. CD19 CAR-T cells of defined CD4+:CD8+ composition in adult B cell ALL patients. J Clin Invest. 2016;126:2123–38.

77. Wang Y, Zhang WY, Han QW, Liu Y, Dai HR, Guo YL, et al. Effective response and delayed toxicities of refractory advanced diffuse large B-cell lymphoma treated by CD20-directed chimeric antigen receptor-modified T cells. Clin Immunol. 2014;155:160–75.

78. Rouce RH, Heslop HE. Forecasting cytokine storms with new predictive biomarkers. Cancer Discov. 2016;6:579–80.

79. Zhang W-y, Wang Y, Guo Y-l, Dai H-r, Yang Q-m, Zhang Y-j, et al. Treatment of CD20-directed Chimeric antigen receptor-modified T cells in patients with relapsed or refractory B-cell non-Hodgkin lymphoma: an early phase IIa trial report. Signal Transduct Target Ther. 2016;1:16002.

80. Turtle CJ, Hay KA, Gust J, Hanafi L-A, Li D, Liles WC, et al. Cytokine release syndrome (CRS) and neurotoxicity (NT) after CD19-specific chimeric antigen receptor- (CAR-) modified T cells. J Clin Oncol. 2017;35:3020.

81. Park JH, Riviere I, Wang XY, Purdon T, Sadelain M, Brentjens RJ. Impact of disease burden on long-term outcome of 19-28z CAR modified T cells in adult patients with relapsed B-ALL. J Clin Oncol. 2016;34:7003.

82. Porter DL, Levine BL, Kalos M, Bagg A, June CH. Chimeric antigen receptor-modified T cells in chronic lymphoid leukemia. N Engl J Med. 2011;365:725–33.

83. Feng K, Liu Y, Guo Y, Qiu J, Wu Z, Dai H, et al. Phase I study of chimeric antigen receptor modified T cells in treating HER2-positive advanced biliary tract cancers and pancreatic cancers. Protein Cell; 2017. https://doi.org/10.1007/s13238-017-0440-4.

84. Turtle CJ, Hanafi LA, Berger C, Hudecek M, Pender B, Robinson E, et al. Immunotherapy of non-Hodgkin's lymphoma with a defined ratio of CD8+ and CD4+ CD19-specific chimeric antigen receptor-modified T cells. Sci Transl Med. 2016;8:355ra116.

85. Xu Y, Zhang M, Ramos CA, Durett A, Liu E, Dakhova O, et al. Closely related T-memory stem cells correlate with in vivo expansion of CAR.CD19-T cells and are preserved by IL-7 and IL-15. Blood. 2014;123:3750–9.

86. Hoyos V, Savoldo B, Quintarelli C, Mahendravada A, Zhang M, Vera J, et al. Engineering CD19-specific T lymphocytes with interleukin-15 and a suicide gene to enhance their anti-lymphoma[sol]leukemia effects and safety. Leukemia. 2010;24:1160.

87. Waldmann TA. Interleukin-15 in the treatment of cancer. Expert Rev Clin Immunol. 2014;10:1689.

88. Kochenderfer JN, Somerville RPT, Lu T, Shi V, Bot A, Rossi J, et al. Lymphoma remissions caused by anti-CD19 Chimeric antigen receptor T cells are associated with high serum Interleukin-15 levels. J Clin Oncol. 2017;35:1803–13.

89. Turtle CJ, Hay KA, Juliane G, Hanafi LA, Li D, Chaney C, et al. Biomarkers of cytokine release syndrome and neurotoxicity after CD19 CAR-T cells and mitigation of toxicity by cell dose. Blood. 2016;128:1852.

90. Gardner R, Leger KJ, Annesley CE, Summers C, Rivers J, Gust J, et al. Decreased rates of severe CRS seen with early intervention strategies for CD19 CAR-T cell toxicity management. Blood. 2016;128:586.

91. Locke FL, Neelapu SS, Bartlett NL, Lekakis LJ, Jacobson CA, Braunschweig I, et al. Preliminary results of prophylactic Tocilizumab after Axicabtageneciloleucel (axi-cel; KTE-C19) treatment for patients with Refractory,Aggressive non-Hodgkin lymphoma (NHL). Blood. 2017;130:–1547.

92. Wang Z, Wu Z, Liu Y, Han W. New development in CAR-T cell therapy. J Hematol Oncol. 2017;10:53.

93. Lichtman EI, Dotti G. Chimeric antigen receptor T-cells for B-cell malignancies. Transl Res; 2017. https://doi.org/10.1016/j.trsl.2017.06.011.

94. Di Stasi A, Tey SK, Dotti G, Fujita Y, Kennedy-Nasser A, Martinez C, et al. Inducible apoptosis as a safety switch for adoptive cell therapy. N Engl J Med. 2011;365:1673–83.

95. Wang X, Chang WC, Wong CW, Colcher D, Sherman M, Ostberg JR, et al. A transgene-encoded cell surface polypeptide for selection, in vivo tracking, and ablation of engineered cells. Blood. 2011;118:1255–63.

96. Philip B, Kokalaki E, Mekkaoui L, Thomas S, Straathof K, Flutter B, et al. A highly compact epitope-based marker/suicide gene for easier and safer T-cell therapy. Blood. 2014;124:1277–87.

97. Qasim W, Zhan H, Samarasinghe S, Adams S, Amrolia P, Stafford S, et al. Molecular remission of infant B-ALL after infusion of universal TALEN gene-edited CAR T cells. Sci Transl Med; 2017. https://doi.org/10.1126/scitranslmed.aaj2013.

23

Overexpression and cytoplasmic localization of caspase-6 is associated with lamin A degradation in set of ovarian cancers

Callinice D Capo-chichi[1,2]* (ID), Kathy Q Cai[3] and Xiang-Xi Xu[2]

Abstract

Background: In most women with ovarian cancer, the diagnosis occurs after dissemination of tumor cells beyond ovaries. Several molecular perturbations occur ahead of tumor initiation including loss of lamin A/C. Our hypothesis was that the loss of nuclear structural proteins A type lamins (lamin A/C) transcribed from LMNA gene and substrate for active caspase-6 maybe one of the molecular perturbations. Our objective is to investigate the association between the loss of lamin A/C and the overexpression of caspase-6 in ovarian cancer cells.

Method: Western blotting and immunofluorescence were used to analyze the expression of lamin A/C and active caspase-6 in normal human ovarian surface epithelial (HOSE) cells, immortalized human ovarian surface epithelial cells and a set of seven ovarian cancer cell lines (including OVCAR3, OVCAR5, and A2780). The activity of caspase-6 was measured by densitometry, fluorescence and flow cytometry. Immunohistochemistry was used to evaluate the expression of caspase-6 in set of ovarian cancer tissues previously reported to have lost lamin A/C.

Results: The results showed that HOSE cells expressed lamin A/C and no or low level of active caspase-6 while cancer cells highly expressed caspase-6 and no or low level of lamin A/C. The inhibition of caspase-6 activity in OVCAR3 cells increased lamin A but has no effect on lamin C; active caspase-6 was localized in the cytoplasm associated with the loss of lamin A.

Conclusion: Overexpression and cytoplasmic localization of caspase-6 in ovarian cancer cells may be involved in lamin A degradation and deficiency observed in some ovarian cancer cells.

Keywords: Ovarian cancer, Active caspase-6, Cytoplasmic localization, Lamin A/C degradation, Immunofluorescence, Flow cytometry

Background

Ovarian cancer is the most lethal gynecological neoplasm and cause of death associated to cancer among women worldwide. Treatment for ovarian cancer is complex and the outcome after diagnosis is not satisfactory because the diagnosis occurs often after cancer cells had spread beyond the ovaries [1, 2]. It was reported that failure in ovarian cancer therapy occurs in 90% of cases [2]. It is becoming obvious that focusing on molecular abnormalities leading to cancer will help saving more women. Our former studies showed that lamin A/C expression was lost in ovarian cancer cell prior to nuclear deformation, chromosomal numerical instability, polyploidy and aneuploidy; all of which are hallmark for ovarian cancer [3, 4]. Lamin A was reported to be a substrate for caspase-6 [5–7]. As matter of fact, cleavage of lamin A/C was utilized as method to measure caspase-6 activity in whole cell assay [7]. Caspase-6 was reported to be activated by caspase-3

---

* Correspondence: callinice.capochichi@gmail.com;
dcapochichi@med.miami.edu
[1]Institute of Applied Biomedical Sciences (ISBA), Unit of Biochemistry and Molecular Biology, Division of Molecular Biomarkers in Cancer and Nutrition, University of Abomey-Calavi, Abomey-Calavi, Benin
[2]Sylvester Cancer Center (SCCC), Ovarian Cancer Program, University of Miami, Miami, Florida, USA
Full list of author information is available at the end of the article

during apoptotic event [8–12]. To the best of our ac-knowledges, the link between cytoplasmic localization of activated caspase-6 and the loss of the nuclear structural protein lamin A in ovarian cancer was not yet reported. Our investigation demonstrated an inverse association between active caspase-6 and lamin A in ovarian cancer cell lines and tissues. We hypothesized that active caspase-6 may be involved in lamin A/C degradation leading to the loss of nuclear structural proteins A type lamins (lamin A/C) prior to nuclear anomalies leading to carcinogenesis.

Methods

Reagents

Tris-Base, glycine, sodium dodecyl sulfate, bis-acrylamide, nitrocellulose membrane, were purchased from Bio-Rad. Inc. (USA). NaCl, KCl, Tween-20, protease inhibitor PMSF, 2-mercaptoethanol, DTT, methanol, ethanol, EDTA, glycerol, sodium azide, sodium fluoride. The primary antibodies made in rabbit against lamin A/C, lamin A and cleaved lamin A were from Transduction Lab (USA). The primary rabbit antibodies for simultaneous detection of procaspase-6 and caspase-6 were from Sigma-Aldrich (USA) and Cell signaling. Peroxidase (HRP)-conjugated secondary antibody (anti-rabbit) made in goat was from Bio-Rad Inc. (USA). A Super Signal West Dura Extended Duration Substrate made by PIERCE was purchased from Thermo Scientific (Rockford, IL USA). Caspase-6 specific inhibitor drug A6339 (N-Acetyl-Val-Glu-Ile-Asp-aldehyde, Synonym: Ac-VEID-CHO) was purchased from Sigma-Aldrich, USA.

Human ovarian surface epithelial and cancer cell cultures

- Human ovarian surface epithelial (HOSE) cells were established from ovaries obtained from prophylactic oophorectomies [13]. Specimen of fresh intact whole ovary was immersed in medium and send to the laboratory where the ovarian surface was gently scraped with a rubber policeman to collect cells. The ovarian tissues were then analyzed by pathologists to confirm the absence of microscopic tumors. HOSE cells were cultured in 105 + 199 media containing 15% FBS, streptomycin, and insulin.
- To prepare human "immortalized" ovarian (HIO) cells, HOSE cells were transfected with SV40 T-antigen and cultured in 105 + 199 (V/V) media containing 15% FBS, streptomycin, and insulin. HIO cells had a longer lifespan in culture and can be cultured up to 50 passages before undergoing senescence unlike HOSE cells that can only be maintained in culture up to 7 passages [3, 13].
- The OVCAR lines were previously established by Thomas Hamilton [3, 13] and the others (A1847,

A2780, and ES2) were obtained from American Type Culture Collection. Ovarian epithelial cancer cell lines were cultured in DMEM with 10% FBS and streptomycin as previously reported [3].

Western blot of ovarian primary surface epithelial, immortalized and cancer cells

Cells were cultured in six well dishes in respective media. Cells were washed with ice cold PBS and lysate with 200 µl RIPA buffer (Santa Cruz Biotechnology) in ice for 30 min. Aliquot of 2 µl was used for protein quantification with the Bio-Rad protein assay kit. Protein denaturation was achieved with 4× SDS buffer containing β-mercaptoethanol (2%) and glycerol (40%). Cell lysates were boiled for 5 min and stored at – 20 °C until needed for western blot analysis. Samples were loaded on 4–12% gradient SDS-polyacrylamide gels (Invitrogen) and run at 100 V for 2 h in tris-glycine buffer. Proteins were transferred from the gels to nitrocellulose membranes with transfer buffer containing tris-glycine and 20% methanol. The membranes were blocked with 5% milk in 1X TBS containing 0.1% Tween-20 (TBST) for 30 min at room temperature before incubation in primary antibody in 1% milk/TBST for 1 h at room temperature. The blots were washed 4 times for 10 min with TBST before incubation with HRP-conjugated secondary antibody in 1% milk/TBST for 1 h. The blots were washed 4 times for 15 min with TBST and the membranes were the incubated 3 min in Super Signal West Dura Extended Duration Substrate and exposed to x-ray film and a film developer for the detection of caspase-6 and lamin A/C. The same protocol was performed for the detection of ß-actin as loading control.

Immunofluorescence microscopy

Cells were cultured on plastic slide up to 90% confluence in a six well plate. Cells were washed twice with PBS and fixed with 4% paraformaldehyde for 15 min. Fixed cells were washed three times with PBS, permeabilized with 0.5% Triton X-100 for 5 min and blocked with 3% BSA in PBS containing 0.1% Tween-20 for 30 min. For double staining of activated caspase-6 (p20) and lamin A, the slides were incubated for 1 h at 37 °C with primary antibody rabbit anti caspase-6 (p20) from Santa-Cruz biotechnology and with primary antibody mouse anti lamin A/C from Cell Signaling (USA). Subsequently slides were washed three times with 1% BSA in PBS and incubated in 1% BSA/PBS solution with secondary antibodies conjugated with AlexaFluor 488 (green fluorescence) and AlexaFluor 594 (red fluorescence) (Invitrogen, Carlsbad, CA). The nuclei were stained with DAPI (Invitrogen, Carlsbad, CA). Cells were mounted on glass slide and sealed in anti-fade reagent containing 0.1 M n-propyl gallate (pH 7.4) and 90% glycerol in PBS. A Zeiss microscope and AxioCam Camera and Axio Vision software 4.8 were used for image acquisition and processing [3].

Flow cytometry analysis

The detection of caspase-6 activity was achieved using an APO LOGIX Carboxyfluorescein caspase-6 specific detection Kit. For the evaluation of caspase-6 activity, FAM-VEID-FMK Caspase-6 detection kit was used as recommended by the manufacturer. Cells were cultured in 96 well dishes in respective media for 24 h before the addition of Carboxyfluorescein (FAM) labeled peptide (VEID)-fluoromethyl Ketone (FMK) reagent for 2 h. FAM-VEID-FMK is a cell permeable probe that enters each cell and covalently binds to the reactive cysteine residue on the large subunit of the caspase-6 heterodimer (FAM- VEID-FMK-Caspase-6). The probe is sequestered and accumulated inside the cell while inhibiting further caspase-6 activity. Cells bounds to FAM-peptide-FMK can be detected by a flow cytometer, or a fluorescence microscope with the green fluorescent channel (488 nm). Cell sorting and flow analyses were performed on LSR Fortessa driven by BD's FACS Diva software version 6.1.3 (Becton Dickinson, San Jose, CA).

Caspase-6 mRNA suppression with siRNA

Caspase-6 down regulation was achieved with siRNA against caspase-6 was purchased from Santacruz biotechnology (USA). Cell were plated in 6 well dish 24 h prior to siRNA transfection with lipofectamine 2000 according to the manufacturer protocol (Invitrogen).

Cells were washed twice with PBS and processed for immunoblotting as previously described [3, 13].

Tumor specimen's acquisition and immunohistochemistry

Tumor specimens processing and immunohistochemistry protocol were previously described [3]. In brief, our current study utilized archived tumor tissue microarrays and cell lines prepared from human ovaries obtained from prophylactic surgeries. Cancer tissues and cells lines were obtained from Fox Chase Cancer Center tumor bank, for research purpose. The use of the tumor tissues for research was approved by the Institutional Review Board (IRB) of both Fox Chase Cancer Center and of the University of Miami, Miller School of Medicine [3, 13]. The ovarian tumor tissue microarrays (duplicate core of 120 tumor tissues and 5 controls) and 20 prophylactic oophorectomies were provided by the Tumor Bank of Fox Chase Cancer Center as previously described in detail [3]. Immunostaining was performed using primary antibodies anti active caspase-6 made in rabbit along with the rabbit DAKO Envision TM+ System and the Peroxidase (DAB) Kit (Dako Carpinteria, CA) as previously described [3]. Negative controls were performed by replacing the primary antibodies with non-immunized IgG.

Result and discussion

Procaspase-6 and caspase-6 expression in ovarian normal, immortalized and cancer cells

Licor-Odyssey immunofluorescence blot system was used to analyze Caspase-6 expressions in human primary surface epithelial cells (HOSE), in human immortalized surface epithelial cells (HIO80) and in ovarian cancer cell lines OVCAR5, OVCAR4, OVCAR2 and A2780 as shown in Fig. 1. After immunofluorescence revelation, OVCAR3 and

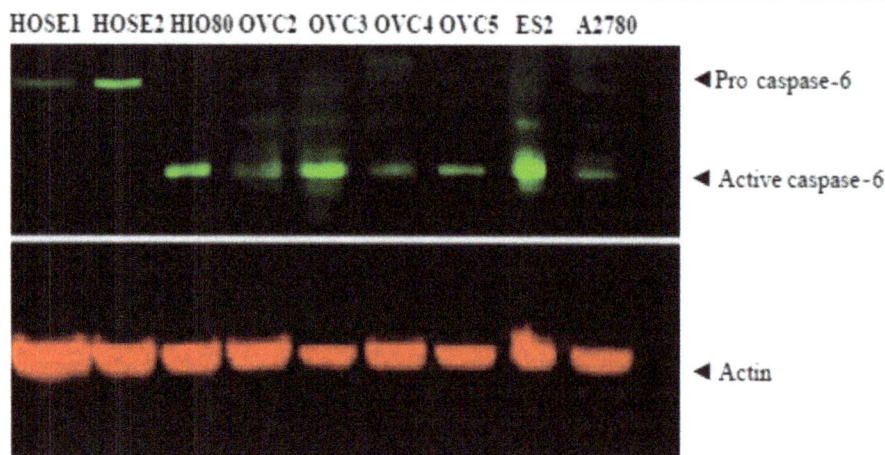

Fig. 1 Immunofluorescence blot showing the expression of procaspase-6 and active caspase-6 in human primary surface epithelial cells (HOSE1 HOSE2), in human immortalized surface epithelial cells (HIO80) and in ovarian cancer cell lines OVCAR2, OVCAR3, OVCAR4, OVCAR5 and A2780. HOSE cells had constitutive procaspase-6 while proliferating HIO and cancer cells had constitutive active caspase-6

ES2 had more activated caspase-6 (Fig. 1). The expressions of procaspase-6 was present in HOSE cells but not active caspase-6. In contrast, active caspase-6 was present in immortalized cells HIO80, in ovarian cancer cell lines OVCAR2–5, ES2 and A2780 but not in normal HOSE cells (Fig. 1). HOSE cells had constitutive procaspase-6 while proliferating HIO in culture and cancer cells had constitutive active caspase-6; actin was used as loading control (Fig. 1).

Analysis of active or cleaved caspase-6 and cleaved Lamin A profile in ovarian normal, immortalized and cancer cells

The profile of cleaved lamin A and cleaved caspase-6 (active caspase-6) in normal HOSE cells, immortalized HIO80, HIO118, in ovarian cancer cell lines OVCAR3, OVCAR5, OVCAR10, ES2, A2780 and A1847 was shown on immuno-chemoluminescence blot (Fig. 2a). HOSE and HIO (passages < 10) cell lines had low or no active caspase-6 nor cleaved lamin A/C in contrast to most of ovarian cancer cell lines with high expression of active caspase-6 and cleaved lamin A (Fig. 2a). ES2 had less cleaved lamin A than the other cancer cells although its active caspase-6 level was higher (Fig. 2a).

Analysis of active or cleaved caspase-6 and lamin A/C profile in ovarian normal, immortalized and cancer cells

Immuno-chemoluminescence blot showing the expression of lamin A/C, active caspase-6 and β-actin in human primary surface epithelial cells (HOSE) in human immortalized surface epithelial cells (HIO80) and in ovarian cancer cell lines ES2, OVCAR2, OVCAR3, OVCAR4, OVCAR5 and A2780, is shown in Fig. 2b. HOSE cells had high lamin A/C and no active caspase-6 (cleaved caspase-6) while proliferating HIO and cancer cells ES2 had active caspase-6 and weak expression of lamin A/C. Exceptionally for OVCAR2 with weak active caspase-6 and lamin A/C and active caspase-6 all other ovarian cancer cell lines had high expression of cleaved caspase-6 and weak expression of lamin A/C (Fig. 2b). The β-actin was used as loading control.

Evaluation of active caspase-6 dynamic in normal and some ovarian cancer cells by immunofluorescence

The detection of caspase-6 activity was achieved using Carboxyfluorescein Caspase-6 Detection Kit, FAM-VEID-FMK caspase-6 (APO LOGIX). The assay was done according to the manufacturer protocol. Carboxyfluorescein (FAM)_labeled peptide fluoromethyl Ketone (FMK)-caspase-6 inhibitor [caspase-6 FAM-VEID-FMK Caspase-6 detection kit] is cell permeable compound that enter each cell and covalently binds to the reactive cysteine residue on the large subunit of the caspase heterodimer. The probe is sequestered and accumulate inside cell while inhibiting further

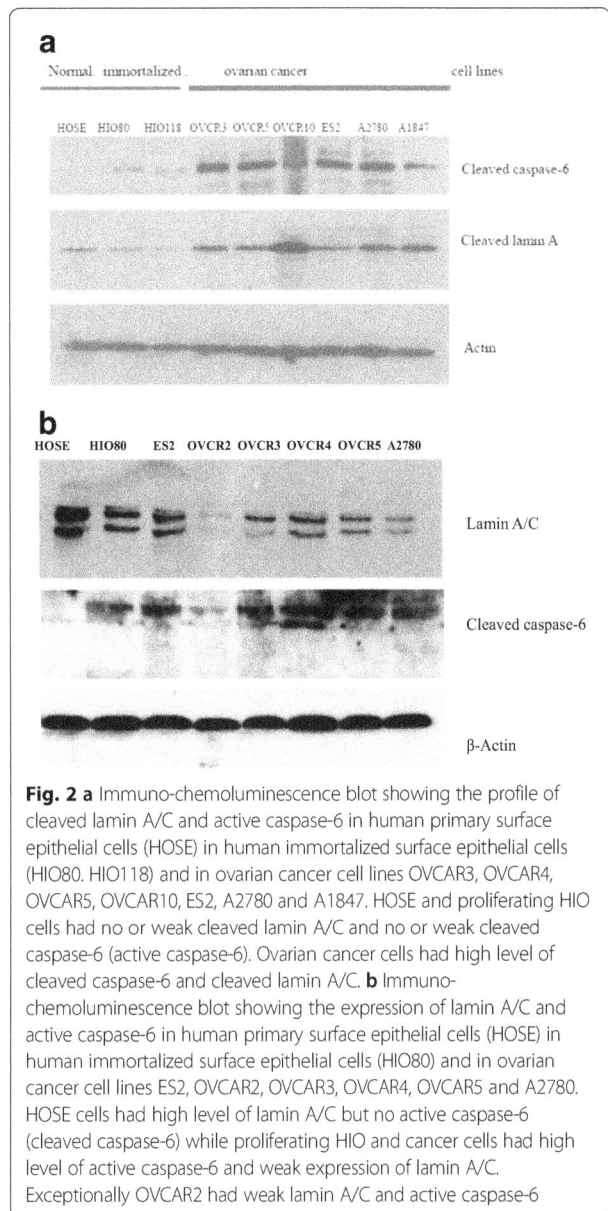

Fig. 2 a Immuno-chemoluminescence blot showing the profile of cleaved lamin A/C and active caspase-6 in human primary surface epithelial cells (HOSE) in human immortalized surface epithelial cells (HIO80. HIO118) and in ovarian cancer cell lines OVCAR3, OVCAR4, OVCAR5, OVCAR10, ES2, A2780 and A1847. HOSE and proliferating HIO cells had no or weak cleaved lamin A/C and no or weak cleaved caspase-6 (active caspase-6). Ovarian cancer cells had high level of cleaved caspase-6 and cleaved lamin A/C. **b** Immuno-chemoluminescence blot showing the expression of lamin A/C and active caspase-6 in human primary surface epithelial cells (HOSE) in human immortalized surface epithelial cells (HIO80) and in ovarian cancer cell lines ES2, OVCAR2, OVCAR3, OVCAR4, OVCAR5 and A2780. HOSE cells had high level of lamin A/C but no active caspase-6 (cleaved caspase-6) while proliferating HIO and cancer cells had high level of active caspase-6 and weak expression of lamin A/C. Exceptionally OVCAR2 had weak lamin A/C and active caspase-6

caspase activity. Cells bounds to FAM-peptide-FMK can be detected by a fluorescence microscope (GFP Chanel) or a flow cytometer. For our experiment to detect active caspase-6 in cancer cells and HOSE controls, cells were plated in 12 well dish for 24 h and then incubated with FAM-VEID-FMK reagent for 2 h. Cells were fixed and cells with green fluorescence were counted among 100 cells. The results are shown in Fig. 3. All ovarian cancer cells displayed more cells with active caspase-6 than control HOSE C1 and HOSE C2. This experiment was repeated three times. The results are displayed in histogram (Fig. 3) as mean ± SD and are HOSEC1 5 ± 0.14; HOSEC2 6.2 ± 1.97; OVCAR3 32.2 ± 4.80; OVCAR5 33.56 ± 7.15; ES2 51.2 ± 9.61; A1847 26.55 ± 4.91 and A2780 33.6 ± 2.54. Flow

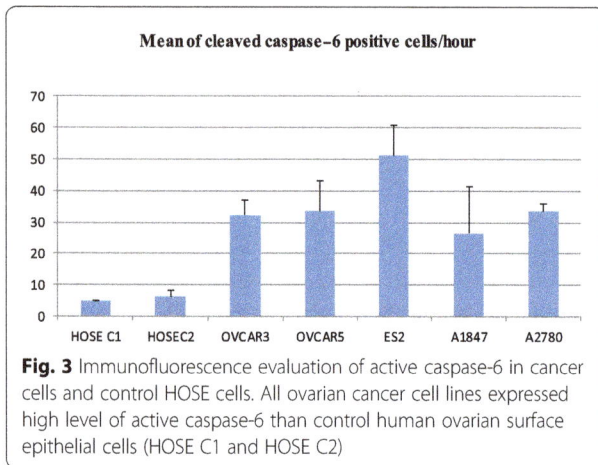

Fig. 3 Immunofluorescence evaluation of active caspase-6 in cancer cells and control HOSE cells. All ovarian cancer cell lines expressed high level of active caspase-6 than control human ovarian surface epithelial cells (HOSE C1 and HOSE C2)

fluorescence emission of FAM-VEID-FMK covalently bound to the reactive cysteine residue on the large subunit of the caspase-6 heterodimer while inhibiting further caspase-6 activity, was detected by flow cytometry. Cell population with green fluorescence indicating cell entry of FAM-VEID-FMK covalently bound to active caspase-6 cysteine residue was counted in a population of 10000 cells (events). Flow analyses performed with two control human ovarian surface epithelial cells (HOSE1 and HOSE2) and three ovarian cancer cells lines (OVCAR3, A1847 and A2780) are shown in Fig. 4. Active caspase-6 is weak in HOSE1 and HOSE2 (4.6% and 3.4%) compared to cancer cell lines OVCAR3, A1847 and A2780 (36.6%, 15.5% and 30.2% respectively).

cytometry also was used to evaluate caspase-6 activity in a set of HOSE and ovarian cancer cell lines. The results are displayed in Fig. 4.

Evaluation of activated caspase-6 in normal and a set ovarian cancer cells by flow cytometer

The detection of caspase-6 activity was achieved using Carboxyfluorescein Caspase-6 Detection Kit, FAM-VEID-FMK Caspase-6 (APO LOGIX). The assay was done according to the manufacturer protocol. Cells were plated in 12 well dish for 24 h and then incubated with FAM-VEID-FMK reagent for 2 h. Green

Inhibition of caspase-6 activity and the effect on Lamin a/ C expression in OVCAR3 cell line

We treated OVCAR3 cell line plated in 6 well culture dish with caspase-6 specific inhibitor drug A6339 for 24 h according to the manufacturer protocol. Cells were harvested and processed for immunoblotting with anti lamin A/C antibody as described above. The results showed an increase in lamin A/ C expression after inhibition of caspase-6 activity with drug A6339, actin was used as loading control (Fig. 5). This drug did not show restoration of lamin A/C in OVCAR5 cell line (data not shown).

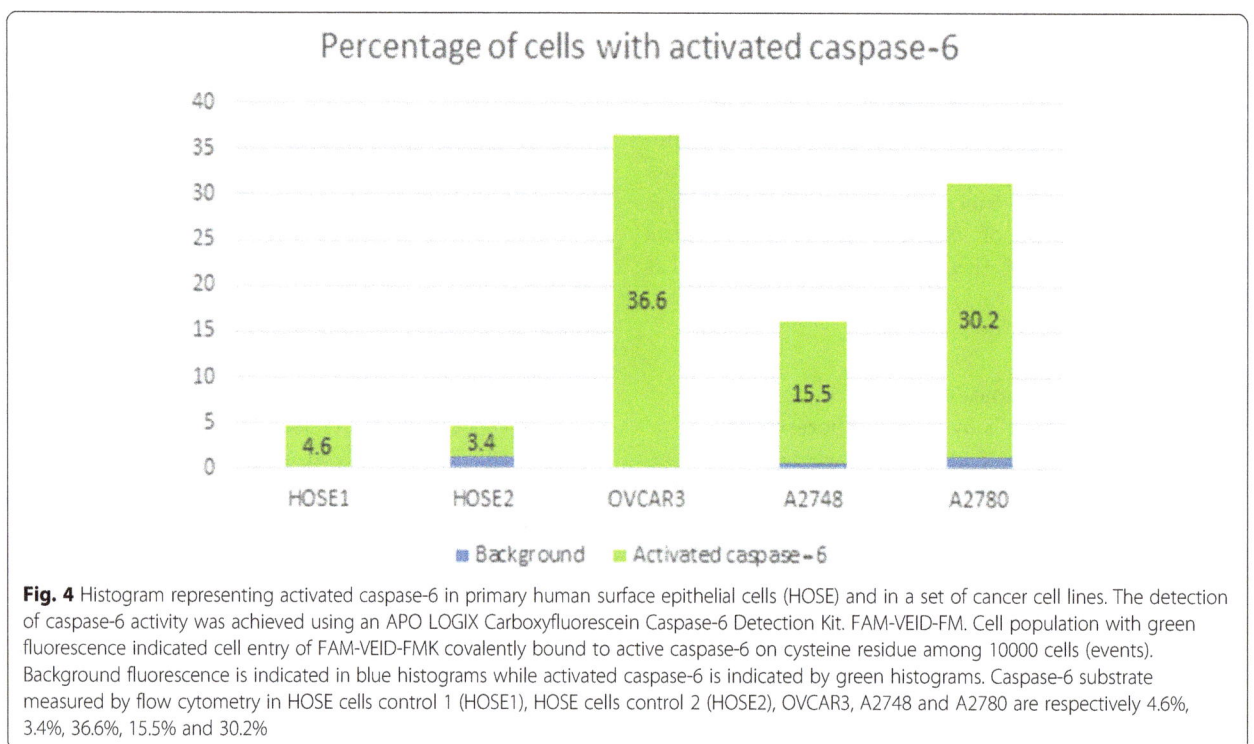

Fig. 4 Histogram representing activated caspase-6 in primary human surface epithelial cells (HOSE) and in a set of cancer cell lines. The detection of caspase-6 activity was achieved using an APO LOGIX Carboxyfluorescein Caspase-6 Detection Kit. FAM-VEID-FM. Cell population with green fluorescence indicated cell entry of FAM-VEID-FMK covalently bound to active caspase-6 on cysteine residue among 10000 cells (events). Background fluorescence is indicated in blue histograms while activated caspase-6 is indicated by green histograms. Caspase-6 substrate measured by flow cytometry in HOSE cells control 1 (HOSE1), HOSE cells control 2 (HOSE2), OVCAR3, A2748 and A2780 are respectively 4.6%, 3.4%, 36.6%, 15.5% and 30.2%

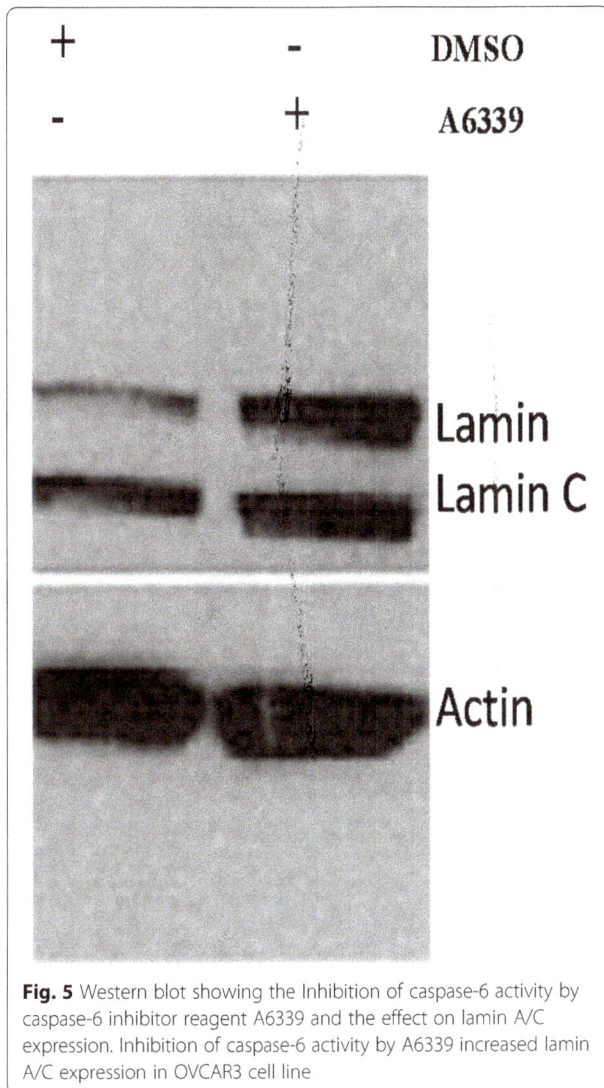

Fig. 5 Western blot showing the Inhibition of caspase-6 activity by caspase-6 inhibitor reagent A6339 and the effect on lamin A/C expression. Inhibition of caspase-6 activity by A6339 increased lamin A/C expression in OVCAR3 cell line

Immunofluorescence staining of active caspase-6 (p20) and lamin A in ovarian cancer cell line OVCAR3

Double staining of active caspase-6 (p20) and lamin A specific antibodies was realized with OVCAR3 cell line and fluorescence microscopy images are displayed in Fig. 6. Image of lamin A immunofluorescence staining (green) along with nuclear counter stain with Dapi (blue) is displayed in Fig. 6a. Merged image of OVCAR3 stained with lamin A (green), caspase-6 (p20) in red and nuclear stain with Dapi (blue) is represented in Fig. 6b. All OVCAR3 cells expressed caspase-6 (p20) while most of cells had lost lamin A. Pictures were taken with 60× oil objective on ZEISS microscope.

Immunofluorescence staining of caspase-6 (p20) and lamin a in ovarian cancer cell line OVCAR5

In OVCAR5 cell line, active caspase-6 (p20) and lamin A expressions were displayed in Fig. 7. Figure 7a represented OVCAR5 stained with lamin A (red); Fig. 7b represented OVCAR5 stained caspase-6 (green); Fig. 7c represented OVCAR5 stained with Dapi (blue) while Fig. 7d represented merged image of OVCAR5 stained with lamin A (red), caspase-6 (green) and Dapi (blue). All OVCAR5 cells expressed caspase-6 (p20) while most cells had lost lamin A. The loss of lamin A was associated with the presence of caspase-6 in the cytoplasm as indicated by white arrows (Fig. 7a-d). Pictures were taken with 100× oil objective on ZEISS microscope.

Immunostaining of caspase-6 in ovarian epithelial transition to neoplasia and ovarian cancer tissues

Active caspase-6 staining by immunohistochemistry in ovarian epithelium transition to ovarian neoplasia is displayed in Fig. 8; caspase-6 staining picture was taken

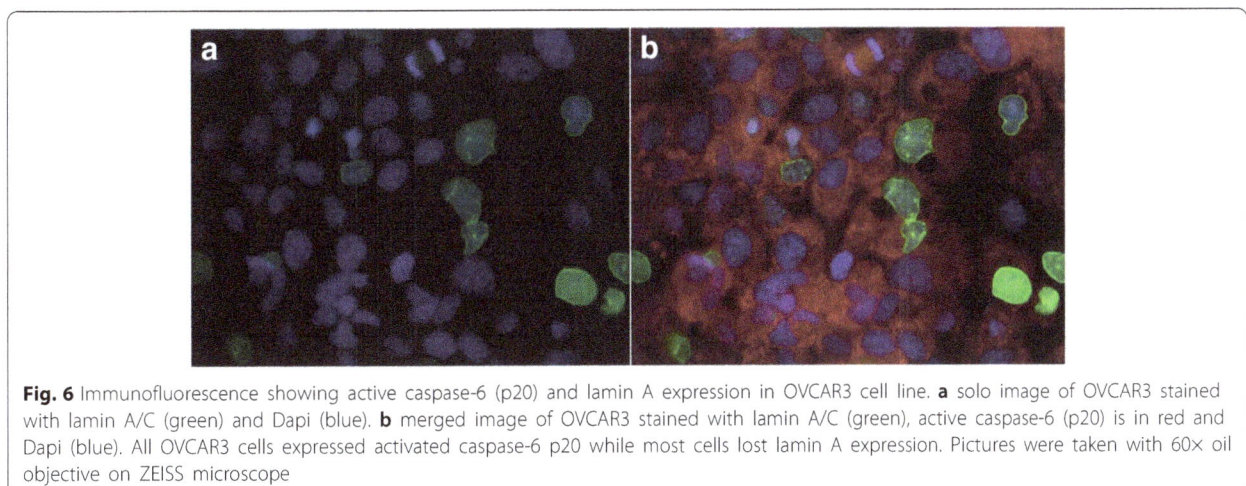

Fig. 6 Immunofluorescence showing active caspase-6 (p20) and lamin A expression in OVCAR3 cell line. a solo image of OVCAR3 stained with lamin A/C (green) and Dapi (blue). b merged image of OVCAR3 stained with lamin A/C (green), active caspase-6 (p20) is in red and Dapi (blue). All OVCAR3 cells expressed activated caspase-6 p20 while most cells lost lamin A expression. Pictures were taken with 60× oil objective on ZEISS microscope

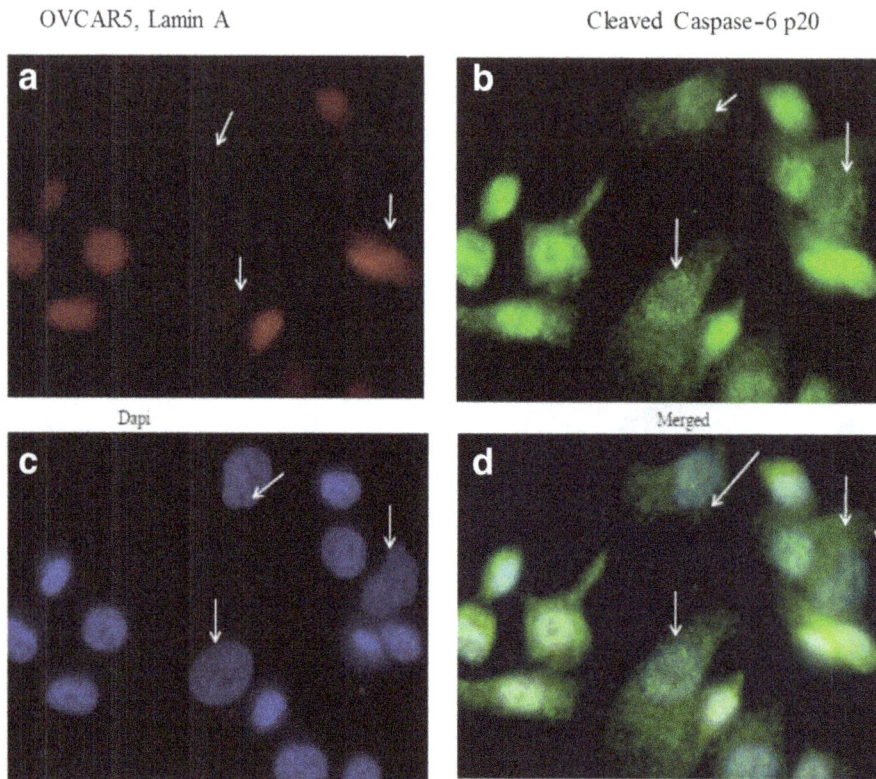

Fig. 7 Immunofluorescence showing activated caspase-6 (p20) and lamin A expression in OVCAR5 cell line. (**a**) OVCAR5 stained with antibody against lamin A (red), and caspase-6 (p20) (**b**). Nuclear counter was stained with Dapi (**c**) and merged image of lamin A, caspase-6 (p20) and Dapi are shown in (**d**). The loss of lamin A is associated with the presence of caspase-6 in the cytoplasm as indicated by white arrows (**a-d**). Pictures were taken with 100× oil objective on ZEISS microscope

with 10× (Fig. 8a) and 40× magnification (Fig. 8b). In normal epithelium active caspase-6 is absent or weak as indicated by green arrows (Fig. 8b). In contrast neoplastic, cells with enlarged nuclei displayed active caspase-6 in the cytoplasm (Fig. 8b). Thus, active caspase-6 expression is absent in normal tissue (green arrows) and over expressed in the adjacent tumorous section.

Immunostaining of caspase-6 and lamin A in human ovarian surface epithelial, fallopian tube and ovarian cancer tissues

Active caspase-6 and lamin A stainings are carried out in human ovarian surface epithelium, fallopian tube, epithelial inclusion cyst and high grade ovarian serous carcinoma and immunohistochemical images are displayed

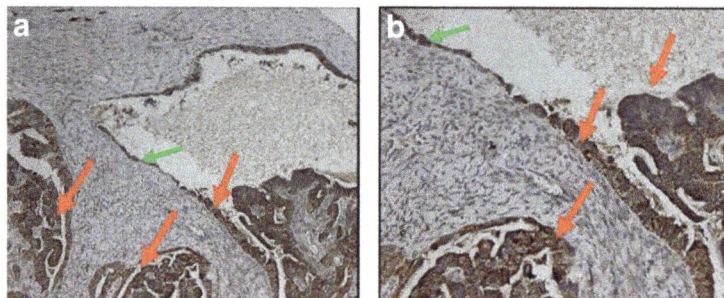

Fig. 8 a Immunohistochemistry showing caspase-6 staining in ovarian epithelium transition to ovarian tumor. (**a**) Caspase-6 staining with 10× magnification; (**b**) Caspase-6 staining with 40× magnification. Activated caspase-6 is absent or weakly expressed in normal looking ovarian surface epithelial cells with normal nuclei (green arrow) while it is overexpressed in the cytoplasm of tumor cells with large nuclei (red arrow). Thus, active caspase-6 expression is absent in normal tissue (green arrows) and over expressed in the adjacent tumorous section

in Fig. 9. Immunohistochemistry with cleaved caspase-6 and lamin A antibodies on human ovarian surface epithelial tissue (Fig. 9a, b), fallopian tube (Fig. 9c, d), epithelial inclusion cyst (Fig. 9e, f) and ovarian high grade serous carcinoma (Fig. 9g, h). No cleaved caspase-6 expression was observed in human ovarian surface epithelial and fallopian tube cells (Fig. 9a, c) in contrast lamin A expression was observed (Fig. 9b, d). Human epithelial inclusion cyst did not express cleaved caspase-6 but still expressing lamin A (Fig. 9e, f). Human high grade serous carcinoma showed overexpression of cleaved caspase-6 in the cytoplasm (Fig. 9g) while the expression of lamin A is lost in the majority of cells (Fig. 9h) as indicated by red arrows. Seemingly

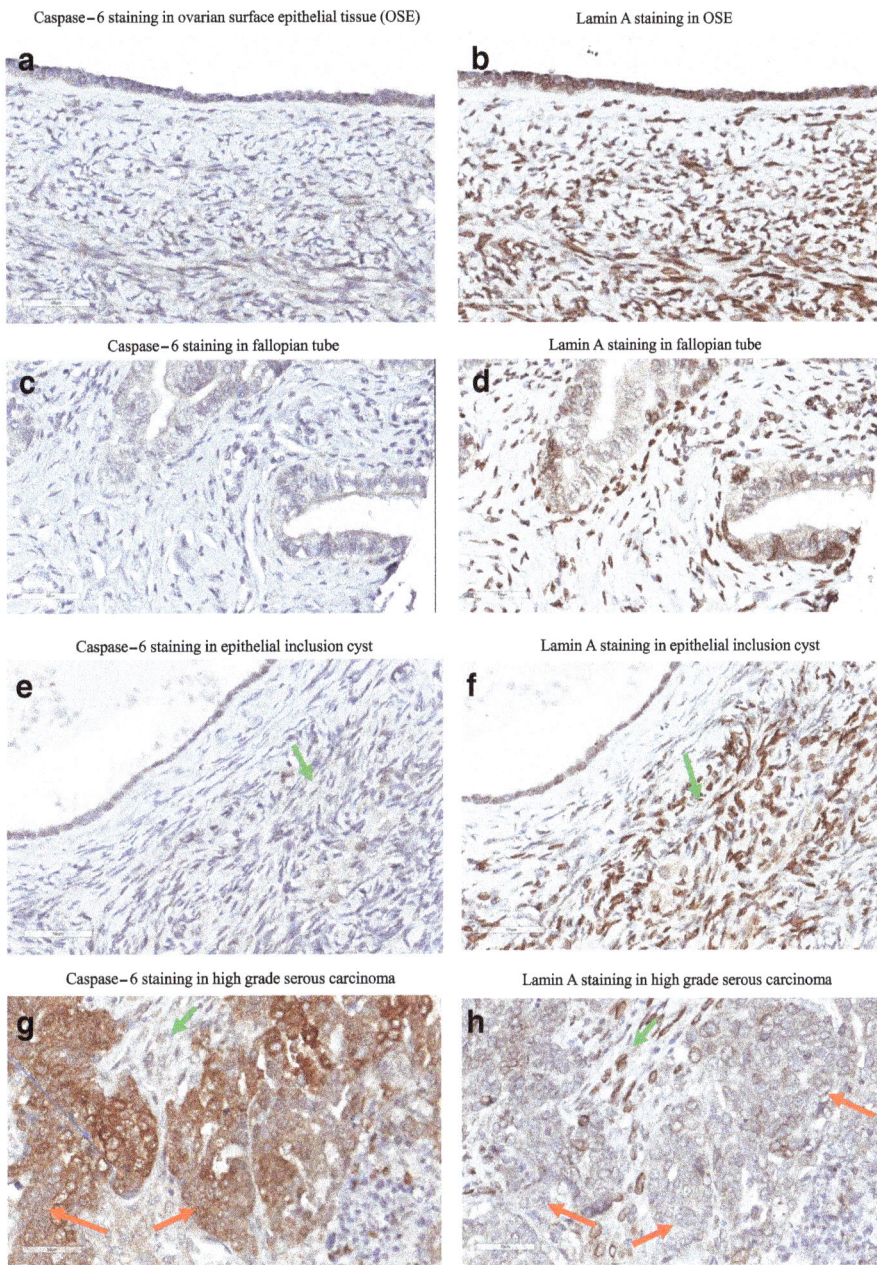

Fig. 9 Immunohistochemistry with cleaved caspase-6 and lamin A antibody in human ovarian surface epithelial tissue (**a**, **b**), fallopian tube (**c**, **d**), epithelial inclusion cyst (**e**, **f**) and ovarian high grade serous carcinoma (**g**, **h**). No cleaved caspase-6 expression was observed in human ovarian surface epithelial and fallopian tube cells (**a**, **c**) in contrast lamin A expression was observed (**b**, **d**). Human epithelial inclusion cyst did not express cleaved caspase-6 but still expression lamin A (**e**, **f**). Human high grade serous carcinoma showed overexpression of cleaved caspase-6 in the cytoplasm (**g**) while the expression of lamin A is lost in the majority of cells (**h**) as indicated by red arrows. Seemingly normal epithelial cells with no cleaved caspase-6 expression still expressing lamin A as indicated by green arrows

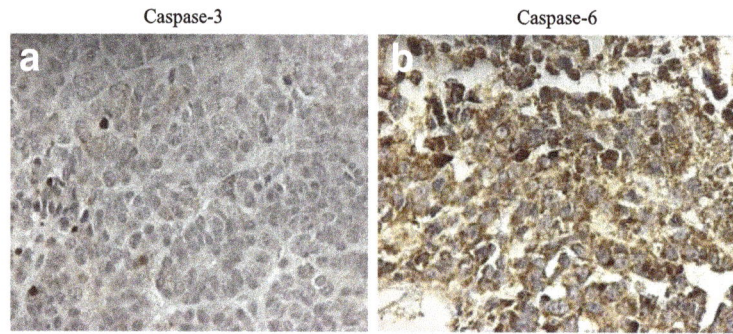

Fig. 10 Immunostaining of caspase-6 and caspase-6 in human ovarian in high grade serous carcinoma. Caspase-3 is absent in ovarian carcinoma (**a**) while caspase-6 is heterogeneously expressed in the cytoplasm and in the nucleus in ovarian carcinoma (**b**). Down regulation of caspase-3 in ovarian carcinoma (**a**) is associated to the upregulation and cytoplasmic localization of caspase-6 (**b**)

normal epithelial cells with no cleaved caspase-6 expression still expressing lamin A as indicated by green arrows. caspase-6 is mostly expressed in the cytoplasm of cancer cells; pictures were taken with 40× magnification. Overall, ovarian cancer cells with abnormal nuclei had high level of active caspase-6 in the cytoplasm while normal looking ovarian epithelial cells with normal nuclei had low or no expression of active caspase-6.

Immunostaining of caspase-3 and caspase-6 in human ovarian high grade serous carcinoma

Figure 10 displayed ovarian high grade serous carcinoma immunohistochemistry images of caspase-3 and cleaved caspase-6 staining. Caspase-3 is absent in ovarian carcinoma (a) while caspase-6 is heterogeneously expressed in the cytoplasm and in the nucleus in ovarian carcinoma (b). Down regulation of caspase-3 in ovarian carcinoma (a) is associated to the upregulation and cytoplasmic localization of caspase-6 (b).

Caspase-3 is absent in OVCAR cell lines but can be restored with anti-cancer drug suberoyl bis-hydroxamis acid

Western blot showed the absence of caspase-3 in ovarian cancer cell lines OVCAR3, OVCAR5 and OVCAR10 is displayed Fig. 11. Selected OVCAR cell line were treated to restore the apoptosis executioner caspase-3. The anti-cancer drug suberoyl bis-hydroxamic acid (SBHA) and a histone deacetylase inhibitor was able to restore caspase-3 in OVCAR3 (line 2, 3) but not in OVCAR5 (lines 5, 6) and OVCAR10 (lines 8, 9) cell lines. DMSO was used as mock treatment (lines 1, 4 and 7). Different mechanisms are involved in apoptotic failure of OVCAR cell lines.

Suppression of caspase-6 with siRNA did not restored lamin A in OVCAR5 and A2780 cell lines

Primary human ovarian surface epithelial cells (HOSE) displayed prominent expression of lamin A/C and weak expression of active caspase-6 while ovarian cancer

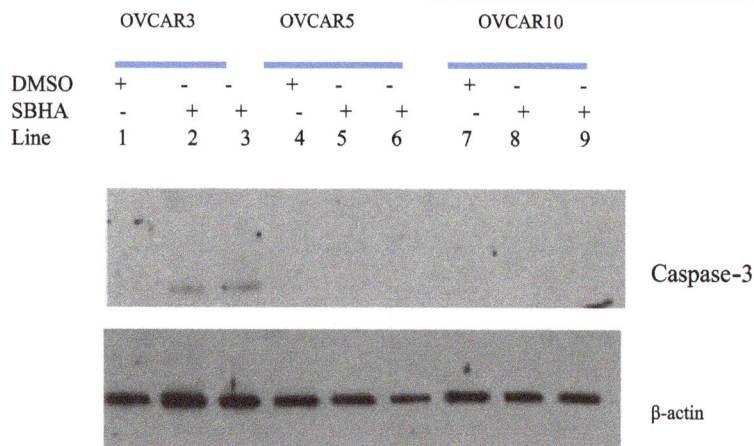

Fig. 11 Western blot showed the absence of caspase-3 in ovarian cancer cell lines OVCAR3, OVCAR5 and OVCAR10. The anti-cancer drug suberoyl bis-hydroxamic acid (SBHA) was able to restore caspase-3 in OVCAR3 (line 2, 3) but not in OVCAR5 (lines 5, 6) and OVCAR10 (lines 8,9) cell lines. DMSO was used as mock treatment (lines 1, 4 and 7)

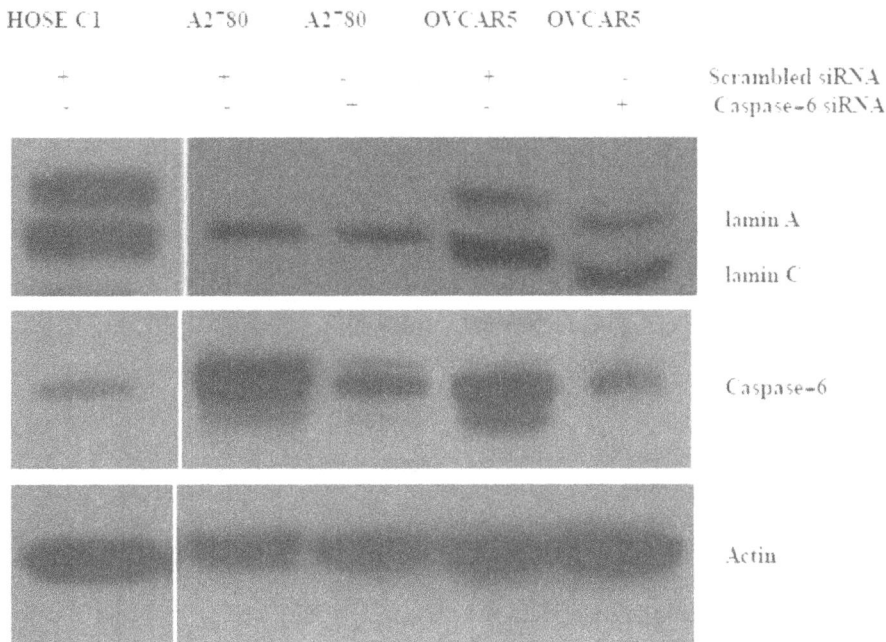

Fig. 12 Immunoblot showing caspase-6 downregulation with siRNA. Primary human ovarian surface epithelial cells (HOSE), A2780 and OVCAR5 cell lines were transfected with siRNA for 72 h before cell lysates were collected for western blot analysis. HOSE cells displayed prominent levels of lamin A/C and low level of caspase-6 expression in contrast to cancer cell lines A2780 and OVCAR5. Caspase-6 downregulation was observed in A2780 and OVCAR5 cell lines but no effect was observed on lamin A/C expression

cells lines displayed prominent expression of active caspase-6 and low lamin A/C. The suppression of caspase-6 was achieved following transfection of siRNA in cancer cell lines OVCAR5 and A2780 for 72 h. The suppression of caspase-6 with siRNA did not restore the level of lamin A/C in OVCAR5 and A2780 cells; actin was used as loading control (Fig. 12).

Conclusion

Lamin A/C expression is important for the maintenance and the integrity of nuclear envelope structure and nuclear morphology [3]. The destruction of lamin A/C in cancer including ovarian cancer is a complex molecular process which is not fully elucidated [3, 4]. From our study, we showed by immunoblotting, immunofluorescence, flow cytometry and immunohistochemistry that active caspase-6 was highly present in most ovarian cancer cell and tissues unlike normal ovarian epithelial cells or tissues. It was reported that lamin A showed proteolytic processing when incubated with recombinant active caspase-6 [14]. The nuclear localization of caspase-6 was commonly associated with the cleavage of nuclear lamin A and cell death (apoptosis) while cytoplasmic localization of active caspase-6 was not associated with instantaneous apoptosis [14, 15]. Our study showed that in ovarian cancer cell lines and in tumor tissues most of cleaved caspase-6 (active caspase-6) was localized to the cytoplasm while the

expression of lamin A/C is absent. Our study also showed in some cancer cell lines the degradation of lamin A is related to active caspase-6 and can be abolished with caspase-6 inhibitor in OVCAR3 (Fig. 5) but not in OVCAR5 nor A2780 cell lines (data not shown). In these cell lines the downregulation of caspase-6 with siRNA did not restore lamin A/C either (Fig. 12) as observed for OVCAR2 cell line (Fig. 2b). Thus, the degradation of lamin A appears to be independent of caspase-6 in some ovarian cancer cell lines (A2780, OVCAR5 and OVCAR2) and suggested the existence of another route for lamin A degradation through phosphorylation by kinases perhaps [15]. Lamin A/C proteins are target for serine/threonine (SER/THR) kinases that are overexpressed in cancer cells [15]. These results will be displayed in a separate publication. Ovarian clear carcinoma ES2 cell line was the exception with low cleaved lamin A/C while active caspase-6 was high. Recent study reported that caspase-6 activation and lamin A degradation may dependent on high glucose metabolism [16]. Thus, ES2 cells may have failure in glucose uptake which may reduce lamin A degradation by caspase-6. It was shown that in normal cells, the apoptosis executioner caspase-3 cleaves caspase-6 which in turn cleaves lamin A/C prior to apoptosis ([5–11]). In our study, caspase-3 is absent while caspase-6 is overexpressed in ovarian carcinoma (Figs. 10 and 11). In cancer cells the concept of lamin A/C cleavage by caspase-6 prior to apoptosis is no longer applicable due to the absence of lamin A. Indeed, in cancer cells, there is an alteration of cell proliferation and apoptotic markers [12]. From our investigation active caspase-3 was absent in cells expressing cleaved caspase-6 as shown in some ovarian cancer cell lines or tumor tissues analyzed (Figs. 10 and 11); meaning that caspase-6 activity initiates caspase-3 activation in cell apoptosis is disrupted in cancer [9]. Treatment with anti-cancer drug suberoyl bis-hydroxamic acid (SBHA) can restore caspase-3 in OVCAR3 cell lines but not in OVCAR5 or OVCAR10. Thus, the mechanism leading to the loss of caspase-3 and overexpression of caspase-6 is different in each cell line and will be further investigated.

Overall, the overexpression and cytoplasmic localization of caspase-6 as well as degradation of lamin A/C in cancer cells seemed to be more associated to nuclear abnormalities initiating polyploidy, aneuploidy and chromosomal instability all of which are hallmarks for ovarian cancer [3, 4]. Further studies are needed to elucidate the switch from apoptotic pathways involving caspase-3, cleaved caspase-6 and lamin A/C degradation, to carcinogenesis pathways linking active caspase-6 and lamin A/C degradation. Thus, molecular events linking cleaved caspase-6 and lamin A/C degradation to apoptosis is uncoupled in most ovarian cancer cells probably due to the absence of caspase-3.

In most of ovarian cancer cell lines and tissues, the presence of active caspase-6 in the cytoplasm is associated with the loss of lamin A/C. This association suggested that an increased expression of caspase-6 and localization to cytoplasm may be involved in lamin A/C degradation prior to nuclear envelope structural defects, aneuploidy and chromosomal instability involved in tumor cell initiation. Beside caspase-6 activity, other molecular events (lamin A phosphorylation) may be involved in lamin A/C degradation and deficiency.

Abbreviations
GFP: Green fluorescence protein; HIO: Human immortalized ovarian cells; HOSE: Human ovarian surface epithelial cells; HRP: Horseradish peroxidase; KCl: Potassium chloride; NaCl: Sodium chloride; NaF: Sodium fluoride; NaN3: Sodium azide; PBS: Phosphate buffered saline; PMSF: Phenyl-methyl-sulfonyl fluoride; SBHA: Suberoyl bis-hydroxamic acid; SDS: Sodium dodecyl sulfate; siRNA: Small interfering ribonucleotide acid; TBS: Tris buffer saline; TBST: Tris buffer saline plus Tween20; Tris-HCl: Tris-hydrochloride

Acknowledgements
We Acknowledge

- The PhD. Students Blanche Aguida and Jeanne Alladagbin from the Institute of Biomedical Sciences and Applications (ISBA), Faculty of Sciences and Technology (FAST), University Abomey Calavi (UAC), Benin.
- The colleagues of Xu's laboratory at the University of Miami, Miller School of Medicine.

Funding
NIH-NCI: 7R01CA079716–10 (PI: Xu), 12/10/1998–11/30/2015.

Authors' contributions
CC PhD, MPH, is a co-investigator who designed, performed bench works and wrote the manuscript. CKC MD, PhD; is a pathologist who carried out immunohistochemistry in ovarian cancer tissue arrays. XX PhD, is a co-investigator and collaborator in the university of Miami who oversaw and financed the study. All authors read and approved the final manuscript.

Competing interests
No competing interest is to be reported by the authors. This study was carried out in laboratory of Dr. Callinice D. Capo-chichi in the university of Abomey Calavi (UAC) in Benin and in the laboratory of Dr. Xiang-Xi Xu in the University of Miami (UM) Miller Medical School in Miami, Florida, USA .

Author details
[1]Institute of Applied Biomedical Sciences (ISBA), Unit of Biochemistry and Molecular Biology, Division of Molecular Biomarkers in Cancer and Nutrition, University of Abomey-Calavi, Abomey-Calavi, Benin. [2]Sylvester Cancer Center (SCCC), Ovarian Cancer Program, University of Miami, Miami, Florida, USA. [3]Department of Pathology, Fox Chase Cancer Center, Philadelphia, PA, USA.

References
1. Ozols RF, Bookman MA, Connolly DC, Daly MB, Godwin AK, Schilder RJ, Xu X, Hamilton TC. Focus on epithelial ovarian cancer. Cancer Cell. 2004;5:19–24.
2. Agarwal R, Kaye SB. Ovarian cancer: strategies for overcoming resistance to chemotherapy. Nat Rev Cancer. 2003;3:502–516.34.
3. Capo-chichi CD, Kathy CQ, Simpkins F, Ganjei-Azar P, Godwin AK, Xu XX. Nuclear envelope structural defects cause chromosomal numerical instability and aneuploidy in ovarian cancer. BMC Med. 2011;9:28.
4. Capo-chichi CD, Yeasky TM, Smith ER, Xu XX. Nuclear envelope structural defect underlies the main cause of aneuploidy in ovarian carcinogenesis. BMC Cell Biol. 2016;17:37 Erratum 2017 18:1.
5. Lee SC, Chan J, Clement MV, Pervaiz S. Functional proteomics of resveratrol-induced colon cancer cell apoptosis: caspase-6-mediated cleavage of Lamin a is a major signaling loop. Proteomics. 2006;6:2386–94.
6. Shahzidi S, Brech A, Sioud M, Li X, Suo Z, Nesland JM, Peng Q. Lamin a/C cleavage by caspase-6 activation is crucial for apoptotic induction by photodynamic therapy with hexaminolevulinate in human B-cell lymphoma cells. Cancer Lett. 2013;339(1):25–32. https://doi.org/10.1016/j.canlet.2013.07.026. Epub 2013.
7. Mintzer R, Ramaswamy S, Shah K, Hannoush RN, Pozniak CD, Cohen F, Zhao X, Plise E, Lewcock JW, Heise CE. A whole cell assay to measure caspase-6 activity by detecting cleavage of Lamin a/C. PLoS One. 2012;7(1):e30376. https://doi.org/10.1371/journal.pone.0030376. Epub 2012.
8. Kang JJ, Schaber MD, Srinivasula SM, Alnemri ES, Litwack GG, Hall DJ, Bjornsti MA. Cascades of mammalian caspase activation in the yeast Saccharomyces cerevisiae. J Biol Chem. 1999;274:3189–98.
9. Allsopp TE, McLuckie J, Kerr LE, Macleod M, Sharkey J, Kelly JS. Caspase 6 activity initiates caspase 3 activation in cerebellar granule cell apoptosis. Cell Death Differ. 2000;7(10):984–93.
10. Fischer U, Janicke RU, Schulze-Osthoff K. Many cuts to ruin: a comprehensive update of caspase substrates. Cell Death Differ. 2003;10:76–100.
11. Sonnemann J, Gänge J, Pilz S, Stötzer C, Ohlinger R, Belau A, Lorenz G, Beck J. Comparative evaluation of the treatment efficacy of suberoylanilide hydroxamic acid (SAHA) and paclitaxel in ovarian cancer cell lines and primary ovarian cancer cells from patients. BMC Cancer. 2006;6:183. https://doi.org/10.1186/1471-2407-6-183.

12. Ananthanarayanan V, Deaton RJ, Yang XJ, Pins MR, Gann PH. Alteration of proliferation and apoptotic markers in normal and premalignant tissue associated with prostate cancer. BMC Cancer. 2006;6:73. https://doi.org/10.1186/1471-2407-6-73.
13. Capo-chichi CD, Roland IH, Vanderveer L, Bao R, Yamagata T, Hirai H, Cohen C, Hamilton TC, Godwin AK, Xu XX. Anomalous expression of epithelial differentiation-determining GATA factors in ovarian tumorigenesis. Cancer Res. 2003;63:4967–77.
14. Klaiman G, Champagne N, LeBlanc AC. Self-activation of Caspase-6 in vitro and in vivo: Caspase-6 activation does not induce cell death in HEK293T cells. Biochim Biophys Acta. 2009;1793:592–601.
15. Capo-chichi CD. Promising personalized anti-Cancer therapy: the hidden molecular paths for Lamin A/C deficiency and restoration. Cell Mol Med. 2015;2:1, ISSN 2573–5365. https://doi.org/10.21767/2573-5365.100011 .
16. Khadija S, Veluthakal R, Sidarala V, Kowluru A. Glucotoxic and diabetic conditions induce caspase 6-mediated degradation of nuclear Lamin a in human islets, rodent islets and INS-1 832/13 cells. Apoptosis. 2014;19(12):1691–701. https://doi.org/10.1007/s10495-014-1038-4 .

24

Associations of single nucleotide polymorphisms with mucinous colorectal cancer: genome-wide common variant and gene-based rare variant analyses

Michelle E. Penney[1], Patrick S. Parfrey[2], Sevtap Savas[1,3] and Yildiz E. Yilmaz[1,2,4*]

Abstract

Background: Colorectal cancer has significant impact on individuals and healthcare systems. Many genes have been identified to influence its pathogenesis. However, the genetic basis of mucinous tumor histology, an aggressive subtype of colorectal cancer, is currently not well-known. This study aimed to identify common and rare genetic variations that are associated with the mucinous tumor phenotype.

Methods: Genome-wide single nucleotide polymorphism (SNP) data was investigated in a colorectal cancer patient cohort ($n = 505$). Association analyses were performed for 729,373 common SNPs and 275,645 rare SNPs. Common SNP association analysis was performed using univariable and multivariable logistic regression under different genetic models. Rare-variant association analysis was performed using a multi-marker test.

Results: No associations reached the traditional genome-wide significance. However, promising genetic associations were identified. The identified common SNPs significantly improved the discriminatory accuracy of the model for mucinous tumor phenotype. Specifically, the area under the receiver operating characteristic curve increased from 0.703 (95% CI: 0.634–0.773) to 0.916 (95% CI: 0.873–0.960) when considering the most significant SNPs. Additionally, the rare variant analysis identified a number of genetic regions that potentially contain causal rare variants associated with the mucinous tumor phenotype.

Conclusions: This is the first study applying both common and rare variant analyses to identify genetic associations with mucinous tumor phenotype using a genome-wide genotype data. Our results suggested novel associations with mucinous tumors. Once confirmed, these results will not only help us understand the biological basis of mucinous histology, but may also help develop targeted treatment options for mucinous tumors.

Keywords: Colorectal cancer, Mucinous adenocarcinoma, Genome-wide association study, Common single nucleotide polymorphisms, Rare single nucleotide polymorphisms

Background

Colorectal cancer is a global health problem and contributes substantially to worldwide cancer mortality [1]. In 2012, this disease was the 3rd most common cancer worldwide with higher rates occurring in developed countries [1]. In Canada, colorectal cancer is expected to cause 26,800

new cases and 9400 deaths in 2017. Newfoundland and Labrador, in particular, have the highest age-standardized rates of incidence and mortality in the country [2].

Mucins are a family of high-molecular-weight glycoproteins that are widely expressed by epithelial tissues [3]. According to the HGNC database [4], there are 22 members in this family that can be expressed in various tissues. They have been identified in two forms: cell surface (transmembrane), such as MUC1 and MUC4, and fully released (gel-forming) [3, 5, 6]. The gel-forming mucin-encoding genes are clustered at chromosome

* Correspondence: yyilmaz@mun.ca
[1]Discipline of Genetics, Faculty of Medicine, Memorial University of Newfoundland, St. John's, Canada
[2]Discipline of Medicine, Faculty of Medicine, Memorial University of Newfoundland, St. John's, Canada
Full list of author information is available at the end of the article

11p15.5 [5, 7, 8]. These mucins, including MUC2, MUC5AC, MUC5B, and MUC6, constitute the major macromolecular components of mucus [5, 7, 9]. Among them, MUC2 is the most highly expressed one in the colorectum and is the predominant component of colorectal mucus [10–12]. MUC5B and MUC6 are highly expressed in the upper gastrointestinal (GI) tract, but low levels of both have been reported in the normal colon [12, 13]. MUC5AC is highly expressed in the upper GI tract and is not expressed in the normal colon, however, abnormal expression is observed in colorectal cancer [14–16].

Mucinous adenocarcinoma is a distinct form of colorectal cancer with the defining characteristic of a high mucin component (more than 50% of the tumor volume). This subtype accounts for 5–15% of colorectal cancer cases. Compared to non-mucinous colorectal cancer, mucinous adenocarcinoma patients are typically younger and are often at an advanced stage at diagnosis [17–23]. Mucinous tumors are more likely to occur in the proximal colon [20, 21, 24, 25] and tend to have an inferior response to systemic therapies [25, 26].

Specific molecular distinctions are also seen in mucinous compared to non-mucinous colorectal tumors, for example, increased rates of *BRAF* mutations and CpG island methylator phenotype (CIMP) [27]. In addition, overexpression of MUC2, strong ectopic expression of gastric MUC5AC, and decreased p53 expression in mucinous tumors are reported in the literature [28, 29]. Mucinous and non-mucinous tumors also appear to have differences in genome-wide gene expression patterns [23]. Some of the upregulated genes in mucinous tumors are involved in cellular differentiation and mucin metabolism, which are characteristics biologically relevant to the phenotype [23]. While the differences between mucinous and non-mucinous colorectal cancers are well recognized, the prognostic importance of a high mucin component has been controversial [19–21, 25, 26, 30–35].

Most studies investigating characteristics of mucinous colorectal tumors examined single or a limited number of candidate genes [10, 36, 37]. This study aimed to comprehensively identify common and rare genetic polymorphisms that may be influencing the production of mucin or formation of the mucinous tumor phenotype. To do so, we applied a genome-wide approach to identify genes and genetic regions that are associated with the risk of developing the mucinous tumor phenotype.

Methods

Patient cohort

The study cohort was a subgroup of the Newfoundland Colorectal Cancer Registry (NFCCR) and consisted of 505 Caucasian patients. Both the NFCCR and the study cohort were described in detail in other publications [38, 39]. In short, the NFCCR recruited 750 colorectal cancer patients in Newfoundland and Labrador collected between 1999 and 2003. All diagnoses were confirmed by pathological examination. Out of 750 patients, 505 patients constituted the study cohort as explained below.

Genotype data

The genotype data used in this study was explained in Xu et al. (2015) [39]. In short, DNA samples of 539 patients were subject to whole-genome single nucleotide polymorphism (SNP) genotyping using the Illumina Omni1-Quad human SNP genotyping platform (Centrillion Bioscience, USA). These patients were included into the genetic analysis because of the availability of their outcome and clinical data as well as the germline DNAs extracted from peripheral blood samples. The quality control analysis and filtering for this data included removing SNPs whose frequencies deviated from Hardy-Weinberg equilibrium, SNPs that had >5% missing values, and patients with discordant sex information, accidental duplicates, divergent or non-Caucasian ancestry, and first, second, or third degree relatives [39]. In Xu et al. (2015) [39], 505 patients were examined to investigate associations between overall and disease-free survival times after colorectal cancer diagnosis and genetic polymorphisms with a minor allele frequency (MAF) of at least 5%. In our study, there were 505 patients with 729,373 common SNPs (MAF ≥ 0.05) and 275,645 rare SNPs (MAF < 0.05) that were included. No SNP was excluded due to high or perfect linkage disequilibrium (LD) with other SNPs. During this study, management and handling of these genotype data was done using PLINK v. 1.07 [40].

Statistical analysis

The response variable is a binary variable indicating existence of mucinous tumor histology or non-mucinous tumor histology.

Common SNP analysis

Univariable logistic regression analysis

Univariable logistic regression analysis was performed on each common SNP (MAF $\geq 5\%$) to determine if individual SNPs were significantly associated with mucinous tumor phenotype (i.e. mucinous versus non-mucinous tumor histology). For each SNP, the additive, co-dominant, dominant, and recessive genetic models were applied. Consequently, we report the 10 SNPs without excluding those in high LD with the highest level of significance in each genetic model (Additional file 1: Tables S1-S4).

Selection of baseline variables and multivariable logistic regression analysis

In order to select significant baseline factors to adjust for in the multivariable analyses, we first examined the variables shown in Table 1 using univariable logistic regression

Table 1 Baseline features of the study cohort and the results of univariable logistic regression analysis

Characteristics		Mucinous No. (%)	Non-mucinous No. (%)	OR (95% CI)	p-value
Age[a]	≤60	20 (9)	203 (91)		
	60–65	17 (18)	78 (82)	2.21 (1.09–4.44)	0.025
	>65	20 (11)	167 (89)	1.22 (0.63–2.34)	0.558
Sex	Female	29 (15)	169 (85)		
	Male	28 (9)	279 (91)	0.58 (0.34–1.02)	0.057
Location	Colon	47 (14)	287 (86)		
	Rectum	10 (6)	161 (94)	0.38 (0.18–0.74)	0.007
Stage	I	3 (3)	90 (97)		
	II	27 (14)	169 (86)	4.79 (1.64–20.45)	0.012
	III	19 (11)	147 (89)	3.88 (1.28–16.83)	0.033
	IV	8 (16)	42 (84)	5.71 (1.57–27.09)	0.013
Grade	Well/moderately diff.	48 (10)	416 (90)		
	Poorly diff.	7 (19)	30 (81)	2.02 (0.78–4.62)	0.115
	Unknown	2	2		
MSI status	MSI-low/MSS	49 (11)	382 (89)		
	MSI-high	6 (11)	47 (89)	1.00 (0.37–2.29)	0.992
	Unknown	3	18		
Lymphatic invasion	Absent	31 (10)	267 (90)		
	Present	23 (14)	144 (86)	1.38 (0.77–2.44)	0.278
	Unknown	3	37		
BRAF V600E mutation	Absent	45 (11)	366 (89)		
	Present	9 (19)	38 (81)	1.93 (0.83–4.09)	0.104
	Unknown	3	44		

[a]The age at diagnosis was separated into 3 groups: ≤60, 60–65, and >65 since the odds ratio does not remain constant for each year increase in age at diagnosis under the logistic regression model and this particular grouping gave the most efficient odds ratio estimates with no significant change in the results when considering slightly different groupings. CI confidence interval, diff. Differentiated, MSI microsatellite instability, MSS microsatellite stable, No number, OR odds ratio (compares the odds of having mucinous tumors with the corresponding factor level to the odds of having mucinous tumors with the reference factor level)

models. These variables were selected for inclusion into the selection process based on previous studies investigating mucinous colorectal tumors [27, 33]. Factors that had a p-value less than 0.1 were then included in a forward stepwise variable selection method. In addition, although there appeared to be a non-significant association between tumor histology and grade in the univariable analysis, tumor grade was still included in the multivariable model as has been shown to be linked to tumor histology [30, 41]. As a result, the baseline characteristics in the final models were sex, age at diagnosis, stage, and tumor location based on the 0.1 level of significance, and tumor grade (Additional file 1: Table S5). The 10 SNPs with the highest level of significance under each genetic model in the univariable logistic regression analysis were analyzed using the multivariable logistic regression model adjusting for the selected baseline characteristics (Additional file 1: Tables S1-S4).

Plausibility of the genetic models

It is common in genetic association studies that only one genetic model is applied. In this study, we applied all four genetic models and assessed the plausibility of the genetic model under which the SNP was identified. To do this, we used the Akaike Information Criterion (AIC) calculations to compare the fit of four different genetic models per SNP under the multivariable logistic regression model. The genetic model with the smallest AIC estimate was considered to be the most plausible genetic model (i.e. the best fitting model). We first ranked the SNPs based on their p-value obtained in the multivariable model with the genetic model under which the SNP was identified (Additional file 1: Table S6). Then, we excluded those SNPs that were not identified in their plausible genetic model. Of note, we present in this manuscript only the 10 SNPs that have the highest association significance levels under the multivariable logistic regression models that were identified in their most plausible genetic model. We refer to these SNPs as "the top 10 SNPs". The LD between SNPs was not taken into account when listing the top 10 SNPs.

Assessing the discriminatory accuracy of the estimated models

We aimed to check the ability of the multivariable models of the top 10 SNPs to discriminate between mucinous and non-mucinous phenotypes. A well-known method for assessing the discriminatory accuracy of a model is using a receiver operating characteristic (ROC) curve [42–44]. Calculating the area under the curve (AUC) of the ROC curve for the given models provides a single numeric representation for the performance of the model [43, 45, 46]. Comparing the AUC values and their corresponding confidence intervals provides a method for determining if one model is significantly superior to another in discriminatory accuracy [44, 47].

ROC curve analysis was performed by calculating the AUC using the pROC package in R [48]. The AUC estimates for (i) the model conditioning only on the baseline characteristics, (ii) the model conditioning on only the top SNPs, and (iii) the model conditioning on the baseline characteristics and the top SNPs. Comparing the AUC, specifically the 95% confidence intervals, between these three models can quantify the differences in the capacity of the models to distinguish mucinous and non-mucinous phenotypes.

Rare variant analysis
SKAT-O analysis

SKAT-O [49] test statistic was used to test the associations between the rare variants and the mucinous tumor phenotype. For this analysis, we prioritized gene-based regions including 5 kb long sequences before and after each gene. To do so, we first obtained genome location information for genome-wide gene-based regions (for the reference genome GRCh37.p13) using the biomaRt tool [50] in the Ensembl database [51]. The SNP information within these regions were then retrieved from the patient genome-wide data and used as the region-based SNP-sets in SKAT-O. During this analysis, each SNP was assigned to one gene-based region only. As a result, when a gene is located in close proximity to another gene, the second gene-based region does not include the SNPs that are analyzed in the first gene-based region. This limits redundancy since no SNP is analyzed more than once. For this analysis, only the additive genetic model was considered as using multiple genetic models is not a practical option for SKAT-O. The associations of gene regions were examined in multivariable models, adjusting for the significant baseline characteristics sex, age at diagnosis, stage, tumor location, and tumor grade.

All statistical analysis was performed using R v. 3.1.3 [52]. Correction for multiple testing was not applied to the results as this is an exploratory study and we did not want to increase false negative rate due to conservative corrections. While this increases the chances of obtaining false positives, we believe replication of these results in other studies will assist in reducing the potential false positive findings.

Bioinformatics analysis

Potential regulatory consequences of the identified SNPs were examined through RegulomeDB (http://www.regulomedb.org/) [53]. Ensembl [51] database was used to retrieve information related to the genes identified in the common and rare variant analysis.

Results

The demographic and clinicopathological information for the sample population is shown in Table 1. We observed a non-significant association of histology with age at diagnosis (>65 versus ≤60), grade, microsatellite instability (MSI) status, lymphatic invasion (LI), and *BRAF* V600E mutation; a moderately significant association with stage, sex, and age at diagnosis between 60 and 65 versus ≤60; and a strongly significant association with tumor location (Table 1). In this cohort, there was a trend for female sex having increased risk of mucinous tumors. As expected, the proportion of mucinous tumors was higher in colon cancer patients compared to rectum cancer patients and in stage II-IV patients compared to stage I patients (Table 1).

Common SNP analysis

None of the associations in this analysis reached the traditional genome-wide significance level ($P < 5 \times 10^{-8}$), but each genetic model identified promising associations.

After the univariable analysis, there were 33 SNPs that were nominally associated with the mucinous tumor phenotype (Additional file 1: Tables S1-S4). Associations of two SNPs (rs11216624 & rs17712784) were identified in both the dominant and co-dominant genetic models; one SNP (rs7314811) was detected in the additive, recessive, and co-dominant genetic models; and three SNPs (rs4843335, rs10511330, & rs16822593) were detected in both the additive and dominant genetic models. The estimates obtained in the univariable analysis did not change significantly when the models were adjusted for the baseline characteristics (Additional file 1: Tables S1-S4).

As explained in the Methods section, the AIC estimates (Additional file 1: Table S6) were used to determine the most plausible genetic models for each of 33 SNPs. Ten SNPs with the smallest *p*-value in the multivariable analysis under the most plausible genetic models were further prioritized (i.e., the top 10 SNPs). The results of the univariable and the multivariable logistic regression analyses for these top 10 SNPs are summarized in Table 2. Seven

Table 2 Top ten promising SNPs identified in univariable analysis and the subsequent multivariable analysis under their plausible genetic models

Genomic location	SNP ID (Genotype[a])	Gene[b]	Information in RegulomeDB	Plausible model[c]	Univariable OR (95% CI)	Univariable p-value	Multivariable[e] OR (95% CI)	Multivariable[e] p-value
Chr6:110750552	rs9481067 (GG)	SLC22A16	ND	Recessive	4.17 (2.33–7.43)	1.24E-06	4.75 (2.53–8.95)	1.24E-06
Chr3:114121019	rs10511330 (CT + CC)	ZBTB20	Minimal binding evidence	Dominant	3.77 (2.06–6.81)	1.24E-05	4.85 (2.54–9.23)	1.40E-06
Chr3:114117327	rs16822593 (AG + AA)	ZBTB20	ND	Dominant	3.70 (2.02–6.68)	1.59E-05	4.83 (2.53–9.20)	1.50E-06
Chr2:179860562	rs13019215 (TC + TT)	CCDC141	ND	Dominant	0.27 (0.14–0.48)	1.56E-05	0.23 (0.12–0.43)	8.20E-06
Chr2:179867985	rs12471607 (TC + TT)	CCDC141	ND	Dominant	0.27 (0.14–0.48)	1.65E-05	0.23 (0.12–0.43)	8.42E-06
Chr5:80483574	rs716897 (CT + CC)	RASGRF2	Minimal binding evidence	Dominant	0.27 (0.15–0.47)	5.33E-06	0.26 (0.14–0.47)	1.12E-05
Chr16:86077637	rs4843335 (AG + AA)	intergenic	Minimal binding evidence	Dominant	4.11 (2.11–7.79)	2.06E-05	4.67 (2.98–9.34)	1.48E-05
Chr6:118634698	rs11968293 (CA + CC)	SLC35F1	Minimal binding evidence	Dominant	0.28 (0.16–0.50)	1.27E-05	0.26 (0.14–0.48)	1.48E-05
Chr9:131923949	rs4837345 (TT)	intergenic	Minimal binding evidence	Recessive	4.72 (2.40–9.05)	4.00E-06	4.56 (2.24–9.11)	1.97E-05
Chr9:131930494	kgp10457679/ rs10819474[d] (CC)	intergenic	Likely to affect binding and linked to expression of a gene target	Recessive	4.72 (2.40–9.05)	4.00E-06	4.56 (2.24–9.11)	1.97E-05

[a]Risk increasing/decreasing genotype. [b]Based on Ensembl [51] or dbSNP databases [61]. [c]Under the recessive genetic model, minor allele homozygous patients are compared to major allele homozygous and heterozygous patients combined. Under the dominant genetic model, minor allele homozygous and heterozygous patients are combined and compared to major allele homozygous patients. [d]The rs number for the kgp10457679 polymorphism was obtained from the UCSC genome browser [62]. [e]Multivariable models adjusted for sex, age at diagnosis, stage, tumor location, and tumor grade. Patients with missing/unknown data for any of these variables were excluded from the analysis. *Chr* chromosome, *CI* confidence interval, *ND* data not available at RegulomeDB, *OR* odds ratio (compares the odds of having mucinous tumors with the specified genotype(s)[a] to the odds of having mucinous tumors with the reference (other) genotype(s))

of these SNPs were located within gene sequences. These genes were quite diverse and belong to a variety of biological processes and pathways (Table 3).

Before the ROC analysis, the LD among the top 10 SNPs were assessed using patient genotype data. These calculations indicated that rs13019215 and rs12471607 were in complete pairwise LD ($r^2 = 1$). The SNPs rs4837345 and kgp10457679 were also in high LD with each other, as well as rs10511330 and rs16822593 ($0.99 \leq r^2 \leq 1.0$). Therefore, we kept one SNP per SNP set in high LD, which left the following SNPs for the ROC analysis: rs9481067, rs10511330, rs13019215, rs716897, rs4843335, rs11968293, and kgp10457679.

Figure 1 shows the ROC curves comparing the accuracy of the models to discriminate mucinous and non-mucinous tumor phenotypes. The model (iii) including both the baseline characteristics and the SNPs (AUC = 0.916, CI: 0.873–0.960) had the most discriminatory accuracy followed by model (ii) including only the SNPs (AUC = 0.868, CI: 0.813–0.923) and model (i) including only the baseline characteristics (AUC = 0.703, 95% CI: 0.634–0.773). Since the confidence intervals of models (i) and (iii) do not overlap, we can confidently claim that there is a statistically significant improvement in the discriminating accuracy of the model containing the SNPs [44, 47]. This also suggests that these SNPs explain some of the

variation between the mucinous and non-mucinous tumor phenotypes.

Rare SNP analysis

In the gene region-based rare variant analysis, we investigated 29,966 regions in the patient cohort using the multivariable SKAT-O method. Table 3 and Table 4 summarize the most significant regions ($P < 10^{-4}$) that potentially contain causal rare variants associated with the mucinous tumor phenotype. The number of variants aggregated in these gene-based regions varied from 5 to 10. While three of these regions (including the *SEC24B*, *SEC24B-AS1*, and *CCDC109B* regions) were located close to each other on chromosome 4, other regions come from different parts of the genome (Table 4).

Discussion

Mucinous tumors are considered an aggressive type of colorectal tumors that are poorly understood [22, 24, 54]. While their role in prognosis is not well established, several studies suggested these tumors are associated with poorer prognosis when compared to non-mucinous tumors [25, 26, 32, 33, 35]. Identification of genes and genetic variations that can have a role in mucinous tumor development, therefore, has both scientific (e.g. dissecting the biology behind the mucinous tumor histology) as well

Table 3 Genes identified in the common and rare analyses

Gene symbol[a]	Gene name[b]	Function
SLC22A16	solute carrier family 22 member 16	codes for a human L-carnitine transporter protein hCT2. hCT2 has been shown to have undetectable expression in a colon cancer cell line. [63, 64]
CCDC141	coiled-coil domain containing 141	codes for a protein that plays a critical role in centrosome positioning and movement, particularly radial migration. Centrosome aberrations have been shown to be present in early-stage colorectal cancers and could contribute to chromosomal instability. [65, 66]
SLC35F1	solute carrier family 35 member F1	codes for a member of the solute carrier family 35, a family of nucleotide sugar transporters. [67]
ZBTB20	zinc finger and BTB domain containing 20	codes for a transcriptional repressor. Upregulation of ZBTB20 has been shown to promote cell proliferation in non-small cell lung cancer and is a potential druggable target for the disease. Similarly, overexpression of ZBTB20 has been associated with poor prognosis in patients with hepatocellular carcinoma. [68–70]
RASGRF2	Ras protein specific guanine nucleotide releasing factor 2	codes for a signalling molecule. RasGRF2 contains regulatory domains for both Ras and Rho GTPases, suggesting it can influence both pathways. The Rho pathway has been thought to be involved in cell migration, while the Ras pathway has been thought to be involved in cell proliferation and survival, which are all processes related to cancer. [71, 72]
SEC24B	SEC24 homolog B, COPII coat complex component	codes for a protein that is a part of the COPII vesicle coat, facilitating molecular transport from the endoplasmic reticulum to the Golgi apparatus. It has been suggested that alterations in vesicle trafficking proteins may be facilitators of epithelial carcinogenesis. [73, 74]
CCDC109b	coiled-coil domain containing 109B	also known as MCUb. This gene codes a protein that interacts with the mitochondrial calcium transporter protein, CCDC109a/MCU, reducing the activity of the transporter. Calcium homeostasis in mitochondria may regulate cell death pathways. [75, 76]
LINC00596	long intergenic non-protein coding RNA 596	no literature data available.
SEC24B-AS1	SEC24B antisense RNA 1	long non-coding RNA (lncRNA) that is involved in gene expression regulation. [77]
RP11-564A8.8	NA	no literature data available.
FAM87A	family with sequence similarity 87 member A	no literature data available.

[a]According to Ensembl database [51]. [b]According to HUGO Gene Nomenclature Committee (HGNC) [4]. *NA* Not available

as clinical value (e.g. biological information gained may assist with development of targeted treatment for this cancer subtype). Accordingly, for the first time with this study, we examined associations of both common and rare variants with the risk of developing the mucinous tumor phenotype using a genome-wide dataset.

While our results did not reach the conservative genome-wide significance level, promising associations were detected in both the common and rare variant analyses. In common SNP analysis, we identified seven unlinked polymorphisms that significantly increased our capacity to discriminate between mucinous and non-mucinous tumor phenotypes (Fig. 1, Table 2). Their effects on tumor histology were independent from the effects of the baseline variables (Fig. 1, Table 2). It is possible these polymorphisms (or others in high LD with them (Additional file 1: Table S7), including three additional SNPs shown in Table 2) are biologically linked to tumor histology or mucin production. Since there was no reported functional consequence of these SNPs in the literature, we searched the RegulomeDB database [53] for their potential biological characteristics. As of March 2018, the only SNP with a predicted/reported regulatory function in this database was kgp10457679

(rs10819474) (RegulomeDB score = 1f). This intergenic SNP is categorized as an expression quantitative trait locus (eQTL)/Transcription Factor (TF) binding/DNAse peak site, with a likely role of influencing the expression of target genes (Additional file 1: Table S8). Specifically, PPP2R4 is noted as the eQTL for this SNP. PPP2R4 is a tumor suppressor protein [55] which has been shown to have low activity in a large portion of a small cohort of colorectal tumors [56] and is associated with shorter survival times in metastatic colorectal cancer patients [57]. A potential link of PPP2R4 to mucinous tumor phenotype risk should be examined in further studies. Interestingly, one GWAS identified a SNP within the sequences of *ZBTB20*, other than the one reported in this study, that is significantly associated with the risk of non-cardia gastric cancer in the Han Chinese population [58]. Overall, all the novel loci identified by the common variant analysis are interesting candidates in examination of mucinous tumor development.

Typical association studies, such as the common variant analysis, focus on a variant-by-variant approach, which is underpowered for rare variants. It has been suggested that gene/region-based approaches can be useful in increasing the power under these circumstances where the direct

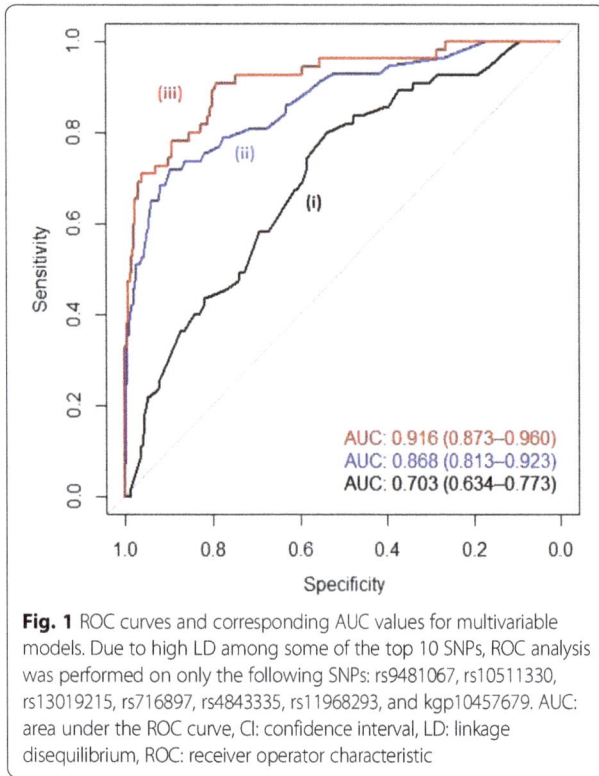

Fig. 1 ROC curves and corresponding AUC values for multivariable models. Due to high LD among some of the top 10 SNPs, ROC analysis was performed on only the following SNPs: rs9481067, rs10511330, rs13019215, rs716897, rs4843335, rs11968293, and kgp10457679. AUC: area under the ROC curve, CI: confidence interval, LD: linkage disequilibrium, ROC: receiver operator characteristic

effects of multiple variants on a phenotype can be examined [59]. Hence, in this study, we performed the first rare variant analysis to explore gene regions that may have a role in mucinous tumor formation using SKAT-O [49]. SKAT-O is a multi-marker association test which has reasonable type I error rate and is a powerful test under many scenarios [49]. In our study, this method identified a number of gene-based regions that may harbor rare variants associated with mucinous phenotype (Tables 3 and 4). Interestingly, three of the gene-based regions in Table 4 (*SEC24B*, *SEC24B-AS1*, and *CCDC109B*-based regions) were located in a 341,243 bp long genomic region on chromosome 4q. Since we assigned each SNP to only one gene region, these results suggest that these three gene regions are associated with the mucinous phenotype independent of each other. A search on the RegulomeDB database [53] indicated that one of the SNPs in *LINC00596* (rs8005541) could have a strong regulatory function (RegulomeDB score = 1f). This variant is located in an eQTL and seems to affect the expression of two nearby genes; *DHRS4* and *DHRS4L2*. These two genes are a part of a gene cluster on chromosome 14 that code for dehydrogenases/reductases [60] and have not been previously linked to mucinous tumors. Similarly, none of the genes in Table 4 had a previously identified connection to the risk of developing mucinous tumors. In conclusion, these regions, genes, or SNPs, alone or in combination, may be influential on the mucinous tumor phenotype and should be explored further.

Table 4 Most significant gene regions identified from SKAT-O multivariable analysis

Genomic location[a]	Gene[b]	Description[c]	Other genes in the gene-based region[d]	# of SNPs	SNPs	P-value
Chr4:110349928–110467052	SEC24B	protein coding	SEC24B-AS1 (partial sequence)	5	rs10516557, kgp21293502, rs10003981, rs17040515, rs17040519	1.81E-05
Chr4:110476361–110614874	CCDC109B	protein coding	CDC42P4 (pseudogene; partial sequence), HIGD1AP14 (pseudogene; full length), CASP6 (partial sequence)	6	rs17619262, rs7654187, rs6831048, rs17619310, rs9997940, rs1053680	3.29E-05
Chr14:24386456–24408777	LINC00596	long intergenic non-protein coding RNA	DHRS4-AS1 (partial sequence)	6	rs8010486, rs1159372, rs10135026, rs8005541, rs8019962, kgp19564619	3.34E-05
Chr4:110263631–110359973	SEC24B-AS1	noncoding RNA; antisense RNA	RBMXP4 (pseudogene; full length), SEC24B (partial sequence)	7	rs10031399, rs17040364, rs17040369, rs11098033, rs17040401, rs12648138, rs11098035	4.21E-05
Chr1:207074273–207084738	RP11-564A8.8	pseudogene	IL24 (partial sequence), FAIM3 (partial sequence), FCMR (partial sequence)	10	rs3093428, kgp15249933, kgp15191074, rs3093447, kgp22852559, rs3093434, rs3093437, rs3093438, rs3093440, rs41304091	5.47E-05
Chr8:320931–338174	FAM87A	non-coding RNA	–	7	rs4527844, kgp20525414, kgp20198205, rs11785854, rs7461388, rs17064450, rs17064458	6.58E-05

[a]These genomic locations describe the region containing the gene as well as 5 kb long sequences before and after the gene. [b]Based on the information in the UCSC database [62]. [c]NCBI's Gene Entrez database [77]. [d]In some cases, the gene regions examined also contained sequences of other genes. *Chr* chromosome

Several strengths and limitations of this study should be mentioned. Studying the mucinous tumor phenotype is inherently challenging since it is not frequently detected. Despite this and the large number of SNPs/gene-based regions investigated, this study identified promising genetic variants and genomic regions that may have a biological connection to the mucinous tumor phenotype. We are aware that our results need to be replicated in independent cohorts and remain to be verified. Of note, SNPs and genetic regions we report are different than the MUC genes, which are the typical candidate genes for mucin production and mucinous phenotype. In the common variant analysis, the recessive and co-dominant models yielded some high odds ratio estimates but also wide confidence intervals (as expected, as these are the models with relatively low power). Consequently, the interpretation of these results should be made with caution. SKAT-O is a robust test and an attractive choice for rare variant analysis, however, it cannot determine which SNPs or how many SNPs within a SNP-set are truly associated with the phenotype. Also, in the rare variant analysis, due to the assignment of one SNP to one gene region, there could be some genes whose associations may have been missed. In addition, in contrast to previous studies, we used a comprehensive genome-wide SNP genotype data, however, analysis of a more comprehensive data (such as those obtained by whole genome sequencing) would be desirable. This is particularly true for rare variants as most genotyping technologies target primarily common SNPs.

Conclusions

In this study, we performed the first genome-wide association study on common and rare SNPs in colorectal cancer patients to identify novel genetic associations with the mucinous tumor phenotype. We identified novel, promising, and independent associations of specific SNP genotypes with the risk of developing mucinous tumors. In the common and rare variant analysis, we reported SNPs within the sequences of genes encoding transporter proteins, such as SLC22A16 and SLC35F1, which may have a role in transporting molecules related to excessive mucin production. In addition, the rare variant analysis reported associations with several regulating RNA molecules, which may influence the expression of genes related to mucin production. Finally, the common SNP analysis reports genes whose protein products are involved in DNA replication (CCDC141) and transcription (ZBTB20) that could have downstream effects on the mucin genes. Furthermore, the common SNPs reported in this study significantly improved the discriminatory accuracy of the multivariable model to distinguish between mucinous and non-mucinous tumors. In addition, we detected novel promising associations between gene-based sets of rare SNPs and mucinous tumors. The results of this study, once replicated in other cohorts, can contribute further information to the molecular characteristics of this understudied but clinically important colorectal cancer subtype.

Abbreviations

AIC: Akaike information criterion; AUC: Area under the curve; CI: Confidence interval; DNA: Deoxyribonucleic acid; eQTL: Expression quantitative trait loci; GI: Gastrointestinal; LD: Linkage disequilibrium; LI: Lymphatic invasion; MAF: Minor allele frequency; MSI: Microsatellite instability; NFCCR: Newfoundland Colorectal Cancer Registry; ROC: Receiver operating characteristic; SNP: Single nucleotide polymorphism; TF: Transcription factor; USA: United States of America

Acknowledgements

We thank the patients and families that participated in NFCCR and all the NFCCR personnel and investigators who contributed to NFCCR.

Funding

This work was funded by the Research and Development Corporation (RDC) Newfoundland and Labrador (NL) [5404.1723.101] and the Faculty of Medicine of Memorial University of Newfoundland (awarded to Y.E. Yilmaz). M.E. Penney is partly supported by a Translational and Personalized Medicine Initiative (TPMI)/NP SUPPORT fellowship. The funding sources were not involved in the study design; in the collection, analysis or interpretation of data; in the writing of the report; or in the decision to submit the paper for publication.

Authors' contributions

MP, SS, and YY designed the study and revised the manuscript. PP provided patient characteristics and disease outcome data. SS provided the genome-wide SNP genotype data and the patient cohort investigated. MP conducted the statistical analysis, interpreted the results, wrote the first draft of the manuscript, and prepared the figure and Tables. SS and YY reviewed the results and their interpretation, and supervised the study. All authors reviewed the manuscript. All authors read and approved the final manuscript.

Competing interests

The authors declare that they have no competing interests.

Author details

[1]Discipline of Genetics, Faculty of Medicine, Memorial University of Newfoundland, St. John's, Canada. [2]Discipline of Medicine, Faculty of Medicine, Memorial University of Newfoundland, St. John's, Canada. [3]Discipline of Oncology, Faculty of Medicine, Memorial University of Newfoundland, St. John's, Canada. [4]Department of Mathematics and Statistics, Faculty of Science, Memorial University of Newfoundland, St. John's, Canada.

References

1. Ferlay J, Soerjomataram I, Dikshit R, Eser S, Mathers C, Rebelo M, et al. Cancer incidence and mortality worldwide: sources, methods and major patterns in GLOBOCAN 2012. Int J Cancer. 2015;136(5):E359–86.
2. Canadian Cancer Society's Advisory Committee on Cancer Statistics. Canadian Cancer Statistics 2017. Toronto, ON: Canadian Cancer Society; 2017.
3. Moniaux N, Escande F, Porchet N, Aubert JP, Batra SK. Structural organization and classification of the human mucin genes. Front Biosci. 2001;6:d1192–206.
4. Gray KA, Yates B, Seal RL, Wright MW, Bruford EA. Genenames.org: the HGNC resources in 2015. Nucleic Acids Res. 2014;43:D1079–85.
5. Desseyn J, Aubert J, Porchet N, Laine A. Evolution of the large secreted gel-forming mucins. Mol Biol Evol. 2000;17(8):1175–84.
6. Dhanisha SS, Guruvayoorappan C, Drishya S, Abeesh P. Mucins: structural diversity, biosynthesis, its role in pathogenesis and as possible therapeutic targets. Crit Rev Oncol Hematol. 2018;122:98–122.
7. Desseyn J, Buisine M, Porchet N, Aubert J, Degand P, Laine A. Evolutionary history of the 11p15 human mucin gene family. J Mol Evol. 1998;46(1):102–6.
8. Gosalia N, Leir S, Harris A. Coordinate regulation of the gel-forming mucin genes at chromosome 11p15.5. J Biol Chem. 2012;288(9):6717–25.
9. Corfield AP. Mucins: a biologically relevant glycan barrier in mucosal protection. Biochim Biophys Acta Gen Sub. 2015;1850(1):236–52.
10. Okudaira K, Kakar S, Cun L, Choi E, Wu Decamillis R, Miura S, et al. MUC2 gene promoter methylation in mucinous and non-mucinous colorectal cancer tissues. Int J Oncol. 2010;36(4):765–75.
11. Johansson MEV, Larsson JMH, Hansson GC. The two mucus layers of colon are organized by the MUC2 mucin, whereas the outer layer is a legislator of host-microbial interactions. Proc Natl Acad Sci U S A. 2010;108:4659–65.
12. Ho SB, Niehans GA, Lyftogt C, Yan PS, Cherwitz DL, Gum ET, et al. Heterogeneity of mucin gene expression in normal and neoplastic tissues. Cancer Res. 1993;53(3):641–51.
13. Toribara NW, Roberton AM, Ho SB, Kuo WL, Gum E, Hicks JW, et al. Human gastric mucin. Identification of a unique species by expression cloning. J Biol Chem. 1993;268(8):5879–85.
14. Biemer-Hüttmann A, Walsh MD, McGuckin MA, Ajioka Y, Watanabe H, Leggett BA, et al. Immunohistochemical staining patterns of MUC1, MUC2, MUC4, and MUC5AC mucins in hyperplastic polyps, serrated adenomas, and traditional adenomas of the colorectum. J Histochem Cytochem. 1999;47(8):1039–48.
15. Bartman AE, Serson SJ, Ewing SL, Niehans GA, Wiehr CL, Evans MK, et al. Aberrant expression of MUC5AC and MUC6 gastric mucin genes in colorectal polyps. Int J Cancer. 1999;80(2):210–8.
16. Amini A, Masoumi-Moghaddam S, Ehteda A, Liauw W, Morris DL. Depletion of mucin in mucin-producing human gastrointestinal carcinoma: results from in vitro and in vivo studies with bromelain and N-acetylcysteine. Oncotarget. 2015;6(32):33329–44.
17. Wu C, Tung S, Chen P, Kuo Y. Clinicopathological study of colorectal mucinous carcinoma in Taiwan: a multivariate analysis. J Gastroenterol Hepatol. 1996;11(1):77–81.
18. Odone V, Chang L, Caces J, George SL, Pratt CB. The natural history of colorectal carcinoma in adolescents. Cancer. 1982;49(8):1716–20.
19. Chew M, Yeo SE, Ng Z, Lim K, Koh P, Ng K, et al. Critical analysis of mucin and signet ring cell as prognostic factors in an Asian population of 2,764 sporadic colorectal cancers. Int J Color Dis. 2010;25(10):1221–9.
20. Papadopoulos VN, Michalopoulos A, Netta S, Basdanis G, Paramythiotis D, Zatagias A, et al. Prognostic significance of mucinous component in colorectal carcinoma. Tech Coloproctol. 2004;8(1):s123–5.
21. Kang H, O'Connell BJ, Maggard AM, Sack J, Ko YC. A 10-year outcomes evaluation of mucinous and signet-ring cell carcinoma of the colon and rectum. Dis Colon Rectum. 2005;48(6):1161–8.
22. Consorti F, Lorenzotti A, Midiri G, Di Paola M. Prognostic significance of mucinous carcinoma of colon and rectum: a prospective case-control study. J Surg Oncol. 2000;73(2):70–4.
23. Melis M, Hernandez J, Siegel EM, McLoughlin JM, Ly QP, Nair RM, et al. Gene expression profiling of colorectal mucinous adenocarcinomas. Dis Colon Rectum. 2010;53(6):936–43.
24. Nozoe T, Anai H, Nasu S, Sugimachi K. Clinicopathological characteristics of mucinous carcinoma of the colon and rectum. J Surg Oncol. 2000;75(2):103–7.
25. Catalano V, Loupakis F, Graziano F, Torresi U, Bisonni R, Mari D, et al. Mucinous histology predicts for poor response rate and overall survival of patients with colorectal cancer and treated with first-line oxaliplatin- and/or irinotecan-based chemotherapy. Br J Cancer. 2009;100(6):881–7.

26. Negri FV, Wotherspoon A, Cunningham D, Norman AR, Chong G, Ross PJ. Mucinous histology predicts for reduced fluorouracil responsiveness and survival in advanced colorectal cancer. Ann Oncol. 2005;16(8):1305–10.
27. Tanaka H, Deng G, Matsuzaki K, Kakar S, Kim GE, Miura S, et al. BRAF mutation, CpG island methylator phenotype and microsatellite instability occur more frequently and concordantly in mucinous than non-mucinous colorectal cancer. Int J Cancer. 2006;118(11):2765–71.
28. Hanski C, Tiecke F, Hummel M, Hanski M, Ogorek D, Rolfs A, et al. Low frequency of p53 gene mutation and protein expression in mucinous colorectal carcinomas. Cancer Lett. 1996;103(2):163–70.
29. Park SY, Lee HS, Choe G, Chung JH, Kim WH. Clinicopathological characteristics, microsatellite instability, and expression of mucin core proteins and p53 in colorectal mucinous adenocarcinomas in relation to location. Virchows Arch. 2006;449(1):40–7.
30. Farhat MH, Barada KA, Tawil AN, Itani DM, Hatoum HA, Shamseddine AI. Effect of mucin production on survival in colorectal cancer: a case-control study. World J Gastroenterol. 2008;14(45):6981–5.
31. Nitsche U, Zimmermann A, Späth C, Müller T, Maak M, Schuster T, et al. Mucinous and signet-ring cell colorectal cancers differ from classical adenocarcinomas in tumor biology and prognosis. Ann Surg. 2013;258(5):775–83.
32. Numata M, Shiozawa M, Watanabe T, Tamagawa H, Yamamoto N, Morinaga S, et al. The clinicopathological features of colorectal mucinous adenocarcinoma and a therapeutic strategy for the disease. World J Surg Oncol. 2012;10:109.
33. Verhulst J, Ferdinande L, Demetter P, Ceelen W. Mucinous subtype as prognostic factor in colorectal cancer: a systematic review and meta-analysis. J Clin Pathol. 2012;65(5):381–8.
34. Nitsche U, Friess H, Agha A, Angele M, Eckel R, Heitland W, et al. Prognosis of mucinous and signet-ring cell colorectal cancer in a population-based cohort. J Cancer Res Clin Oncol. 2016;142(11):2357–66.
35. Park JS, Huh JW, Park YA, Cho YB, Yun SH, Kim HC, et al. Prognostic comparison between mucinous and nonmucinous adenocarcinoma in colorectal cancer. Medicine. 2015;94(15):e658.
36. Hanski C. Is mucinous carcinoma of the colorectum a distinct genetic entity? Br J Cancer. 1995;72(6):1350–6.
37. Kim DH, Kim JW, Cho JH, Baek SH, Kakar S, Kim GE, et al. Expression of mucin core proteins, trefoil factors, APC and p21 in subsets of colorectal polyps and cancers suggests a distinct pathway of pathogenesis of mucinous carcinoma of the colorectum. Int J Oncol. 2005;27:957–64.
38. Woods MO, Hyde AJ, Curtis FK, Stuckless S, Green JS, Pollett AF, et al. High frequency of hereditary colorectal cancer in Newfoundland likely involves novel susceptibility genes. Clin Cancer Res. 2005;11(19):6853.
39. Xu W, Xu J, Shestopaloff K, Dicks E, Green J, Parfrey P, et al. A genome wide association study on Newfoundland colorectal cancer patients' survival outcomes. Biomarker Res. 2015;3(1):6.
40. Purcell S, Neale B, Todd-Brown K, Thomas L, Ferreira M, Bender D, et al. PLINK: a tool set for whole-genome association and population-based linkage analyses. Am J Hum Genet. 2007;81(3):559–75.
41. Leopoldo S, Lorena B, Cinzia A, Gabriella D, Angela Luciana B, Renato C, et al. Two subtypes of mucinous adenocarcinoma of the colorectum: clinicopathological and genetic features. Ann Surg Oncol. 2008;15(5): 1429–39.
42. Lasko TA, Bhagwat JG, Zou KH, Ohno-Machado L. The use of receiver operating characteristic curves in biomedical informatics. J Biomed Inform. 2005;38(5):404–15.
43. Zhou X, Obuchowski NA, McClish DK. Chapter 2. Measures of diagnostic accuracy. In: Statistical methods in diagnostic medicine. 2nd ed. Hoboken: Wiley; 2011. p. 13–57.
44. Søreide K. Receiver-operating characteristic curve analysis in diagnostic, prognostic and predictive biomarker research. J Clin Pathol. 2008;62(1):1.
45. Hanley JA, McNeil BJ. The meaning and use of the area under a receiver operating characteristic (ROC) curve. Radiology. 1982;143(1):29–36.
46. Kumar R, Indrayan A. Receiver operating characteristic (ROC) curve for medical researchers. Indian Pediatr. 2011;48(4):277–87.
47. Zweig MH, Campbell G. Receiver-operating characteristic (ROC) plots: a fundamental evaluation tool in clinical medicine. Clin Chem. 1993;39(4):561.
48. Robin X, Turck N, Hainard A, Tiberti N, Lisacek F, Sanchez J, et al. pROC: an open-source package for R and S+ to analyze and compare ROC curves. BMC Bioinformatics. 2011;12(1):77.

49. Lee S, Wu MC, Lin X. Optimal tests for rare variant effects in sequencing association studies. Biostatist. 2012;13(4):762–75.

50. Kinsella RJ, Kähäri A, Haider S, Zamora J, Proctor G, Spudich G, et al. Ensembl BioMarts: a hub for data retrieval across taxonomic space. Database. 2011:bar030.

51. Flicek P, Amode MR, Barrell D, Beal K, Billis K, Brent S, et al. Ensembl 2014. Nucleic Acids Res. 2014;42(D1):D749–55.

52. Core Team R. R: a language and environment for statistical computing. R Foundation for Statistical Computing 2013.

53. Boyle AP, Hong EL, Hariharan M, Cheng Y, Schaub MA, Kasowski M, et al. Annotation of functional variation in personal genomes using RegulomeDB. Genome Res. 2012;22(9):1790–7.

54. Yamamoto S, Mochizuki H, Hase K, Yamamoto T, Ohkusa Y, Yokoyama S, et al. Assessment of clinicopathologic features of colorectal mucinous adenocarcinoma. Am J Surg. 1993;166(3):257–61.

55. Janssens V, Goris J, Van Hoof C. PP2A: the expected tumor suppressor. Curr Opin Genet Dev. 2005;15(1):34–41.

56. Cristóbal I, Rincón R, Manso R, Madoz-Gúrpide J, Caramés C, del Puerto-Nevado L, et al. Hyperphosphorylation of PP2A in colorectal cancer and the potential therapeutic value showed by its forskolin-induced dephosphorylation and activation. Biochim Biophys Acta Mol Basis Dis. 2014;1842(9):1823–9.

57. Cristóbal I, Manso R, Rincón R, Caramés C, Zazo S, del Pulgar TG, et al. Phosphorylated protein phosphatase 2A determines poor outcome in patients with metastatic colorectal cancer. Br J Cancer. 2014;111(4):756–62.

58. Shi Y, Hu Z, Wu C, Dai J, Li H, Dong J, et al. A genome-wide association study identifies new susceptibility loci for non-cardia gastric cancer at 3q13.31 and 5p13.1. Nat Genet. 2011;43:1215.

59. Li B, Leal SM. Methods for detecting associations with rare variants for common diseases: application to analysis of sequence data. Am J Hum Genet. 2008;83(3):311–21.

60. Gabrielli F, Tofanelli S. Molecular and functional evolution of human DHRS2 and DHRS4 duplicated genes. Gene. 2012;511(2):461–9.

61. Sherry ST, Ward MH, Kholodov M, Baker J, Phan L, Smigielski EM, et al. dbSNP: the NCBI database of genetic variation. Nucleic Acids Res. 2001;29(1):308–11.

62. Kent WJ, Sugnet C,W., Furey TS, Roskin KM, Pringle TH, Zahler AM, et al. The human genome browser at UCSC. Genome Res 2002;12(6):996–1006.

63. Enomoto A, Wempe MF, Tsuchida H, Shin HJ, Cha SH, Anzai N, et al. Molecular identification of a novel carnitine transporter specific to human testis: insights into the mechanism of carnitine recognition. J Biol Chem. 2002;277(39):36262–71.

64. Aouida M, Poulin R, Ramotar D. The human carnitine transporter SLC22A16 mediates high affinity uptake of the anticancer polyamine analogue bleomycin-A5. J Biol Chem. 2009;285(9):6275–84.

65. Fukuda T, Sugita S, Inatome R, Yanagi S. CAMDI, a novel disrupted in schizophrenia 1 (DISC1)-binding protein, is required for radial migration. J Biol Chem. 2010;285(52):40554–61.

66. Kayser G, Gerlach U, Walch A, Nitschke R, Haxelmans S, Kayser K, et al. Numerical and structural centrosome aberrations are an early and stable event in the adenoma-carcinoma sequence of colorectal carcinomas. Virchows Arch. 2005;447(1):61–5.

67. Ishida N, Kawakita M. Molecular physiology and pathology of the nucleotide sugar transporter family (SLC35). Pflugers Arch. 2004;447(5):768–75.

68. Xie Z, Zhang H, Tsai W, Zhang Y, Du Y, Zhong J, et al. Zinc finger protein ZBTB20 is a key repressor of alpha-fetoprotein gene transcription in liver. Proc Natl Acad Sci U S A. 2008;105(31):10859–64.

69. Zhao J, Ren K, Tang J. Zinc finger protein ZBTB20 promotes cell proliferation in non-small cell lung cancer through repression of FoxO1. FEBS Lett. 2014; 588(24):4536–42.

70. Wang Q, Tan Y, Ren Y, Dong L, Xie Z, Tang L, et al. Zinc finger protein ZBTB20 expression is increased in hepatocellular carcinoma and associated with poor prognosis. BMC Cancer. 2011;11(1):271.

71. Fan W, Koch CA, de Hoog CL, Fam NP, Moran MF. The exchange factor Ras-GRF2 activates Ras-dependent and Rac-dependent mitogen-activated protein kinase pathways. Curr Biol. 1998;8(16):935–9.

72. Crespo P, Calvo F, Sanz-Moreno V. Ras and rho GTPases on the move: the RasGRF connection. BioArchitecture. 2011;1(4):200–4.

73. Wendeler MW, Paccaud J, Hauri H. Role of Sec24 isoforms in selective export of membrane proteins from the endoplasmic reticulum. EMBO Rep. 2006;8(3):258–64.

74. Goldenring JR. A central role for vesicle trafficking in epithelial neoplasia: intracellular highways to carcinogenesis. Nat Rev Cancer. 2013;13(11):813–20.

75. Raffaello A, De Stefani D, Sabbadin D, Teardo E, Merli G, Picard A, et al. The mitochondrial calcium uniporter is a multimer that can include a dominant-negative pore-forming subunit. EMBO J. 2013;32(17):2362–76.

76. Duchen MR. Mitochondria and calcium: from cell signalling to cell death. J Physiol. 2000;529:57–68.

77. Brown GR, Hem V, Katz KS, Ovetsky M, Wallin C, Ermolaeva O, et al. Gene: a gene-centered information resource at NCBI. Nucleic Acids Res. 2014;43:D36–42.

78. Green RC, Green JS, Buehler SK, Robb JD, Daftary D, Gallinger S, et al. Very high incidence of familial colorectal cancer in Newfoundland: a comparison with Ontario and 13 other population-based studies. Familial Cancer. 2007;6(1):53–62.

25

Molecular landscape and targeted therapy of acute myeloid leukemia

Runxia Gu, Xue Yang and Hui Wei*

Abstract

For decades, genetic aberrations including chromosome and molecular abnormalities are important diagnostic and prognostic factors in acute myeloid leukemia (AML). ATRA and imatinib have been successfully used in AML and chronic myelogenous leukemia, which proved that targeted therapy by identifying molecular lesions could improve leukemia outcomes. Recent advances in next generation sequencing have revealed molecular landscape of AML, presenting us with many molecular abnormalities. The individual prognostic information derived from a specific mutation could be modified by other molecular lesions. Therefore, the genomic complexity in AML poses a huge challenge to successful translation into more accurate risk stratification and targeted therapy. Herein, a summary of these mutations and targeted therapies are described. We focus on the prognostic information of recent identified molecular lesions and emerging targeted therapy.

Keywords: Acute myeloid leukemia, Molecular landscape, Targeted therapy

Background

Acute myeloid leukemia (AML) is a heterogeneous disease, characterized by multiple somatically acquired driver mutations, coexisting competing clones, and disease evolution over time [1, 2]. Specific chromosomal aberrations and translocations have provided fundamental information in the evaluation of patients and guide for rational management. With advances in Next-generation sequencing (NGS) technologies, a detailed knowledge of the molecular landscape of AML has been discovered, with a better understanding in disease pathogenesis, classification and new therapeutic strategies [3–5]. More recently, German–Austrian AML Study Group revealed the cytogenetics and clinical data in 1540 patients with AML from three prospective trials (AML-HD98A, AML-HD98B and AMLSG-07-04). A total of 5234 AML driven mutations were identified and classified into non-overlapping 11 subtypes, which enabled us a better understanding of genomic landscape of AML from a macro perspective [1]. Encouraging efficacy of targeted therapy have brought about huge advance to AML treatment (details in Table 1) [6, 7]. A summary of these mutations and targeted therapy is described in the following sections (Fig. 1). Since fusion genes like PML-RARα, AML-ETO, CBFβ-MYH11 and MLL have been investigated for a long time, we wouldn't discuss them here in our review.

Nucleophosmin 1 (NPM1)

NPM1 mutations are reported in approximately one-third of AML adults, and more than half of them are with normal cytogenetics (CN-AML). It often co-occurs with mutations in epigenetic modifiers such as DNA methyltransferase 3A (DNMT3A), Ten-eleven translocation gene-2(TET2) and Isocitrate dehydrogenase1/2 (IDH1/2) mutations [6]. Numerous studies have confirmed that NPM1 mutations are an independent predictor of high CR rate and favorable prognosis in younger adults with AML, specifically in those without FMS-related tyrosine kinase 3-internal tandem duplications (FLT3-ITD) mutations [8, 9]. Recent studies have indicated that AML patients with NPM1 mutation and FLT3-ITD low allelic ratio may also have a more favorable prognosis regardless of chromosomal status, who should not be routinely assigned to allogeneic hematopoietic stem cell transplant (allo-HSCT) in the first complete remission [10, 11]. Patients harboring NPM1 mutations, even with high allelic ratio FLT3-ITD mutations have better prognosis than those with FLT3-ITD mutations alone [12]. In this setting, the latest ELN and NCCN risk stratification systems both classify NPM1 mutations with high allelic ratio FLT3-ITD mutations as intermediate risk group [13, 14]. However, the coexisting

* Correspondence: weihui@ihcams.ac.cn
Leukemia Center, Institute of Hematology and Blood Diseases Hospital, Chinese Academy of Medical Sciences & Peking Union Medical College, Tianjin 300020, People's Republic of China

Table 1 therapeutic targeting of individual AML mutations

Mutation	Therapeutic target	Inhibitors (phase of clinical trials)
FLT3	FLT3	FLT3 tyrosine kinase inhibitors: sorafenib (III), midostaurin (approved), quizartinib (III), crenolanib (III), gilteritinib (III), lestaurtinib (III) Other TKIs: ponatinib (I/II)
IDH1/2	IDH1	Ivosidenib (approved), IDH-305(I), BAY1436032(I), FT-2102(I/II), AG-881(I)
	IDH2	Enasidenib (approved), AG-881(I)
	BCL-2	venetoclax (III)
KIT	KIT	TKIs: imatinib, dasatinib (III), ponatinib
		sorafenib, sunitinib, quizartinib
TP53	TP53	PANDAS
	BCL-2	venetoclax
	MDM2	MDM2 inhibitors: RG7112 (I)
	Others	decitabine
SF3B1	SF3b complex	H3B-8800 (I)

MDM2 mouse double minute 2 homolog, *SF3B1* splicing factor 3B subunit 1

DNMT3A and FLT3-ITD mutations may predict the worst prognosis among AML patients with NPM1 mutation [1, 15]. It remains confirmed whether high NPM1-mutant allele burden at diagnosis predicts unfavorable outcomes in large prospective cohorts [16]. In elderly patients, NPM1 mutations are associated with a better CR rate, the prognosis of which has not been systematically confirmed. Most trials showed older CN-AML patients with NPM1 mutations have favorable treatment response and survival rate, while the prognosis of them is inferior to younger patients on the whole [17, 18]. However, several researches did not find favorable outcome of NPM1 mutation in older patients. Which may be related to different treatment regimens [19]. As for therapies, in the E1900 trial, patients with NPM1 mutant AML exposed to high dose daunorubicin (90 mg/m^2) derived an increase in median overall survival (OS) compared with Standard dose daunorubicin (45 mg/m^2) therapy

(16.9 m vs 75.9 m) [20]. Besides, whether patients with NPM1 mutation will benefit from all-trans retinoic acid or arsenic acid treatment remains further discussion [21, 22].

Signaling and kinase pathway mutations

In addition to mutations in NPM1, mutations leading to aberrant activation and proliferation of cellular signaling pathways, including FLT3, KRAS, NRAS, PTPN11, NF1, and KIT, are present in approximately two-thirds of AML cases.

FLT3

Mutations in FLT3 mostly involves internal tandem duplications within the juxta membrane region (FLT3-ITD) and point mutations in the tyrosine kinase domain (FLT3-TKD). Previous studies have confirmed that, FLT3-ITD mutations are associated with higher relapse rate and poorer overall survival, particularly with a high ratio of mutant allelic

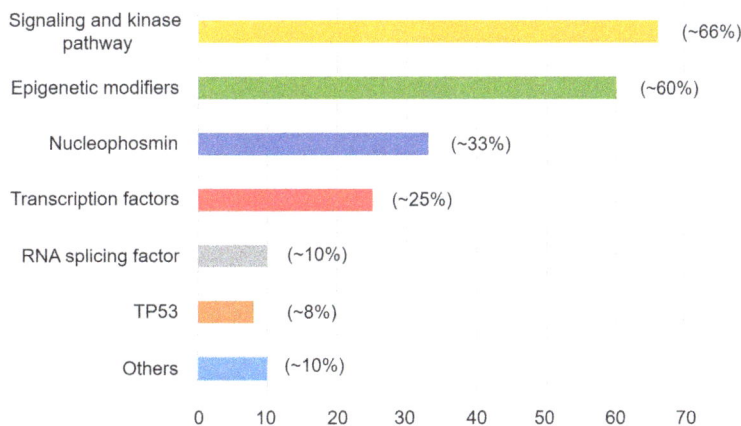

Fig. 1 Distribution of recurrent AML mutations by functional group. A summary of the most frequent recurrent mutations in AML are listed in this figure. Other mutation as Cohesin complex are not discussed in detail in the manuscript. Mutational frequencies of each subgroup are derived from integration of data from several researches [1, 6, 8]

burden [23, 24]. In recent years, with great efforts in developing protein kinase inhibitors targeting FLT3 mutations the prognosis of patients with FLT3-ITD mutation has been significantly improved. Generally, the first generation of FLT3 inhibitors mainly include sorafenib, sunitinib, midostaurin and lestaurtinib. Because of having broad inhibiting targets besides FLT3-ITD mutation, it may improve the prognosis in AML without FLT3-ITD mutation. A phase II SORMAL clinical trial from Germany demonstrated that sorafenib could improve 3-year EFS in full set of primary AML (40% vs 22%, HR = 0.64, n = 267) [25]. A phase III international prospective RATIFY study confirmed that, addition of midostaurin to standard induction chemotherapy could significantly increase OS vs placebo among AML adults with FLT3 mutation (median OS of 74.7 m vs 25.6 m, HR = 0.78, n = 717) [26]. These results attribute a lot on the approval of midostaurin by FDA in newly diagnoses AML with FLT3-ITD mutation. According to the latest ELN and NCCN guideline for AML, midostaurin combining with chemotherapy was recommended as the first line treatment in adult FLT3 mutated AML [13, 14]. Second-generation small molecule FLT3 inhibitors such as quizartinib (AC-220), crenolanib (CP-868596), and gilteritinib (ASP-2215), have shown potent activity. Overall response for single agent FLT3 kinase inhibitor in treating FLT3-ITD mutated relapsed or refractory (R/R) AML is 40-50% in phase I and II clinical trials [27–29]. The efficacy of quizartinib was tested in patients with R/R FLT3-ITD mutated AML compared to salvage chemotherapy in a QuANTUM-R Trial. The median OS was 27 weeks and 20.4 weeks for patients treated with quizartinib and salvage chemotherapy, respectively [30]. It is the first phase III trial to demonstrate improved OS with FLT3 inhibitors in the R/R FLT3-ITD mutated AML setting. Also encouraging, interim study results of a phase I study of the combination of gilteritinib with induction chemotherapy reported an composite complete remission rate of 91.3% in newly diagnosed AML with FLT3-mutation (n = 23) [31]. Adding crenolanib to standard induction chemotherapy in patients with FLT3-mutated AML may be associated with low relapse rate when HSCT is routinely taken. In addition, for the patients did not undergo HSCT, only one (1/7) of them has relapsed, suggesting that standard chemotherapy plus crenolanib may also provide durable remissions without HSCT [32]. FLT3 inhibitors such as quizartinib and sorafenib target the inactive conformation of the kinase domain and only inhibit FLT3-ITD. Other inhibitors such as crenolanib, gilteritinib, and midostaurin target both the active and inactive conformation and show activity against both FLT3-ITD and TKD mutations [33]. Currently, several trials have been initiated to investigate the role of FLT3 inhibitors in maintenance therapy, eradiating MRD, and the combination regimen with chemotherapy (NCT02421939, NCT02752035, NCT02927262, NCT0307 0093).

Kit

The receptor tyrosine kinase KIT is frequently mutated in Core-binding factor AML (CBF-AML), which is defined by the occurrence of t (8;21) or inv.(16)/t (16;16) rearrangements. It has been demonstrated that the frequency of inv.(16)/t (16;16) AML in CBF leukemia is higher in Caucasian than in Chinese and Japanese [34]. The main mutational clusters in CBF-AML are commonly observed in KIT exon 8 and exon 17. It has been reported that mutations in KIT exon 17 or delayed reduction of RUNX1-RUNX1T1 transcripts conferred a higher risk of relapse and inferior OS in AML with t (8;21) [35]. Recently, several researches confirmed that t (8;21) AML patients with KIT mutations have a lower responsive rate after relapse. The prognostic impact of KIT mutations in inv.(16)/t (16;16) AML remains controversial [36]. Our recent study found that t (8;21) AML patients bearing KIT-D816 mutations have lower remission rates than those with wild-type KIT [37]. Patients with CBF-AML may benefit from high dose Cytarabine [38]. That is quite different from patients with NPM1 mutation who benefited from escalating dosage of anthracyclines, which have been mentioned above. The CALGB10801 trial indicated that adding multikinase inhibitors with activity against KIT mutations to chemotherapy, like dasatinib, could result in the similar 2 years DFS and OS in CBF-AML patients with kit mutation compared to those without, suggesting that dasatinib might improve the prognosis of in CBF-AML patients with KIT mutations [39]. Unfortunately, for patients with high-risk CBF-AML in CR1, dasatinib alone failed to prevent relapse due to molecular primary resistance or recurrence. Clinical trials about dasatinib undertaken by Shanghai Ruijin Hospital and our hospitial in China (ChiCRT-IPR-15006862 and NCT03560908) and other centers (NCT00850382) are ongoing.

Mutations in transcription factors

Mutations in transcription factors occur in 20- 25% of patients with AML, including myeloid transcription factors, Runt-related transcription factor 1 (RUNX1) and CCAAT/enhancer binding protein α (CEBPA).

RUNX1

RUNX1 mutations were reported in 5% to 10% of AML, and more in patients with secondary AML evolving from myelodysplastic syndrome [40, 41]. The 2016 revised WHO AML classification system has added mutated RUNX1 as a provisional entity [42]. Studies have confirmed RUNX1 mutations an independent predictor of poorer prognosis [40, 41]. Concomitant mutations with ASXL1, SF3B1, SRSF2, PHF6 have been reported to have negative impact on OS, whereas patients with the genotype RUNX1mut/IDH2mut had better clinical outcome

[40]. In addition, mutation burden and wild-type allele loss of RUNX1 as well as additional mutations also have impact on prognosis of adult RUNX1-mutated AML. Both wild-type loss and > 1 RUNX1mut showed adverse impact on prognosis compared with 1 RUNX1mut (OS 5 m vs 22 m, P = 0.002; 14 m vs 22 m, P = 00.048). Concomitant ASXL1 mutation and ≥ 2 additional mutations correlated with shorter OS (10 m vs 18 m, P = 0.028; 12 m vs 20 m, P = 0.017) [43].

CEBPA

Mutated CEBPA gene occur in 5-14% of AML patients, mainly in CN-AML, and was related to better prognosis. Recent studies showed that, the favorable impact of mutant CEBPA on prognosis is associated with biallelic mutations [44, 45]. The 2016 revision to the WHO classification system redefined the provisional WHO 2008 entity AML with CEBPA mutations to those with biallelic mutations [42]. Although the response rate for CEBPA double mutants is up to 90%, with estimated 5 years OS ranging between 50 and 70%, relapse still remains the major cause of treatment failure. The estimated cumulative incidence of relapse (CIR) of CEBPA dm patients after 5 years is up to 58% for intensive chemotherapy [46]. Richard, et al. analyzed 124 AML patients with CEBPA dm who achieved CR1. They found that the relapse-free survival (RFS) was significantly higher in patients receiving HSCT in CR1 compared with chemotherapy, whereas the OS was not different, which might be associated with a high second CR rate after salvage therapy [46].

Mutations in epigenetic modifiers: Regulation of DNA methylation and chromatin modification

In recent years, the discovery of epigenetic regulators has provided great insight into the pathogenesis of AML. Mutations in these genes such as IDH1/2, DNMT3A, TET2, Additional sex comb-like 1(ASXL1), and Enhancer of zeste homolog 2(EZH2), which appear to impact on DNA methylation or histone posttranslational modifications, may serve as prognostic markers for risk stratification and therapeutic decision [47–49].

IDH1/2

Mutations in genes encoding IDH1 and IDH2 gene mainly involves IDH1-R132, IDH2-R140, and IDH2-R172, and IDH1 and IDH2 mutations rarely co-occur. IDH1-R132 or IDH2-R140 frequently occur in AML patients with normal cytogenetics and advanced age, with concurrent mutations of NPM1 [50]. While IDH2-R172 may represent a distinct genomic subgroup, which mutual exclusivity with NPM1 and with a distinct DNA methylation profile [51]. Experimental evidence demonstrates that IDH1/2 mutation occurs in the origin of clone, which is insufficient to induce

leukemic transformation alone. Early data suggested that IDH mutations were associated with adverse prognosis, while recent results from a large cohort suggested that IDH mutations of different sites and additional co-occurring mutations may result in different outcomes [2, 51]. Several evidences showed that IDH1 and IDH2-R172 mutation may predict a worse clinical outcome especially in CN-AML, while the IDH2-R140 concomitant NPM1 mutation may be associated with better prognosis in AML [51–53]. Clearly, the prognostic impact of IDH1/2 mutations in AML has far been conflicting, and more efforts are needed for further study. Several small molecule inhibitors of IDH (AG-120, IDH-305 and FT-2102 for IDH1; AG-221 for IDH2; AG-881 for IDH1/2) have demonstrated potent preclinical activity, most of which are currently undergoing clinical trials and the early results are promising. The first-in-human phase I/II clinical trial of AG-221 (NCT01915498) for patients with IDH2-mutant advanced hematologic malignancies reported an objective response rate (ORR) of 40.3% (71/176) in R/R AML patients, with 19.3% CR rate and a median response duration of 5.8 months [54]. Interim study results of AG-120 reported an 41.9% ORR, including a 24.0% CR in IDH1-mutant R/R AML (n = 179) [55]. Based on its convincing therapeutic effects and great tolerance, ivosidenib (AG-120) and enasidenib (AG-221) had been approved by FDA for treatment in adult patients with R/R IDH1 and IDH2 mutant AML respectively. Studies investigating IDH inhibitors as monotherapy or combination regimen are still ongoing (NCT02632708, NCT02677922, NCT01915498, NCT02577406, NCT02719574, NCT03127 -735, NCT02492737). Moreover, patients with IDH mutations are found to be more responsive to B-cell CLL/lymphoma 2 (BCL-2) inhibitor [56].

DNMT3A, TET2 and ASXL1

Mutations in epigenetic regulators also include DNMT3A, TET2 and ASXL1, namely DTA mutations. These mutations are most common in people harboring age-related clonal hematopoiesis. Nowadays, no consensus has been reached on the prognosis of DNMT3a mutation. Some studies reported its poor prognosis [57], while others failed to find adverse impact [58]. Current researches suggested that DNMT3a mutation conferred adverse prognosis in AML patients with NPM1 mutation [59]. AML patients harboring NPM1, FLT3-ITD and DNMT3a mutations are associated with the worst prognosis [1]. Most recently, the latest ELN and NCCN risk stratification systems both classify ASXL1 mutations as adverse-risk AML subtypes. However, ASXL1 mutations should not be used as an adverse prognostic marker if they cooccur with favorable-risk AML subtypes [14, 60]. A recent series of studies demonstrated that, DNMT3A, occurred at a very early stage among genetic abnormalities, possessing a selective proliferative advantage which might be preleukemic events [61–63].

And in vivo experiments showed that mutated ASXL1 lowered the threshold of meningioma-1 driven engraftment, although it was insufficient to lead to blood malignancies [64]. Results from a systematic study involving 482 AML patients younger than 65 years old showed that DTA mutations remained detectable even during CR, and the persisting rates were 78.7% for DNMT3A, 54.2% for TET2, and 51.6% for ASXL1. The detection of persistent mutations did not correlate with an increased relapse rate with in a follow up period of 4 years ($P = 0.29$) [65, 66]. But a recent report revealed that the persistence of pre-leukemic mutation including DNMT3a might contribute to the inferior outcome of AML patients. Thus, the role of DNMT3a mutation during CR still needs further investigation [67].

RNA splicing factor mutations

RNA splicing factor mutations

Mutations in splicing factors accounts for 10% of AML patients, which are defined by mutations in genes regulating RNA splicing (SF3B1, SRSF2, U2AF1 and ZRSR2). They are likely to cause aberrant splicing, affecting the transcriptome and proteome of cells. Accumulating evidence shows that spliceosome mutations are associated with older age, less proliferative disease, low response rate to standard treatment, and poorer survival [68]. Recent data suggested that many spliceosome inhibitors showed therapeutic potential in spliceosome mutant cancers. An orally available modulator of SF3b complex, H3B-8800, exhibits therapeutic potential of splicing modulation in spliceosome-mutant cancers in preclinical studies [69]. One phase I trial of H3B-8800 for patients with hematologic malignancies is currently ongoing (NCT02841540).

Mutations in tumor suppressor genes

TP53

Although a lot of mutations are predicted to be activating or neomorphic, many of them have been demonstrated to be loss-of-function mutations, such as mutation in tumor protein 53(TP53), rendering them less tractable targets. TP53 is a key tumor suppressor gene. TP53 mutations accounts for 8% of patients with AML, and are associated with complex cytogenetics, therapy-related AML, chemoresistance, high relapse rates and poor survival [6, 58, 70]. Considering the fact that most of targeted drugs are gene inhibitors, as loss-of-function mutations, TP53 mutation is difficult to target. Although treat with intensive chemotherapy, the overall survival time is around 4.6 months [71]. It has been reported that decitabine, which decreases mutp53 levels, may improve the prognosis of patients with TP53 mutation, with a median survival of 12.7 months [72]. Besides, TP53 mutations have been described to be predictive for a favorable response to MDM2 inhibitors and BCL-2 inhibitors in hematologic malignancies [73–75]. Recently, Lu and his colleagues

from Shanghai Jiaotong University identified a small molecule from thousands of compounds that can restore mutant TP53 with anti-cancer effect, which is named as PANDAS. Compared with previous TP53-targeting agents, PANDAS stabilizes molecular architecture of mutant TP53, restores its activity and promotes tumor cell apoptosis. The efficacy and tolerability of PANDAS, particularly in synergistic combinations, are keenly awaited.

Conclusion and prospects

The discovery of the molecular landscape of AML not only provides us a chance to better understand the pathogenesis of the disease, but also refines the risk stratification and management of patients. However, evolving evidence demonstrated that the individual prognostic information derived from a specific mutation could be modified by other molecular characteristic and clinical parameters. Therefore, development of risk group classification schemes based on comprehensive genomic assessment should be considered a work in future. Targeted therapy to these mutations achieved huge progress in recent years. For instance, both IDH1/2 and FLT3 inhibitors showed promising results. And the combination of venetoclax with azacitidine produced a median OS longer than 12 months in older AML patients with a favorable safety profile [76, 77]. Considering the promising preliminary results of venetoclax, we can reasonably expect that the clinical outcomes for AML in older patients will be further improved in the foreseeable future.

In addition to genetic aberrations, epigenetics or posttranscriptional regulations may also play a pivotal role in determining the biological behavior of AML. Current researches demonstrated that DNA methylation patterns and long noncoding RNAs contribute to many critical signaling pathways in AML development, even exert effects on diagnosis classification and outcome of AML [78, 79]. And a further understanding of the relationship among genetic aberrations, DNA methylation, and long noncoding RNAs action might pave the way to better understand and treat AML patients.

In addition, encouraging efficacy of immunotherapeutic agents, especially the chimeric antigen receptor T (CAR-T) cell therapy, has brought huge advance to ALL treatment in the past decade [80–83]. However, previous trials of CAR-T therapy for AML did not result in long-term responses and exhibited the likelihood of hematopoietic toxicity, mainly due to the lack of AML-specific targeted antigens [84]. Currently, Liu and her colleagues reported on the robust anti-tumor activity and high safety of CAR-T cells targeting two different antigens simultaneously (CLL1-CD33 cCAR-T cells) [85]. This research unveiled a new strategy to circumvent unwanted off-target toxicity and contributed a significant step forward in AML immunotherapy. We believe that rational combination of targeted and immunotherapeutic agents will provide new insight into AML therapies and continue to accelerate progress in AML outcomes within the coming years.

Abbreviations

allo-HSCT: Allogeneic hematopoietic stem cell transplant; AML: Acute myeloid leukemia; ASXL1: Additional sex comb-like 1; BCL-2: B-cell CLL/lymphoma 2; CAR-T: Chimeric antigen receptor T; CBF-AML: Core-binding factor AML; CEBPA: CCAAT/enhancer binding protein α; CIR: Cumulative incidence of relapse; CN-AML: Normal cytogenetics; DNMT3A: DNA methyltransferase 3A; EZH2: Enhancer of zeste homolog 2; FLT3-ITD: FMS-related tyrosine kinase 3-internal tandem duplications; FLT3-TKD: FMS-related tyrosine kinase 3-tyrosine kinase domain; IDH1/2: Isocitrate dehydrogenase1/2; MDM2: Mouse double minute 2 homolog; NGS: Next-generation sequencing; OS: Overall survival; R/R AML: Relapsed or refractory AML; RFS: Relapse-free survival; RUNX1: Runt-related transcription factor 1; SF3B1: Splicing factor 3B subunit 1; TET2: Ten-eleven translocation gene-2; TP53: Tumor protein 53

Funding

This study was supported by National Natural Science Foundation of China (81670159), CAMS Innovation Fund for Medical Sciences (CIFMS 2016-I2M-3-004), Peking Union Medical College Youth Fund (2017320022).

Authors' contributions

RG and XY wrote the paper. HW revised the paper. All authors collected the data, read and approved the final manuscript.

Competing interests

The authors declare that they have no competing interests.

References

1. Papaemmanuil E, Gerstung M, Bullinger L, Gaidzik VI, Paschka P, Roberts ND, et al. Genomic classification and prognosis in acute myeloid leukemia. N Engl J Med. 2016;374:2209–21.
2. Patel JP, Gonen M, Figueroa ME, Fernandez H, Sun Z, Racevskis J, et al. Prognostic relevance of integrated genetic profiling in acute myeloid leukemia. N Engl J Med. 2012;366:1079–89.
3. Grimwade D, Hills RK, Moorman AV, Walker H, Chatters S, Goldstone AH, et al. Refinement of cytogenetic classification in acute myeloid leukemia: determination of prognostic significance of rare recurring chromosomal abnormalities among 5876 younger adult patients treated in the United Kingdom Medical Research Council trials. Blood. 2010;116:354–65.
4. Grimwade D, Mrozek K. Diagnostic and prognostic value of cytogenetics in acute myeloid leukemia. Hematol Oncol Clin North Am. 2011;25:1135–61.
5. Lichtenegger FS, Krupka C, Haubner S, Kohnke T, Subklewe M. Recent developments in immunotherapy of acute myeloid leukemia. J Hematol Oncol. 2017;10:142.
6. Grimwade D, Ivey A, Huntly BJ. Molecular landscape of acute myeloid leukemia in younger adults and its clinical relevance. Blood. 2016;127:29–41.
7. Liu B, Song Y, Liu D. Clinical trials of CAR-T cells in China. J Hematol Oncol. 2017;10:166.
8. DiNardo DC, JE C. In: Tallman MS, McCrae KR, Sonali S, Crowther MA, editors. Mutations in AML: prognostic and therapeutic implications: Hematology, Washington: American Society of Hematology. 2016. p. 348–55.
9. Schnittger S, Schoch C, Kern W, Mecucci C, Tschulik C, Martelli MF, et al. Nucleophosmin gene mutations are predictors of favorable prognosis in acute myelogenous leukemia with a normal karyotype. Blood. 2005;106: 3733–9.
10. Pratcorona M, Brunet S, Nomdedeu J, Ribera JM, Tormo M, Duarte R, et al. Favorable outcome of patients with acute myeloid leukemia harboring a low-allelic burden FLT3-ITD mutation and concomitant NPM1 mutation: relevance to post-remission therapy. Blood. 2013;121:2734–8.
11. Haferlach C, Mecucci C, Schnittger S, Kohlmann A, Mancini M, Cuneo A, et al. AML with mutated NPM1 carrying a normal or aberrant karyotype show overlapping biologic, pathologic, immunophenotypic, and prognostic features. Blood. 2009;114:3024–32.
12. Versluis J, In 't Hout FE, Devillier R, van Putten WL, Manz MG, Vekemans MC, et al. Comparative value of post-remission treatment in cytogenetically normal AML subclassified by NPM1 and FLT3-ITD allelic ratio. Leukemia. 2017;31:26–33.
13. Döhner H, Estey E, Grimwade D, Amadori S, Appelbaum FR, Büchner T, et al. Diagnosis and management of AML in adults: 2017 ELN recommendations from an international expert panel. Blood. 2017;129:424–47.
14. O' Donnell MR. Tallman MS. Abboud CN. Altman JK. Appelbaum FR. Bhatt VR, et al. NCCN clinical practice Guilelines in oncology: acute meyloid leukemia. Version 2. 2018. https://www.nccn.org/professionals/physician_gls/default.aspx#site. Accessed 1 Aug 2018.
15. Loghavi S, Zuo Z, Ravandi F, Kantarjian HM, Bueso-Ramos C, Zhang L, et al. Clinical features of de novo acute myeloid leukemia with concurrent DNMT3A, FLT3 and NPM1 mutations. J Hematol Oncol. 2014;7:74.
16. Patel SS, Kuo FC, Gibson CJ, Steensma DP, Soiffer RJ, Alyea EP 3rd, et al. High NPM1-mutant allele burden at diagnosis predicts unfavorable outcomes in de novo AML. Blood. 2018;131:2816–25.
17. Becker H, Marcucci G, Maharry K, Radmacher MD, Mrozek K, Margeson D, et al. Favorable prognostic impact of NPM1 mutations in older patients with cytogenetically normal de novo acute myeloid leukemia and associated gene- and microRNA-expression signatures: a Cancer and leukemia group B study. J Clin Oncol. 2010;28:596–604.
18. Ostronoff F, Othus M, Lazenby M, Estey E, Appelbaum FR, Evans A, et al. Prognostic significance of NPM1 mutations in the absence of FLT3-internal tandem duplication in older patients with acute myeloid leukemia: a SWOG and UK National Cancer Research Institute/Medical Research Council report. J Clin Oncol. 2015;33:1157–64.
19. Lazenby M, Gilkes AF, Marrin C, Evans A, Hills RK, Burnett AK. The prognostic relevance of flt3 and npm1 mutations on older patients treated intensively or non-intensively: a study of 1312 patients in the UK NCRI AML16 trial. Leukemia. 2014;28:1953–9.
20. Luskin MR, Lee JW, Fernandez HF, Abdel-Wahab O, Bennett JM, Ketterling RP, et al. Benefit of high-dose daunorubicin in AML induction extends across cytogenetic and molecular groups. Blood. 2016;127:1551–8.
21. Schlenk RF, Frohling S, Hartmann F, Fischer JT, Glasmacher A, del Valle F, et al. Phase III study of all-trans retinoic acid in previously untreated patients 61 years or older with acute myeloid leukemia. Leukemia. 2004;18:1798–803.
22. El Hajj H, Dassouki Z, Berthier C, Raffoux E, Ades L, Legrand O, et al. Retinoic acid and arsenic trioxide trigger degradation of mutated NPM1, resulting in apoptosis of AML cells. Blood. 2015;125:3447–54.
23. Schlenk RF, Kayser S, Bullinger L, Kobbe G, Casper J, Ringhoffer M, et al. Differential impact of allelic ratio and insertion site in FLT3-ITD-positive AML with respect to allogeneic transplantation. Blood. 2014;124:3441–9.
24. Wang Y, Xu Y, Li S, Liu J, Xing Y, Xing H, et al. Targeting FLT3 in acute myeloid leukemia using ligand-based chimeric antigen receptor-engineered T cells. J Hematol Oncol. 2018;11:60.
25. Rollig C, Serve H, Huttmann A, Noppeney R, Muller-Tidow C, Krug U, et al. Addition of sorafenib versus placebo to standard therapy in patients aged 60 years or younger with newly diagnosed acute myeloid leukaemia (SORAML): a multicentre, phase 2, randomised controlled trial. Lancet Oncol. 2015;16:1691–9.
26. Stone RM, Mandrekar SJ, Sanford BL, Laumann K, Geyer S, Bloomfield CD, et al. Midostaurin plus chemotherapy for acute myeloid leukemia with a FLT3 mutation. N Engl J Med. 2017;377:454–64.
27. Cortes JE, Kantarjian H, Foran JM, Ghirdaladze D, Zodelava M, Borthakur G, et al. Phase I study of quizartinib administered daily to patients with relapsed or refractory acute myeloid leukemia irrespective of FMS-like tyrosine kinase 3-internal tandem duplication status. J Clin Oncol. 2013;31:3681–7.
28. Perl AE, Altman JK, Cortes J, Smith C, Litzow M, Baer MR, et al. Selective inhibition of FLT3 by gilteritinib in relapsed or refractory acute myeloid leukaemia: a multicentre, first-in-human, open-label, phase 1-2 study. Lancet Oncol. 2017;18:1061–75.
29. Yang X, Wang J. Precision therapy for acute myeloid leukemia. J Hematol Oncol. 2018;11:3.

30. Cortes J, Khaled S, Martinelli G, Perl AE, Ganguly S, Russell N, et al. Quizartinib significantly prolongs overall survival in patients with FLT3-internal tandem duplication-mutated (Mut) relapsed/refractory AML in the phase 3, randomized, controlled quantum-r trial. European Hematology Association Congress Abstract. 2018:LB2600. https://learningcenter.ehaweb.org/eha/2018/stockholm/218882/jorge.cortes.quizartinib.significantly.prolongs.overall.survival.in.patients.htmlf=menu=6*ce_id=1346*ot_id=19045*media=3*browseby=8. Accessed 16 July 2018.

31. Pratz K, Cherry M, Altman JK, Cooper BW, Cruz JC, Jurcic JG, et al. Preliminary results from a phase 1 study of gilteritinib in combination with induction and consolidation chemotherapy in subjects with newly diagnosed acute myeloid leukemia (AML). Blood. 2017;130:722.

32. Walter RB, Collins RH, Stone RM, Tallman MS, Karanes C, Vigil CE, et al. Addition of crenolanib to standard induction and consolidation therapies improved long-term outcomes in newly diagnosed FLT3 mutant AML patients ≤ 60 years old. European Hematology Association Congress Abstract. 2018:PF227. https://learningcenter.ehaweb.org/eha/2018/stockholm/214713/roland.b.walter.addition.of.crenolanib.to.standard.induction.and.consolidation.html?f=menu=6*ce_id=1346*ot_id=19045*media=3*browseby=8. Accessed 16 July 2018.

33. Saygin C, Carraway HE. Emerging therapies for acute myeloid leukemia. J Hematol Oncol. 2017;10:93.

34. Wei H, Wang Y, Zhou C, Lin D, Liu B, Liu K, et al. Distinct genetic alteration profiles of acute myeloid leukemia between Caucasian and eastern Asian population. J Hematol Oncol. 2018;11:18.

35. Qin YZ, Wang Y, Xu LP, Zhang XH, Chen H, Han W, et al. The dynamics of RUNX1-RUNX1T1 transcript levels after allogeneic hematopoietic stem cell transplantation predict relapse in patients with t (8;21) acute myeloid leukemia. J Hematol Oncol. 2017;10:44.

36. Paschka P, Marcucci G, Ruppert AS, Mrozek K, Chen H, Kittles RA, et al. Adverse prognostic significance of KIT mutations in adult acute myeloid leukemia with inv (16) and t (8;21): a Cancer and leukemia group B study. J Clin Oncol. 2006;24:3904–11.

37. Gong BF, Tan YH, Liao AJ, Li J, Mao YY, Lu N, et al. Impact of KIT D816 mutation on salvage therapy in relapsed acute myeloid leukemia with t (8; 21) translocation. Zhonghua Xue Ye Xue Za Zhi. 2018;39:460–4. https://doi.org/10.3760/cma.j.issn.0253-2727.2018.06.004.

38. Miyawaki S, Ohtake S, Fujisawa S, Kiyoi H, Shinagawa K, Usui N, et al. A randomized comparison of 4 courses of standard-dose multiagent chemotherapy versus 3 courses of high-dose cytarabine alone in postremission therapy for acute myeloid leukemia in adults: the JALSG AML201 study. Blood. 2011;117:2366–72.

39. Marcucci G, Geyer S, Zhao W, Caroll AJ, Bucci D, Uy GL, et al. Adding KIT inhibitor Dasatinib (DAS) to chemotherapy overcomes the negative impact of KIT mutation/over-expression in core binding factor (CBF) acute myeloid leukemia (AML): results from CALGB 10801(Alliance). Blood. 2014;124:8.

40. Gaidzik VI, Teleanu V, Papaemmanuil E, Weber D, Paschka P, Hahn J, et al. RUNX1 mutations in acute myeloid leukemia are associated with distinct clinico-pathologic and genetic features. Leukemia. 2016;30:2160–8.

41. Gaidzik VI, Bullinger L, Schlenk RF, Zimmermann AS, Rock J, Paschka P, et al. RUNX1 mutations in acute myeloid leukemia: results from a comprehensive genetic and clinical analysis from the AML study group. J Clin Oncol. 2011; 29:1364–72.

42. Arber DA, Orazi A, Hasserjian R, Thiele J, Borowitz MJ, Le Beau MM, et al. The 2016 revision to the World Health Organization classification of myeloid neoplasms and acute leukemia. Blood. 2016;127:2391–405.

43. Stengel A, Kern W, Meggendorfer M, Nadarajah N, Perglerova K, Haferlach T, et al. Number of RUNX1 mutations, wild-type allele loss and additional mutations impact on prognosis in adult RUNX1-mutated AML. Leukemia. 2018;32:295–302.

44. Taskesen E, Bullinger L, Corbacioglu A, Sanders MA, Erpelinck CA, Wouters BJ, et al. Prognostic impact, concurrent genetic mutations, and gene expression features of AML with CEBPA mutations in a cohort of 1182 cytogenetically normal AML patients: further evidence for CEBPA double mutant AML as a distinctive disease entity. Blood. 2011;117:2469–75.

45. Wouters BJ, Lowenberg B, Erpelinck-Verschueren CA, van Putten WL, Valk PJ, Delwel R. Double CEBPA mutations, but not single CEBPA mutations, define a subgroup of acute myeloid leukemia with a distinctive gene expression profile that is uniquely associated with a favorable outcome. Blood. 2009;113:3088–91.

46. Schlenk RF, Taskesen E, van Norden Y, Krauter J, Ganser A, Bullinger L, et al. The value of allogeneic and autologous hematopoietic stem cell

47. Dang L, White DW, Gross S, Bennett BD, Bittinger MA, Driggers EM, et al. Cancer-associated IDH1 mutations produce 2-hydroxyglutarate. Nature. 2009;462:739–44.

48. Figueroa ME, Abdel-Wahab O, Lu C, Ward PS, Patel J, Shih A, et al. Leukemic IDH1 and IDH2 mutations result in a hypermethylation phenotype, disrupt TET2 function, and impair hematopoietic differentiation. Cancer Cell. 2010; 18:553–67.

49. Hackl H, Astanina K, Wieser R. Molecular and genetic alterations associated with therapy resistance and relapse of acute myeloid leukemia. J Hematol Oncol. 2017;10:51.

50. Abbas S, Lugthart S, Kavelaars FG, Schelen A, Koenders JE, Zeilemaker A, et al. Acquired mutations in the genes encoding IDH1 and IDH2 both are recurrent aberrations in acute myeloid leukemia: prevalence and prognostic value. Blood. 2010;116:2122–6.

51. Marcucci G, Maharry K, Wu YZ, Radmacher MD, Mrozek K, Margeson D, et al. IDH1 and IDH2 gene mutations identify novel molecular subsets within de novo cytogenetically normal acute myeloid leukemia: a Cancer and leukemia group B study. J Clin Oncol. 2010;28:2348–55.

52. Green CL, Evans CM, Zhao L, Hills RK, Burnett AK, Linch DC, et al. The prognostic significance of IDH2 mutations in AML depends on the location of the mutation. Blood. 2011;118:409–12.

53. Boissel N, Nibourel O, Renneville A, Gardin C, Reman O, Contentin N, et al. Prognostic impact of isocitrate dehydrogenase enzyme isoforms 1 and 2 mutations in acute myeloid leukemia: a study by the acute leukemia French association group. J Clin Oncol. 2010;28:3717–23.

54. Stein EM, DiNardo CD, Pollyea DA, Fathi AT, Roboz GJ, Altman JK, et al. Enasidenib in mutant IDH2 relapsed or refractory acute myeloid leukemia. Blood. 2017;130:722–31.

55. Pollyea DA, DiNardo CD, Botton SD, Stein EM, Roboz GJ, Mims AS, et al. Ivosidenib (AG-120) in mutant IDH1 relapsed/refractory Acute myeloid leukemia:results of a phase 1 study. European Hematology Association Congress Abstract. 2018:S1560. https://learningcenter.ehaweb.org/eha/2018/stockholm/214479/daniel.a.pollyea.ivosidenib.28ag-12029.in.mutant.idh1.relapsed.refractory.acute.html?f=menu=6*ce_id=1346 *ot_id=19045*media=3*browseby=8. Accessed 16 July 2018.

56. Wei A, Strickland SA, Roboz GJ, Hou J-Z, Fiedler W, Lin TL, et al. Safety and efficacy of venetoclax plus low-dose cytarabine in treatment-naive patients aged ≥65 years with acute myeloid leukemia. Blood. 2016;128:102.

57. Yuan XQ, Peng L, Zeng WJ, Jiang BY, Li GC, Chen XP. DNMT3A R882 mutations predict a poor prognosis in AML: a meta-analysis from 4474 patients. Medicine. 2016;95:e3519.

58. Gaidzik VI, Schlenk RF, Paschka P, Stolzle A, Spath D, Kuendgen A, et al. Clinical impact of DNMT3A mutations in younger adult patients with acute myeloid leukemia: results of the AML study group (AMLSG). Blood. 2013;121: 4769–77.

59. Gale RE, Lamb K, Allen C, El-Sharkawi D, Stowe C, Jenkinson S, et al. Simpson's paradox and the impact of different DNMT3A mutations on outcome in younger adults with acute myeloid leukemia. J Clin Oncol. 2015;33:2072–83.

60. Micol JB, Duployez N, Boissel N, Petit A, Geffroy S, Nibourel O, et al. Frequent ASXL2 mutations in acute myeloid leukemia patients with t(8;21)/RUNX1-RUNX1T1 chromosomal translocations. Blood. 2014;124:1445–9.

61. Shlush LI, Zandi S, Mitchell A, Chen WC, Brandwein JM, Gupta V, et al. Identification of pre-leukaemic haematopoietic stem cells in acute leukaemia. Nature. 2014;506:328–33.

62. Tan Y, Liu H, Chen S. Mutant DNA methylation regulators endow hematopoietic stem cells with the preleukemic stem cell property, a requisite of leukemia initiation and relapse. Front Med. 2015;9:412–20.

63. Jan M, Snyder TM, Corces-Zimmerman MR, Vyas P, Weissman IL, Quake SR, et al. Clonal evolution of preleukemic hematopoietic stem cells precedes human acute myeloid leukemia. Sci Transl Med. 2012;4:149ra18.

64. Hsu YC, Chiu YC, Lin CC, Kuo YY, Hou HA, Tzeng YS, et al. The distinct biological implications of Asxl1 mutation and its roles in leukemogenesis revealed by a knock-in mouse model. J Hematol Oncol. 2017;10:139.

65. Jongen-Lavrencic M, Grob T, Hanekamp D, Kavelaars FG, Al Hinai A, Zeilemaker A, et al. Molecular Minimal Residual Disease in Acute Myeloid Leukemia. N Engl J Med. 2018;378:1189–99.

66. Jongen-Lavrencic M, Tim Grob FG, ASA K, Al Hinai AZ, CAJ E-V, Yvette Norden RM, et al. Prospective mlecular MRD dtection by NGS: a powerful

transplantation in prognostically favorable acute myeloid leukemia with double mutant CEBPA. Blood. 2013;122:1576–82.

independent predictor for relapse and survival in adults with newly diagnosed AML. Blood. 2017;130:LBA-5.

67. Rothenberg-Thurley M, Amler S, Goerlich D, Kohnke T, Konstandin NP, Schneider S, et al. Persistence of pre-leukemic clones during first remission and risk of relapse in acute myeloid leukemia. Leukemia. 2018;32:1598–608.

68. Lindsley RC, Mar BG, Mazzola E, Grauman PV, Shareef S, Allen SL, et al. Acute myeloid leukemia ontogeny is defined by distinct somatic mutations. Blood. 2015;125:1367–76.

69. Seiler M, Yoshimi A, Darman R, Chan B, Keaney G, Thomas M, et al. H3B-8800, an orally available small-molecule splicing modulator, induces lethality in spliceosome-mutant cancers. Nat Med. 2018;24:497–504.

70. Devillier R, Mansat-De Mas V, Gelsi-Boyer V, Demur C, Murati A, Corre J, et al. Role of ASXL1 and TP53 mutations in the molecular classification and prognosis of acute myeloid leukemias with myelodysplasia-related changes. Oncotarget. 2015;6:8388–96.

71. Grossmann V, Schnittger S, Kohlmann A, Eder C, Roller A, Dicker F, et al. A novel hierarchical prognostic model of AML solely based on molecular mutations. Blood. 2012;120:2963–72.

72. Welch JS, Petti AA, Miller CA, Fronick CC, O'Laughlin M, Fulton RS, et al. TP53 and Decitabine in acute myeloid leukemia and myelodysplastic syndromes. N Engl J Med. 2016;375:2023–36.

73. Andreeff M, Kelly KR, Yee K, Assouline S, Strair R, Popplewell L, et al. Results of the phase I trial of RG7112, a small-molecule MDM2 antagonist in leukemia. Clin Cancer Res. 2016;22:868–76.

74. Irish JM, Anensen N, Hovland R, Skavland J, Borresen-Dale AL, Bruserud O, et al. Flt3 Y591 duplication and Bcl-2 overexpression are detected in acute myeloid leukemia cells with high levels of phosphorylated wild-type p53. Blood. 2007;109:2589–96.

75. Stilgenbauer S, Eichhorst B, Schetelig J, Coutre S, Seymour JF, Munir T, et al. Venetoclax in relapsed or refractory chronic lymphocytic leukaemia with 17p deletion: a multicentre, open-label, phase 2 study. Lancet Oncol. 2016; 17:768–78.

76. DiNardo CD, Pratz K, Potlur J, Pullarkat V, Jonas BA, Wei AH, et al. Durable response with venetoclax in combination with decitabine or azacitadine in elderly patients with acute myeloid leukemia. European Hematology Association Congress Abstract. 2018:S15630. https://learningcenter.ehaweb. org/eha/2018/stockholm/214482/courtney.d.dinardo.durable.response.with. venetoclax.in.combination.with.htmlf=menu=6*ce_id=1346*ot_id= 19045*media=3*browseby=8. Accessed 16 July 2018.

77. DiNardo CD, Pratz KW, Letai A, Jonas BA, Wei AH, Thirman M, et al. Safety and preliminary efficacy of venetoclax with decitabine or azacitidine in elderly patients with previously untreated acute myeloid leukaemia: a non-randomised, open-label, phase 1b study. Lancet Oncol. 2018;19:216–28.

78. Li Y, Xu Q, Lv N, Wang L, Zhao H, Wang X, et al. Clinical implications of genome-wide DNA methylation studies in acute myeloid leukemia. J Hematol Oncol. 2017;10:41.

79. Wei S, Wang K. Long noncoding RNAs: pivotal regulators in acute myeloid leukemia. Exp Hematol Oncol. 2016;5:30.

80. Zhang C, Liu J, Zhong JF, Zhang X. Engineering CAR-T cells. Biomark Res. 2017;5:22.

81. Park JH, Riviere I, Gonen M, Wang X, Senechal B, Curran KJ, et al. Long-term follow-up of CD19 CAR therapy in acute lymphoblastic leukemia. N Engl J Med. 2018;378:449–59.

82. Ghelli Luserna di Rora A, Iacobucci I, Martinelli G. The cell cycle checkpoint inhibitors in the treatment of leukemias. J Hematol Oncol. 2017;10:77.

83. Gokbuget N, Dombret H, Bonifacio M, Reichle A, Graux C, Faul C, et al. Blinatumomab for minimal residual disease in adults with B-cell precursor acute lymphoblastic leukemia. Blood. 2018;131:1522–31.

84. Fan M, Li M, Gao L, Geng S, Wang J, Wang Y, et al. Chimeric antigen receptors for adoptive T cell therapy in acute myeloid leukemia. J Hematol Oncol. 2017;10:151.

85. Liu F, Pinz K, Ma Y, Wada M, Chen K, Ma G, et al. First in human CLL1-CD33 compound CAR T cells as a two-pronged approach for the treatment of refractory acute myeloid leukemia. European Hematology Association Congress Abstract. 2018:S149. https://learningcenter.ehaweb.org/eha/2018/ stockholm/215925/fang.liu.first-in-huma n.cll1-cd33.compound.car.t.cells.as.a. two-pronged.html?f=menu=6*ce_id=1346*ot_id=19045*media= 3*browseby=8. Accessed 16 July 2018.

26

Sphingosine kinase 2 supports the development of BCR/ABL-independent acute lymphoblastic leukemia in mice

Vicki Xie[1], Daochen Tong[1], Craig T. Wallington-Beddoe[1,3,4,5], Ken F. Bradstock[2] and Linda J. Bendall[1]* ⓘ

Abstract

Background: Sphingosine kinase (SphK) 2 has been implicated in the development of a range of cancers and inhibitors of this enzyme are currently in clinical trial. We have previously demonstrated a role for SphK2 in the development of acute lymphoblastic leukemia (ALL).

Methods: In this and our previous study we use mouse models: in the previous study the disease was driven by the proto-oncogene BCR/ABL1, while in this study cancer risk was elevated by deletion of the tumor suppressor ARF.

Results: Mice lacking ARF and SphK2 had a significantly reduced incidence of ALL compared mice with wild type SphK2.

Conclusions: These results show that the role of SphK2 in ALL development is not limited to BCR/ABL1 driven disease extending the potential use of inhibitors of this enzyme to ALL patients whose disease have driver mutations other than BCR/ABL1.

Keywords: Acute lymphoblastic leukemia, Sphingosine kinase 2, Mouse models

Background

There are two forms of sphingosine kinase (SphK), SphK1 and SphK2. SphK1 has an established role in malignant biology with overexpression being associated with poor survival in patients with solid tumors [1–10] and resistance to therapy [11–14]. Furthermore, inhibitors of SphK1 have demonstrated preclinical activity in acute myeloid leukemia (AML) [15, 16]. The role of SphK2 has been more controversial but it is increasingly being shown to play a role in malignant disease and has been associated with poor patient outcome [17]. Knockdown of SphK2 expression increases the sensitivity of cancer cells to chemotherapy [18–20], while chemical inhibition can reduce cancer cell growth in vitro [21–28] and in pre-clinical animal models [21, 24, 26]. SphK2 inhibitors are now in phase II clinical trials for a number of cancers including B cell malignancies, following successful completion of phase I studies [29]. We have recently shown that chemical inhibition of SphK2 can reduce acute lymphoblastic leukemia (ALL) cell growth, induce cell death in vitro and extend the survival of mice bearing human ALL xenografts. Furthermore, cells lacking SphK2 had a reduced capacity to induce ALL driven by the BCR/ABL1 fusion gene in WT mice, while SphK2 inhibition synergized with imatinib treatment of BCR/ABL1+ ALL in vitro and in vivo [30].

Mice deficient in the tumor suppressor gene ARF are prone to malignancies, with undifferentiated sarcomas predominating (~ 38%), followed by lymphomas (~ 23%), carcinomas (~ 15%) and neurological tumors (~ 10%), with a latency of around 266 days [31]. Genetic loss of material at the 9p21 locus, which includes ARF, is common in ALL, being reported in up to 45% of B lineage disease [32–34], making this a biologically relevant model. The development of tumors in these mice appears to be dependent on the aquisition of additional genetic changes as treatment with radiation or the mutagen DMBA significantly reduces latency. Here we show that blockade of T and B cell maturation by crossing ARF deficient mice onto a Rag1$^{-/-}$ background [35] resulted in an incidence of ALL of over 60%. Further crossing of these mice onto SphK2 deficient animals [36]

* Correspondence: linda.bendall@sydney.edu.au
[1]Centre for Cancer Research, The Westmead Institute for Medical Research, The University of Sydney, Sydney, Australia
Full list of author information is available at the end of the article

permitted the examination of the role of SphK2 in the development of ALL, demonstrating a significant reduction in disease incidence.

Methods

Development of mouse model

Mice lacking the p19ARF product of the INK4a/ARF locus (ARF$^{-/-}$) develop malignancies at a high penetrance with 80% of animals dying within the first year of life [31]. To facilitate breeding we used mice where the ARF gene had been floxed (ARF$^{fl/fl}$) (B6.129-Cdkn2atm4Cjs/Nci, [37]) obtained from Graham Walker (QIMR, Queensland Australia). In order to produce an ALL model we crossed these mice with those lacking Rag1^{tm1Mom} from The Jackson Laboratory (Bar Harbour, ME, USA) [35]. The resulting Mx1.Cre.ARF$^{fl/fl}$.Rag1$^{-/-}$ (MAR) mice were then crossed onto animals lacking SphK2 (Richard Proia (Bethesda, USA) [36]) to produce Mx1.Cre.ARF$^{fl/fl}$.Rag1$^{-/-}$.SphK2$^{-/-}$ animals (MARS2 mice). The deletion of the ARF gene was undertaken at 6 weeks of age by intraperitoneal injection of 15 mg/kg of PolyI:polyC every second day for a total of 3 doses and confirmed by PCR (Additional file 1: Figure S1). All mice were obtained or were backcrossed onto on a C57Bl6 background. Experimental mice were monitored for up to 400 days. Mice were defined as having ALL when at the time of death the bone marrow and spleen primarily consisted of B220$^+$CD19$^+$Gr1$^-$ cells. Survival was analysed using the Kaplan-Meier method and SPSS Statistics software.

Mice were genotyped by PCR on genomic DNA obtained from ear punches using DirectPCR Lysis Reagent (Ear) (Viagen Biotech, Los Angeles CA) with 0.4 mg/mL proteinase K (Promega, Alexandria, NSW, Australia) (complete lysis solution). Ear punches from mice were incubated in complete lysis solution for 2 h at 56 °C and proteinase K was inactivated for 30 min at 85 °C prior to PCR. Deletion of ARF was detected in genomic DNA obtained from spleen cells recovered from culled mice. PCR reactions were performed using MyTaq DNA polymerase (Bioline, Eveleigh NSW Australia) and specific primers as indicated in Additional file 1: Table S1. The IL-2 PCR was used as a positive DNA control for the Mx1.Cre reaction. The PCR conditions were 95 °C for 1″, then 95 °C for 15″, 58 °C for 15″, 72 °C for 20″ for 35 cycles, 72 °C for 5′. Amplified products were separated on a 2% agarose (Sigma-Aldrich) gel stained with Midori Green Nucleic Acid solution (Bulldog Bio Inc., Portsmouth NH) and visualised using ChemiDoc MP Imaging System (Bio-Rad, Hercules, CA).

Flow cytometry

Flow cytometry was performed using a FACSCanto 6-colour flow cytometer (BD Biosciences, San Jose CA).

The following antibodies were purchased: Sca-1-PE-Cy7, c-Kit-APC, CD43-APC, IgM-PCP.Cy5.5, IgM-Biotin (Australian Biosearch, WangarraWA, Australia); B220-APC.Cy7, B220 PE-Cy5, CD11b-PE, CD11b-FITC, CD19-PE, CD19-APC.Cy7, Gr1-FITC, Streptavidin APC and Lineage Cocktail of biotinylated CD3, Gr-1, Ter119, B220 and CD11b (BD Biosciences, San Jose CA), and Streptavidin Pacific Blue (Thermofisher Scientific, North Ryde, NSW, Australia). Cells were labelled with antibodies as previously described [30].

Histology and image acquisition

Blood films were prepared and stained with a Romanowsky stain. Tissues were fixed in 10% formalin, embedded, sectioned and stained as previously described [38]. Femurs were decalcified prior to embedding as previously described [38]. Images were obtained using a NanoZoomer Slide Scanner (SDR Scientific, Sydney Australia) or an Olympus BX51 microscope with images captured using a Spot RT slider camera (Diagnostic Instruments, Sterling Heights, MI) and SPOT Advanced software. Composite figures prepared using Adobe Photoshop software.

Results

Deletion of ARF in Rag1 deficient mice predisposes to ALL

Mice lacking ARF are known to develop malignancies with an increased incidence [31]. To generate an ALL model we bred Mx1.Cre.ARF$^{fl/fl}$ mice with Rag1$^{-/-}$ mice to generate Mx1.Cre.ARF$^{fl/fl}$.Rag1$^{-/-}$ mice. At 6 weeks of age mice received 3 injections of polyI:polyC to delete the ARF gene producing Mx1.Cre.ARF$^{-/-}$.Rag1$^{-/-}$ (MAR) mice.

Rag1$^{-/-}$ mice with deleted ARF (MAR mice) survived for up to 304 days (median 193 days) (Fig. 1a). The most common cause of death was B lineage ALL, which occurred in 61% of mice between 119 and 243 days with a median of 192 days. The remaining animals succumbed to a number of causes including other haematological malignancies, with the most common feature of non-ALL deaths being massively enlarged pale livers that sometimes contained defined tumors (Fig. 1b). However the origin of the tumors could not be determined with certainty. Many appeared to be haematological in origin based on morphology but the bone marrows mostly appeared normal (Additional file 1: Figure S2). Flow cytometric analysis of cells recovered from the bone marrow and spleens of these animals was generally uninformative.

Mice that developed ALL were easily identified, demonstrating weight loss, reduced activity and/or impaired use of hind limbs and tail. One displayed hydrocephaly, with fitting. Necropsy findings were consistent with B lineage ALL with enlarged spleens and often enlarged livers, without evidence of tumors and a normal dark

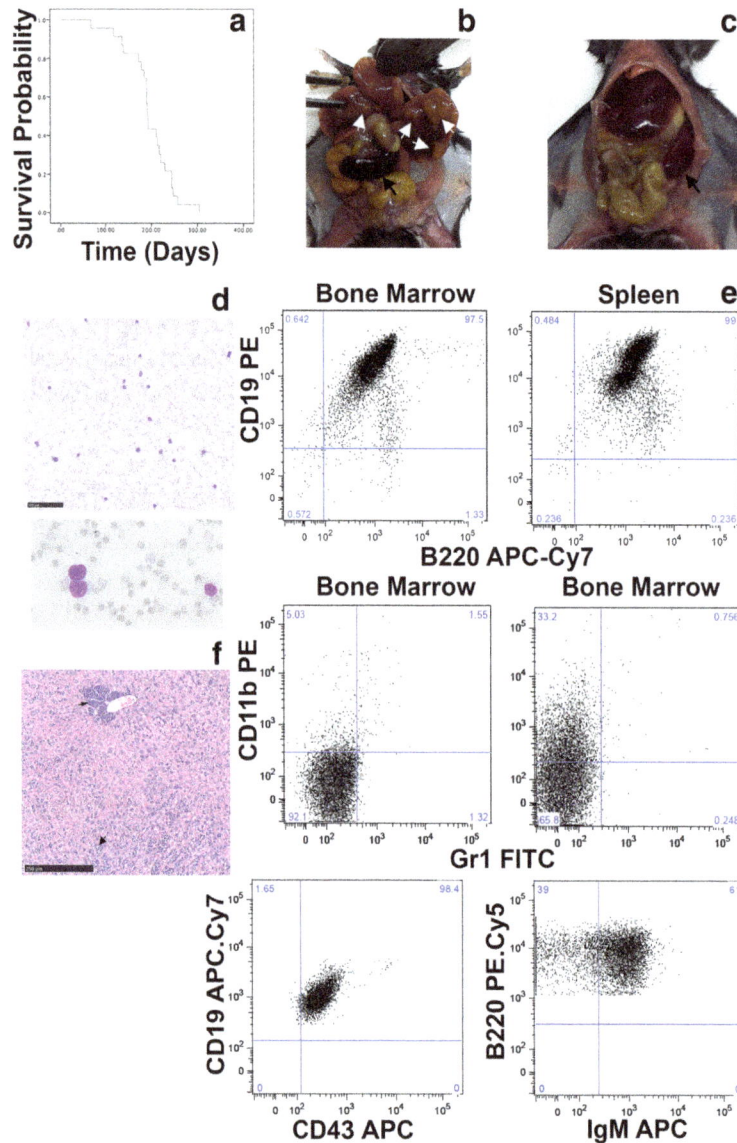

Fig. 1 MAR mice develop malignancies with B lineage ALL predominating. **a** Kalpan-Meyer analysis showing the survival of MAR mice. **b** Mouse culled due to disease other than ALL showing tumors in the liver (white arrows) and an enlarged spleen (black arrow). **c** Mouse culled due to ALL showing enlarged spleen (black arrow). **d** Blood film from a mouse with ALL showing circulating lymphoblasts. Image acquired using a slide scanner and size bar represents 100 μm. Lower imaged taken on a Spot camera, original magnification 600×. **e** Flow cytometric analysis of bone marrow and spleen cells from mice culled due to ALL. Upper panels are from the same mouse. Central panels show the lowest and highest CD11b expression detected. Lower panels show typical expression of maturation markers B220, CD19, CD43 and surface IgM. Quadrants were set based on control stained cells from the same animal. **f** Section of liver from a mouse culled due to ALL showing both perivascular (thin arrow) and diffuse (thick arrow) infiltration by ALL cells. The degree of infiltration in this animal was typical. Image acquired using slide scanner and size bar indicates 250 μm

red colour (Fig. 1c). Mice with ALL also had elevated WBC for immune-compromised mice (median 15.2, range 2.1-286.5 cells/mL) with significant numbers of lymphoblasts present in blood smears (Fig. 1d). Lymph nodes were rarely involved with only 2 mice having visible nodes on cull and only 1 of those having significant lymphadenopathy (Additional file 1: Figure S3). Cells in the spleen and bone marrow were mostly B220 and CD19 positive (average of 73%, range 56-87 and 86%, range 73-97 respectively), lacking staining for the myeloid marker Gr1 and the T cell marker CD3, however CD11b was detected on cells from some animals (Fig. 1e). Cells from all mice with ALL were positive for immature marker CD43 and most expressed IgM on at least a proportion of the cells (Fig. 1e). The lack of lymph node involvement in the vast majority of animals, near complete replacement of the bone marrow by lymphoblasts as well as the expression of the immature marker CD43 and low expression of IgM indicate a proto-pre-B classification of these leukemias. Other organs, primarily the liver, were infiltrated with lymphoblasts (Fig. 1f). ALL induced death tended to be earlier compared to non-ALL deaths, with the latter occurring between 68 and 304 days with a median of 229 days, although this was not statistically significant, $p = 0.06$ (Additional file 1: Figure S4). Animals that did not develop ALL mostly presented with solid tumors at a slightly later time point.

Deletion of SphK2 reduced the incidence of B ALL

A cohort of mice lacking ARF and Rag1 was also generated using the same methodology on an SphK2$^{-/-}$ background (MARS2 mice). ARF was similarly deleted at 6 weeks of age by 3 injections of polyI:polyC. These mice also largely succumbed to conditions consistent with malignant diseases but compared to MAR mice had significantly increased overall survival with deaths occurring between 120 and > 400 days (one mouse was electively culled disease free at 400 days) with a median of 234 days ($p < 0.05$) (Fig. 2a). Notably there were fewer deaths resulting from ALL in MARS2 animals with only 43% of deaths being due to ALL, resulting in a significant increase in leukemia free survival in MARS2 mice ($p = 0.044$) (Fig. 2b).

The absence of SphK2 did not alter the nature of the ALL that developed, with latency, phenotype and disease dissemination being similar. Death due to ALL was slightly delayed in MARS2 mice (range 169 – 253, median 219.5 days), however this was not significantly different from that of MAR mice (Fig. 2c). Interestingly the WBC in the leukemic MARS2 mice was significantly lower than in the MAR mice, as was the number of circulating blasts (Fig. 2d), however the blast percentage was similar between the two groups. Otherwise the disease was identical in MARS2 and MAR mice, with similar enlargement of spleen and liver and infiltration of other organs (Fig. 2e–g).

Discussion

Inhibition of sphingosine kinases has recently become of interest for the treatment of a number of conditions including malignant disease [39]. Clinical trials for the SphK2 inhibitor ABC294640, are well under way with phase I studies complete [29] and phase I/II and phase II trials examining hepatocellular carcinoma, Kaposi sarcoma as well as the haematological malignancies multiple myeloma and diffuse large B cell lymphoma ongoing (NCT02229981, NCT02939807 and NCT02757326). These trials have been supported by recent preclinical data from a number of groups [23, 24, 26, 30, 40–44]. The majority of these studies have focussed on solid tumors, however there are reports in haematological malignancies including multiple myeloma [26] and T-ALL [45], and we have previously reported a role for SphK2 in B lineage

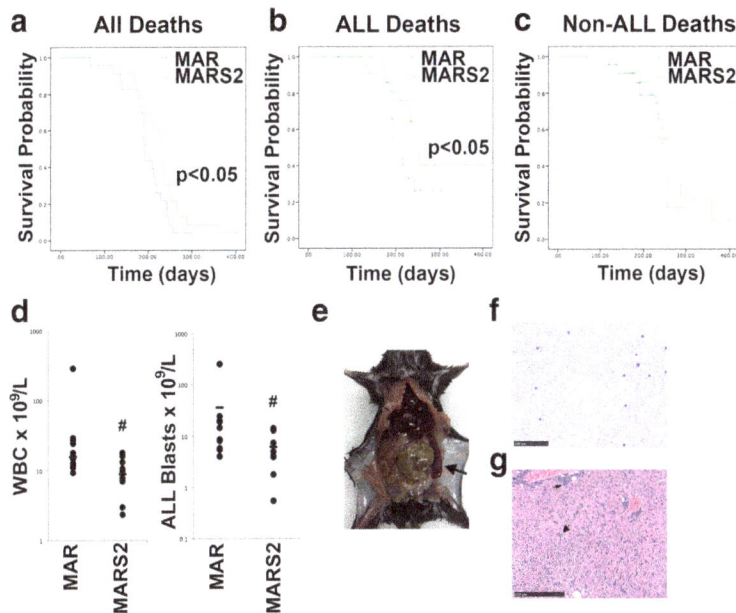

Fig. 2 Loss of SphK2 reduces the incidence of B lineage ALL. **a-c** Kaplan-Meier plots showing all (**a**) and ALL-induced (**b**) deaths. Deaths due to causes other than ALL are illustrated in (**c**). Total WBC (**d**, left panel) and ALL blast counts (**d**, right panel) at the time of sacrifice are shown. # indicates $p < 0.05$. **e** Mouse culled due to ALL showing enlarged spleen (black arrow). **f** Blood film from a mouse with ALL showing circulating lymphoblasts. Image acquired using a slide scanner and size bar represents 100 μm. **g** Section of liver from a mouse culled due to ALL showing both perivascular (thin arrow) and diffuse (thick arrow) infiltration by ALL cells. The degree of infiltration in this animal was typical. Image acquired using slide scanner and size bar indicates 250 μm

ALL [30] using a BCR/ABL1-dependent model. In this study, we examined the effects of SphK2 gene deletion on the development of ALL in a model that is not dependent on forced expression of BCR/ABL1 and demonstrated that genetic deletion of SphK2 also inhibits the development of B lineage ALL independent of BCR/ABL1 expression. The similar latency and features of the disease in MAR and MARS2 mice suggests that the principal effect of SphK2 loss was on leukemia initiation rather than rate of disease progression. However, we previously demonstrated that the SphK2 inhibitor ABC294640 impedes disease progression in a xenograft model of Ph$^-$ human ALL, suggesting that SphK2 loss/inhibition has some effect on disease progression [30].

The reason why loss of SphK2 decreases the incidence of ALL is not entirely clear. However SphK2 has a well-established role in promoting malignant cell survival [46] making it possible that in the absence of SphK2, cells with newly acquired potentially oncogenic changes are more susceptible to cell death. While precise mechanisms are yet to be determined, one potential explanation relates to CDKN1A expression. CDKN1A is an inhibitor of apoptosis induced in response to DNA damage whose expression is increased by SphK2-mediated effects on histone acetylation [47]. In the absence of SphK2, induction of CDKN1A expression following DNA damage could be reduced increasing the probability of cell death. Another possible mechanism relating loss of SphK2 to the reduced incidence of ALL concerns the localization of SphK2 to the endoplasmic reticulum (ER) membrane and its involvement in sphingolipid metabolism at this site. We have recently demonstrated that inhibition of SphK2 induces unrecoverable ER stress leading to apoptosis of multiple myeloma cells and this ER stress-inducing mechanism is most likely also applicable to a range of cell types, including those of ALL, thus impacting on its development in our model [48].

The lower WBC in leukemic MARS2 was interesting and although altered trafficking of lymphoid cells in SphK2$^{-/-}$ animals might be an explanation for this observation, previous reports have demonstrated increased plasma sphingosine-1-phosphate (S1P) and resultant increased lymphocyte mobilization in SphK2$^{-/-}$ mice [49]. All but one MARS2 mouse that did not develop ALL went on to develop solid tumors at a time closer to the previously reported latency (median of 266 days) for solid tumors in ARF deficient animals [31]. Since the tumors that emerged in this study could not be definitively classified, it is not possible to comment on the effects of SphK2 loss on the development of other malignancies.

Conclusions

We have previously demonstrated the role of SphK2 in ALL driven by BCR/ABL1 and the potential therapeutic application of SphK2 inhibitors in this disease. In this study we demonstrate that SphK2 also plays a role in the development of BCR/ABL1 negative ALL with genetic deletion of SphK2 reducing disease incidence. These findings further support and broaden the potential application of SphK2 inhibitors in the treatment of ALL.

Abbreviations

ALL: Acute lymphoblastic leukemia; AML: Acute myeloid leukemia; ARF$^{-/-}$: Mice lacking the p19ARF product of the INK4a/ARF locus; ARF$^{fl/fl}$: Mice where the ARF gene had been floxed; ER: Endoplasmic reticulum; MAR: Mx1.Cre.ARF$^{fl/fl}$.Rag1$^{-/-}$; MARS2: Mx1.Cre.ARF$^{fl/fl}$.Rag1$^{-/-}$.SphK2$^{-/-}$; S1P: Sphingosine-1-phosphate; SphK: Sphingosine kinase

Acknowledgements

Flow cytometry was performed in the Flow Cytometry Core Facility that is supported by Westmead Institute for Medical Research, Westmead Research Hub, Cancer Institute New South Wales and National Health and Medical Research Council. Histology was performed in the Histology Platform at Westmead Institute for Medical Research with the assistance of Virginia James.

Funding

This work was supported by an NHMRC Senior Research Fellowship (1042305) and Cancer Institute NSW Fellowship.

Authors' contributions

LB, CW-B and KB made substantial contributions to conception and design of the study. DT, LB and CW-B designed the breeding strategies required for the development of the animals used in this study. VX and LB were responsible for data acquisition, analysis and interpretation of data. LB drafted the manuscript and all authors made significant contributions to revising the final document. All authors read and approved the final manuscript.

Competing interests

The authors declare that they have no competing interests.

Author details

^{1}Centre for Cancer Research, The Westmead Institute for Medical Research, The University of Sydney, Sydney, Australia. ^{2}Haematology Department, Westmead Hospital, Westmead, NSW, Australia. ^{3}Centre for Cancer Biology, University of South Australia and SA Pathology, Adelaide, Australia. ^{4}College of Medicine and Public Health, Flinders University, Adelaide, Australia. ^{5}School of Medicine, University of Adelaide, Adelaide, Australia.

References

1. Cai H, Xie X, Ji L, Ruan X, Zheng Z. Sphingosine kinase 1: a novel independent prognosis biomarker in hepatocellular carcinoma. Oncol Lett. 2017;13(4):2316–22.
2. Chen MH, Yen CC, Cheng CT, Wu RC, Huang SC, Yu CS, et al. Identification of SPHK1 as a therapeutic target and marker of poor prognosis in cholangiocarcinoma. Oncotarget. 2015;6(27):23594–608.
3. Facchinetti MM, Gandini NA, Fermento ME, Sterin-Speziale NB, Ji Y, Patel V, et al. The expression of sphingosine kinase-1 in head and neck carcinoma. Cells Tissues Organs. 2010;192(5):314–24.
4. Kim HS, Yoon G, Ryu JY, Cho YJ, Choi JJ, Lee YY, et al. Sphingosine kinase 1 is a reliable prognostic factor and a novel therapeutic target for uterine cervical cancer. Oncotarget. 2015;6(29):26746–56.
5. Li W, Yu CP, Xia JT, Zhang L, Weng GX, Zheng HQ, et al. Sphingosine kinase 1 is associated with gastric cancer progression and poor survival of patients. Clin Cancer Res. 2009;15(4):1393–9.
6. Liu G, Zheng H, Zhang Z, Wu Z, Xiong H, Li J, et al. Overexpression of sphingosine kinase 1 is associated with salivary gland carcinoma progression and might be a novel predictive marker for adjuvant therapy. BMC Cancer. 2010;10:495.
7. Meng XD, Zhou ZS, Qiu JH, Shen WH, Wu Q, Xiao J. Increased SPHK1 expression is associated with poor prognosis in bladder cancer. Tumour Biol. 2014;35(3):2075–80.
8. Li J, Guan HY, Gong LY, Song LB, Zhang N, Wu J, et al. Clinical significance of sphingosine kinase-1 expression in human astrocytomas progression and overall patient survival. Clin Cancer Res. 2008;14(21):6996–7003.
9. Ruckhaberle E, Rody A, Engels K, Gaetje R, von Minckwitz G, Schiffmann S, et al. Microarray analysis of altered sphingolipid metabolism reveals prognostic significance of sphingosine kinase 1 in breast cancer. Breast Cancer Res Treat. 2008;112(1):41–52.
10. Van Brocklyn JR, Jackson CA, Pearl DK, Kotur MS, Snyder PJ, Prior TW. Sphingosine kinase-1 expression correlates with poor survival of patients with glioblastoma multiforme: roles of sphingosine kinase isoforms in growth of glioblastoma cell lines. J Neuropathol Exp Neurol. 2005;64(8):695–705.
11. Salas A, Ponnusamy S, Senkal CE, Meyers-Needham M, Selvam SP, Saddoughi SA, et al. Sphingosine kinase-1 and sphingosine 1-phosphate receptor 2 mediate Bcr-Abl1 stability and drug resistance by modulation of protein phosphatase 2A. Blood. 2011;117(22):5941–52.
12. Bonhoure E, Lauret A, Barnes DJ, Martin C, Malavaud B, Kohama T, et al. Sphingosine kinase-1 is a downstream regulator of imatinib-induced apoptosis in chronic myeloid leukemia cells. Leukemia. 2008;22(5):971–9.
13. Baran Y, Salas A, Senkal CE, Gunduz U, Bielawski J, Obeid LM, et al. Alterations of ceramide/sphingosine 1-phosphate rheostat involved in the regulation of resistance to imatinib-induced apoptosis in K562 human chronic myeloid leukemia cells. J Biol Chem. 2007;282(15):10922–34.
14. Sobue S, Nemoto S, Murakami M, Ito H, Kimura A, Gao S, et al. Implications of sphingosine kinase 1 expression level for the cellular sphingolipid rheostat: relevance as a marker for daunorubicin sensitivity of leukemia cells. Int J Hematol. 2008;87(3):266–75.
15. Paugh SW, Paugh BS, Rahmani M, Kapitonov D, Almenara JA, Kordula T, et al. A selective sphingosine kinase 1 inhibitor integrates multiple molecular therapeutic targets in human leukemia. Blood. 2008;112(4):1382–91.
16. Powell JA, Lewis AC, Zhu W, Toubia J, Pitman MR, Wallington-Beddoe CT, et al. Targeting sphingosine kinase 1 induces MCL1-dependent cell death in acute myeloid. Leukemia. 2017;129(6):771–82.
17. Wang Q, Li J, Li G, Li Y, Xu C, Li M, et al. Prognostic significance of sphingosine kinase 2 expression in non-small cell lung cancer. Tumour Biol. 2014;35(1):363–8.
18. Sankala HM, Hait NC, Paugh SW, Shida D, Lepine S, Elmore LW, et al. Involvement of sphingosine kinase 2 in p53-independent induction of p21 by the chemotherapeutic drug doxorubicin. Cancer Res. 2007;67(21):10466–74.
19. Nemoto S, Nakamura M, Osawa Y, Kono S, Itoh Y, Okano Y, et al. Sphingosine kinase isoforms regulate oxaliplatin sensitivity of human colon cancer cells through ceramide accumulation and Akt activation. J Biol Chem. 2009;284(16):10422–32.
20. Schnitzer SE, Weigert A, Zhou J, Brune B. Hypoxia enhances sphingosine kinase 2 activity and provokes sphingosine-1-phosphate-mediated chemoresistance in A549 lung cancer cells. Mol Cancer Res. 2009;7(3):393–401.
21. Weigert A, Schiffmann S, Sekar D, Ley S, Menrad H, Werno C, et al. Sphingosine kinase 2 deficient tumor xenografts show impaired growth and fail to polarize macrophages towards an anti-inflammatory phenotype. Int J Cancer. 2009;125(9):2114–21.
22. Beljanski V, Knaak C, Smith CD. A novel sphingosine kinase inhibitor induces autophagy in tumor cells. J Pharmacol Exp Ther. 2010;333(2):454–64.
23. French KJ, Zhuang Y, Maines LW, Gao P, Wang W, Beljanski V, et al. Pharmacology and antitumor activity of ABC294640, a selective inhibitor of sphingosine kinase-2. J Pharmacol Exp Ther. 2010;333(1):129–39.
24. Beljanski V, Lewis CS, Smith CD. Antitumor activity of sphingosine kinase 2 inhibitor ABC294640 and sorafenib in hepatocellular carcinoma xenografts. Cancer Biol Ther. 2011;11(5):524–34.
25. White MD, Chan L, Antoon JW, Beckman BS. Targeting ovarian cancer and chemoresistance through selective inhibition of sphingosine kinase-2 with ABC294640. Anticancer Res. 2013;33(9):3573–9.
26. Venkata JK, An N, Stuart R, Costa LJ, Cai H, Coker W, et al. Inhibition of sphingosine kinase 2 downregulates the expression of c-Myc and Mcl-1 and induces apoptosis in multiple myeloma. Blood. 2014;124(12):1915–25.
27. Chu JH, Gao ZH, Qu XJ. Down-regulation of sphingosine kinase 2 (SphK2) increases the effects of all-trans-retinoic acid (ATRA) on colon cancer cells. Biomed Pharmacother. 2014;68(8):1089–97.
28. Yang J, Yang C, Zhang S, Mei Z, Shi M, Sun S, et al. ABC294640, a sphingosine kinase 2 inhibitor, enhances the antitumor effects of TRAIL in non-small cell lung cancer. Cancer Biol Ther. 2015;16(8):1194–204.
29. Britten CD, Garrett-Mayer E, Chin SH, Shirai K, Ogretmen B, Bentz TA, et al. A phase I study of ABC294640, a first-in-class sphingosine kinase 2 inhibitor, in patients with advanced solid tumors. Clin Cancer Res. 2017;23(16):4642–50.
30. Wallington-Beddoe CT, Powell JA, Tong D, Pitson SM, Bradstock KF, Bendall LJ. Sphingosine kinase 2 promotes acute lymphoblastic leukemia by enhancing MYC expression. Cancer Res. 2014;74(10):2803–15.
31. Kamijo T, Bodner S, van de Kamp E, Randle DH, Sherr CJ. Tumor spectrum in ARF-deficient mice. Cancer Res. 1999;59(9):2217–22.
32. Faderl S, Estrov Z, Kantarjian HM, Thomas D, Cortes J, Manshouri T, et al. The incidence of chromosome 9p21 abnormalities and deletions of tumor suppressor genes p15(INK4b)/p16(INK4a)/p14(ARF) in patients with acute lymphoblastic leukemia. Cytokines Cell Mol Ther. 1999;5(3):159–63.
33. Bertin R, Acquaviva C, Mirebeau D, Guidal-Giroux C, Vilmer E, Cave H. CDKN2A, CDKN2B, and MTAP gene dosage permits precise characterization of mono- and bi-allelic 9p21 deletions in childhood acute lymphoblastic leukemia. Genes Chromosomes Cancer. 2003;37(1):44–57.
34. Gardiner RB, Morash BA, Riddell C, Wang H, Fernandez CV, Yhap M, et al. Using MS-MLPA as an efficient screening tool for detecting 9p21 abnormalities in pediatric acute lymphoblastic leukemia. Pediatr Blood Cancer. 2012;58(6):852–9.
35. Mombaerts P, Iacomini J, Johnson RS, Herrup K, Tonegawa S, Papaioannou VE. RAG-1-deficient mice have no mature B and T lymphocytes. Cell. 1992;68(5):869–77.
36. Mizugishi K, Yamashita T, Olivera A, Miller GF, Spiegel S, Proia RL. Essential role for sphingosine kinases in neural and vascular development. Mol Cell Biol. 2005;25(24):11113–21.
37. Gromley A, Churchman ML, Zindy F, Sherr CJ. Transient expression of the Arf tumor suppressor during male germ cell and eye development in Arf-Cre reporter mice. Proc Natl Acad Sci U S A. 2009;106(15):6285–90.
38. Crazzolara R, Cisterne A, Thien M, Hewson J, Baraz R, Bradstock KF, et al. Potentiating effects of RAD001 (Everolimus) on vincristine therapy in childhood acute lymphoblastic leukemia. Blood. 2009;113(14):3297–306.
39. Pyne S, Adams DR, Pyne NJ. Sphingosine 1-phosphate and sphingosine kinases in health and disease: recent advances. Prog Lipid Res. 2016;62:93–106.
40. Antoon JW, White MD, Driver JL, Burow ME, Beckman BS. Sphingosine kinase isoforms as a therapeutic target in endocrine therapy resistant luminal and basal-A breast cancer. Exp Biol Med (Maywood). 2012;237(7):832–44.
41. Liu K, Guo TL, Hait NC, Allegood J, Parikh HI, Xu W, et al. Biological characterization of 3-(2-amino-ethyl)-5-[3-(4-butoxyl-phenyl)-propylidene]-thiazolidine-2,4-dione (K145) as a selective sphingosine kinase-2 inhibitor and anticancer agent. PLoS One. 2013;8(2):e56471.
42. Xun C, Chen MB, Qi L, Tie-Ning Z, Peng X, Ning L, et al. Targeting sphingosine kinase 2 (SphK2) by ABC294640 inhibits colorectal cancer cell growth in vitro and in vivo. J Exp Clin Cancer Res. 2015;34:94.
43. Schrecengost RS, Keller SN, Schiewer MJ, Knudsen KE, Smith CD. Downregulation of critical oncogenes by the selective SK2 inhibitor ABC294640 hinders prostate cancer progression. Mol Cancer Res. 2015;13(12):1591–601.

44. Venant H, Rahmaniyan M, Jones EE, Lu P, Lilly MB, Garrett-Mayer E, et al. The sphingosine kinase 2 inhibitor ABC294640 reduces the growth of prostate cancer cells and results in accumulation of dihydroceramides in vitro and in vivo. Mol Cancer Ther. 2015;14(12):2744–52.

45. Evangelisti C, Evangelisti C, Teti G, Chiarini F, Falconi M, Melchionda F, et al. Assessment of the effect of sphingosine kinase inhibitors on apoptosis, unfolded protein response and autophagy of T-cell acute lymphoblastic leukemia cells; indications for novel therapeutics. Oncotarget. 2014;5(17):7886–901.

46. Wallington-Beddoe CT, Bradstock KF, Bendall LJ. Oncogenic properties of sphingosine kinases in haematological malignancies. Br J Haematol. 2013; 161(5):623–38.

47. Hait NC, Allegood J, Maceyka M, Strub GM, Harikumar KB, Singh SK, et al. Regulation of histone acetylation in the nucleus by sphingosine-1-phosphate. Science. 2009;325(5945):1254–7.

48. Wallington-Beddoe CT, Bennett MK, Vandyke K, Davies L, Zebol JR, Moretti PAB, et al. Sphingosine kinase 2 inhibition synergises with bortezomib to target myeloma by enhancing endoplasmic reticulum stress. Oncotarget. 2017;8(27):43602–16.

49. Adamiak M, Chelvarajan L, Lynch K, Santos W, Abdel-Latif A, Ratajczak M. Mobilization studies in mice deficient in sphingosine kinase 2 support a crucial role of the plasma level of sphingosine-1-phosphate in the egress of hematopoietic stem progenitor cells. Oncotarget. 2017;8(39):65588–600.

27

SALL4 as a transcriptional and epigenetic regulator in normal and leukemic hematopoiesis

Jianchang Yang

Abstract

In recent years, there has been substantial progress in our knowledge of the molecular pathways by which stem cell factor SALL4 regulates the embryonic stem cell (ESC) properties, developmental events, and human cancers. This review summarizes recent advances in the biology of SALL4 with a focus on its regulatory functions in normal and leukemic hematopoiesis. In the normal hematopoietic system, expression of SALL4 is mainly enriched in the bone marrow hematopoietic stem/progenitor cells (HSCs/HPCs), but is rapidly silenced following lineage differentiation. In hematopoietic malignancies, however, SALL4 expression is abnormally re-activated and linked with deteriorated disease status in patients. Further, SALL4 activation participates in the pathogenesis of tumor initiation and disease progression. Thus, a better understanding of SALL4's biologic functions and mechanisms will facilitate development of advanced targeted anti-leukemia approaches in future.

Keywords: Pluripotency, Hematopoietic stem and progenitor cells, Apoptosis, Transgenic, Wnt/β-catenin signaling, Mixed-lineage leukemia, Chromatin modification

Background

SALL4 is one of four human homologues (SALL1, 2, 3, and 4) of the Drosophila region-specific homeotic gene *spalt* (*sal*) [1–4]. SALL4 encodes multiple Cys2His2 zinc finger (C2H2-ZF) domain-containing transcription factor that either activates or represses gene transcription depending on cell context. In mammals, expression of SALL4 has been primarily detected in ESCs and adult tissue "stem-like" cell populations, where it acts as a core controller regulating cell "stemness" in developmental events and also in tumor growth [5–9]. To date, aberrant SALL4 expression in humans has been observed in over 10 types of solid tumors and in several common types of leukemia (see review [8–11]), and SALL4 has been considered a biomarker for the diseases. In addition, studies suggest that SALL4 may be a useful therapeutic target in combating human leukemia in clinic [10, 11]. For these reasons, it will be important to understand, how SALL4 as a stem cell factor exerts its effects in different cell contexts, and how we can

effectively translate our gained knowledge into treatment breakthroughs in future.

Sall4 stem cell gene

The stem cell factor SALL4 is required for ESC pluripotency and for early embryonic development. It is an essential component of the 'stemness' regulatory circuit involving OCT4, SOX2, NANOG and other factors in maintaining ESC self-renewal and pluripotency [12–17]. In ESCs, a well-controlled SALL4/OCT4 transcription regulatory loop balances proper expression dosage of SALL4 and OCT4; and like OCT4, reduction of SALL4 results in re-specification of ESCs to the trophoblast lineage [18–20]. SALL4 is also a critical regulator in reprogramming of somatic cells to pluripotency. Shu et al. recently reported that GATA family members GATA4 and GATA6 can substitute for OCT4 in mouse somatic reprogramming, and identified SALL4 as a major target gene of the GATA members, serving as a bridge linking the lineage-specifying GATA family to the pluripotency circuit [21]. In fact, ectopic expression of SALL4, NANOG, ESRRB, and LIN28 [22], or the combination of SALL4, SALL1, UTF1, NANOG and MYC

Correspondence: jianchay@bcm.edu
Department of Surgery and Medicine, Baylor College of Medicine, Houston, TX 77030, USA

[23] in embryonic fibroblasts reprogram them into induced pluripotent stem cells (iPSCs) in the absence of OCT4.

In murine development, significant zygotic SALL4 transcription occurs at as early as the 4-cell stage. At the blastocyst stage, SALL4 expression becomes enriched in the inner cell mass (ICM) and the trophectoderm [12, 24–26]. Reduction of SALL4 in oocytes and ESCs results in early embryo defects, and disruption of both *Sall4* alleles causes embryonic lethality during peri-implantation [27–29]. SALL4 is also expressed in extraembryonic endoderm (XEN) cells, where it participates in cell fate decision by simultaneously activating key pluripotency maintaining factors and silencing endoderm lineage-associated factors such as GATA6, GATA4, and SOX17 [30, 31]. During subsequent stages, heterozygous disruption of *Sall4* allele leads to multi-organ malformations including limb and heart defects, which model human disease [27, 29]. It has been reported that TBX5, a gene encoding a T-box transcription factor, regulates SALL4 expression in the developing forelimb and heart, and interacts with SALL4 to synergistically regulate downstream gene expression [28, 29, 32].

In both humans and mice, SALL4 proteins exist at least in three isoforms termed A, B and C, with A and B isoforms being the most studied [32–36]. In ESCs, the SALL4 proteins are sequestered into the nuclear foci and bind to heterochromatin, where they participate in chromatin structure remodeling during transcription repression [37, 38]. SALL4 has also been shown to interact with the histone H3 lysine 36 (H3K36me3)-specific methyltransferase Wolf-Hirschhorn syndrome candidate 1 (WHSC1), which affects histone modification and thus regulate the expression of their target genes [39–41].

Functions of Sall4 and its regulated networks in normal hematopoiesis

Given SALL4's prominent roles in ESCs, development, and its specific expression patterns in the hematopoietic system, our research group previously investigated SALL4's functions in the self-renewal of HSCs/HPCs. We demonstrated that the SALL4 isoforms are robust stimulators for human CD34+ HSCs/HPCs expansion [42, 43]. Of note, we reported that the SALL4-driven ex vivo expansion of HSCs/HPCs is dependent on excessive special cytokines, and does not affect mature colony formation in colony-forming unit (CFU) assays [42]. In another study, Tatetsu et al. report that ex vivo culture of mobilized peripheral blood CD34+ cells with histone deacetylase (HDAC) inhibitors leads to expansion of a CD34+ CD90+ population, and SALL4 is identified as a key transcription factor responsible for the process [44]. In mouse model studies, forced overexpression of SALL4 in Lineage⁻ Sca-1⁺c-Kit⁺ (LSK) bone marrow (BM) cells likewise leads to sustained cell proliferation, as well as

enhanced marrow-repopulating potential [45]. Transcripts assays showed that the increased HSC/HPC growth was associated with upregulation of multiple HSC regulatory genes including HOXB4, NOTCH1, BMI1, RUNX1, CMYC, MEIS1 and NF-YA [45]. Further, in a myeloid progenitor cell line (32D cells), overexpression of SALL4 blocked granulocyte-colony stimulating factor (G-CSF)-induced granulocytic differentiation, and permitted expansion of undifferentiated cells in the presence of defined cytokines [42, 45]. Thus, the SALL4 isoforms stimulate HSC/HPC proliferation by activating important self-renewal regulators and simultaneously inhibiting differentiation. Recently, Mossahebi-Mohammadi et al. reported that the CD133⁺ umbilical cord blood HSCs/HPCs are also efficiently expanded following SALL4 lentivirus transduction, and the SALL4-expanded CD133⁺ cells retain self-renewal and differentiation capacities with no chromosomal aberrations [46]. In another study, it is further reported that SALL4 in CD34+ cells was downregulated by microRNAs miR-15b and miR-219-5p, and inhibition of miR-15b, –which activates SALL4 expression, significantly increased the number of CD34⁺ HSCs/HPCs in culture [47].

In elucidating the SALL4 regulated networks, Gao et al. sorted human CD34+ BM cells and performed chromatin immunoprecipitation followed by microarray hybridization (ChIP-on-chip), together with gene expression assays [48]. These works identified that CD34, RUNX1, HOXA9, and PTEN are SALL4-directed target genes. In particular, HOXA9 is being characterized as a major SALL4 target in hematopoiesis. Moreover, downregulation of SALL4 or HOXA9 expression in CD34+ cells results in similar effects, i.e., reduced in vitro myeloid colony formation and impaired in vivo engraftment [48]. In another study [49], the polycomb complex protein BMI-1 as a critical SALL4 downstream target has been documented. Chromatin immunoprecipitation coupled with quantitative PCR (ChIP-qPCR) in 32D cells reveals that SALL4 binds to a specific region of *Bmi-1* gene promoter, and heterozygous disruption of *Sall4* allele significantly reduced BMI-1 expression in BM cells. Further, in transgenic mice that constitutively overexpress human SALL4B, there is up-regulated expression of BMI-1, and the levels of BMI-1 in these mice increase as they progress from normal to preleukemic (myelodysplastic syndrome [MDS]) and leukemic (acute myeloid leukemia [AML]) stages.

Very recently, SALL4's functions in normal hematopoiesis have been further explored using conditional gene targeting approaches [50]. Surprisingly, wild type *Sall4^{f/f}*/CreER^{T2} mice that are treated with tamoxifen, or Vav-Cre-mediated (hematopoietic-specific) *Sall4^{-/-}* mice are all healthy and display no significant hematopoietic defects, which is in contrast to previous human CD34+ cell studies. Reasons for this discrepancy have not been fully addressed. To be noted however, some genes may exert aberrant functions only when cells encounter transplantation or replicative stress (see review [51]), and some Vav-Cre knockout models may demonstrate hematopoietic defects at late stages [52]. Thus it may be necessary to perform serial transplantation and/or stress induction (such as 5-fluorouracil injury) assays with SALL4-deficient cells to fully clarify SALL4 effect and mechanisms in maintaining normal HSCs.

Functions of Sall4 and its regulated networks in leukemia

SALL4 as a diagnostic marker in human leukemia

Aberrant expression of SALL4 has been detected in MDS patients and its expression levels are correlated with disease progression [34, 53]. Also, SALL4 and BMI-1 share a similar expression pattern in the patients with both expressions increase in high-grade morphology and high International Prognostic Scoring System (IPSS) score cases [53]. In addition, higher SALL4 protein levels are associated with the complex karyotype (equal to or more than three aberrant karyotypes), and SALL4 appears to be involved in the DNA damage response in patients [54], as supported by their roles in the ESC system [38]. In AML cases, immunohistochemistry staining reveals that SALL4 proteins are present in nearly all the patient samples that are examined (n = 81, subtypes M1 to M5, the French-American-British [FAB] classification) [34], and SALL4 expression in patients with complex karyotype is significantly higher than that in MDS patients with normal karyotype [54]. Similarly, variable transcript levels of SALL4A and SALL4B expression are reported in pediatric AML patients [55]. In other leukemia cases, aberrant SALL4 expression has been reported in ALK positive anaplastic large cell lymphoma (ALK[+] ALCL) [56], B cell acute lymphocytic leukemia (B-ALL), –most prominently in B-ALL patients with TEL-AML1 translocation, which is the most common genetic abnormality in pediatric B-ALL [57, 58]. SALL4 expression is also detected in patient samples from blastic stage of chronic myeloid leukemia (CML), as contrast to the chronic phase, and CML patients who have achieved complete remission or those who have tyrosine kinase inhibitor resistance [59–61]. Lastly, constitutive SALL4 expression has been documented in various human myeloid and lymphoid leukemia cell lines including KG1a (AML-M0), KASUMI-1 (AML-M2), HL-60 (AML-M2/M3), NB-4 (AML M3), THP1 (AML-M5), TEX (FUS/TLS-ERG oncogene immortalized AML), K562 (CML/AML M6), RPMI-8226 (myeloma), LAMA84 (CML-acute phase), BV173 (B-ALL), REH (ALL), NALM6 (ALL), 697 (pre-B ALL), BLIN-1 (pre-B ALL) and JURKAT (T cell leukemia) [34, 58, 61–65].

Interestingly, the SALL4 expression appears to be selectively enriched in leukemia side-population (SP) cells (defined by low Hoechst 33,342 blue/red fluorescence intensity), –a fraction specifically involved in cancer initiation and drug resistance [66], which supports the SALL4 expression features observed in above clinical cases, and suggests a role of SALL4 in maintaining the leukemia "initiating or stem" cell (LIC/LSC) populations.

Leukemogenesis induction by SALL4B in a transgenic model

In 2006, our research group reported the first SALL4-mediated leukemogenesis model [34]. We investigated transgenic mice that overexpress human SALL4A or SALL4B proteins, controlled by a universal CMV promoter. All the SALL4B mice from 6 founders developed MDS-like features at 2 months of age, and 9 of them (53%) progressed to AML. By contrast, none of the SALL4A mouse exhibits leukemia formation during the test period [34, 67]. These groups of studies suggest that SALL4B, but not SALL4A, is a novel oncogene in inducing leukemogenesis. As an adding note, however, while forced overexpression of either SALL4A or SALL4B isoform fails to transform primary BM cells, nor induces leukemia formation in transplanted mice [43, 67, 68], one may deduce that in the SALL4B transgenic mice, an abnormal "niche" resulting from aberrant SALL4B expression in various mouse tissues throughout the mouse development may play a role, and/or SALL4B may bear oncogenic potential during the dysregulated hematopoiesis. Further in-depth studies are needed to elucidate the associated mechanisms.

Role of SALL4 in mixed lineage leukemia (MLL)-rearranged (MLL-r) leukemogenesis

Considering the strong association of SALL4 expression with tumor initiation and leukemia survival, our group recently explored its effects in the pathogenesis of leukemia mediated by MLL-AF9, –one of the most common MLL-r oncoproteins found in leukemia patients [69–71]. MLL-r leukemias have been very challenging in therapy and associated with poor outcomes [70, 72, 73]. Further, a previous study has shown that the MLL wild type protein physically interacts with SALL4 in regulating HOXA9 expression [74]. We report that SALL4 expression is essentially required for MLL-AF9-mediated myeloid transformation in primary BM cells. Cre recombinase or shRNA mediated SALL4 knockdown in MLL-AF9-transformed cells induced apoptotic death and cell cycle arrest at G1. Consistently, disruption of both Sall4 alleles in transplanted mouse models completely prevented leukemia initiation and also attenuated pre-existing disease progression [50]. These studies support that the SALL4 pathway may not only be used as a useful biomarker or therapeutic target, proper inhibition of the SALL4 pathway may also effectively prevent disease initiation in patients at early stages.

SALL4 as a therapeutic target in human leukemic cells

SALL4 as a key regulator of survival has been widely documented in different subtypes of leukemias and in various human cancers [8, 10, 54, 75, 76]. In these malignancies, downregulation of SALL4 prominently causes increased apoptosis and cell cycle arrest [50, 62, 75–78]. In AMLs, aberrant SALL4 has also been shown to block all-trans retinoic acid (ATRA)-mediated myeloid differentiation in both ATRA-sensitive and ATRA-resistant AML subtypes [62]. Thus, these studies support that SALL4 maintains leukemic growth by protecting their proper proliferation and also inhibiting their differentiation. Not surprisingly, in recent years, SALL4-targeted anti-leukemia strategies have gained increasing interest and been elaborately explored (see review [11]). In a study by Gao et al., a SALL4- derived peptide blocking its protein-protein interaction with the nucleosome remodeling and histone deacetylation (NuRD) complex results in notable leukemic cell death, but causes no cytotoxic effects on normal CD34+ HSCs/HPCs [64]. Gao et al., also reported that SALL4 knockdown in combination with BCL-2 inhibitor treatment increased the apoptotic AML cells to 2 to 3 fold as compared to cells treated with each alone [77]. Our research group reported that while SALL4 and its interacting epigenetic factor LSD1 inhibited ATRA-induced granulocytic differentiation, co-inhibition of SALL4, LSD1, plus ATRA treatment severely disrupted ATRA-resistant AML cell growth, and blocked HL60 AML xenograft tumors by ~91%, while the treated mice exhibit no signs of illness [62, 79]. Considering that *Sall4* depletion in mice minimally affects adult hematopoiesis [50], these separate works collectively suggest that the SALL4 regulation-targeted approaches, which induce leukemia apoptosis and differentiation but spare normal cells, likely represent clinically effective and novel anti-leukemia strategies.

SALL4 regulated pathways in leukemia

ChIP-on-chip assays with a promyelocytic leukemic cell line, NB4 reveal that SALL4-binding genes are involved in more than 30 different signaling pathways [75]. Most prominent of these pathways are WNT/β-catenin, apoptosis, NOTCH signaling, the polycomb complex protein BMI-1, PTEN, and nuclear factor-kB. Further, SALL4 expression in these cells represses important apoptosis-inducing genes (*CARD9, CARD11, CYCS, LTA, TNF, TP53, PTEN*) but promotes apoptosis suppressor genes (*BMI-1, BCL2, DAD1, TEGT, XIAP*). In *SALL4B* transgenic mouse studies, the SALL4A and SALL4B isoforms have been found to bind β-catenin protein, and

interaction of these factors synergistically activates the WNT/β-catenin pathway, –which plays critical roles in controlling LSC self-renewal [34, 80–82]. The interaction domain between SALL4 and β-catenin was not determined. However, it was deduced that the C-terminal portion of SALL4 may play a role, based on binding data between SALL1 and β-catenin [8, 83]. Intriguingly, in a recent study by Kode et al., transgenic activation of a mutated *β-catenin* allele in murine osteoblasts, –one of the key HSC/HPC niches in BM [84, 85], induced MDS and AML in mice at very early ages via dysregulated NOTCH ligand JAG1 [86–88]. Since *SALL4B* transgenic mice also develop MDS/AML, and SALL4B-overexpressed BM cells do not induce leukemia formation in transplanted mice, an interesting question will be in the *SALLB* mouse, if/how SALL4B potentially activates β-catenin signaling, which synergistically dysregulate the HSC/HPC osteoblastic niche and thus promote leukemogenesis. Further detailed transgenic studies are required to address this probability.

ChIP assays with sequencing (ChIP-Seq) assays with mouse MLL-AF9 transformed leukemic cells are also performed [50], which identified that SALL4 binds to 451 genes including MLL-AF9 targets (*Meis1, Hoxa9*), MLL-r leukemia-related genes (*Cebpα, Id2, Elf1, Evl, Flt3, Nf1, Tal1, Tcf7l1, Nkx2–3*), HOX factors (*Hoxa-9, –10, –11, –13*), Notch ligand *Jag2*, and Wnt/β-catenin regulator *Wnt7b*. Further, loss of SALL4 downregulated the expression levels of *Bmi1, cMyb, Runx1, Meis1*, and HOX factors. In the same MLL-AF9 transformed cells, mRNA microarrays assays following early *Sall4* deletion identified upregulated genes including cell cycle inhibitors *Cdkn1a* (*p21*), *Trp53inp1*; HSC/HPC colony-forming repressor *Slfn2*; and hematopoietic differentiation markers *Col5a1, Fyb, Irf8* and *Pira6*. In contrast, downregulated genes included multiple TGFβ signaling components *Tgfβ2, Tgfβ3* and *Tgfβr3*; genes related to chemo-resistance or leukemia aggressiveness such as *Thbs1, Tgm2, Ambp*, and the AF9 regulator *Sgk1*, –which negatively regulates the DOT1A-AF9 complex-mediated transcriptional repression [50, 89]. Taken together, these studies suggest that SALL4 may regulate MLL-AF9 mediated leukemogenesis via multiple HSC/HPC- and LSC-related signaling pathways.

To date, upstream regulators of SALL4 expression in leukemia remain poorly understood, although OCT4, GATA4, GATA6, STAT3, TBX5, the WNT/β-catenin signaling factors, and micorRNAs such as miR-98, miR-33b and miR-294 are reported in other cell systems [8–10, 76, 90, 91]. Of note, DNA methylation modifications of the *SALL4* promoter may play a role, –studies using B-ALL cell lines and patient samples detected hypomethylation of the *SALL4* CpG islands spanning the exon1-intron1 region [57], which has also been observed in

MDS and AML patients, and this hypomethylation correlates with high SALL4 expression [92, 93]. Some other studies have documented SALL4-repressing compounds, such as apigenin, matrine, indole and its derivative 2-(1-((2, 4-Aril)imino)-2,2,2-trifluoroethyl) phenyl-1H Indole-3- carbaldehyde (TFPHC) are documented [10, 94]. Such works suggest that the SALL4 regulatory pathway may be potentially disrupted by clinically applicable drugs, and more such related ongoing works are expected to promote translation of cutting-edge SALL4 knowledge into clinical practice in future.

Epigenetic mechanisms involved in Sall4's regulatory functions in normal and leukemic hematopoiesis

Multiple chromatin modification regulators have been identified involving in SALL4's regulatory functions. So far the reported SALL4-interacting epigenetic factors include: DNA methyltransferases DNMT-1, –3A, -3B, –3 L, methyl-CpG-binding domain 2 protein (MBD2) [95]; NuRD complex that contains histone deacetylases HDAC1/2 [64, 96]; H3K4 methyltransferase MLL1 [74, 97]; H3K79 methyltransferase DOT1L [50, 98]; H3K36 methyltransferase WHSC1 [39, 99], and lysine-specific histone demethylase LSD1/KDM1A [50, 62, 79]. All of these are critical regulators in normal blood development and are frequent targets for dysregulation in hematological malignancies [100–103]. Of note, the SALL4 proteins seem to interact with these epigenetic factors at different sites. For example, while the amino-terminal 174 amino acid sequence of SALL4 is critical for SALL4-DNMT1 or -HDAC interaction, it seems less relevant to SALL4-LSD1 interaction. This is important in designing protein-protein interaction based anti-SALL4 strategies. Noteworthily, clinical epigenetic remedies inhibiting such SALL4-interacting epigenetic factors have been shown effective in treating leukemia [104–108]. Indeed, in MLL-AF9-mediated mouse AML studies, inhibition of either SALL4, DNMT1, LSD1, or DOT1L completely blocked leukemia initiation and significantly delayed disease progression in vivo [109–111].

By dynamically recruiting each specific epigenetic factor, SALL4 expression can directly affect DNA and histone methylation/acetylation status at important genes that control hematopoietic differentiation, apoptosis, tumor induction or suppression. For example, in NB4 AML cells transduced with lentiviral SALL4, there was an overall increased percentage of DNA methylation (a range of 1.2 to 2-fold) at various CpG sites of tumor suppression gene PTEN promoter, which co-relates with a down-regulated gene transcription [95]. In mouse BM LSK cells, overexpression of the SALL4 isoforms also induces increased percentage of methylation (1.2 to 6-fold) at the CpG sites of early B-cell factor 1 (Ebf1) promoter, as well as the Sall4 gene promoter itself, which

facilitates an undifferentiated cellular status [95]. Similarly, SALL4 overexpression or Cre-induced Sall4 gene deletion affected LSD1 binding and altered H3K4me2 levels at the promoter regions of tumor necrosis factor (Tnf) and differentiation-related genes Ebf1, Gata1 (up to ~300 and ~700 fold changes), which are associated with relevantly altered gene transcription levels [79]. Further, in 32D myeloid progenitor cells following lentiviral SALL4 transduction, the H3K4me3 and H3K79me2/3 levels at SALL4-occupied regions of Bmi1 promoter were increased [49]. Additionally, expression levels of SALL4 protein affect H3K4me3 and H3K79me3 amounts at promoter regions of Meis1 and multiple HOX family genes in normal or leukemic BM cells, as we and others reported [48, 50, 74]. Also, in the functional study by Gao et al., while SALL4 interacts with the HDAC complex, and silences PTEN promoter via reduced acetylation of histone H3 at its binding sites, the SALL4-derived peptide blocks this interaction and leads to reactivated PTEN expression, which induces leukemia cell death that can be rescued by a PTEN-specific inhibitor [64, 96].

Evidence suggests that SALL4 may compensatively recruit different epigenetic regulators. For example, LSD1 has been shown to contribute to global DNA methylation via stabilizing DNMT1 [112], while in the absence of LSD1 proteins, SALL4 seems to compensatively recruit DNMT1 or DNMT3L to downstream genes (such as EBF1, TNF) and modulate their expression [79]. Also, co-inhibition of DNMTs and HDACs can synergistically block SALL4's regulatory effects in cultured cells, which induces differentiation and cell growth arrest in human leukemia [113]. In addition, LSD1 has been shown to interact with the SALL4/CDX4 (a master regulator of the HOX genes) circuit and affect granulocytic/erythroid maturation [114, 115]. SALL4 also appears to confer cell resistance to DNA double-stranded break (DSB)-induced cytotoxicity by collaborating with HDAC-1 and -2 [38, 116].

It is important to note that SALL4's regulation of specific epigenetic modification programs is strictly dependent on the cellular contexts. Analysis of the ChIP-on-chip data from NB4 AML cells and normal CD34+ HSCs/HPCs reveals distinct SALL4 binding patterns between these two cell types, which reflect a cell type-specific epigenetic signature and SALL4 function [48, 75]. This finding is supported by ChIP-Seq data analysis of ESCs and extra-embryonic endoderm cell studies [30]. In ESCs, the SALL4-bound genomic loci are largely enriched for activating marker H3K4me3, which indicates an association of SALL4 with non-repressed genes. In XEN cells, however, the SALL4-binding loci display significantly less H3K4me3 enrichment. Instead, over 60% of these regions are either accompanied with H3K27me3 or lacking both H3K4me3 and H3K27me3, –the "epi-markers" frequently associated with gene repression. In our MLL-AF9 leukemia model studies

[50], SALL4 appears to recruit both DOT1L and LSD1 to specific downstream target genes and modulate their H3K79me2/3 and H3K4me3 levels, thereby maintaining proper gene expression and leukemic survival (see Fig. 1). As reported in previous studies, however, some non-MLL-r human AMLs may not rely on DOT1L-regulated H3K79 methylation, and DOT1L recruitment to MLL-AF9 is further associated with the level of leukemic transformation [117–120]. Thus, we may anticipate that in normal hematopoiesis and such different subtypes of human leukemias, SALL4 should differentially interact with such epigenetic factors during regulation of gene expression, thereby exerting a disease/subtype–dependent regulatory effect. In-depth functional and epigenetic studies are required to prove this assumption.

Conclusions

This review summarized recent advances in the biology of the stem cell factor SALL4 with a focus on its regulatory functions in normal and leukemic hematopoiesis. In recent years, there have been gains in our understanding of SALL4-regulated molecular mechanisms and SALL4-targeted strategy in killing tumor cells. Understanding how SALL4 mechanisms maintain normal HSCs/HPCs vs. leukemic cells will facilitate development of newer, more efficient anti-leukemia strategies.

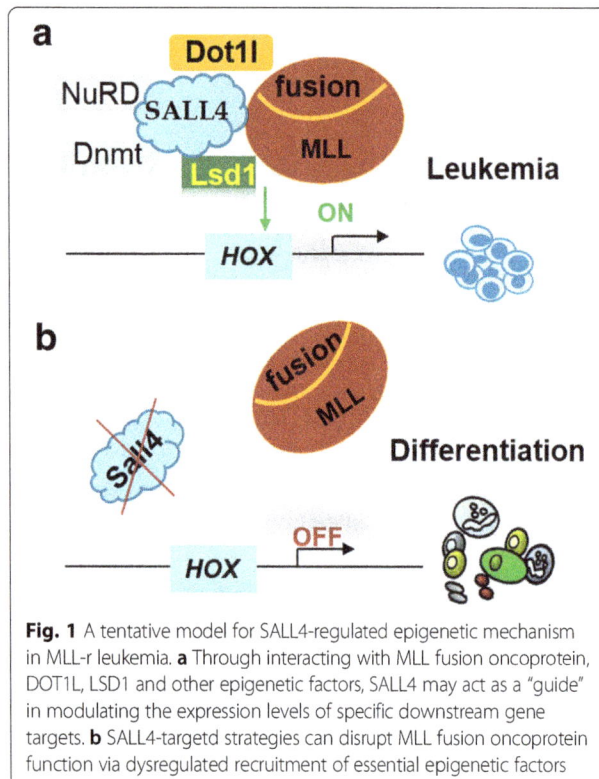

Fig. 1 A tentative model for SALL4-regulated epigenetic mechanism in MLL-r leukemia. **a** Through interacting with MLL fusion oncoprotein, DOT1L, LSD1 and other epigenetic factors, SALL4 may act as a "guide" in modulating the expression levels of specific downstream gene targets. **b** SALL4-targetd strategies can disrupt MLL fusion oncoprotein function via dysregulated recruitment of essential epigenetic factors

Abbreviations
ALK+ ALCL: ALK positive anaplastic large cell lymphoma; AML: Acute myeloid leukemia; ATRA: All-trans retinoic acid; B-ALL: B cell acute lymphocytic leukemia; BM: Bone marrow; C2H2-ZF: Cys2His2 zinc finger; CFU: Colony-forming unit; ChIP-on-chip: Chromatin immunoprecipitation followed by microarray hybridization; ChIP-PCR: Chromatin immunoprecipitation coupled with quantitative PCR; ChIP-Seq: ChIP assays with sequencing; CML: Chronic myeloid leukemia; Ebf1: Early B-cell factor 1; ESC: Embryonic stem cell; FAB: The French-American-British classification; G-CSF: Granulocyte-colony stimulating factor; HDAC: Histone deacetylase; HSPs/HPCs: Hematopoietic stem/progenitor cells; ICM: Inner cell mass; iPSCs: Induced pluripotent stem cells; IPSS: International Prognostic Scoring System; LIC/LSC: Leukemia "initiating or stem" cell; LSK: Lineage- Sca-1+ c-kit+; MBD2: Methyl-CpG-binding domain 2 protein; MDS: Myelodysplastic syndrome; MLL-r: Mixed lineage leukemia (MLL)-rearranged; NuRD: Nucleosome remodeling and deacetylase; SP: Side-population; TFPHC: 2-(1-((2, 4-Aril)imino)-205 2,2,2-trifluoroethyl) phenyl-1H Indole-3- carbaldehyde; Tnf: Tumor necrosis factor; WHSC1: Wolf-Hirschhorn syndrome candidate 1; XEN: Extraembryonic endoderm

Acknowledgments
I would like to thank all my colleagues who have provided support in related research program. I would also like to thank Kimberly Macellaro, PhD, a member of the Baylor College of Medicine Michael E. DeBakey Department of Surgery Research Core Team, for her editorial assistance.

Funding
This project was supported by American Cancer Society Research Scholar Grant RSG-12-216-01-LIB (to J. Y.).

Author contributions
J.Y. wrote the paper.

Competing interests
The author declares that he has no competing interests.

References
1. Kohlhase J, Schuh R, Dowe G, Kuhnlein RP, Jackle H, Schroeder B, Schulz-Schaeffer W, Kretzschmar HA, Kohler A, Muller U. Isolation, characterization, and organ-specific expression of two novel human zinc finger genes related to the drosophila gene spalt. Genomics. 1996;38
2. Eildermann K, Aeckerle N, Debowski K, Godmann M, Christiansen H, Heistermann M, Schweyer S, Bergmann M, Kliesch S, Gromoll J, et al. Developmental expression of the pluripotency factor sal-like protein 4 in the monkey, human and mouse testis: restriction to premeiotic germ cells. Cells Tissues Organs. 2012;196(3):206–20.
3. Sweetman D, Munsterberg A. The vertebrate spalt genes in development and disease. Dev Biol. 2006;293(2):285–93.
4. de Celis JF, Barrio R. Regulation and function of Spalt proteins during animal development. Int J Dev Biol. 2009;53(8–10):1385–98.
5. Yang J, Liao W, Ma Y. Role of SALL4 in hematopoiesis. Curr Opin Hematol. 2012;19
6. Kohlhase J, Heinrich M, Schubert L, Liebers M, Kispert A, Laccone F, Turnpenny P, Winter RM, Reardon W. Okihiro syndrome is caused by SALL4 mutations. Hum Mol Genet. 2002;11(23):2979–87.

7. Kohlhase J: SALL4-Related Disorders. In: *GeneReviews(R)*. edn. Edited by Adam MP, Ardinger HH, Pagon RA, Wallace SE, Bean LJH, Mefford HC, Stephens K, Amemiya A, Ledbetter N. Seattle (WA); 1993.

8. Tatetsu H, Kong NR, Chong G, Amabile G, Tenen DG, Chai L. SALL4, the missing link between stem cells, development and cancer. Gene. 2016;584

9. Xiong J. SALL4: engine of cell Stemness. Current gene therapy. 2014;

10. Zhang X, Yuan X, Zhu W, Qian H, Xu W. SALL4: an emerging cancer biomarker and target. Cancer Lett. 2015;357(1):55–62.

11. Wang F, Zhao W, Kong N, Cui W, Chai L. The next new target in leukemia: the embryonic stem cell gene SALL4. Mol Cell Oncol. 2014;1(4):e969169.

12. Elling U, Klasen C, Eisenberger T, Anlag K, Treier M. Murine inner cell mass-derived lineages depend on Sall4 function. Proc Natl Acad Sci U S A. 2006; 103(44):16319–24.

13. Zhang J, Tam WL, Tong GQ, Wu Q, Chan HY, Soh BS, Lou Y, Yang J, Ma Y, Chai L, et al. Sall4 modulates embryonic stem cell pluripotency and early embryonic development by the transcriptional regulation of Pou5f1. Nat Cell Biol. 2006;8(10):1114–23.

14. Wang J, Rao S, Chu J, Shen X, Levasseur DN, Theunissen TW, Orkin SH. A protein interaction network for pluripotency of embryonic stem cells. Nature. 2006;444(7117):364–8.

15. Yang J, Chai L, Fowles TC, Alipio Z, Xu D, Fink LM, Ward DC, Ma Y. Genome-wide analysis reveals Sall4 to be a major regulator of pluripotency in murine-embryonic stem cells. Proc Natl Acad Sci U S A. 2008;105

16. Wu Q, Chen X, Zhang J, Loh YH, Low TY, Zhang W, Sze SK, Lim B, Ng HH. Sall4 interacts with Nanog and co-occupies Nanog genomic sites in embryonic stem cells. J Biol Chem. 2006;281

17. Tan MH, KF A, Leong DE, Foygel K, Wong WH, Yao MW. An Oct4-Sall4-Nanog network controls developmental progression in the pre-implantation mouse embryo. Mol Syst Biol. 2013;9:632.

18. Zhang J, Tam WL, Tong GQ, Wu Q, Chan HY, Soh BS, Lou Y, Yang J, Ma Y, Chai L. Sall4 modulates embryonic stem cell pluripotency and early embryonic development by the transcriptional regulation of Pou5f1. Nat Cell Biol. 2006;8

19. Yang J, Gao C, Chai L, Ma Y. A novel SALL4/OCT4 transcriptional feedback network for pluripotency of embryonic stem cells. PLoS One. 2010;5(5): e10766.

20. Nosi U, Lanner F, Huang T, Cox B. Overexpression of trophoblast stem cell-enriched MicroRNAs promotes trophoblast fate in embryonic stem cells. Cell Rep. 2017;19(6):1101–9.

21. Shu J, Zhang K, Zhang M, Yao A, Shao S, Du F, Yang C, Chen W, Wu C, Yang W, et al. GATA family members as inducers for cellular reprogramming to pluripotency. Cell Res. 2015;25(2):169–80.

22. Buganim Y, Markoulaki S, van Wietmarschen N, Hoke H, Wu T, Ganz K, Akhtar-Zaidi B, He Y, Abraham BJ, Porubsky D, et al. The developmental potential of iPSCs is greatly influenced by reprogramming factor selection. Cell Stem Cell. 2014;15(3):295–309.

23. Mansour AA, Gafni O, Weinberger L, Zviran A, Ayyash M, Rais Y, Krupalnik V, Zerbib M, Amann-Zalcenstein D, Maza I, et al. The H3K27 demethylase Utx regulates somatic and germ cell epigenetic reprogramming. Nature. 2012; 488(7411):409–13.

24. Xu K, Chen X, Yang H, Xu Y, He Y, Wang C, Huang H, Liu B, Liu W, Li J, et al. Maternal Sall4 is indispensable for epigenetic maturation of mouse oocytes. J Biol Chem. 2017;292(5):1798–807.

25. Sakaki-Yumoto M, Kobayashi C, Sato A, Fujimura S, Matsumoto Y, Takasato M, Kodama T, Aburatani H, Asashima M, Yoshida N, et al. The murine homolog of SALL4, a causative gene in Okihiro syndrome, is essential for embryonic stem cell proliferation, and cooperates with Sall1 in anorectal, heart, brain and kidney development. Development. 2006;133(15):3005–13.

26. Miller A, Gharbi S, Etienne-Dumeau C, Nishinakamura R, Hendrich B: Transcriptional control by Sall4 in blastocysts facilitates lineage commitment of inner cell mass cells. *bioRxiv* 2017.

27. Warren M, Wang W, Spiden S, Chen-Murchie D, Tannahill D, Steel KP, Bradley A. A Sall4 mutant mouse model useful for studying the role of Sall4 in early embryonic development and organogenesis. Genesis. 2007;45(1): 51–8.

28. Harvey SA, Logan MP. sall4 acts downstream of tbx5 and is required for pectoral fin outgrowth. Development. 2006;133(6):1165–73.

29. Koshiba-Takeuchi K, Takeuchi JK, Arruda EP, Kathiriya IS, Mo R, Hui CC, Srivastava D, Bruneau BG. Cooperative and antagonistic interactions between Sall4 and Tbx5 pattern the mouse limb and heart. Nat Genet. 2006;38(2):175–83.

30. Lim CY, Tam WL, Zhang J, Ang HS, Jia H, Lipovich L, Ng HH, Wei CL, Sung WK, Robson P. Sall4 regulates distinct transcription circuitries in different blastocyst-derived stem cell lineages. Cell Stem Cell. 2008;3

31. Oikawa T, Kamiya A, Kakinuma S, Zeniya M, Nishinakamura R, Tajiri H, Nakauchi H. Sall4 regulates cell fate decision in fetal hepatic stem/progenitor cells. Gastroenterology. 2009;136(3):1000–11.

32. Bohm J, Heinritz W, Craig A, Vujic M, Ekman-Joelsson BM, Kohlhase J, Froster U. Functional analysis of the novel TBX5 c.1333delC mutation resulting in an extended TBX5 protein. BMC Med Genet. 2008;9:88.

33. Rao S, Zhen S, Roumiantsev S, McDonald LT, Yuan GC, Orkin SH. Differential roles of Sall4 isoforms in embryonic stem cell pluripotency. Mol Cell Biol. 2010;30(22):5364–80.

34. Ma Y, Cui W, Yang J, Qu J, Di C, Amin HM, Lai R, Ritz J, Krause DS, Chai L. SALL4, a novel oncogene, is constitutively expressed in human acute myeloid leukemia (AML) and induces AML in transgenic mice. Blood. 2006;108

35. Uez N, Lickert H, Kohlhase J, de Angelis MH, Kuhn R, Wurst W, Floss T. Sall4 isoforms act during proximal-distal and anterior-posterior axis formation in the mouse embryo. Genesis. 2008;46(9):463–77.

36. Gassei K, Orwig KE. SALL4 expression in gonocytes and spermatogonial clones of postnatal mouse testes. PLoS One. 2013;8(1):e53976.

37. Hobbs RM, Fagoonee S, Papa A, Webster K, Altruda F, Nishinakamura R, Chai L, Pandolfi PP. Functional antagonism between Sall4 and Plzf defines germline progenitors. Cell Stem Cell. 2012;10(3):284–98.

38. Xiong J, Todorova D, NY S, Kim J, Lee PJ, Shen Z, Briggs SP, Xu Y. Stemness factor Sall4 is required for DNA damage response in embryonic stem cells. J Cell Biol. 2015;208(5):513–20.

39. Nimura K, Ura K, Shiratori H, Ikawa M, Okabe M, Schwartz RJ, Kaneda Y. A histone H3 lysine 36 trimethyltransferase links Nkx2-5 to wolf-Hirschhorn syndrome. Nature. 2009;460(7252):287–91.

40. Kim JY, Kee HJ, Choe NW, Kim SM, Eom GH, Baek HJ, Kook H, Kook H, Seo SB. Multiple-myeloma-related WHSC1/MMSET isoform RE-IIBP is a histone methyltransferase with transcriptional repression activity. Mol Cell Biol. 2008; 28(6):2023–34.

41. Yu C, Yao X, Zhao L, Wang P, Zhang Q, Zhao C, Yao S, Wei Y. Wolf-Hirschhorn syndrome candidate 1 (whsc1) functions as a tumor suppressor by governing cell differentiation. Neoplasia. 2017;19(8):606–16.

42. Aguila JR, Liao W, Yang J, Avila C, Hagag N, Senzel L, Ma Y. SALL4 is a robust stimulator for the expansion of hematopoietic stem cells. Blood. 2011;118(3):576–85.

43. Liao W, Aguila JR, Yao Y, Yang J, Zieve G, Jiang Y, Avila C, Senzel L, Lai R, Xu D, et al. Enhancing bone marrow regeneration by SALL4 protein. J Hematol Oncol. 2013;6:84.

44. Tatetsu H, Wang F, Gao C, Ueno S, Tian X, Armant M, Federation A, Qi J, Bradner JE, Tenen DG, et al. SALL4 is a key factor in HDAC inhibitor mediated ex vivo expansion of human peripheral blood mobilized stem/progenitor CD34+CD90+ cells. Blood. 2014;124(21):1566–6.

45. Yang J, Aguila JR, Alipio Z, Lai R, Fink LM, Ma Y. Enhanced self-renewal of hematopoietic stem/progenitor cells mediated by the stem cell gene Sall4. J Hematol Oncol. 2011;4:38.

46. Mossahebi-Mohammadi M, Atashi A, Kaviani S, Soleimani M. Efficient expansion of SALL4-transduced umbilical cord blood derived CD133 +hematopoietic stem cells. Acta Med Iran. 2017;55(5):290–6.

47. Akhavan Rahnama M, Movassaghpour AA, Soleimani M, Atashi A, Anbarlou A, Shams Asenjan K. MicroRNA-15b target Sall4 and diminish in vitro UCB-derived HSCs expansion. EXCLI J. 2015;14:601–10.

48. Gao C, Kong NR, Li A, Tatetu H, Ueno S, Yang Y, He J, Yang J, Ma Y, Kao GS. SALL4 is a key transcription regulator in normal human hematopoiesis. Transfusion. 2013;53

49. Yang J, Chai L, Liu F, Fink LM, Lin P, Silberstein LE, Amin HM, Ward DC, Ma Y. Bmi-1 is a target gene for SALL4 in hematopoietic and leukemic cells. Proc Natl Acad Sci U S A. 2007;104(25):10494–9.

50. Yang L, Liu L, Gao H, Pinnamaneni JP, Sanagasetti D, Singh VP, Wang K, Mathison M, Zhang Q, Chen F, et al. The stem cell factor SALL4 is an essential transcriptional regulator in mixed lineage leukemia-rearranged leukemogenesis. J Hematol Oncol. 2017;10(1):159,

51. Rossi L, Lin KK, Boles NC, Yang L, King KY, Jeong M, Mayle A, Goodell MA. Less is more: unveiling the functional core of hematopoietic stem cells through knockout mice. Cell Stem Cell. 2012;11(3):302–17.

52. Damnernsawad A, Kong G, Wen Z, Liu Y, Rajagopalan A, You X, Wang J, Zhou Y, Ranheim EA, Luo HR, et al. Kras is required for adult hematopoiesis. Stem Cells. 2016;34(7):1859–71.

53. Wang F, Guo Y, Chen Q, Yang Z, Ning N, Zhang Y, Xu Y, Xu X, Tong C, Chai L, et al. Stem cell factor SALL4, a potential prognostic marker for myelodysplastic syndromes. J Hematol Oncol. 2013;6(1):73.

54. Wang F, Gao C, Lu J, Tatetsu H, Williams DA, Muller LU, Cui W, Chai L. Leukemic survival factor SALL4 contributes to defective DNA damage repair. Oncogene. 2016;35(47):6087–95.

55. Milanovich S, Peterson J, Allred J, Stelloh C, Rajasekaran K, Fisher J, Duncan SA, Malarkannan S, Rao S: Sall4 overexpression blocks murine hematopoiesis in a dose-dependent manner. *Experimental hematology* 2015, 43(1):53–64 e51–58.

56. Wang P, Zhang JD, Wu F, Ye X, Sharon D, Hitt M, McMullen TP, Hegazy SA, Gelebart P, Yang J, et al. The expression and oncogenic effects of the embryonic stem cell marker SALL4 in ALK-positive anaplastic large cell lymphoma. Cell Signal. 2012;24(10):1955–63.

57. Ueno S, Lu J, He J, Li A, Zhang X, Ritz J, Silberstein LE, Chai L. Aberrant expression of SALL4 in acute B cell lymphoblastic leukemia: mechanism, function, and implication for a potential novel therapeutic target. Exp Hematol. 2014;42(4):307–16. e308

58. Cui W, Kong NR, Ma Y, Amin HM, Lai R, Chai L. Differential expression of the novel oncogene, SALL4, in lymphoma, plasma cell myeloma, and acute lymphoblastic leukemia. Modern pathology : an official journal of the United States and Canadian Academy of Pathology, Inc. 2006;19(12):1585–92.

59. Lu J, Ma Y, Kong N, Alipio Z, Gao C, Krause DS, Silberstein LE, Chai L. Dissecting the role of SALL4, a newly identified stem cell factor, in chronic myelogenous leukemia. Leukemia. 2011;25(7):1211–3.

60. Shen Q, Liu S, Hu J, Chen S, Yang L, Li B, Wu X, Ma Y, Yang J, Ma Y, et al. The differential expression pattern of the BMI-1, SALL4 and ABCA3 genes in myeloid leukemia. Cancer Cell Int. 2012;12(1):42.

61. Hupfeld T, Chapuy B, Schrader V, Beutler M, Veltkamp C, Koch R, Cameron S, Aung T, Haase D, Larosee P, et al. Tyrosinekinase inhibition facilitates cooperation of transcription factor SALL4 and ABC transporter A3 towards intrinsic CML cell drug resistance. Br J Haematol. 2013;161(2):204–13.

62. Liu L, Liu L, Leung E, Cooney AJ, Chen C, Rosengart TK, Ma Y, Yang J. Knockdown of SALL4 enhances all-trans retinoic acid-induced cellular differentiation in acute myeloid leukemia cells. J Biol Chem. 2015;

63. Yang F, Yao Y, Jiang Y, Lu L, Ma Y, Dai W. Sumoylation is important for stability, subcellular localization, and transcriptional activity of SALL4, an essential stem cell transcription factor. J Biol Chem. 2012;287(46):38600–8.

64. Gao C, Dimitrov T, Yong KJ, Tatetsu H, Jeong HW, Luo HR, Bradner JE, Tenen DG, Chai L. Targeting transcription factor SALL4 in acute myeloid leukemia by interrupting its interaction with an epigenetic complex. Blood. 2013;121

65. Schenk T, Chen WC, Gollner S, Howell L, Jin L, Hebestreit K, Klein HU, Popescu AC, Burnett A, Mills K, et al. Inhibition of the LSD1 (KDM1A) demethylase reactivates the all-trans-retinoic acid differentiation pathway in acute myeloid leukemia. Nat Med. 2012;18(4):605–11.

66. Jeong HW, Cui W, Yang Y, Lu J, He J, Li A, Song D, Guo Y, Liu BH, Chai L. SALL4, a stem cell factor, affects the side population by regulation of the ATP-binding cassette drug transport genes. PLoS One. 2011;6

67. Aguila JR, Liao W, Yang J, Avila C, Hagag N, Senzel L, Ma Y. SALL4 is a robust stimulator for the expansion of hematopoietic stem cells. Blood. 2011;118

68. Yang J, Aguila JR, Alipio Z, Lai R, Fink LM, Ma Y. Enhanced self-renewal of hematopoietic stem/progenitor cells mediated by the stem cell gene Sall4. J Hematol Oncol. 2011;4

69. Prange KHM, Mandoli A, Kuznetsova T, Wang SY, Sotoca AM, Marneth AE, van der Reijden BA, Stunnenberg HG, Martens JHA. MLL-AF9 and MLL-AF4 oncofusion proteins bind a distinct enhancer repertoire and target the RUNX1 program in 11q23 acute myeloid leukemia. Oncogene. 2017;36(23):3346–56.

70. Winters AC, Bernt KM. MLL-rearranged Leukemias-an update on science and clinical approaches. Front Pediatr. 2017;5:4.

71. Zhu N, Chen M, Eng R, DeJong J, Sinha AU, Rahnamay NF, Koche R, Al-Shahrour F, Minehart JC, Chen CW, et al. MLL-AF9- and HOXA9-mediated acute myeloid leukemia stem cell self-renewal requires JMJD1C. J Clin Invest. 2016;126(3):997–1011.

72. Marschalek R. MLL leukemia and future treatment strategies. Arch Pharm (Weinheim). 2015;348(4):221–8.

73. de Boer J, Walf-Vorderwulbecke V, Williams O. Focus: MLL-rearranged leukemia. Leukemia. 2013;27(6):1224–8.

74. Li A, Yang Y, Gao C, Lu J, Jeong HW, Liu BH, Tang P, Yao X, Neuberg D, Huang G, et al. A SALL4/MLL/HOXA9 pathway in murine and human myeloid leukemogenesis. J Clin Invest. 2013;123(10):4195–207.

75. Yang J, Chai L, Gao C, Fowles TC, Alipio Z, Dang H, Xu D, Fink LM, Ward DC, Ma Y. SALL4 is a key regulator of survival and apoptosis in human leukemic cells. Blood. 2008;112

76. Zhou W, Zou B, Liu L, Cui K, Gao J, Yuan S, Cong N. MicroRNA-98 acts as a tumor suppressor in hepatocellular carcinoma via targeting SALL4. Oncotarget. 2016;7(45):74059–73.

77. Gao C, Kong NR, Chai L. The role of stem cell factor SALL4 in leukemogenesis. Crit Rev Oncog. 2011;16(1–2):117–27.

78. Li A, Jiao Y, Yong KJ, Wang F, Gao C, Yan B, Srivastava S, Lim GS, Tang P, Yang H, et al. SALL4 is a new target in endometrial cancer. Oncogene. 2015;34(1):63–72.

79. Liu L, Souto J, Liao W, Jiang Y, Li Y, Nishinakamura R, Huang S, Rosengart T, Yang VW, Schuster M. Histone lysine-specific demethylase 1 (LSD1) protein is involved in Sal-like protein 4 (SALL4)-mediated transcriptional repression in hematopoietic stem cells. J Biol Chem. 2013;288

80. Reya T, Clevers H. Wnt signalling in stem cells and cancer. Nature. 2005;434(7035):843–50.

81. Wang Y, Krivtsov AV, Sinha AU, North TE, Goessling W, Feng Z, Zon LI, Armstrong SA. The Wnt/beta-catenin pathway is required for the development of leukemia stem cells in AML. Science. 2010;327(5973):1650–3.

82. Heidel FH, Mar BG, Armstrong SA. Self-renewal related signaling in myeloid leukemia stem cells. Int J Hematol. 2011;94(2):109–17.

83. Sato A, Kishida S, Tanaka T, Kikuchi A, Kodama T, Asashima M, Nishinakamura R. Sall1, a causative gene for Townes-brocks syndrome, enhances the canonical Wnt signaling by localizing to heterochromatin. Biochem Biophys Res Commun. 2004;319(1):103–13.

84. Yin T, Li L. The stem cell niches in bone. J Clin Invest. 2006;116(5):1195–201.

85. Levesque JP, Helwani FM, Winkler IG. The endosteal 'osteoblastic' niche and its role in hematopoietic stem cell homing and mobilization. Leukemia. 2010;24(12):1979–92.

86. Kode A, Manavalan JS, Mosialou I, Bhagat G, Rathinam CV, Luo N, Khiabanian H, Lee A, Murty VV, Friedman R, et al. Leukaemogenesis induced by an activating beta-catenin mutation in osteoblasts. Nature. 2014;506(7487):240–4.

87. Weber JM, Calvi LM. Notch signaling and the bone marrow hematopoietic stem cell niche. Bone. 2010;46(2):281–5.

88. Pajcini KV, Speck NA, Pear WS. Notch signaling in mammalian hematopoietic stem cells. Leukemia. 2011;25(10):1525–32.

89. Zhang W, Xia X, Reisenauer MR, Rieg T, Lang F, Kuhl D, Vallon V, Kone BC. Aldosterone-induced Sgk1 relieves Dot1a-Af9-mediated transcriptional repression of epithelial Na+ channel alpha. J Clin Invest. 2007;117

90. Lin Y, Liu AY, Fan C, Zheng H, Li Y, Zhang C, Wu S, Yu D, Huang Z, Liu F, et al. MicroRNA-33b inhibits breast cancer metastasis by targeting HMGA2, SALL4 and Twist1. Sci Rep. 2015;5:9995.

91. Melton C, Judson RL, Blelloch R. Opposing microRNA families regulate self-renewal in mouse embryonic stem cells. Nature. 2010;463(7281):621–6.

92. Ma JC, Qian J, Lin J, Qian W, Yang J, Wang CZ, Chai HY, Li Y, Chen Q, Qian Z. Aberrant hypomethylation of SALL4 gene is associated with intermediate and poor karyotypes in acute myeloid leukemia. Clin Biochem. 2013;46(4–5):304–7.

93. Lin J, Qian J, Yao DM, Qian W, Yang J, Wang CZ, Chai HY, Ma JC, Deng ZQ, Li Y, et al. Aberrant hypomethylation of SALL4 gene in patients with myelodysplastic syndrome. Leuk Res. 2013;37(1):71–5.

94. Sheikhrezaei Z, Heydari P, Farsinezhad A, Fatemi A, Khanamani Falahati-pour S, Darakhshan S, Noroozi Karimabad M, Darekordi A, Khorramdelazad H, Hassanshahi G. A new indole derivative decreased SALL4 gene expression in acute Promyelocytic leukemia cell line (NB4). Iran Biomed J. 2017;

95. Yang J, Corsello TR, Ma Y. Stem cell gene SALL4 suppresses transcription through recruitment of DNA methyltransferases. J Biol Chem. 2012;287(3):1996–2005.

96. Lu J, Jeong HW, Kong N, Yang Y, Carroll J, Luo HR, Silberstein LE, Yupoma, Chai L. Stem cell factor SALL4 represses the transcriptions of PTEN and SALL1 through an epigenetic repressor complex. PLoS One. 2009;4(5):e5577.

97. Dou Y, Milne TA, Ruthenburg AJ, Lee S, Lee JW, Verdine GL, Allis CD, Roeder RG. Regulation of MLL1 H3K4 methyltransferase activity by its core components. Nat Struct Mol Biol. 2006;13(8):713–9.

98. Nguyen AT, Zhang Y. The diverse functions of Dot1 and H3K79 methylation. Genes Dev. 2011;25(13):1345–58.

99. Campos-Sanchez E, Deleyto-Seldas N, Dominguez V, Carrillo-de-Santa-Pau E, Ura K, Rocha PP, Kim J, Aljoufi A, Esteve-Codina A, Dabad M, et al. Wolf-

Hirschhorn syndrome candidate 1 is necessary for correct hematopoietic and B cell development. Cell Rep. 2017;19(8):1586–601.

100. Rice KL, Hormaeche I, Licht JD. Epigenetic regulation of normal and malignant hematopoiesis. Oncogene. 2007;26(47):6697–714.

101. Goyama S, Kitamura T. Epigenetics in normal and malignant hematopoiesis: an overview and update 2017. Cancer Sci. 2017;108(4):553–62.

102. Ding LW, Sun QY, Tan KT, Chien W, Mayakonda A, Yeoh AEJ, Kawamata N, Nagata Y, Xiao JF, Loh XY, et al. Mutational landscape of pediatric acute lymphoblastic leukemia. Cancer Res. 2017;77(2):390–400.

103. Feng Z, Yao Y, Zhou C, Chen F, Wu F, Wei L, Liu W, Dong S, Redell M, Mo Q, et al. Pharmacological inhibition of LSD1 for the treatment of MLL-rearranged leukemia. J Hematol Oncol. 2016;9:24.

104. Wouters BJ, Delwel R. Epigenetics and approaches to targeted epigenetic therapy in acute myeloid leukemia. Blood. 2016;127(1):42–52.

105. Gallipoli P, Giotopoulos G, Huntly BJ. Epigenetic regulators as promising therapeutic targets in acute myeloid leukemia. Ther Adv Hematol. 2015;6(3): 103–19.

106. Bernt KM, Armstrong SA. Targeting epigenetic programs in MLL-rearranged leukemias. Hematology / the Education Program of the American Society of Hematology American Society of Hematology Education Program. 2011; 2011:354–60.

107. Saygin C, Carraway HE. Emerging therapies for acute myeloid leukemia. J Hematol Oncol. 2017;10(1):93.

108. Song Y, Wu F, Wu J. Targeting histone methylation for cancer therapy: enzymes, inhibitors, biological activity and perspectives. J Hematol Oncol. 2016;9(1):49.

109. Trowbridge JJ, Sinha AU, Zhu N, Li M, Armstrong SA, Orkin SH. Haploinsufficiency of Dnmt1 impairs leukemia stem cell function through derepression of bivalent chromatin domains. Genes Dev. 2012;26(4):344–9.

110. Kuntimaddi A, Achille NJ, Thorpe J, Lokken AA, Singh R, Hemenway CS, Adli M, Zeleznik-Le NJ, Bushweller JH. Degree of recruitment of DOT1L to MLL-AF9 defines level of H3K79 di- and tri-methylation on target genes and transformation potential. Cell Rep. 2015;11(5):808–20.

111. Harris WJ, Huang X, Lynch JT, Spencer GJ, Hitchin JR, Li Y, Ciceri F, Blaser JG, Greystoke BF, Jordan AM, et al. The histone demethylase KDM1A sustains the oncogenic potential of MLL-AF9 leukemia stem cells. Cancer Cell. 2012; 21(4):473–87.

112. Wang J, Hevi S, Kurash JK, Lei H, Gay F, Bajko J, Su H, Sun W, Chang H, Xu G, et al. The lysine demethylase LSD1 (KDM1) is required for maintenance of global DNA methylation. Nat Genet. 2009;41(1):125–9.

113. Thurn KT, Thomas S, Moore A, Munster PN. Rational therapeutic combinations with histone deacetylase inhibitors for the treatment of cancer. Future Oncol. 2011;7(2):263–83.

114. Kerenyi MA, Shao Z, Hsu YJ, Guo G, Luc S, O'Brien K, Fujiwara Y, Peng C, Nguyen M, Orkin SH. Histone demethylase Lsd1 represses hematopoietic stem and progenitor cell signatures during blood cell maturation. elife. 2013;2:e00633.

115. Paik EJ, Mahony S, White RM, Price EN, Dibiase A, Dorjsuren B, Mosimann C, Davidson AJ, Gifford D, Zon LI. A Cdx4-Sall4 regulatory module controls the transition from mesoderm formation to embryonic hematopoiesis. Stem Cell Reports. 2013;1(5):425–36.

116. Miller KM, Tjeertes JV, Coates J, Legube G, Polo SE, Britton S, Jackson SP. Human HDAC1 and HDAC2 function in the DNA-damage response to promote DNA nonhomologous end-joining. Nat Struct Mol Biol. 2010;17(9): 1144–51.

117. Bernt KM, Zhu N, Sinha AU, Vempati S, Faber J, Krivtsov AV, Feng Z, Punt N, Daigle A, Bullinger L, et al. MLL-rearranged leukemia is dependent on aberrant H3K79 methylation by DOT1L. Cancer Cell. 2011;20(1):66–78.

118. Bernt KM, Armstrong SA. A role for DOT1L in MLL-rearranged leukemias. Epigenomics. 2011;3(6):667–70.

119. Chen CW, Armstrong SA. Targeting DOT1L and HOX gene expression in MLL-rearranged leukemia and beyond. Exp Hematol. 2015;43(8):673–84.

120. Bernt KM, Zhu N, Sinha AU, Vempati S, Faber J, Krivtsov AV, Feng Z, Punt N, Daigle A, Bullinger L. MLL-rearranged leukemia is dependent on aberrant H3K79 methylation by DOT1L. Cancer Cell. 2011;20

Permissions

All chapters in this book were first published in BR, by BioMed Central; hereby published with permission under the Creative Commons Attribution License or equivalent. Every chapter published in this book has been scrutinized by our experts. Their significance has been extensively debated. The topics covered herein carry significant findings which will fuel the growth of the discipline. They may even be implemented as practical applications or may be referred to as a beginning point for another development.

The contributors of this book come from diverse backgrounds, making this book a truly international effort. This book will bring forth new frontiers with its revolutionizing research information and detailed analysis of the nascent developments around the world.

We would like to thank all the contributing authors for lending their expertise to make the book truly unique. They have played a crucial role in the development of this book. Without their invaluable contributions this book wouldn't have been possible. They have made vital efforts to compile up to date information on the varied aspects of this subject to make this book a valuable addition to the collection of many professionals and students.

This book was conceptualized with the vision of imparting up-to-date information and advanced data in this field. To ensure the same, a matchless editorial board was set up. Every individual on the board went through rigorous rounds of assessment to prove their worth. After which they invested a large part of their time researching and compiling the most relevant data for our readers.

The editorial board has been involved in producing this book since its inception. They have spent rigorous hours researching and exploring the diverse topics which have resulted in the successful publishing of this book. They have passed on their knowledge of decades through this book. To expedite this challenging task, the publisher supported the team at every step. A small team of assistant editors was also appointed to further simplify the editing procedure and attain best results for the readers.

Apart from the editorial board, the designing team has also invested a significant amount of their time in understanding the subject and creating the most relevant covers. They scrutinized every image to scout for the most suitable representation of the subject and create an appropriate cover for the book.

The publishing team has been an ardent support to the editorial, designing and production team. Their endless efforts to recruit the best for this project, has resulted in the accomplishment of this book. They are a veteran in the field of academics and their pool of knowledge is as vast as their experience in printing. Their expertise and guidance has proved useful at every step. Their uncompromising quality standards have made this book an exceptional effort. Their encouragement from time to time has been an inspiration for everyone.

The publisher and the editorial board hope that this book will prove to be a valuable piece of knowledge for researchers, students, practitioners and scholars across the globe.

List of Contributors

Sabrina Tosi, Yasser Mostafa Kamel and Temitayo Owoka
Leukaemia and Chromosome Research Laboratory, Division of Biosciences, Brunel University London, Middlesex UB8 3PH, UK

Concetta Federico and Salvatore Saccone
Dipartimento di Scienze Biologiche, Geologiche e Ambientali, Sezione di Biologia Animale, University of Catania, Catania, Italy

Tony H. Truong
Division of Pediatric Oncology, Blood and Marrow Transplant, Alberta Children's Hospital, University of Calgary, Calgary, Canada

Nicolai Aagaard Schultz and Carsten Palnæs Hansen
Department of Surgical Gastroenterology and Transplantation, Rigshospitalet, Copenhagen University Hospital, Copenhagen, Denmark

Christian Dehlendorff
Danish Cancer Society Research Center, Danish Cancer Society, Copenhagen, Denmark

Mogens K. Boisen
Department of Oncology, Herlev and Gentofte Hospital, Copenhagen University Hospital, Herlev, Denmark

Jane Preuss Hasselby
Department of Pathology, Rigshospitalet, Copenhagen University Hospital, Copenhagen, Denmark

Jens Werner
Department of General, Visceral, and Transplant Surgery, LMU, University of Munich, Munich, Germany

Heike Immervoll
Gade Laboratory for Pathology, Department of Clinical Medicine, University of Bergen, Bergen, Norway
Department of Pathology, Ålesund Hospital, Ålesund, Norway

Anders Molven
Gade Laboratory for Pathology, Department of Clinical Medicine, University of Bergen, Bergen, Norway
Department of Pathology, Haukeland University Hospital, Bergen, Norway

Julia S. Johansen
Department of Oncology, Herlev and Gentofte Hospital, Copenhagen University Hospital, Herlev, Denmark
Department of Medicine, Herlev and Gentofte Hospital, Copenhagen University Hospital, Herlev, Denmark
Institute of Clinical Medicine, Faculty of Health and Medical Sciences, University of Copenhagen, Copenhagen, Denmark

Dan Calatayud
Department of Surgical Gastroenterology and Transplantation, Rigshospitalet, Copenhagen University Hospital, Copenhagen, Denmark
Department of Oncology, Herlev University Hospital, Herlev Ringvej 75, DK-2730 Herlev, Denmark

David Borg, Charlotta Hedner, Alexander Gaber, Björn Nodin, Richard Fristedt, Karin Jirström, Jakob Eberhard and Anders Johnsson
Department of Clinical Sciences Lund, Division of Oncology and Pathology, Lund University, Skåne University Hospital, 221 85 Lund, Sweden

Wu Zhang and Jie Xu
State Key Laboratory for Medical Genomics, Shanghai Institute of Hematology, Rui-Jin Hospital affiliated to Shanghai Jiao-Tong University School of Medicine, 197 Rui Jin Er Road, 200025 Shanghai, China

Rosalia de Necochea-Campion and Saied Mirshahidi
Biospecimen Laboratory, Loma Linda University Cancer Center, Loma Linda University School of Medicine, 11175 Campus Street, Chan Shun Pavilion 11017, Loma Linda, CA 92354, USA

Lee M. Zuckerman
Department of Orthopaedic Surgery, Loma Linda University Medical Center, 11406 Loma Linda Drive, Suite 218, Loma Linda, CA 92354, USA

Hamid R. Mirshahidi
Division of Hematology/Oncology, Loma Linda University School of Medicine, 11175 Campus Street, Chan Shun Pavilion 11015, Loma Linda, CA 92354, USA

Shahrzad Khosrowpour
Chapman University, One University Drive, Orange, CA 92866, USA

Chien-Shing Chen
Biospecimen Laboratory, Loma Linda University Cancer Center, Loma Linda University School of Medicine, 11175 Campus Street, Chan Shun Pavilion 11017, Loma Linda, CA 92354, USA
Division of Hematology/Oncology, Loma Linda University School of Medicine, 11175 Campus Street, Chan Shun Pavilion 11015, Loma Linda, CA 92354, USA

Md. T Anam and Md. B Hossain
Department of Statistics, Biostatistics and Informatics, University of Dhaka, Dhaka 1000, Bangladesh

Alokta Ishika and Jesmin
Department of Genetic Engineering and Biotechnology, University of Dhaka, Dhaka 1000, Bangladesh

Tasleem Katchi and Delong Liu
Division of Hematology and Oncology, New York Medical College and Westchester Medical Center, Valhalla, NY 10595, USA

Eugene Lin
Graduate Institute of Biomedical Sciences, China Medical University, Taichung, Taiwan
Vita Genomics, Inc, Taipei, Taiwan
TickleFish Systems Corporation, Seattle, WA, USA

Hsien-Yuan Lane
Graduate Institute of Biomedical Sciences, China Medical University, Taichung, Taiwan Department of Psychiatry, China Medical University Hospital, Taichung, Taiwan

David L. Wang
Department of Biology, Vanderbilt University, Nashville, TN, USA

Chuanguang Xiao and Liang Li
Zibo Central Hospital, Zibo, China

Guofeng Fu and Xing Wang
Array Bridge Inc., 4320 Forest Park Ave, Suite 303, St. Louis, MO 63108, USA

Jing Huang and Jianzhou Liu
School of Pharmaceutical Science and Technology, Dalian University of Technology, Dalian 116024, China

Gary Guishan Xiao
School of Pharmaceutical Science and Technology, Dalian University of Technology, Dalian 116024, China
Harbor-University of California Los Angeles Research and Education Institute, UCLA School of Medicine, Torrance, CA 90502, USA
Genomics and Functional Proteomics Laboratories, Creighton University Medical Center, Omaha, NE 68131, USA

Kevin Chen-Xiao, Xuemei Zhang, W. N. Paul Lee and Vay Liang W. Go
Harbor-University of California Los Angeles Research and Education Institute, UCLA School of Medicine, Torrance, CA 90502, USA

Erik Rahimi and Jen-Jung Pan
Division of Gastroenterology, Hepatology and Nutrition, University of Texas Medical School at Houston, 6431 Fannin Street, MSB 4.234, Houston, TX 77030, USA

Laurence P. Diggs and Eddy C. Hsueh
Division of General Surgery, Department of Surgery, Saint Louis University, 3635 Vista at Grand Blvd., St. Louis, MO 63110, USA

William Kofi Anyan, Kofi Owusu Baffour-Awuah and Kwabena Mante Bosompem
Noguchi Memorial Institute for Medical Research (NMIMR), College of Health Sciences, University of Ghana, Accra, Ghana

Veronique Penlap Beng
Laboratory for Tuberculosis Research and Pharmacology, Biotechnology Centre, Nkolbisson, University of Yaoundé 1, Yaoundé, Cameroon

Daniel Boamah
Centre for Plant Medicine Research (CPMR), Akwapim, Mampong, Ghana

Stephanie Keyetat Tekwu
Yaounde Emergency Centre (CURY), Yaoundé, Cameroon

Alexander Kwadwo Nyarko
School of Pharmacy, College of Health sciences, University of Ghana, Accra, Ghana

Emmanuel Mouafo Tekwu
Noguchi Memorial Institute for Medical Research (NMIMR), College of Health Sciences, University of Ghana, Legon, Accra, Ghana Laboratory for Tuberculosis Research and Pharmacology, Biotechnology Centre, Nkolbisson, University of Yaoundé 1, Yaoundé, Cameroon

Bernard Klein and Jerome Moreaux
Laboratory for Monitoring Innovative Therapies, Department of Biological Hematology, Hôpital Saint-Eloi - CHRU de Montpellier, 80, av. Augustin Fliche, 34295 Montpellier, Cedex 5, France
Institute of Human Genetics, CNRS-UPR1142, Montpellier F-34396, France
University of Montpellier 1, UFR de Médecine, Montpellier, France

Philippe Pasero and Elena Viziteu
Institute of Human Genetics, CNRS-UPR1142, Montpellier F-34396, France

Alboukadel Kassambara
Laboratory for Monitoring Innovative Therapies, Department of Biological Hematology, Hôpital Saint-Eloi - CHRU de Montpellier, 80, av. Augustin Fliche, 34295 Montpellier, Cedex 5, France
Institute of Human Genetics, CNRS-UPR1142, Montpellier F-34396, France

Steffen Koerdt, Nadine Tanner, Niklas Rommel, Nils H. Rohleder, Gesche Frohwitter, Klaus-Dietrich Wolff and Marco R. Kesting
Department of Oral and Maxillofacial Surgery, Technical University of Munich (TUM), Ismaninger Str. 22, D-81675 Munich, Germany

Oliver Ristow
Department of Oral and Maxillofacial Surgery, Heidelberg University Hospital, Im Neuenheimer Feld 400, D-69120 Heidelberg, Germany

Elisabeth Hofmann, Nico Jacobi, Christian Klein, Christoph Wiesner, Harald Hundsberger and Andreas Eger
Department Life Sciences, IMC University of Applied Sciences Krems, Piaristengasse 1, A-3500 Krems, Austria

Kamil Oender
Research Program for Rational Drug Design in Dermatology and Rheumatology, Department of Dermatology, Paracelsus Medical University of Salzburg, Müllner Hauptstraße 48, A-5020 Salzburg, Austria

Peter Obrist and Samuel Huter
Pathology Laboratory Obrist and Brunhuber, Klostergasse 1, A-6511 Zams, Austria

Rita Seeboeck
Department Life Sciences, IMC University of Applied Sciences Krems, Piaristengasse 1, A-3500 Krems, Austria
Pathology Laboratory Obrist and Brunhuber, Klostergasse 1, A-6511 Zams, Austria

Wataru Goto, Shinichiro Kashiwagi, Yuka Asano, Koji Takada, Tsutomu Takashima, Kosei Hirakawa and Masaichi Ohira
Department of Surgical Oncology, Osaka City University Graduate School of Medicine, 1-4-3 Asahi-machi, Abeno-ku, Osaka 545-8585, Japan

Katsuyuki Takahashi and Shuhei Tomita
Department of Pharmacology, Osaka City University Graduate School of Medicine, 1-4-3 Asahi-machi, Abeno-ku, Osaka 545-8585, Japan

Takaharu Hatano and Hisashi Motomura
Department of Plastic and Reconstructive Surgery, Osaka City University Graduate School of Medicine, 1-4-3 Asahi-machi, Abeno-ku, Osaka 545-8585, Japan

Masahiko Ohsawa
Department of Diagnostic Pathology, Osaka City University Graduate School of Medicine, 1-4-3 Asahi-machi, Abeno-ku, Osaka 545-8585, Japan

Ryan F. Coates, Abiy Ambaye and Juli-Anne Gardner
Department of Pathology and Laboratory Medicine, University of Vermont Medical Center, 111 Colchester Avenue, Burlington, VT, USA

Richard Zubarick
Gastroenterology, University of Vermont Medical Center, 111 Colchester Avenue, Burlington, VT, USA

Yuan Gao
Department of Gastrointestinal Surgery, Nanjing Medical University affiliated Changzhou 2nd People's Hospital, Changzhou, Jiangsu, China

Joan Skelly
University of Vermont Medical Biostatistics Department, Burlington, VT, USA

James G. Liu
Applied Pathology Systems, Worcester, MA, USA

Mari Mino-Kenudson
Department of Pathology, Massachusetts General Hospital, Boston, MA, USA

Michelle X. Yang
Department of Pathology and Laboratory Medicine, University of Vermont Medical Center, 111 Colchester Avenue, Burlington, VT, USA
Present address: Department of Pathology, University of Massachusetts Medical Center, 1 Innovation Drive, Worcester, MA 01605, USA

Yuki Nagata, Kouichi Ozaki and Shumpei Niida
Medical Genome Center, National Center for Geriatrics and Gerontology, 7-430 Morioka-cho, Obu, Aichi 474-8511, Japan

Akiyoshi Hirayama, Satsuki Ikeda, Aoi Shirahata, Futaba Shoji, Midori Maruyama and Tomoyoshi Soga
Institute for Advanced Biosciences, Keio University, 246-2 Mizukami, Kakuganji, Tsuruoka, Yamagata 997-0052, Japan

Mitsunori Kayano
Research Center for Global Agromedicine, Obihiro University of Agriculture and Veterinary Medicine, 2-11 Inada-cho, Obihiro, Hokkaido 080-8555, Japan

Masahiko Bundo
Department of Experimental Neuroimaging, National Center for Geriatrics and Gerontology, Obu, Aichi 474-8511, Japan

Kotaro Hattori, Sumiko Yoshida and Yu-ichi Goto
Medical Genome Center, National Center of Neurology and Psychiatry, Kodaira, Tokyo 187-8551, Japan

Katsuya Urakami
Department of Biological Regulation, School of Health Science, Faculty of Medicine, Tottori University, Yonago, Tottori 683-8503, Japan

Yuan Ling, Qing Xie, Zikang Zhang and Hua Zhang
Guangdong Provincial Key Laboratory of Medical Molecular Diagnostics, Institute of Laboratory Medicine, Guangdong Medical University, Dongguan 523808, China

Sandeep Kondisetty and Ginil Kumar Pooleri
Department of Urology, Amrita Institute of Medical Sciences, Amrita Vishwa Vidyapeetham, Ponekkara, Kochi, Kerala, India

Krishnakumar N. Menon
Center for Nanosciences and Molecular Medicine, Amrita Institute of Medical Sciences, Amrita Vishwa Vidyapeetham, Ponekkara, Kochi, Kerala, India

Zhenguang Wang and Weidong Han
Molecular and Immunological Department, Bio-therapeutic Department, Chinese PLA General Hospital, No. 28 Fuxing Road, Beijing 100853, China

Callinice D Capo-chichi
Institute of Applied Biomedical Sciences (ISBA), Unit of Biochemistry and Molecular Biology, Division of Molecular Biomarkers in Cancer and Nutrition, University of Abomey-Calavi, Abomey-Calavi, Benin
Sylvester Cancer Center (SCCC), Ovarian Cancer Program, University of Miami, Miami, Florida, USA

Kathy Q Cai
Department of Pathology, Fox Chase Cancer Center, Philadelphia, PA, USA

Xiang-Xi Xu
Sylvester Cancer Center (SCCC), Ovarian Cancer Program, University of Miami, Miami, Florida, USA

Michelle E. Penney
Discipline of Genetics, Faculty of Medicine, Memorial University of Newfoundland, St. John's, Canada

Patrick S. Parfrey
Discipline of Medicine, Faculty of Medicine, Memorial University of Newfoundland, St. John's, Canada

Sevtap Savas
Discipline of Genetics, Faculty of Medicine, Memorial University of Newfoundland, St. John's, Canada
Discipline of Oncology, Faculty of Medicine, Memorial University of Newfoundland, St. John's, Canada

Yildiz E. Yilmaz
Discipline of Genetics, Faculty of Medicine, Memorial University of Newfoundland, St. John's, Canada
Discipline of Medicine, Faculty of Medicine, Memorial University of Newfoundland, St. John's, Canada
Department of Mathematics and Statistics, Faculty of Science, Memorial University of Newfoundland, St.John's, Canada

Runxia Gu, Xue Yang and Hui Wei
Leukemia Center, Institute of Hematology and Blood Diseases Hospital, Chinese Academy of Medical Sciences and Peking Union Medical College, Tianjin 300020, People's Republic of China

Vicki Xie, Daochen Tong and Linda J. Bendall
Centre for Cancer Research, The Westmead Institute for Medical Research, The University of Sydney, Sydney, Australia

Ken F. Bradstock
Haematology Department, Westmead Hospital, Westmead, NSW, Australia

Craig T. Wallington-Beddoe
Centre for Cancer Research, The Westmead Institute for Medical Research, The University of Sydney, Sydney, Australia
Centre for Cancer Biology, University of South Australia and SA Pathology, Adelaide, Australia
College of Medicine and Public Health, Flinders University, Adelaide, Australia
School of Medicine, University of Adelaide, Adelaide, Australia

Jianchang Yang
Department of Surgery and Medicine, Baylor College of Medicine, Houston, TX 77030, USA

Index

www.ingramcontent.com/pod-product-compliance
Lightning Source LLC
Chambersburg PA
CBHW061303190326
41458CB00011B/3753